Blood Stasis
China's classical concept in modern medicine

For Elsevier:

Commissioning Editor: Karen Morley
Development Editor: Louise Allsop
Project Manager: Andrew Palfreyman
Design Direction: Andy Chapman

Blood Stasis

China's classical concept in modern medicine

Including a translation of the seminal work of Wang Qing-Ren 'Corrections of mistakes in the medical world'.

Gunter R. Neeb

Translated by:
Maximilian Beer and Julia Kaiser

Foreword from the German edition by:
Professor Zhang Bo-Li, PhD, MD (Chinese and Western medicine)

Foreword by:
Steven Clavey B.A., Dip Ac.

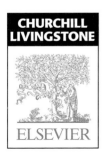

CHURCHILL
LIVINGSTONE

ELSEVIER

EDINBURGH   LONDON   NEW YORK   OXFORD   PHILADELPHIA   ST LOUIS   SYDNEY   TORONTO   2007

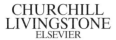

An imprint of Elsevier Limited
© Elsevier Ltd 2007. All rights reserved.

Originally published in German as *Das Blutstasesyndrom*
Copyright © 2001 Verlag für Ganzheitliche Medizin Dr. Erich Wühr GmbH

First published 2007

ISBN 0-443-10185-X
ISBN 13: 978 0 443 10185 4

British Library Cataloguing in Publication Data
A catalogue record for this book is available from the British Library

Library of Congress Cataloging in Publication Data
A catalog record for this book is available from the Library of Congress

---

Notice

Knowledge and best practice in this field are constantly changing. As new research and experience broaden our knowledge, changes in practice, treatment and drug therapy may become necessary or appropriate. Readers are advised to check the most current information provided (i) on procedures featured or (ii) by the manufacturer of each product to be administered, to verify the recommended dose or formula, the method and duration of administration, and contraindications. It is the responsibility of the practitioner, relying on their own experience and knowledge of the patient, to make diagnoses, to determine dosages and the best treatment for each individual patient, and to take all appropriate safety precautions. To the fullest extent of the law, neither the publisher nor the author assumes any liability for any injury and/or damage to persons or property arising out of or related to any use of the material contained in this book.

Printed in China

Contents

About the author

Gunter Ralf Neeb MD TCM (China) was born in Wiesbaden, Germany in 1959. He became interested in Chinese culture at an early stage. As a student he read translations of Chinese philosophers and later on during 3 years of studying naturopathy he became deeply involved with Chinese acupuncture and Western phytotherapy.

After his Heilpraktiker examination (German equivalent of naturopath; apart from that of medical doctors, the only profession entitled to practise medicine – Translator's note) he carried out a study on the comparison of herbs used in traditional Chinese and traditional Western medicine. In order to study Chinese medicine in China himself, in 1987 and 1988 he successfully completed the three-stage Chinese language course at the Sinikum, University of Bochum, and then went on to Taiwan in 1988.

For 3 years at the Taiwan National Normal University he studied the traditional characters of modern and classical Chinese to the highest level, and was awarded two scholarships by the Chinese Ministry of Education in Taiwan, which are only available to the top 3% of all students.

From 1991 to 1993 he also worked as an acupuncturist in the clinic of Professor Chang Cung-Gwo PhD, MD, and completed a 2 years' training in Qi Gong and Taoist techniques with Master Li Feng-Shan in Taipei.

In 1994 he first studied at the College for Chinese Medicine in Yunnan province and later on commenced his Master's degree at the International College for Traditional Chinese Medicine of Tianjin. In 1998 he graduated as the first non-Chinese with a Master's degree in Chinese Internal Medicine. His thesis was titled 'Physiology and pathology of acute and chronic Blood stasis and its treatment'. From 1996 he worked as a doctor of Chinese medicine in the clinical centre of the Research Institute of Tianjin University and in addition, has translated many classical texts into German.

In January 2001 he finished his doctoral thesis on geomedical aspects of Chinese medicine and thus concluded his 12 years of studies in Taiwan and China and returned to Germany, being the first non-Chinese with a doctor's degree in Chinese medicine. Following his teaching activities at the University of Tianjin he was accepted into the university's teaching staff as a lecturer, and is now instructing at the Universität Witten-Herdicke and various other medical institutions in Germany, Switzerland, Sweden, the Netherlands and Spain.

So far, he has published articles on Chinese medicine in English and Chinese and several articles and book contributions in German, amongst which is *Das Blutstasesyndrom*. His well-known homepage www.TCMinter.net publishes extensive amounts of new material from modern scientific as well as classical sources of Chinese medicine.

He believes in his aim of combining the traditional experience of classical sources with the latest findings of research and science into one system of medicine, which is able to meet the requirements of the third millennium.

Foreword

This is less a book than a banquet, a banquet with a theme: the understanding and treatment of blood stasis. Its various interwoven courses include Chinese and Western, theory and practice, single herbs and formulae, sprinkled with illuminating case histories, with the main course being a full translation of the seminal work on blood stasis in Chinese medicine, Wang Qing-Ren's *Yi Lin Gai Cuo* from the Qing dynasty. This is followed by a rich dessert in the appendices. All in all, not something to be attempted in one sitting, but rather to be savoured over time.

Ten years ago I met Dr. Gunter Neeb in Rothenburg on the Tauber river in Bavaria, and was immediately impressed. Here was a Westerner living and practicing Chinese medicine in Beijing, with several scholarly research articles already published in Chinese, not to mention German, and some in English. But he did not seem to regard this as anything particularly special, and was soon entertaining me with his gentle quirky humour. Having enjoyed his writings that have since occasionally appeared in European and Australian journals, it is a pleasure to greet the English translation of this comprehensive book, which was published in German in 2001.

Blood stasis is an area where Western medicine appears, at first sight, to be more advanced than TCM, an appearance due primarily to the presentation of impressively technical measurements. However technology is only as good as the conceptual principles which guide it, and – as Dr. Neeb shows throughout this book – in this fundamental arena Western medicine is only beginning to approach the sophistication of Chinese medicine.

My own field of gynaecology is a good example. Clinical observation and analysis of successful treatments over twenty years have shown unequivocally that clotting during menstruation is not only abnormal, but significantly related to a wide variety of disorders such as endometriosis, menorrhagia, infertility, dysmenorrhea, and many others. The sad fact is that many instances of these conditions could have been prevented by early attention to the appearance of clots in the menstrual blood, but in the West all is confusion. On the one hand, it is recognised that normal menstrual blood should not clot. On the other it is felt that some degree of clotting is 'normal.' "And besides, trying to clear up clotting just isn't worth the trouble!" one doctor confessed, when tackled on why he thought clotting was acceptable. Blood coagulation factors, platelet function, fibrinolysis, plasma proteins – repeated measurement and investigation of these cell-level factors are ineffective without a firm guiding conceptual principle: clotting is not normal or acceptable during menstruation.

Doctors of Chinese medicine (and most women!) have known for centuries that clotting during menstruation is abnormal. Women know it because often they can feel it for themselves; one type of severe dysmenorrhea is directly due to the pain of clots passing, when the clots are cleared, the pain goes too. The aetiology of endometriosis, which is by definition a disease of blood stasis in the Chinese conception, may again be related at least in part to menstrual clotting. How does endometrial tissue end up outside the uterus? I believe it may be a result of failure of endometrial debris to pass efficiently down and out vaginally, due to obstruction from excessive clotting. This of course encourages discharge out through the only other exit from the uterus, via the fallopian tubes, into the pelvis where the free floating endometrial cells implant, bleed, and form the disease endometriosis.

My teacher in gynaecology, Professor Song Guang-Ji, told me that the main causes for heavy menstrual bleeding were three: heat, qi deficiency, and blood stasis, in that order. After many years of practicing in the West, it has become apparent to me that for us, the order is different: blood stasis is primary. And the reason this should be so is that, unlike Chinese doctors, Western doctors accept menstrual clotting as normal, or at least acceptable, and do nothing about it. In many cases of menorrhagia, the heavy bleeding attributed to uterine myoma (fibroids) has been reduced to normal when the menstrual clotting was cleared – even though the fibroids themselves had not reduced. This again demonstrates the crucial role blood stasis plays in disturbing the functioning of the body, and points to the importance of Dr. Neeb's work.

Gynaecology of course is only one discipline in which blood stasis is a significant aetiological factor. Any system, any area of the body nourished by the blood – in short, all areas – can be affected by the obstruction of this essential nourishment, with a wide variety of consequences. This broad area is well covered in this book, along with a wealth of case histories that illustrate the flexibility of approach that is the hallmark of Chinese medicine.

It may be, however, that the true significance of *Blood Stasis Syndrome: China's classical concept in modern medicine* will lie in its rich potential for cross-fertilisation, the sparking-off of new ideas that so often follows an apparent clash of paradigms. Let us hope that it is not only Chinese doctors who read this inspiring work. In the last century Chinese medicine has been strongly influenced in a variety of ways by Western medicine: perhaps we are ready for the tide to turn.

Steven Clavey
B.A. (USA), Dip Ac. (Nanjing),
Cert. Gynaecology (Zhejiang)
Registered Chinese herbalist
(Melbourne, Australia)

Foreword from the German edition

Prof Zhang Bo-Li, PhD MD (Chinese and Western medicine)

Nowadays, Blood stasis is a commonly diagnosed syndrome in China. As a concept of Chinese medicine it is characterized by an abnormal blood flow within the blood vessels. The successful treatment of this disease is based upon extensive experience accumulated in the course of more than 2000 years. Within the past 30 years the theory and treatment in the field of Blood stasis has been complemented and expanded by China's promotion of pharmacological research regarding Blood invigorating medicinals and by practical contributions in the field of haemorheology.

Further progress in the comprehension of the aetiology, the course of disease and the clinical picture of Blood stasis was achieved by the methods of integrated Chinese and Western medicine. This was also the case for the therapeutic indications of Blood invigorating medicinals, and finally for research into the characteristics of Blood stasis. Through the combination of these two medical systems, researching Blood stasis has become one of the most attractive fields in Chinese medicine. The results have stirred the interest of scholars in Japan, Korea, the USA, South-East Asia and Europe.

Although Blood stasis and high blood viscosity are derived from two different sciences, both have a good deal in common as regards content and pathological relevance. Both are the causes and mechanisms for ischemic heart and brain disease, geriatric diseases, formation of tumours and many other illnesses. Great progress in medical science can come about through comparing and mutually complementing traditional knowledge concerning Blood stasis and modern insights into high blood viscosity.

The author Gunter Neeb, MSc PhD (TCM) (Chinese name: Nei Long-Dao) is a research student from Germany with a great interest in Chinese medicine and herbal pharmacology. For more than a decade, with determination and persistence, he has spared no effort to study the classical language, philosophy and later the medicine of China in a systematic and comprehensive way. In doing so he has developed a thorough understanding of the theory and practice of Chinese Medicine. He is extremely well-read, has a keen spirit of inquiry, and achieved good grades.

As supervisor for his PhD I particularly appreciate his open and sharp mind, which he successfully employs in making comparative analyses between Chinese and Western medicine as well as Western phytotherapy and Chinese medicinals. He stands at what is just the beginning of an even more profound integration in a field of research which I regard as most important for further progress and success.

Moreover, it is admirable to note how he has used the time remaining after his studies and clinical practice to integrate into this book his processing and systematizing of the theory, diagnosis and clinical picture of Blood stasis along with his translation of related classical texts. This contribution is of great value. All material used has been suitably selected and accurately described. Explanations are coherent and precise in giving an authentic and trustworthy account of the meaning of Blood stasis.

I hope that this book can add to a better cultural and medical understanding between Germany and China, and that Chinese medicine can make a contribution to improved healthcare for all mankind.

Prof Zhang Bo-Li, PhD MD
(Chinese and Western medicine)
Summer 1997, International Academy
of Traditional Chinese Medicine, Tianjin
Research Institute of Tianjin City
(2006) Director of the University of Chinese
Medicine, Tianjin

Preface

Wang Qing-Ren and chaos theory

SOME THOUGHTS ON THE AIM AND CONTENTS OF THIS BOOK

This book is intended to provide comprehensive insight for those practitioners interested in Chinese medicine, both into the ancient concept of Blood stasis and its modern scientific aspects. These often overlap to a considerable extent with Western medicine concepts such as high blood viscosity, reduced blood cell plasticity, diminished blood flow and increased blood cell aggregation. Diseases in direct relationship to Blood stasis are arteriosclerosis, apoplexy, cardiac infarction, heart failure and angina pectoris, cor pulmonale, acute renal failure, respiratory arrest, chronic hepatitis, diabetes, numerous skin diseases, dementia, all kinds of haemorrhagic and menstrual diseases, tinnitus and deafness, insomnia, low immunity and formation of tumours, rheumatic and arthritic conditions and many more. This may appear to be a rather comprehensive list, yet it is obvious that long-term decreased blood supply and the subsequently arising problems can entail further conditions. Functional impairment and patho-morphological changes, which chronic Blood stasis can generate in the heart, brain, blood vessels, liver, kidney and other organs, can already be detected at an earlier stage by clinical investigation. This was proved for the first time in experiments conducted within my own research project at the research division of Tianjin TCM University in 1998, published in my doctoral thesis 'Experimental long-term study on chronic Blood stasis/hyperviscosity syndrome – patho-morphology and functional impairment of internal organs'.

First, this book presents a description of the concept of Blood stasis, background knowledge, causes and diagnosis from the viewpoint of Chinese and conventional medicine. This is then clarified by means of case studies. Subsequently, individual medicinals necessary for treatment are listed, with their combinations, including acupuncture and herbal medicine prescriptions, and a classification of treatment principles. Finally, important classical texts dealing with the topic are presented to facilitate an immediate view of thought and practice in China.

As a complement, the appendices contain an extensive glossary explaining technical terms, references and bibliographies, comparative lists and a general index. In this way, the concept of Blood stasis will be illuminated from the point of view of both traditional Chinese medicine (TCM) and modern science.

One might wonder why we need to look to China given all the current accomplishments possessed by conventional medicine which are put into use in treating the above-mentioned conditions. This is due to the fact that the study of the causes of these conditions is still in the fledgling stage in the West, where treatment only starts once organic damage has already occurred. Conversely, TCM concentrates primarily on the functional disturbances and applies centuries' worth of experience in the treatment of those conditions. Although the science of haemorheology is still in its infancy, it allows us to diagnose signs of Blood stasis by scientific and verifiable means. However, regarding treatment, there is still a long way to go.

This is where Chinese medicine comes into play: it provides us with medicinals and formulas that have been tried and tested on patients for centuries. And for those who are in doubt and require scientific proof, during the last 30 years Chinese medicinals have also been subjected to analysis by Western research and tested for pharmacological efficacy.

Concerning the material at hand, there is a great deal of 'buried treasure' within Chinese medicine which has been ignored merely because of language barriers. In contrast, the Chinese have accessed Western medical knowledge fully and completely, rendering their conventional medicine equal to our own.

It is lamentable that, unlike the Americans, we have barely got beyond acupuncture, even though there was already an interest in Chinese medicine in the Old World decades ago. As a result, for example in Germany, Chinese herbal plants and medicinals have only been available for a few years, yet they exist without any legal status whatsoever and are priced far higher than necessary.

This may be due to a more conservative European attitude. On the other hand, in the USA it may be due to the higher accessibility of TCM, owing to the Chinese immigrant community. In any case, today's knowledge is open to anybody willing to look for it.

This book, then, is intended to continue to bridge the medical worlds of the East and West. The concept of Blood stasis will be comprehensively elucidated, including all the most essential classical and modern sources. It may well be possible for established conventional doctors to become distracted and confused by the use of a similar nomenclature based on a different meaning. At the same time, purists from the alternative healing community might be bothered by the presence of numerous scientific terms and connections, which are scarcely found in contemporary works of TCM.

For these reasons I ask for tolerance from both sides, which is necessary for everyone willing to learn. If we approach any new concept with a prejudiced mind and preconceived ideas, then there will be nothing to learn except for that already known.

TOLERANCE AND FLEXIBILITY – TWO INDISPENSABLE CHARACTERISTICS WHEN STUDYING TCM

Regarding tolerance, during the translation of Wang Qing-Ren's book, in particular the section on anatomy, I often found myself in doubt as to whether it was worth the trouble, considering the abundant fallacies and ambiguities of that time. He believes food and drink to be digested separately, otherwise the stool would be runny; he also says that if urine is filtered from the food mass in the Small Intestine (as it is according to Chinese medical classics), then in that case it would smell just as strong as the faeces. Thus he 'puts the mistakes right' – and in doing so, he turns the truth upside down.

Initially, I translated statements such as 'Heart not containing any blood' with a certain reluctance, knowing today's correct anatomy as a matter of course. But in the eighteenth century Wang criticized the accepted anatomy taught in the classics. And he criticized the fact that nobody dared to question it.

Wang had his doubts about classical Chinese theories, so he tried to correct them using anatomical studies. This undertaking was as controversial as Einstein's critique on Huygen's popular hypothesis on light propagation, as both had the scientific establishment of their time against them.

Wang was wise enough to describe his findings as mere beginnings, which might not be absolute. He invites ensuing generations to continue his work and to rectify it wherever necessary. Bearing in mind that anatomy books of 1830 contained many flaws, we can pardon his errors, including his greatest: his attempt to mix two systems, that of concrete anatomy from the West with the abstract models of Chinese medicine!

I had the idea of choosing the concept of time to further exemplify the differences between Western and Chinese thought. This comparison acts as a parallel to the concept of the human body, which is also viewed distinctly by both cultures. While it was customary to divide the day into 24 hours and the year into 12 months in the West, it was the other way round in China, where 12 hours made up one day and 24 months of 14 days each added up to 1 year. This means that while in China the year was more precise, so in Europe was the day. Both systems worked perfectly in reference to the same object, time. One might also divide time into decimal units, which we would soon become accustomed to.

Both systems have their pros and cons: for farmers, long-term weather assessment was surely more important than a daily assessment. This created smaller units and thus greater precision for one year. In the West, more precision for one day had its own advantages, thus both systems could coexist without being mutually exclusive.

One of my Tianjin professors suggested that this example may well illustrate the principle of using different models of thought with the same end in view. However, he continued, this comparison would not be accurate as time is abstract in nature, and the human body is concrete. But is this truly so? This caused me to think about the concept of this concrete and seemingly tangible body. What actually is the definition of the body? Where does it start and where does it end? When will the air we breathe, the food we eat, become part of our body? Are the boundaries of our body defined by our optical or tactile cognition? And what about voice? Does it belong to my body or to the air?

For instance, is my body temperature part of my body? Infrared imaging can show the body's radiant warmth, which is perceivable by touch. This by far exceeds the optically visible wave range of the body. Our other senses also permit such further definitions. If we do not want to rely on our senses, resorting to technology with its inherent higher precision would further complicate the issue: are we now measuring boundaries of the body including dead and desquamated skin cells, or do we exclude them? Do those shed gut cells still belong to me? And what about hair, excrement, fertilized ova, phagocytes absorbing foreign bodies etc.? Recently, parts of DNA from cattle and pigs were found in human tissue. Obviously, the DNA had not fully degraded into amino acids, as always assumed: a completely new aspect of the proverb 'You are what you eat'.

So, where does the body begin and where does it end? The apparently very natural idea that our body is clearly distinguished from its environment, is now being challenged: also, due to increasing accuracy in other sciences such as quantum physics, nonlinear biochemistry and complex mathematics, our perception of the body appears to be approaching a more holistic concept, reminiscent of Chinese philosophy.

I have assumed the body to be a concrete object in both schools of thought. But the more I contemplated this, the more blurred this seemingly sharp definition of the body became. It becomes all the more difficult when looking at Wang Qing-Ren's ideas on physiology and pathology. Within these ideas, we cannot expect any precise facts, but rather statistical probabilities such as the most likely position of the appendix, number of vertebrae, symmetry of renal function etc. Eventually, just like Wang Qing-Ren's contemporaries, I assumed familiar facts and ended up with fuzzy logic, chaos theory and the like.

Bit by bit I felt like the hunter in Zhuang-Zi's story: he closely watches a praying mantis, which itself is being stalked by a bird. He in turn is after the bird, but instead gets caught out and chased away by the park ranger.

Whilst trying to be broad-minded in judging the mistakes of Wang, who strived to improve the implicitness of medical theory of his time, I found myself stumbling across some habits of thought of my own. What can be learned from this experience may surely be sound advice to every scientist at any time: *to question our habits is always a good habit*!

A cultural and intellectual exchange has often been beneficial for ensuing ages. In this way, the more function-oriented thought models of Chinese medicine can indeed complement those more substance-oriented models of Western medicine.

Today, after almost 200 years, we can still learn from Wang Qing-Ren's mistakes and apply both models separately to the same object, in accordance with their advantages, in the same sense as we can apply Newton's theories on earth and Einstein's in space. Every model can be justified, without one excluding the other.

On the contrary, this mutual complementation will bring about more individualized treatment for the patient, and a greater choice in therapeutic management for the practitioner. In this respect, China is one step ahead of us. In addition to traditional and conventional medicine, they have a third option: the so-called integrated medicine that combines the best features from both sides. For example, with regard to the classical concept of Blood stasis, China's integrated medicine applies all diagnostic methods, using haemorheology and blood screening protocols in combination with traditional diagnostics. But computer tomography (CT), magnetic resonance imaging (MRI) and other methods may also be employed if necessary. Yet treatment focuses on the use of traditional medicinals[1] which improve not only the composition but also the fluid state of blood. This reflects the pragmatic stance of integrated medicine, which does not see any contradiction in the simultaneous use of modern and traditional medicine.

Coming back to Wang Qing-Ren's book: whilst his anatomical studies are of more historical and methodical importance (which may well be skipped by the more practically minded reader), the second and third parts of his book bear much more significance for us. His indications and formulas can be applied unmodified and are still in popular use in contemporary China, even in very specific fields such as the prevention and treatment of apoplexy, dementia, arteriosclerosis, heart attack, coronary heart disease, diabetes, insomnia, high blood pressure and so on.

Regarding clinical application, and to facilitate a full picture of *Yu Xue* (Blood stasis) in Chinese medicine, I have added translations of relevant classical texts discussing Blood stasis. I have analysed and explained medicinals and formulas appearing in Wang Qing-Ren's book, also including pharmacological effects.

Due to the recent availability of Chinese medicinals in Germany over the past few years,[2] every practitioner can evaluate the effect of the formulas introduced in this book on his own. One should not forget (as for acupuncture) that working with Chinese medicinals requires thorough knowledge of the foundations and basic theories of TCM, as well as diagnostic methods and specific (i.e. not symptomatic) syndrome differentiation (*Bian Zheng*).

The World Health Organization (WHO) is asking for an individualized medicine in the twenty-first century, a request that Chinese medicine is ideally placed to respond to: it is not only able to categorize and assess purely functional disorders that are perceived subjectively by the patient, prior to detectable organic disease, but Chinese medicine also offers tailor-made treatments, allowing patients to receive an individualized therapy for their specific illness.

Whilst fully acknowledging the single human being, TCM does not ignore the individual's position in the bigger picture.

As well as to mental and physical disposition[3] and social background, consideration during the diagnostic procedure is given to climatic, dietary and lifestyle patterns (e.g. sleep, sex, exercise etc.), i.e. the individual in his surroundings. Such a non-linear or integrated perception shows exactly why modern sciences like complex mathematics, chaos theory, quantum physics, non-homeostatic biochemistry, cybernetics etc. have a great advantage over medicine: an integrated mindset. Nearly all sciences have completed this paradigm shift, except for medicine, which is continuing its search for answers in the cul-de-sacs of molecular biology.

Accepting new paradigms does not mean we must abandon old ones: in China, there are efforts to integrate both systems; likewise in Australia and the USA, where the TCM system is also

---

[1] Further information can be found in my doctoral thesis and (Chinese) publications of my supervisor, Professor Zhang Bo-Li.

[2] For addresses see website: www.TCMinter.net

[3] Contrary to Western thought, Chinese philosophy does not separate mind and body, but regards them both as aspects of the body.

gaining more popularity. However, it seems that medical science has not yet woken up to these new developments. This raises the question: Has the pioneering spirit of the Old World left, together with the pioneers, to emigrate to the New World?

Hoping that this is not the case, we can leave aside our prejudices about the alleged inferiority of foreign medical theories; instead, let us be open to unfamiliar views, new ideas and a systemic way of thinking, so that we can further our knowledge and take another step into a more universal future for medicine.

Gunter Ralf Neeb
Tianjin, Feng He Yuan
Summer 1997
ragune@mac.com

Dedication and acknowledgments

'Panta rhei' (Everything flows)

Heraclites

After three years of studying there was no disease under the sky that I could not cure. However, after three years of practice there were not sufficient prescriptions under the sky to cure all the diseases that I encountered.

Sun Si-Miao

This book is dedicated to all those who have journeyed to the Orient, who have returned home with some of the noble spirit of the East, and to all participants of the *Xi You Ji* (voyage to the West), who have come to explore the treasures of the West, as well as to all the bridges that connect the paths of both wanderers and thus make this world a little smaller.

I would like to cordially thank my parents Hartmut and Erika Neeb, my wife Bi-Hsia, my parents-in-law as well as my teachers and lecturers, without whose encouragement and support my own voyage to the East would not have been possible.

GN

Notes on translation style

This book is addressed to all those interested in TCM or practitioners of acupuncture and Chinese medicine who have adequate previous knowledge. A fundamental understanding of Chinese medicine is presumed. For the most part, when new terms are introduced, I will briefly explain their meaning. They are all listed in the Glossary (Appendix 1), which should make understanding as easy as possible for beginners. Additionally, the special features of Chinese medicine will be briefly introduced.

The translation is designed to be useful primarily to those practising and studying Chinese medicine. Therefore, it should be as easily and fluently readable as possible. It implies that the translator must prefer to reflect the gist of a text to a verbatim reproduction. For the benefit of readability, I have abstained from parenthesizing all words not appearing in the original script and which are merely added by the translator. To cite Bob Flaws:[1]

'. . . and (therefore, this disease) cannot be treated in one and the same way. (we) should follow (Liu) He-Jian, who is unquestionably right in ascribing (this disease) to inappropriate nursing and (inadequate) rest with water unable to restrain fire. According to (the cases) available (to me) so far, (although) there is indeed external wind stroke . . .'.

Sentences like these are undoubtedly more detailed than my own informal and more natural style. However, readability suffers gravely. From the experience gained as a translator in my early undergraduate years in Taiwan I have come to conclude that readers require a clear and comprehensible translation in their native language. I therefore ask all expert readers to forgive me for using a more casual style, which is unavoidable as my target group consists predominantly of clinical practitioners of TCM.

Concerning frequently used terms, Chinese medicine has focused on the interpretation of functional relationships at an early stage; in this sense, terms like Wind, Fire or Dampness in fact very rarely stand for the actual substance. They are abstractions of the original substance, like *Yin* and *Yang*, comprising certain qualities in one model of thought. The use of concrete, for example meteorological, phenomena is intended to serve as a memory hook, i.e. a mnemonic, which is why these terms should never be taken literally (compare to conventional medicine: when discussing gouty and rheumatic spheres, nobody will start looking for circles; what's more, nobody will be likely to run for the fire extinguisher if something is 'inflamed'). This fact is constantly emphasized by Porkert, Wiseman[2] and other experts in the field. However, as some laymen and newcom-

[1] Translation from *Dan Xi Zhi Fa Xin* by Yang Shou-Zhong and Bob Flaws, Blue Poppy Press (see Appendix 7).

[2] M Porkert: *Lehrbuch des Chinesischen Diagnostik*, also his other publications (see Appendix 7); N Wiseman, A Ellis 'Translators Foreword' in *Fundamentals of Chinese Medicine*, SMC, Taiwan.

ers in Chinese medicine still become confused, to mention the presence of these abstracted terms should never be neglected.

As regards terminology of Chinese medicinals, Latin and botanical terms have been adopted internationally, as they are (mostly) used in China's foreign language editions. I have also adhered to this practice, drawing my sources either from Porkert's excellent book *Klinische Chinesische Pharmakologie* or occasionally from Bensky and Gamble's *Materia Medica* (1993) (see Appendix 7). Unfortunately, both lack any of the latest developments on pharmacology and mode of action of Chinese medicinals. The research results compiled in *Materia Medica* are taken from the *Encyclopaedia of Chinese Traditional Medicinals* (*Zhong Yao Da Ci Dian*, Shanghai), published in 1977 (see Appendix 7). Since then, a good deal more has been discovered.

The same applies to Paulus and Ding's (1987) *Handbuch der traditionellen Chinesischen Heilpflanzen.* (*Handbook of Traditional Chinese Healing Plants*) (see Appendix 7) which I rarely consult due to its somewhat impractical botanical classification. For the description of those medicinals appearing in my book, I therefore chose to use the latest available sources in China ranging from 1993 to 1998 (see Appendix 7, Bibliography).

Formula names can also be quite a worry to someone who is translating Chinese, as these – Chinese being a monosyllabic language – are mostly quite succinct. When translated into German, the resulting expression either becomes ridiculously long or just turns into a tongue-twister. This makes memorization as hard a task as learning the Chinese term itself.

Most Chinese formula names consist of three to five syllables, which are predominantly derived from names of medicinals. One of the longest with 11 syllables is most certainly *Dang Gui Si Ni Jia Wu Zhu Yu Sheng Jiang Tang*.[3] For instance, Porkert translates it using the Latinized version Decoctum

quatuor Contravectionum cum Angelica sinensis, Evodia et Zingiberi augmentato (32 syllables). *Bu Zhong Yi Qi Tang*[3] (5 syllables) was correspondingly and correctly translated by Stefan Hager into the German version Dekokt zur Kräftigung des mittleren Erwärmers und zur Unterstützung des Qi (21 syllables; English: decoction for fortifying the Middle Burner and to supplement Qi), but not without rendering it four times as long as the original.

In this case, the same principle applies as when acupuncture was introduced in the West. Although in my opinion it is of great value to learn the meaning of acupuncture names (as they can mostly indicate location and action), the majority of Western acupuncturists usually start off with memorizing point numbers (e.g. LI 4 instead of *He Gu* and Joined Valleys respectively) in order simply to manage the vast amount of information.

Looking at the even greater number of medicinals and formulas, a simplified nomenclature should be beneficial to any TCM beginner. Having a nomenclature that varies with the author, and having to learn lengthy and complicated expressions may cause considerable trouble and discouragement to any student. Equally, I am fully aware that most people are simply not able to move to China for a few decades in order to study the language and Chinese medicine. Thus, after long consideration, I have decided to use the approach described below.

Regular Chinese terms will be printed in *Pinyin* (i.e. phonetic spelling, International Organization for Standardization (ISO) standard for the Romanization of Chinese); their meaning and Western equivalent will be mentioned in brackets before or after, according to readability. Medicinals and formulas will be specified in *Pinyin* followed by the respective name in English. The full meaning will be mentioned thereafter.

There are still no accepted standards for translations in spite of increasing efforts made by all parties (this may be the reason for the lack of standards). Most authors still pretty much 'do their own thing', so I have arrived at the following conclusion: I will continue to keep to the rules of translating technical terms into simple and memorable equivalents, nevertheless Chinese

---

[3] The Chinese *Tang* means decoction, colloquially 'soup'. Here in the West 'tea' is commonly used instead of decoction, even when this does not contain any leaves of Thea Sinensis. I recommend memorizing the term *Tang*, which is just as essential to know as *Luo* (collaterals) in acupuncture.

terms in *Pinyin* will be included, as these are the only international standard currently available. This should also facilitate communication with Chinese practitioners. This method is also applied by virtually all well-known English speaking authors.[4]

Another goal to strive for is to keep technical terms in *Pinyin*, or alternatively to supplement the translated term with the *Pinyin* term, and to use this as a standard. In this matter I totally agree with Steven Clavey.[5] Students of Western medicine also need to learn and understand technical terms derived from foreign languages, such as Latin or English. Irrespective of the term, whether e.g. 'haemorrhoids' or 'piles' is used, the implied meaning should be clear.

As used in earlier publications by Jeremy Ross, an exclusively *Pinyin* nomenclature could prevent potential confusion, for example in the TCM organ function of the 'Liver' as compared to the Western 'liver'. Unfortunately, it makes it more difficult to appreciate the mutual relationship of both organ conceptions, especially for beginners.

On the other hand, a complete adaptation into English should not be necessary; Wiseman consents to having clear limits when introducing the number of terms in *Pinyin*,[6] but if this ends at 30 words, then one should not think about studying Chinese medicine. Equally, one can hardly demand the exclusive use of non-technical terms from his lecturers and textbooks, just to save oneself the effort of having to learn them. Therefore, if every term is translated and the original term is put in brackets, the argument put forward by Wiseman to abolish the usage of Chinese terms no longer applies.[7]

Furthermore, all technical terms are explained and mentioned in *Pinyin* within the Glossary. Exceptions are common terms such as *Yin*, *Yang*, *Qi*, Deficiency and Excess, a method also endorsed by Maciocia and others.

In addition, symptoms of a disease have the same meaning as in conventional medicine. Yet, 'syndrome' (*Zheng*) describes a collection of symptoms in Chinese medicine. In extreme cases, sometimes consistency or clarity of the text had to be sacrificed; this means either continue to use one translation for a specific term or changing and selecting a translation according to the actual context. In those cases, I always decided to forego consistency in favour of clarity (see footnote 7), which to me has higher priority.

I am aware of the fact that this methodology might not suit everyone. Future editions will incorporate any necessary modifications that prove useful. Therefore, I am open to and grateful for any suggestions. All translations of Chinese source texts stem from me; potential discrepancies with regard to other translations can all be accounted for.

---

[4] Clavey, Barolet, Bensky, Gamble, Hsu, Kaptchuk, Maciocia, Vangermeersch et al (see Appendix 7).
[5] See Foreword in *Fluid Physiology* by J Clavey (see Appendix 7).
[6] N Wiseman *English–Chinese, Chinese–English Dictionary of Traditional Chinese Medicine*. Introduction: *Pinyin* loans, p 72 (see Appendix 7).
[7] The practice of using Chinese terms exclusively (e.g. Ross: Zang Fu) is repudiated by Wiseman for the following reasons: (Wiseman, ibid. Introduction: Applicability of methods. p 60 bottom) 'The Pinyin rendering obscures for the foreign reader the only definite thing about the nature of the Chinese concept.' However, this applies only if the term is rendered exclusively in *Pinyin*. I can by all means write 'Lacrimation syndrome due to Wind' when referring to the climatic influence Wind, or on the other hand, 'Aversion to Wind' (*Feng*) when referring to the pathogenic factor Wind, which is then explained, for instance, in the Glossary. The opinion that a different translation of the same word interrupts the coherence of the translation is not necessarily warranted: occasionally I have to add to the information hidden within the context in any case to achieve the comprehensibility that the reader would expect. For the Chinese words '*la*' (spicy), '*re*' (hot) and '*tang*' (hot to touch) I cannot always give the English translation 'hot'; to facilitate comprehensibility I need to add or alter something, for example 'spicy-hot' or 'acrid', 'hot' or 'heat' and 'scalding hot' or 'scorching'. Conversely, according to the context, I need to translate the Chinese word '*shang*' into either 'above', 'on top', 'on' or 'over', which adds to the original information not only something about the horizontal or vertical position (on the wall, on top of the table), but also whether the object has direct contact (on top of the table – above the table). Although when translating the fundamental rule applies to add as little as possible of one's own interpretation and to continue using a previously chosen term, this applies only if *greater* clarity is thereby achieved. If it is not, and the information becomes less clear, then an interpretative translation style is appropriate.

Notes on terminology

Even Confucius observes: 'What is necessary is to rectify names' (*Lun Yu*, Chapter 13.3). But this proves to be difficult, as we shall see.

The etymology of the word '*Yu*' gives us the following: *Yu* (first tone) is described as 'extravasated blood' by the (in my opinion, not always accurate) sinologist Wiegert. This rather modern interpretation stems from Tang Zong-Hai (Qing dynasty). The '*Shuo Wen*' (Han dynasty) says: *Yu* is accumulation (*Ji*) of Blood in a disease. *Zhi* means contraction (*Ning*) and *Yu* means obstruction or thicket. We can thus translate *Yu* and *Zhi* freely as stasis and stagnation, the question being which term is used and when.

In Anglo-Saxon countries, the Chinese term '*Yu Xue*' (*Yu* first tone) is translated as Bloodstasis (Maciocia, Wiseman's and Ou Yang's dictionary), Blood-Stasis (Bensky), stagnant blood (Xie Zhufan) and Blood-Stagnation (also but seldom used by Bensky). In Germany, the term is translated as Blut-Stagnation (Unschuld, Kirschbaum, Wühr), Blutstau (Geng Junying, Wühr), Blut-Stase (Hager, Wiesmann, Wühr) and Stase des *Xue* (Porkert). The question is, which term should be used?

Whilst the meaning of Blood stasis has been put down into writing since the '*Nei Jing*', when it came into the nomenclature of Blood stasis syndrome, even Chinese scholars were unable to come to an agreement. Mentioned within the '*Nei Jing*' are 'poor Blood' (*Bei Xue*), blocked vessels, clogged arteries, coagulated Blood etc.

A more precise model for diagnosis and treatment of Blood stasis was developed by Zhang Zhong-Jing in third century AD (Han dynasty): he was the first to use the word '*Yu Xue*' (Blood stasis), but also '*Xu Xue*' (Blood amassment, corresponding to Blood stasis with Heat). For instance, it is mentioned in the '*Shang Han Lun*', clause 237: 'If the patient is forgetful, then there must be Blood stasis'. In the twentieth century, this reference has led to the successful treatment of senile dementia and sequelae of apoplexy with Blood invigorating medicinals. After Zhang Zhong-Jing, it was not until 1500 years later that the term *Yu Xue* was to be established as an official description of a syndrome.

However, even present-day Chinese textbooks allow '*Yu Xue*' and sometimes '*Xue Yu*', which in 1989 at the national research committee for Blood stasis was defined as 'Blood stasis' and 'static Blood', i.e. the former being a syndrome, the latter a state of Blood.

So, is it really necessary for ordinary TCM practitioners to pay attention to this apparent quibbling about minor details? The answer is yes. Consider: as soon as these terms are confused, finding your way through the resulting jungle of terms will be even more difficult.

Problems arise in the first place due to the existence of other types of stagnation in the body: *Qi* and Liver-*Qi* (which is closely related to emotions) can stagnate, identified by the terms *Qi-Zhi* and *Qi-Yu* (fourth tone, different character); food can stagnate; very occasionally, even Blood stagnation 'Xue Zhi' is mentioned as a precursor of Blood stasis (see Bensky in *Formulas and Strategies*, p 311). Thus in Chinese this is a matter of different terms, which should not be translated with the same word. The same applies in German and English. In any case, most standard Chinese textbooks use 'Yu' only in association with Blood, i.e. Blood-stasis or Blood stasis, whereas 'Zhi' can be used for *Qi* and food stagnation. If 'Zhi' is therefore translated as stagnation, then inevitably we have to select another term for 'Yu' – in this case, stasis.

For the above-mentioned etymological, semantic and logical reasons, and considering some already established terms, I suggest the following classification:

1. Blood stasis (*Yu Xue*, *Yu* = first tone)

Retardation or ceased movement of flow of Blood. Exterior causes are trauma, pathogenic Cold and Heat; interior causes are internal deficiency syndromes such as deficiency of Blood due to bleeding, deficiency of *Qi*, deficiency of *Yang*, exhaustion due to prolonged illness and weak condition due to overstrain; internal excess syndromes are *Qi* stagnation, emotional upsets and physical overexertion.

2. Stagnation (*Zhi*)

A flow that is slowed down or even brought to a standstill. Contrary to 'stasis', which is related specifically to Blood, this term is used in China for digested food (food stagnation, *Shi Zhi*) and *Qi* (*Qi* stagnation, *Qi Zhi*).

3. Blood amassment (*Xù Xue*)

This term was originally coined by Zhang Zhong-Jing in the '*Shang Han Za Bing Lun*' (which is now known as '*Shang Han Lun*'). It describes a type of Blood stasis caused by pathogenic Heat in the Lower Burner, showing symptoms like pain in the lower abdomen and some mental disorders (see translation '*Jin Kui*', Chapter 16, and '*Shang Han*', clause 124).

Later on, the term was used as a generic term for all kinds of Blood stasis and Blood depression.

After the time of Wang Qing-Ren and Tang Zhong-Hai the term was used again in its original meaning.

4. Depression (*Yù*)

Digested food, Blood, *Qi* and Body Fluids are all substances that are in constant flux. Any form of obstruction to this flow will impair physiological processes. *Qi* is responsible for the transport of all other substances; if *Qi* is depressed (e.g. due to Liver-*Qi* depression), it provides the basis for all other types of depressions and should therefore always be treated concomitantly. Other types of depression are Blood depression (*Yù Xue*, a type of Blood stasis caused by *Qi* depression), Dampness depression, Heat depression, Phlegm depression and food depression (a type of food stagnation caused by an emotional *Qi* depression).

5. Obstructions (*Bu Tong*)

Generally, obstructions affect the flow of all naturally circulating substances, such as *Qi*, Blood and Body Fluids (*Jin* and *Ye*). The latter can congest and thus produce Phlegm (*Tan*) and Phlegm-Fluids (*Tan Yin*). Any obstructed substance may in the long run bring other substances to a halt, for instance in the relation of Blood stasis and *Qi* stagnation both may be either cause or effect. If the Channels or Collaterals are affected, this is usually associated to *Qi*; however, Blood invigorating medicinals are often prescribed.

In German, the terms '*statisch, stagnieren, stauen*' (static, to stagnate, to accumulate – Translator's note) are all related. The question may arise, why do we say stasis for 'Yu', stagnation for 'Zhi', and depression for 'Yù'. Why not vice-versa? To begin with, I regard Maciocia and Bensky as two very popular and practically minded authors in TCM; then there is Wiseman who has the highest expertise concerning linguistics, and finally there are Hager, Höll and Wiesmann whom I consider to be established and precise translators within the German TCM community. This virtually sets a certain standard. In addition, those authors use these terms consistently. Unfortunately, a precise terminological comparison has never been drawn – until now. Finally, this is the first manual on Blood stasis appearing in a language other than

Chinese. All terms come directly from the author, who in the last 13 years was able to obtain in-depth knowledge and a feel for the Chinese language and writing system. Nevertheless, there may well be the reader who is already used to certain translations. We hope that everyone can accept the above-mentioned terminology which we are striving to formulate as clearly and coherently as possible.

SUMMARY

In this book we will discuss:

- stasis, especially Blood stasis impairing blood flow
- stagnation affecting the flow of *Qi* and digested food
- depression due to emotions and impaired flow of Liver-*Qi*
- Blood amassment in the case of Blood stasis with Heat, as described in the *Shang Han Lun*
- obstructions in the course of unspecified impaired flow, such as obstruction of channels, chest *Bi* syndrome, etc.

Further terms are included in the comprehensive Glossary at the end of the book.

The term 'TCM'

Whenever we are using the abbreviated form 'TCM', the entirety of Traditional Chinese Medicine is implied. The myth of TCM being a new school within Chinese medicine, which Unschuld, Flaws et al brought into being, lacks any basis. In the 1950s, after the integration of Chinese medicine into the Republic's university system, many partly conflicting theories were made subject to restructuring and eventually unified. However, if you look closely, all those theories are still available. Nowadays, learning contents are more logically structured in order to be more plausible to the student, whereas in the past the lack of a proper syllabus resulted in confusion; as a result, students had to make some sense out of disconnected ideas in their minds, relying solely on intuition to organize their information. This method is still in practice in many private clinics in Taiwan. Although it can work, a greater amount of time is needed and but a few chosen ones are accepted. Only a 'preparation for the masses', which is quite normal in the Republic of China, turns the medicine of China into a subject that can be studied systematically by all. Because I was able to learn about both systems in both countries for more than 5 years respectively, I would venture to claim that the above-mentioned 'TCM' is not merely an alternative school of thought within Chinese medicine: it is the Traditional Chinese Medicine taught in all universities, contrary to the TCM taught in the traditional way of master and student. Although methods may differ, the content of both 'TCMs' remains the same.

Consequently, the abbreviated form 'TCM' used within this book embraces all of Traditional Chinese Medicine, regardless of place.

Abbreviations used in the text

A/G	= Albumin/Glutamine
ALT	= Alanine Aminotransferase, GPT (Glutamate Pyruvate Transaminase)
Anti-HBc	= Hepatitis B core antibodies
Anti-HBcIgM	= Hepatitis B core Immunoglobulin M antibodies
Anti-HBs negative	= Hepatitis B antibodies negative
AST	= Aspartate Amino Transferase, GOT (Glutamate Oxalacetate Transaminase)
Bil	= Bilirubin
BP	= Blood pressure
CHD	= Coronary Heart Diseases (angina pectoris, myocardial infarction, coronary heart insufficiency, coronary arrhythmia)
CT	= Computer Tomography
DIC	= Disseminated intravascular coagulation
ECG	= Electrocardiograph
EMG	= Electromyogram
ESR	= Erythrocyte Sedimentation Rate
GGT	= Gamma Glutamyl Transpeptidase
HBe negative	= Hepatitis B envelope negative
HBsAg	= Hepatitis B surface Antigen
HBsAg positive	= Hepatitis B surface Antigen positive
LDL	= Law density lipoprotein
LLT (+)	= Limulus Lysate test positive
MRI	= Magnetic Resonance Imaging
Pt/Pa	= Prothrombin time/Prothrombin agglutination
SOD	= Super Oxide Dismutase
STB	= Stercobilin
TCM	= Traditional Chinese Medicine, in the literal sense, meaning the entire non-Western medicine in China from ancient until present times
TIA	= Transient ischemic attack, temporary disturbance of blood circulation to the brain, similar to apoplexy but without necrosis
TTT	= Thymol Turbidity Test

SECTION 1

Theory and background knowledge

This section presents an introduction to the TCM way of thinking and its models, a description of the concept of Blood stasis from a Western medicine stance, and a more thorough description from the TCM point of view. Within TCM, the physiological functions and pathological changes of Blood, and the aetiology, diagnostics and historical background of Blood stasis are discussed. In addition, case studies taken from contemporary and classical sources are portrayed, to provide practical insight for the reader.

The main sections include a short summary of the aforementioned content.

SECTION CONTENTS

Chapter 1

Introduction: thought models in Chinese medicine

When I resolved to study Chinese – a language that I knew to be totally different from our European languages – I asked myself whether my behaviour would change, whether I would become more 'Chinese', whether I would be able to think in this language day after day. After all, I wanted to learn Chinese so that I could 'live' the philosophy and way of thinking of traditional Chinese medicine (TCM).

Thirteen years later, I still do not have a clear answer to my question, although for years I have been thinking Chinese, and reading and writing Chinese characters on a daily basis. Probably, I will never get an answer. The problem is that I cannot think simultaneously in two languages nor put myself into two different states of mind; similarly, I am incapable of being in two places at the same time. Thus I can only consciously experience one state, like the weather either in Beijing *or* in Frankfurt, but not in both cities at the same time, nor can I observe from a third position and remark on any differences.

It should be obvious that there are definite social and interpersonal differences between Eastern and Western behaviour. To which extent cultural imprint or language are involved remains to be clarified, possibly by ethnologists or anthropologists.

In my opinion, the West is more concerned with asking for the reasons (thus causal-analytical, as described by Porkert), i.e. investigating the background of any given event, whilst in China, events and their mutual relationships are enquired into as they take place. To point out something that appears obvious may sound to us odd or even funny (Riff-Raff: 'You are wet.' Brad: 'Yes. It's raining.'), and so I have heard a number of Western people in China commenting on this with amusement: 'Why do the Chinese always state the obvious?'

On that other side of the planet (i.e. in China), the usual answer one is given is: 'That's the way it is. Live with it. You cannot always know the reasons for everything.' Indeed, this becomes clear to us in the West every time we have to answer a child in its 'why' phase: at some point the question goes too far back, and we arrive at God, the Big Bang, the quarks or we get carried yet further away into the sands of infinity.

On the other hand, the question of 'what' and its relationships can nearly always be fully answered: 'What's in that picture?' A boy, his dog and the leash. 'What else?' The boy's clothes, the dog's hairs . . . etc. Eventually, we will have defined everything, important and unimportant, and clarified all the relationships between them. Note: we do not need to engage in abstract considerations, finding 'invisible' events of the past to explain the picture. No questions remain. Everything has come full circle.

Somebody once wrote that the endless search for reasons, for answers to the big 'why', was precisely the cause of the perpetual 'Faustian quest' in the West. Conversely, Joseph Needham, the famous English Sinologist, proposed the theory in *Science and Civilization* (see Appendix 7) that the simple and satisfactory act of putting all objects into the systematic order of the *I Ching* (*Yi Jing*) for centuries was responsible for preventing Chinese culture from developing research and science in the way the West.[1]

In fact, classical texts have a comparatively lower incidence of the question '*He Gu*', i.e. for what reason, than other interrogative expressions. The 'why' question that *we* have to ask ourselves now is why the study of what exists at this moment should be inferior to the study of those things resulting from the past. It may be that different applications of certain ways of thinking

have led to different findings, every one of which has prompted different findings in various disciplines; therefore, I have no grounds for believing that the Western causal way of thinking is superior to the Chinese.[2]

The reforms that took place in TCM, which demystified it and showed that many of its effects could be proven by means of laboratory experiments and statistics, are justified in that they accommodate Western scientists with TCM's ways of thinking and working, and so contribute to a better understanding – but beyond this the structure of TCM remains unchanged: that is to say, if TCM tried to imitate Western medicine's causal-analytical way of thinking, it would probably only remain a 'second class' medicine.

Numerous explanations of how TCM's scientific practice works have already been published – unfortunately only in Chinese. However, another field that has largely remained unexplored is the effect of Chinese medicinals. A great deal of pharmacological research conducted in earlier decades has meant that the most important active ingredients are now known. When a Chinese doctor prescribes a decoction made up of various plants consisting of a few thousand chemical ingredients for his patient, he doesn't need to know all of them or to be aware of all the biochemical reactions in the body, provided he knows that the decoction leads to a recovery.

And to be honest, does his Western colleague, when administering a mixture of 5–10 drugs in hospital, know what reciprocal effects, side effects, and exactly what biochemical reactions this drug cocktail causes? Or does he too rely on the expe-

---

[1] Which is no less ethnocentric than the question: Why can't the Chinese speak German like we do?

[2] At present in China, I sometimes note that inexperienced, younger TCM doctors seem to be suffering from an inferiority complex with regard to Western medicine, which has now successfully set worldwide standards and can provide scientific evidence for everything. So, is it superior to TCM? If so, in what way? Of course, it is a 'home match': if you have to play by rules that your opponent is allowed to set and change, then you will probably lose every time. In this respect, many more therapists in the West go wrong, because wariness about the unknown involves the least expenditure of energy; in this way, both the xenophobe and the lazy student ('don't want to learn new information') find themselves in agreement over thermodynamics.

rience and knowledge of his profession? It is a matter for ethical debate whether I should recommend to my patient the treatment that is empirically proven to be the best one, or whether I should not, based on the grounds that I cannot tell exactly which principle explains the treatment or why it works.

And so we come to the next point, the question of how things relate together; in other words, the interconnections between everything that exists.

Science, by which I mean *every* science, uses models of explanation that are designed to facilitate easy understanding of any given process. Sometimes these models are replaced by better ones, which are based on more up-to-date knowledge and understanding. By this process, the existence of the ether as a supporting medium for waves was declared a redundant model and the Bohr atomic shell model was abolished in favour of Rutherford's cloud model, and so on. Most scientists know that these models serve as memory hooks to aid understanding, but they are not unalterable dogmas. So this is not about who is right, but about how to grasp something.

When studying physics at school, when I had to learn that a current flows from a positive to a negative pole I protested, remembering that my chemistry teacher had taught us that electric ion exchange always takes place from a negative to a positive pole. But it was explained that taking this concept as a basic in physics would get me further. Later on, in maths and geometry, I also learned that various concepts (in Euler, Einstein, Euclid etc.) exist, which, depending on their application, could be more useful either in normal life or in calculating cosmic measurements.

In the next chapter, we are going to look at particular aspects of Chinese medicine that are especially pertinent for understanding the 'how', in other words the relationship between physical functions and dysfunctions. However, in this process we must not forget that this is also about having a well-functioning theory and not exclusively about physical entities, although these too are part of the picture. For example, regarding the *Zang-Fu* organs, the anatomically present, real organ forms a part of the functional entity of the TCM organ; but we must remember that the latter comprises considerably more than its anatomical part.

As mentioned in Korbinsky, 'The map is not the same as the landscape'. However, in TCM the map in one's hand is also part of the landscape in which one stands. Anyone who finds it hard to accept terms like Fire in the Heart and Wind in the Liver has failed to understand that we are employing a model which works in a different way from the usual causal-analytical one.

To understand Chinese medicine it is not necessary to think in Chinese, but a little less dogmatism and more flexibility helps a great deal. This should be highly recommended as much to members of the esoteric and technology-opposed community as to those in the scientific and anti-mystical TCM community.

SPECIAL FEATURES OF TCM

Chinese medicine can be differentiated from Western medicine in three ways. These are:

1. Its holistic view of man and nature (systemic)
2. Its syndrome differentiation/*Bian Zheng Lun Zhi* (individual)
3. Its consideration of permanent variable factors (dynamic).

These are explained in detail below.

HOLISTIC VIEW OF MAN AND NATURE

The human body is viewed as a complex, interwoven system that in itself interacts with and is linked to its environment (living space, workplace, social and natural surroundings).

Likewise, in TCM it is obvious that the weather can make someone prone to certain diseases, or that one may succumb to other climatic influences such as localized winds (for example the alpine wind in South Germany), dampness, sea winds etc. Different seasons have different effects, too. In a similar way, chronobiology, for example, has been able to conclude that rhythmic variations of the immune system, sleep, body temperature and other cycles are influenced by the season.[3]

---

[3] Moore-Ede: *Clocks that time us*, Meier Knoll: *Chronobiology*, Reiter: *Melatonin*, Orlock: *Inner Time*, as well as articles by Wagner, Emslie, Levy, Zawilska and many more (see Bibliography).

Finally, the inner emotional state is incorporated into the analysis of the present state of the body, and the social environment as part of the human network also belongs here; doctors in China nearly always enquire about family or work-related issues, because aggravation, stress and so on have been proved to have an effect on physical disease processes. This is all part of the first step in TCM, the diagnosis.

For some decades now, such a nonlinear, joined-up and systemic view has been found within the most up-to-date front-line branches of science, starting with non-Newtonian physics and quantum physics, dissipative structures in biochemistry, and going as far as chaos theory and dynamic system theory in complex mathematics. While medicine in the West has traditionally been regarded as the 'unreliable' discipline among the exact sciences, it has now, ironically, become obsessed with detail and precision. As a result, having become a Cartesian-rigid, linear science, it is now lagging behind the new flexibility of its nonlinear siblings. Although first signs of a systemic medicine are emerging, as seen in geomedicine, chronobiological medicine and interdisciplinary systems, they are barely noticed in mainstream medicine and are poorly promoted, because the fundamental structure of medicine today has failed so far to overcome the limits of Cartesian thought. In this respect, integrated Chinese medicine is one step ahead of us.

SYNDROME DIFFERENTIATION (*BIAN ZHENG LUN ZHI*)

Bian Zheng Lun Zhi or syndrome differentiation means discussion of symptoms in order to draw up a treatment concept. All data that was gathered during diagnosis is now arranged in such a way as to obtain a clear picture of the situation that prevails inside the body. Then an appropriate treatment concept is matched with this picture, to restore those functions that were unbalanced to a state of stability. Syndrome differentiation is the second step in TCM. Someone who does not master this will unfortunately only be able to treat symptomatically (e.g. prescription acupuncture) and will fail to achieve good therapeutic results because of the lack of precision. The application of

syndrome differentiation is not based only on the principle of cause and effect (causal analysis) that is commonly used in Western thought, but mainly on a system-linking model, for which one may use the term 'inductive synthesis'.[4]

Using syndrome differentiation allows the physician to treat *not only every disease, but also every patient*; this means the treatment is individually and specifically adapted to every person's present condition.

CONSIDERATION OF PERMANENT VARIABLE FACTORS

Every time a patient goes to see a doctor in China, a new case history is completed (although not in as much detail as the initial one). Treatment is based each time on this up-to-date history. This procedure makes sense as each (successful) treatment should bring about some physical changes which will be apparent in the subsequent consultation. Thus the third step in diagnosis and treatment is consideration of the patient's present condition.

Unfortunately, patients are usually prescribed the same medication in the same dose each time they visit their general practitioner, which is understandable because conventional medicine does not aim to address the whole functional condition of the body but is focused primarily on treating symptoms. However, in TCM if a practitioner believes he is able to cure a patient of a complex condition using only *one* acupuncture combination or *one* herbal prescription, then he has not grasped the concept of TCM.

To give an example, one of the professors who taught me in Tianjin told me that on his 1-year stay in Germany he got to know a therapist. He worked in his practice for a while treating patients. For every new patient the professor's new colleague made some notes about the acupuncture combination, but did not ask about the reasons for the selection of the points. At the patient's second consultation he was astonished and asked the Chinese if he had made a mistake, as he had in part used different points the last

---

[4] M. Porkert: all his work, especially *Theoretische Grundlagen der Chinesischen Medizin*, Stuttgart 1982.

time. Amused, the TCM doctor answered him: 'Yes of course. But that was *last* week!'

This anecdote is a typical representation of the prevalent attitude towards TCM; traditional Chinese medicine *cannot* be applied correctly if its theoretic concepts and foundations are not understood.

This is not about teaching Western medicine a few more prescriptions and tricks to complement its storehouse of therapies. The aim of this book is to present an independent medical system, which is superior to Western medicine in those areas where Western medicine is limited by its own conceptual mode. It cannot be denied that both systems are successful in their respective fields. However, this is only the case as long as they are employed according to their own fundamental logic.

By taking the dynamic aspects of diseases into consideration, which calls for a new syndrome differentiation in every case, it is possible to adjust the treatment to the individual and his present condition in a highly specific way. Furthermore, one is even able to be one step ahead of the disease development and to prevent its progression. For this reason this book is structured systematically, according to the approach in contemporary TCM. Introduction and case history are followed by Western diagnosis (which, in most cases, the patient already has), Chinese aetiology and diagnosis, syndrome differentiation, treatment principle and treatment application.

Chapter 2

History and development of Blood stasis and its pathological mechanisms

Although Wang Qing-Ren was not the first to notice the concept of Blood stasis, he certainly contributed the most towards its development.

Findings from the Stone Age of the first acupuncture needles made from bones and of stone splints point towards their use for blood letting and the therapeutic removal of blood clots, which marks a pre-stage of Blood stasis therapy. Written records can be traced back to as early as the *'Nei Jing'*, the Yellow Emperor's classic work, dating from the Warring States dynasty (475–221 BC). Mentioned within the *'Nei Jing Su Wen'* are 'poor Blood', blocked vessels, clotted arteries, coagulated Blood etc. The condition is classified into four aetiological factors: trauma, Cold-induced coagulation, emotional causes, notably fits of anger, and chronic exhausting diseases. It is described literally as: 'Injury resulting from fall produces poor Blood in the interior, which is hard to clear.' (Chapter 58 *'Ling Shu'*: Thievish Wind) This citation refers to acute Blood stasis with the formation of haematomata. But there are also references to chronic Blood stasis due to disturbed blood circulation and coagulation (Chapter 81: Abscesses): 'If *Ying-Qi* and *Wei-Qi* (Nutritive and Defensive energy) stagnate in the channels and vessels,[1] Blood will clot and not move. If this does not move, *Wei-Qi* (being *Yang* in nature, hence warm) cannot flow through and starts to accumulate, leading to Heat.'

A more accurate account of diagnosis and treatment was developed by Zhang Zhong-Jing in the third century (Han dynasty): in his book *'Shang Han Za Bing Lun'* (known today as *'Shang Han Lun'* and *'Jin Kui Yao Lüe'*), he used the term *'Yu Xue'* (Blood stasis) for the first time. But the term *Xu Xue* (Blood amassment, which is Blood stasis with Heat) is also mentioned in relation to impaired blood flow. For example: 'If the patient is forgetful, then Blood stasis is evident.' (*'Shang Han Lun'*, clause 237). In the twentieth century, this reference has led to the successful treatment of senile dementia and sequelae of apoplexy with Blood invigorating medicinals. After Zhang Zhong-Jing, it was not until 1500 years later that the term *Yu Xue* was to be established as an official description of a syndrome. (All relevant passages are translated in Chapter 10).

First hints of a link between Blood stasis and gynaecological disorders are given by the Sui dynasty practitioner Chao Yuan-Fang, who ascribed dysmenorrhoea as 'static Blood' (*Ji Xue*) and 'confluent Blood' (*Liu Xue*).

In the subsequent Tang dynasty (seventh to tenth centuries) Blood stasis was mentioned using

---

[1] I intentionally prefer the more general term 'blood vessel' (German: 'Ader' – Translator's note) to other anatomical terms like vessel, vein, artery and so on, particularly if there are no distinctions made in the Chinese source texts with regard to channels and blood vessels (*Qi* – Ader and Blutader in German – Translator's note). If information that is missing in the source language is translated into a clearly defined term that suggests different information, then, in my opinion, this is an interpretation that comes close to falsification.

a variety of names: the famous Taoist doctor Sun Si-Miao developed new Blood invigorating formulas for Blood amassment (*Xu Xue*) and Blood that is not moving (*Xue Bu Xing*); also Wang Tao, author of the 'Wai Tai Mi Yao' (*Medical Secrets of an Official*), developed Blood invigorating formulas for internal and external injuries. In the period of the first millennium, when Chinese medicine evolved into many new theories and schools of thought, when specialized branches such as gynaecology and paediatrics emerged, further progress was achieved in diagnosis and treatment of Blood stasis. Chen Wu-Ze, in his great book 'San Yin Ji Yi Bing Fang Lun' (*Treatise on the Three Categories of Disease Causes*, 1174), undertook pioneering work in the classification of diseases according to aetiology; he followed Zhang Zhong-Jing's ideas (in the 'Shang Han Lun') and went into greater detail in his elaborations on the treatment of Blood amassment (for translation see Section 3).

Li Dong-Yuan (Jin dynasty, twelfth and thirteenth centuries) applied *Dang Gui* (Angelica Sinensis) and other Blood invigorating medicinals in his prescriptions. His later contemporary Zhu Dan-Xi (Yuan dynasty, under Mongolian rule, thirteenth and fourteenth centuries) referred to Blood stasis as 'dead Blood' (*Si Xue*) and enhanced the theory of stagnation (*Yù*, fourth tone),[2] which often leads to Blood stasis. Thus he concluded: 'As long as *Qi* and Blood flow together harmoniously, the ten thousand diseases will not appear. But as soon as stagnation arises, disease will be the result. It is for this reason that many diseases afflicting man are derived from stagnation.' He then utilized Blood invigorating medicinals like *Chuan Xiong* (Ligusticum) to treat stagnation of Blood.

In the Qing dynasty (seventeenth century), under Manchurian rule, the most substantial progress in Blood stasis research was eventually achieved: Wang Ken-Tang's encyclopaedic work 'Zheng Zhi Zhung Sheng' (*Standard Manual for Diagnosis and Treatment*, 1602) includes a separate chapter about Blood amassment (*Xu Xue*), also containing the treatment of Blood stasis (for translation see Section 3).

His contemporary, the great scholar Zhang Jing-Yue, who would also publish his monumental complete works 20 years later on, elaborated on the treatment of three degrees of severity for Blood stasis in the chapter on masses (*Ji*): 'If Blood accumulates or becomes 'knotted', then it [stasis] should be broken up or disseminated, using *Tao Ren* (Persica), *Hong Hua* (Carthamus), *Su Mu* (Sappan) etc. . . . If Blood moves hard [literally 'rough'], it should be moved using *Niu Xi* (Achyranthis), *Yi Mu Cao* (Leonuri) etc. . . . If Blood is deficient and stagnant, it should be invigorated and tonified, using *Dang Gui* (Angelica), *Chuan Xiong* (Ligusticum), *Niu Xi* (Achyranthis), *Shou Di* (Rehmanniae Praeparata) etc.'

At the time of the last dynasty, further progress into the investigation of infections was spurred on by the school of 'febrile diseases' (*Wen Bing Xue*). One of its protagonists was the great Ye Tian-Shi (eighteenth century), who was also an excellent clinician, as can be seen from his case study reports. He further developed the theories on Blood stasis by pointing out the purple tongue colour in stasis, and by examining the concept in the 'Nei Jing' claiming that chronic disease always leads to impaired flow of Blood, for which he then also created treatment plans. (Some of his case studies on Blood stasis are presented in Chapter 9.)

Finally, in the nineteenth century, Wang Qing-Ren appeared. After having studied the classics, he came to the conclusion that post-mortem examinations, which were still frowned upon, had to be encouraged in order to further medical knowledge. Having examined many corpses, where blood could be found in all parts of the body, he deduced that diseased blood could lead to illness anywhere in the body. He then went on to specialize in the treatment of Blood stasis and its sequelae. His complete anatomical and clinical experiences were eventually published in his book 'Yin Lin Gai Cuo' (*Corrections of Mistakes in the Medical World*), which more than any other classic contributed profoundly to the theory and practice of Blood stasis. Even though his anatomical views have been outdated for a long time, his prescriptions and contributions on the treatment of apoplexy are still in wide use today. (For a complete translation see Section 3.)

---

[2] For details see Glossary (Appendix 1): Blood stagnation, Blood stasis and Blood amassment.

Wang's contemporary Lin Pei-Qin, a learned practitioner who focused on clinical experience, described nearly all the methods of treatment for Blood stasis at that time. (Excerpts are also included in Section 3, 'Classical texts'.) Later on, at the end of the nineteenth century, Tang Zhong-Hai devoted his life to the specific treatment of bleedings and conditions related to Blood, also including Blood stasis. (All relevant passages are translated in Chapter 11.)

Zang Xi-Chun, who died in 1933, contributed to the treatment of Blood stasis in modern times. Most notably, he emphasized the Blood invigorating function of *San Qi* (Notoginseng) and the combination of *E Zhu* and *San Leng* (Curcuma and Spargani). He conceived some prescriptions noted for the treatment of apoplexy, like *Huo Luo Xiao Ling Dan* (Wondrous Channel-invigorating Pill). (Some of his case studies are mentioned in different sections of this book.)

Since the 1960s, there have been major advances in scientific research on Blood stasis, its diagnosis and treatment, particularly in pharmacology, haemorheology, oncology and vascular diseases. There are still various concepts to classify in the aetiology of Blood stasis. However, it must be noted – as mentioned in the introduction – that TCM aetiology is not strictly causal-analytical, i.e. it is not always possible to make a definite dividing line between cause and effect. This becomes immediately clear with Blood stasis: many of its causes arise together with Blood stasis or they may be the result, for instance long-term Blood stasis may lead to *Qi* deficiency, but *Qi* deficiency may also cause Blood stasis. To the practitioner, however, it is more relevant to know whether *Qi* deficiency is present, and to treat it as well.

Chapter 3

Comprehension and diagnostics of Blood stasis in conventional medicine

BLOOD STASIS IN WESTERN MEDICINE

Note: Unlike throughout the rest of this book, organs mentioned in this chapter, such as heart, liver etc. refer only to the anatomical organ in the narrow sense as defined by conventional medicine.

'Blood stasis,' simply explained, means that the flow of blood is slowed down or even brought to a standstill.

Looking at the physiological function of blood, its circulation and microcirculation, it becomes clear that any minor blockage may entail a plethora of consequences: decreased supply of nutrients and oxygen to *all* tissues, changes in blood pressure, thus affecting blood vessels too, impeded vascular transport of hormones and messenger substances including waste materials that should be eliminated by blood. Thus, there may be pathological changes affecting the endocrine and immune systems, temperature homeostasis, blood clotting and the entire metabolic system. Indeed, it would be easier to list those areas and systems unaffected by stasis.

To the great surprise of the Chinese, who have understood for centuries that Blood stasis is a disease-causing factor, Western research in this area started merely a few decades ago. Based on physics and physiology, this research is concerned with the flow of blood and its disorders, i.e. haemorheology.

Originally, rheology is part of mechanics within physics and is concerned with variations in fluidity of different substances. Haemorheology, being a branch of biological medicine, investigates specifically the fluidity of blood and morphological changes of blood cells.

In the past few years, research has shown that changes in blood and its constituents, for example blood viscosity, blood viscoelasticity, blood plasma viscosity, erythrocyte aggregation (gathering of red blood cells), plasticity of blood cells, thixotropy, fluidity of white blood cells, thrombocyte aggregation and adhesion (gathering, mutual attraction and rejection of blood platelets), all play a very important role in the appearance and development of many dangerous and chronic diseases associated with microcirculation. Examples are apoplexy, diabetes, heart attack, acute renal failure, apnoea, cor pulmonale etc.

There is a direct connection between the scope of haemorheologic changes and the gravity of most critical conditions and their prognosis. Having an understanding of the pathophysiological and therapeutic implications of haemorheology can definitely alter the prognosis and outcome of these diseases.

In the Republic of China, millions of pounds are invested yearly in pharmaceutical and clinical research. The three leading areas of research in medicine, established by the government 40 years ago, are:

1. Traditional Chinese medicine, the effectiveness of which can be explained step by step by modern scientific methods, regarding both acupuncture and herbal medicine.

2. Western conventional medicine; different from our system, this frequently corresponds to and overlaps with the other two areas of medicine.

3. Integrated medicine (*Zhong Xi Yi He Jie*) objectively applies methods from both the above disciplines to find the ideal treatment for the particular type of disease. It is truly a 'holistic' medicine, because it does not reject any therapies, and chooses the most pragmatic way, without following any dogma.

An example is found in research into apoplexy and its therapy. The diagnostic methods of haemorheology (see above) and blood screening are consulted to identify any tendency towards or risk of an imminent stroke. Next, traditional medicinals are administered to avert the risk; a subse-

quent blood test will show the result. However, in the case of an existent stroke, a CT or MRI is employed to obtain information about the type of stroke and the damage. Afterwards, traditional and if necessary also modern drugs are administered to improve blood flow in the ischemic regions, dissolve the thrombus more quickly and prevent any further aggravation. In the event of hemiplegia, acupuncture is used as an adjunct to minimize any signs of paralysis or, if it is present, to treat it as quickly as possible. Thus, conventional and traditional methods cooperate for the benefit of the patient.

Within the last 20 years, two subjects that have attracted interest from all three fields of medicine in China are diagnostic haemorheology and research regarding therapy for Blood stasis.

China is the leading country in Asia, and Germany in Europe with regard to research into haemorheology. Both countries are spearheading haemorheologic research world-wide.

Unfortunately, most medical faculties in Germany mention haemorheology only marginally, if at all, as it is still regarded as an emerging subject. In this text I can only give a brief introduction. Readers who are interested are advised to consult the latest edition of Schmidt and Thews[1] or, for those wanting to dig deeper into research in haemorheology, the first-class journal 'Clinical Hemorheology' or AM Ehrly's *Therapeutic Hemorheology* (published by Springer, 1991). In addition, the essential terms in haemorheology are listed in the Glossary at the end of this book (Appendix 7).

BLOOD STASIS IN HAEMATOLOGY

High viscosity

Viscosity means internal friction resistance in fluids and is influenced by a range of factors. The first one is of course density of a fluid, which increases with a higher ratio of blood cells, blood lipids and platelets (thrombocytes), and decreases with a lower ratio of blood plasma, which for instance may arise from a 'seeping' through leaky vessel walls. Another factor is the state of vessel walls, which when intact cause less friction as

---

[1] Schmidt/Thews: *Physiologie des Menschen*, 26th edition, and *Clinical Hemorheology*, Pergamon Press – Elsevier Publishing.

compared to scarred and damaged ones. In the laboratory haematocrit and blood cholesterol levels (cholesterol, HDL and LDL) are assayed to determine the ratio of highly viscous constituents within blood.

Microcirculation

By using diagnosis on nail bed capillaries and fundoscopy, the velocity and continuity within the smallest capillary vessels can be determined. A high pressure due to inadequate blood drainage can engender convoluted and loop-like vessels. Moreover, there may be signs of tissue haemorrhaging and microscopic thromboses, if a case of Blood stasis exists. During fundoscopy, the presence of papilloedema hints at disturbances within cerebral microcirculation and permeability of the vascular system. This also points to Blood stasis.

Coagulation tendency

Blood clotting is a very complicated process that is influenced and triggered by many factors. In the ordinary scenario of a trauma, rapid clotting makes sense and is useful, as by constricting local vessels and agglutinating blood platelets bleedings can be sealed and further blood loss is avoided. It starts becoming pathological when there is an increased tendency for blood clotting and thrombus formation. Such abnormalities can be determined from clotting time as well as from length and severity of a thrombus, which is generated from a blood sample in the laboratory.

Blood cell plasticity

Usually, erythrocytes have a life expectancy of 120 days. They are filtered from the system when they are too old and unpliable to pass through the fine capillaries of the spleen and thus other capillaries without obstruction.

Decreasing sedimentation rate and increase of its K value also hint at Blood stasis. To simplify matters, any type of impediment or slowdown in the amount and speed of blood that is physiologically necessary marks a situation which can be defined in terms of TCM as Blood stasis.

As shown by the latest research,[2] the following changes can be demonstrated in blood pathology.

---

[2] Xu Zhong-Pei, Zhang Bo-Li et al. *Gao Nian Zhi Xue Zheng De Zhong Yi Bian Zheng Gui Lü Yan Jiu*, 1997, Tianjin.

Table 3.1

Syndrome differentiation in TCM	Haemorheologic changes
Blood stasis with *Qi* deficiency	Intracellular viscosity of erythrocytes ↑, plasticity of erythrocytes ↓
Blood stasis with *Yang* deficiency	Total blood viscosity ↑, coagulation in vitro ↑, plasma viscosity ↑, fibrinogen ↑, haematocrit ↑
Blood stasis with *Yin* deficiency	Plasma viscosity ↑, haematocrit ↑, K value (h/R) erythrocyte agglutination ↑, thrombocyte aggregation ↑, erythrocyte electrophoresis ↓
Blood stasis with Phlegm	Total blood and plasma viscosity ↑, coagulation in vitro ↑, fibrinogen ↑, haematocrit ↑, thrombocyte aggregation ↑
Blood stasis in general	Shear rate ↑, total blood viscosity ↑, reduced viscosity ↑, total haematocrit ↑

BASIC RESEARCH IN THE FIELD OF BLOOD STASIS

In the past decades various research was undertaken to create Blood stasis experimentally. However, this could only simulate acute, aggressive and temporary Blood stasis due to injury (heat, cold, chemical agents, physical impacts etc.). Thus, the research was based on an ideal case scenario with a single pathogenic influence in a high dose, which clinically is barely encountered.

The animal study that I carried out in 1998 (see Appendix 9) is notable both for its length (112 days) and the utilization of 3 different factors (blood viscosity, vasoconstriction and immunological factors) in a low dose to create chronic, multiple Blood stasis in the sense of TCM. In general, this correlates with the type of blood stasis commonly encountered in the clinical practice of human medicine, such as in diabetes mellitus, chronic hepatitis, coronary heart disease (CHD), ischemic apoplexies and so on.

The study was able to show that within the organism Blood stasis first gives rise to functional changes, which could be traced by examining over 70 parameters in the blood and within blood vessels. In particular, metabolic functions (especially of the liver and myocardium), and haemorheologic and immunological changes could be observed, which provided the evidence for the relationship between Blood stasis and hepatitis, CHD and carcinogenic processes.

Furthermore, the results showed that severe chronic Blood stasis generates pathomorphological changes in the liver, kidney and heart, and secondarily in the spleen and lungs. Although the end weight in the experimental group was much lower, the weight of heart, liver, spleen and brain was higher than in the control group, verified microscopically by findings of cardiac wall enlargement, hepatosplenomegaly and brain oedema. Tongue diagnosis, which is strongly weighted in TCM, demonstrated diminishment of tongue vessels and of the vessel density (= purple-cyanotic tongue body, commonly seen in Blood stasis). The results of the study clearly show that Blood stasis syndrome not only plays a role as a background illness and accompanying phenomenon, it is also involved in the subsequent development of functional disorders of the internal organs and is a partial cause for the development of organic, pathomorphologically visible lesions throughout the organism and its prime organs. This also accounts for the broad spectrum of the Blood stasis phenomenon and its relation to many severe diseases.

PATHOLOGY OF BLOOD STASIS

MEDICAL HISTORY

According to Wang Qing-Ren's assumptions and today's findings in TCM, Blood stasis frequently occurs after long-term chronic illnesses. It can also be commonly observed in the aftermath of surgery or external injuries. Jaundice must also be mentioned, especially in the presence of chronic hepatitis.

In female patients, there are often longstanding menstrual disorders (amenorrhoea, dysmenor-rhoea or extreme irregular menses), in many cases accompanied by dark or clotted blood; but menopause, strong lochia or metrorrhagia, as well as infertility of both genders, can also be related to Blood stasis.

Regarding the patients' lifestyle, those who engage in heavy smoking and drinking, eat sweet and fatty foods, and who have either a choleric or timid temper are also predisposed to Blood stasis. In addition, in some cases a history of epilepsy and mental illnesses are also present.

CLINICAL SYMPTOMS

The list below is complete inasmuch as it mentions all symptoms that are present in an ideal case. However, such an 'ideal and typical patient', presenting all signs without exception, does not exist in Chinese medicine, nor in Western medicine.

Temperature

Often, there is an enduring elevated body temperature or fever, or temperature that increases only at particular times. Those affected may sometimes feel heat or heat sensations alternating with cold in locations like the palms of the hands and feet, the chest, abdomen and genitals.

Pain

The typical Blood stasis pain is stabbing and always in a fixed location that is also sensitive to pressure. It is often described as stabbing like a needle or knife and cannot be removed easily or quickly.

Sensory irritations

This is sometimes described as itchiness under the skin that does not abate when scratching, or a prickling sensation as if bitten by ants. Local numbness and even failure to differentiate warm and cold also occur regularly.

Pressure

A feeling of pressure or tension in the head, eyes, breast, hypochondrium area or limbs, along with fullness in the epigastric area, abdomen and back are often described. Typically the sensations are felt on a daily basis and tend to worsen rather than get better.

Stiffness

Limbs and neck are often stiff and hard to move or stretch. The head can only be turned with effort.

Haemorrhages

All types of blood loss, including bruises and injuries that are hard to contain, as well as bloody stool and urine, nose bleeding, vomiting of blood and excessively heavy menstruation, can in the long run lead to Blood stasis. Dark or clotted blood is often found in these cases.

Dryness

Because Blood is a *Yin* (fluid), there are often signs of deficient nutritive fluids in Blood stasis: a dry mouth with a disinclination to drink large amounts of fluids is as typical as dry, sometimes scaly skin and rough, lacklustre hair that falls out easily without growing back.

Sleep and memory

Sleep disorders and being easily woken up or night terrors with many dreams are common, according to Wang Qing-Ren, as are poor memory, being unable to concentrate and in extreme cases also hallucinations.

Head

The face shows a dark colouration, sometimes with a tendency to a dark red, purple or even blackish complexion. There are often spider naevi or reddish vessels on the face, cheeks and nose. The sclera may show a yellowish colouration with many visible arterioles. Dark eye rings may also be present.

Typically, the lips are dark, i.e. of a purple, bluish-cyanotic or dark red complexion. The tongue body is purple, dark and slightly enlarged. The sides often have bluish marks or dots as if there was a localized bleeding. The veins under the tongue are often dark, swollen, crooked and more prominent.

The neck may often have bluish, prominent veins, and its colour may be reddish as seen in cooked crustaceans (crabs, shrimps).

Trunk

Throbbing or pulsating sensations in the breast may sometimes be noticed. The skin is dark red. The cervical and thoracic spine is markedly prominent and painful to pressure.

The abdomen is typically distended, sometimes like a drum, so that the navel protrudes. Convoluted veins may also emerge under the skin. Another sign for Blood stasis is the presence of abdominal masses that are palpable and painful to pressure.

Limbs

The lower limbs may be swollen or dark and sore. Clubbing of the fingers and toes may also be found. Even more typical is pallor of the hands and feet, which feel ice-cold to the touch and feature bluish nails.

SYSTEMATIC PATHOLOGY

Nervous system/mental functions

Becoming easily irritated and experiencing other extremely strong emotions (e.g. jealousy etc.) as well as confusion, depression and mania often go along with Blood stasis. Sudden palpitations that are due to nervousness are also related.

Digestive system

Pain that is worse on pressure, and fullness, have already been described above as typical abdominal symptoms. More common are diarrhoea or constipation and low appetite, nausea, a burning sensation in the epigastrium, a dry throat and hiccups.

Respiratory system

All prolonged respiratory diseases such as chronic cough and asthma, and also shortness of breath and coughing up bloody sputum are associated with Blood stasis.

Genitourinary system

A swelling and distending sensation in the lower abdomen has already been mentioned, as well as infertility in both genders. Moreover, cloudy or increased urine and painful or intermittent urination may also point towards Blood stasis.

Circulation

Palpitations or tachycardia for no reason, breathlessness, oedematous lower limbs and heart pain or a stabbing sensation in the heart hint at Blood stasis.

CLINICAL DIAGNOSIS AND LABORATORY ANALYSIS

Blood screening

Naturally, haemorheologic tests are the first line of investigation: absolute indications for Blood stasis are elevated blood and blood plasma viscosity, also a slowdown in sedimentation rate and an increase in its K value. Increased agglutination of all blood cells and of fibrinogen concentration also suggest Blood stasis.

Microcirculation

Nail bed examination, which was performed more regularly in the past, and also fundus examination may show an increase of convoluted capillaries, local exudation and a slowdown of blood flow. Hyperlipidaemia, elevated cholesterol and bilirubin levels and increased blood cells and platelets are often detected in Blood stasis patients as well. Secondary features of Blood stasis are elevated albumin levels, elevated erythrocyte sedimentation rate and the presence of positive rheumatoid factors, antistreptolysin O and lupus cells in the blood.

Diagnostic imaging

CT and MRI can often show thrombi, haematomata, ischemias and tumours in the brain and internal organs. Electromyogram (EMG) and sonogram occasionally show hepatosplenomegaly, hydronephrosis and hypertrophy of the heart. X-ray can provide evidence for lung infec-

tions or tumours, and also diverticula and polyps. However, these findings are less definite compared with the results from blood screening and, in particular, haemorheology.

SUMMARY

In conventional medicine, blood stasis is characterized by a deteriorated or even arrested blood flow. The following changes can be noted:

- In many cases a standstill of blood flow occurs within the capillaries, as made clearly visible by nail bed examinations. The blood will have a higher tendency for thrombus formation, as clearly demonstrated by blood screening protocols (see below).
- The metabolism produces pathological changes: initially there are changes in the skin and internal tissues such as scleromata and other skin diseases; post-surgical adhesion formation; and all kinds of haemorrhagic diseases. Other common consequences of Blood stasis are endocrinological changes or decrease of body fluids in terms of fluid electrolyte balance and insulin and hormone levels, especially sex hormones.
- Amongst the immunological changes are greater susceptibility to infections and allergies along with weakened immunity and increased formation of neoplasms. Blood screening will show increased blood or blood plasma viscosity, decreasing erythrocyte sedimentation rate and increasing K value and blood cell agglutination, and elevation of fibrinogen and blood platelet levels and frequently of red and white blood cells as well. Further on, hyperlipidaemia is often present.

At the International Congress for Blood stasis Research, held in Beijing in 1998, the research association for integrated Western and Chinese medicine established the following standard criteria for the assessment of Blood stasis, of which one would suffice to strongly suggest Blood stasis:

1. Dark or purple tongue body with the typical blood stasis spots or lines
2. Typical rough pulse or no pulse

3. Pain that is fixed (or also stabbing, sensitive to pressure and chronic)
4. Typical abdominal Blood stasis symptoms
5. Palpable abdominal masses (resistances)
6. Extravasated blood (also through wounds and internal bleedings)
7. Blood vessel changes (curved, thicker) and blood stasis signs on the skin (petechiae, spider naevi, subcutaneous dark blue spots etc.)
8. Dysmenorrhoea with dark, clotted blood or amenorrhoea
9. Dry, scaly or cracked skin
10. Palsies and numbness
11. Irritability, even manic psychosis.

DISEASES RELATED TO BLOOD STASIS ACCORDING TO WESTERN MEDICINE

Chronic Blood stasis can be linked to the following diseases:

- **Cardiology**: Heart attack, cardiac insufficiency and angina pectoris, cor pulmonale, arrhythmias
- **Blood vessels and circulation**: Arteriosclerosis, thromboses, disseminated intravascular coagulation (DIC), all kinds of haemorrhagic diseases
- **Neurology and brain**: Transient ischemic attack (TIA), apoplexies (ischemic and haemorrhagic), memory disorders and senile dementia due to vascular ischemia and multiple infarct dementia, tinnitus and sudden deafness
- **Dermatology**: Psoriasis, neurodermatitis, seborrhoea, ichthyosis, chloasma and many more
- **Gynaecology**: All kinds of menstrual disorders, metrorrhagia, lochial discharges, postpartum disorders
- **Oncology**: All kinds of tumour formations, especially in the abdomen
- **Immunology**: Low immunity and rheumatic-arthritic diseases
- **Genitourinary**: acute renal failure, dysuria, prostatitis
- **Lungs and respiratory tract**: Dyspnoea, asthma and haemoptysis
- **Mind, psyche**: Depression, mania, psychosis, insomnia, senile dementia
- **Liver, metabolism**: chronic hepatitis, liver cirrhosis, diabetes.

In addition, Blood stasis may arise in any place with poor blood supply, where subsequent tissue changes can lead to pathological dysfunctions.

Chapter 4

Aetiology of Blood stasis in Chinese medicine

FOUNDATIONS OF TCM – BLOOD AND *QI*

The Chinese term '*Xue*', translated here as Blood, has a much broader meaning in China.

Blood is derived from the purified essence of food, which after distillation in the Spleen functional entity[1] is sent upwards to the Lung. The *Qi* gained from air directs it to the Heart. Here, under the influence of Kidney-*Qi* and *Yuan-Qi* (Original *Qi*), it is turned into red Blood.

According to this, *Ying* (Nutritive *Qi*) and Blood are always linked to each other. Red Blood forms the more material and gross part and *Qi* the more subtle and energetic. Blood nourishes the *Qi* of all organs. *Qi* provides Blood with its warming and moving energy. Wherever *Qi* flows, Blood will follow. Thus the saying: '*Qi* is the commander of Blood, Blood is the mother of *Qi*.' It is mentioned in the '*Huang Di Nei Jing*' (*The Yellow Emperor's Classic*), in the '*Ling Shu*', Chapter 18:

---

[1] In China, the concept of a functional entity embraces a good deal more than the mere anatomical correspondence. For historical reasons, all functions that are more or less associated with this organ are subsumed. Porkert calls these functional entities 'Orbi' (singular: Orbis). Many other authors choose not to use any additional terms like functional entity because in their opinion everyone who has gone beyond the fundamental concepts of TCM should know that the TCM Heart does not correspond only with the anatomical one. As this book is aimed at the advanced user, I have abstained from emphasizing the Chinese concept in the text that follows.

Blood (Xue) and Qi have different names, but they are both of the same kind. How can one understand this? Qi Bo *(physician of the Yellow Emperor) answers:* 'Ying *and* Wei *(Nutritive and Defensive* Qi*) belong to the* Jing *(Essence-*Qi*), Blood belongs to the* Shen *(Mind-*Qi*).'* Zhang Zhi-Cong *gives the following explanation:* 'Ying *and* Wei *both stem from food essences. Blood (*Xue*) also arises from the purified essences of the Middle Burner but it requires the subtle energy of the Heart (Mind-*Shen*) to be transformed into Blood (*Xue*). Blood,* Ying *and* Wei *are all created from* Jing *(Essence), hence the name is different, but the quality is the same.'* [2]

The functions of Blood are manifold: as a *Yin* fluid it needs to moisturize the entire body and its organs including the Mind. It has to maintain a balance with the *Yang* characteristics of *Qi*. Due to its function in menstruation and childbirth, Blood has a central position in gynaecology.

Blood and *Qi* are like *Yin* and *Yang*; *Qi* provides energy for generating the movement of Blood through the vessels and holds the Blood within them. Conversely, Blood is essential in the formation of *Qi* and provides transportation for *Qi* into all areas of the body. Thus, Zhang Jing-Yue wrote: 'The human being possesses *Yin* and *Yang*, *Qi* and Blood. Yang governs *Qi*. If *Qi* is sufficient, the Mind is empowered. *Yin* governs Blood. If Blood is sufficient, then the body is strong.'

PATHOLOGY OF BLOOD IN TCM

According to the Chinese medicine definition, disorders of Blood can manifest principally in four different ways:

1. Loss of Blood due to excessive Heat, *Qi* deficiency (*Xu*) or *Yin* deficiency, and finally resulting from Blood stasis (*Yu Xue*) and traumas.

2. Blood Heat with symptoms of accelerated pulse, red tongue, signs of inflammation, dryness and heat sensation. Blood Heat presents differently depending on the organ involved.
3. Blood deficiency[3] usually results from Spleen-*Qi* deficiency. It affects predominantly Liver and Heart, but also menstruation and the mind.
4. Blood stasis (*Yu Xue*), a slowing down and obstruction of Blood, which is discussed below.

THE 10 PRINCIPAL SYNDROMES AND CAUSES OF BLOOD STASIS

1. Blood stasis due to *Qi* stagnation

There is a saying in TCM: 'If stagnated *Qi* does not flow – Blood will accumulate and cease flowing.' This cause for Blood stasis is absolutely identical with high blood viscosity, because Blood moves too slowly through the vessels, or it partly stagnates in the capillaries. Conversely, Blood stasis may cause *Qi* stagnation, as Blood transports *Qi*. In this context, stagnated Liver-*Qi*, for example due to frequent or suppressed anger, marks one of the most common pathological mechanisms.

2. Blood stasis due to *Qi* deficiency

'*Qi* is the commander of Blood', as is mentioned in the '*Nei Jing*'. If *Qi* lacks the power to force Blood through the vessels, Blood will stagnate. Chronic and consumptive diseases can at first weaken *Qi*, and later on Blood stasis arises. Chronic hepatitis, neurasthenia and exhaustion, which are all characterized by tiredness and mental or physical weakness, are often in a causal relationship with this type of Blood stasis.

---

[2] Further details would go beyond the scope of this introduction. To the interested reader I recommend becoming familiar with the foundations of Chinese medicine, for example in the works of Giovanni Maciocia or Wiseman and Ellis for English readers, or alternatively M Porkert or CC Schnorrenberger for German readers. For clinicians, I recommend Maciocia's works, which are both detailed and practical.

[3] Deficiency and Excess (*Xu* and *Shi*, pronounced like 'shoe' and 'shi' in 'shimmer'; 'Leere' and 'Fülle' in German), depending on the author, are called Inanitas/Depletion and Repletio/Repletion (Porkert), Deficiency and Excess (Maciocia, Bensky), Vacuity and Repletion (Wiseman), Sthenic and Asthenic (Ou et al). Since Schnorrenberger the terms 'Leere' and 'Fülle' have become widely accepted amongst German practitioners, therefore I will stick with them. I will continue to add the Chinese equivalent in brackets, because since the conversion from Wades-Giles to the internationally accepted *Pinyin*, the Chinese terms are the only ones that are used consistently.

3. Blood stasis due to *Yang* deficiency Cold

The warming function of *Yang-Qi* of the Kidneys, Spleen and Heart provides for the necessary warmth in the body. In the case of *Yang* or *Qi* deficiency, it will be easier for pathogenic Cold to invade. In addition, the body itself lacks warmth. The next cause can lead to a similar scenario: Blood becomes thick and viscous like freezing water, which then results in Blood stasis. Gastrointestinal and gynaecological diseases are commonly associated with this cause.

4. Blood stasis due to exogenous pathogenic Cold

A well-known fact in TCM is that Blood that is warmed by *Wei-Qi* will be able to flow. However, if it becomes cold, it will contract. This may be due to the influence of exogenous pathogenic Cold or due to lack of *Yang-Qi* warming the Blood. In both events Blood 'freezes', which means its flow slows down or stops altogether. Rheumatic diseases are often involved here.

5. Blood stasis due to pathogenic Heat

Pathogenic Heat consumes Body Fluids, therefore, in the presence of Heat, Blood in effect thickens. If there is further Heat, it starts to clot. This is one of the causes of Blood stasis which has already been recognized in the '*Nei Jing*' and '*Shang Han Lun*'. Febrile diseases and a tendency to bleeding due to Blood Heat are closely connected to this cause, as are many types of skin conditions.

6. Blood stasis due to injury

Any kind of trauma involving internal or external bleeding incurs acute Blood stasis, for example in haematomata. Sometimes, the coagulated Blood is not fully reabsorbed. This can be observed in changes of skin colour above large haematomata, which are visible for many years. Chinese medicine attributes these trauma-induced disorders, which are often mere functional disorders but nevertheless disturbing to the patient, to Blood stasis as well. Modern Chinese medicine calls this type 'acute Blood stasis', whereas disturbed blood flow, which is often less obvious in appearance, is ascribed to 'chronic Blood stasis'.

7. Blood stasis due to Blood deficiency (e.g. in the case of blood loss)

Primarily affected by this are the fields of traumatology and gynaecology. All kinds of traumas give rise to acute Blood stasis, causing Blood to extravasate. Blood then either leaks from the wound, which can entail Blood deficiency, or it can accumulate under the skin and become a haematoma. Internal and menstrual bleeding should also be mentioned in this context. Depending on the severity of the Blood loss, Blood stasis can be generated.

8. Blood stasis due to exogenous Dryness or *Yin* deficiency

Skin conditions and senile dementia often come into this category. *Yin* deficiency or insufficient Body Fluids due to a declining sense of thirst in elderly people can lead to high blood viscosity and its consequences, such as arteriosclerosis etc. Since Blood is a part of all *Yin* in the body, long-term *Yin* deficiency leads to Blood Dryness, as the thin fluid constituents that are part of Blood have been diminished. In this type of Blood stasis, cause and effect are hardly separable, as they account for each other.

9. Phlegm combining with Blood stasis

Wang Qing-Ren explains that Phlegm is produced in the throat, instead of the Lung, as suggested in ancient times. However, it should not be forgotten that 'Phlegm' had a common meaning in the sense of the phlegm that was regularly brought up when clearing one's throat. Another meaning is in a medical context, where Phlegm is a generic term for all tenacious and viscous substances that inhibit physiological processes in the body, for example low density lipoprotein (LDL) and cholesterol. Many of the consequences of arteriosclerosis belong to this category, for example cardiac and vascular diseases.

10. Exhaustion causing Blood stasis

Specific repetitive movements or postures (as in certain occupational disorders) or lack of sufficient exercise will restrict the flow of blood and thus engender Blood stasis. The latter often occurs in

Table 4.1

Qi	Cold/Heat	Blood/Yin	Other causes
Qi deficiency	Cold due to Yang-Qi deficiency	Blood deficiency (blood loss, anaemia)	Exhaustion (fatigue)
Qi deficiency due to protracted illness	Pathogenic Cold	Traumas (acute Blood stasis)	Phlegm (due to diet)
Qi stagnation	Pathogenic Heat	Dryness, Yin deficiency (due to diet or exogenous)	Emotional causes (anger, depression)

obese and bedridden patients and is involved in the emergence of Blood stasis in chronic diseases.

Suppressed emotions

Emotional causes, especially anger, may easily lead to Qi stagnation by affecting the smooth flow of Liver-Qi. As a result, on the one hand Qi stagnation can cause Blood stasis, and on the other, the Liver of all *Zang* organs is the most susceptible to emotional stress. This cause is connected to Qi stagnation. Epigastric pain, abdominal masses, Plum Stone Syndrome and menstrual disorders are often related to Blood stasis due to emotions.

Dietary habits

Consuming raw and cold food in excess can exhaust the warming function of Spleen *Yang-Qi*. In combination with Qi deficiency and Cold, this in turn can easily lead to Blood stasis. Luxurious, greasy and sweet food (including alcohol and nicotine) produce Phlegm and internal Heat and as a result lead to Blood stasis. The consequences may be coronary heart disease, angina pectoris etc.

Table 4.1 summarizes the causes of Blood stasis including the syndromes leading to Blood stasis.

CASE STUDIES CLASSIFIED ACCORDING TO AETIOLOGY

The following medical histories stem from classical and modern sources. Cases are described from the point of view of either TCM or integrated Chinese medicine. They correspond to the aforementioned 10 causes of Blood stasis and are designed to elucidate them.

ABBREVIATIONS

Bu. = Bulbus
Cn. = Cornu
Co. = Concha
Cs. = Caulis
Cx. = Cortex
En. = Endothelium
Ex. = Excrementum
Fl. = Flos
Fo. = Folium
Fr. = Fructus
Hb. = Herba
Md. = Medulla
Pc. = Pericarpium
Ps. = Periostracum
Rl. = Ramulus
Rx. = Radix
Rm. = Ramus
Rh. = Rhizoma
Se. = Semen
Su. = Succus
Tu. = Tuber

1. BLOOD STASIS DUE TO *QI* STAGNATION

Case Study 4.1 Ischemic heart disease, sick sinus syndrome

If Qi *is blocked, Blood will also stagnate, so Blood stasis with* Bi *syndromes will gradually develop; if this is allowed to continue further, abdominal masses will also develop.*

(Ye Tian-She)

Case study taken from the medical records of the First University Hospital of the Hua Xi Medical University, Chengdu. Mrs M, 51-year-old worker, single, admission 3.12.83

History

Thirteen years ago the patient suddenly became unconscious. An electrocardiograph (ECG) revealed a large bradycardic abnormal rhythm (dysrhythmia), which normalized within 2 minutes. General health following the incidence was good. Four years ago the patient felt a sudden pain in the heart area, followed by cardiac and respiratory arrest. After 18 minutes of resuscitation the heart started beating again. Breathing, pulse waves and blood pressure returned to normal. An ECG showed arrhythmia in the atrio-ventricular border, ventricular extrasystoles and signs of an acute infarct.

The tongue body was pale, pulse was weak and fine. Syndrome differentiation was *Shao Yin* Heart syncope. The treatment principle was 'Tonify *Qi* and restore *Yang*' using a prescription of *Shen Fu Tang* (Ginseng Aconite Decoction) once daily. Eventually, 5 months later, the patient returned to health.

Three years ago, she suffered repeated Adam-Stokes attacks which were treated by implanting a pacemaker. Due to a problem with the pacemaker two years ago, atropine and isopropyl-noradrenaline were prescribed to stabilize her condition.

A month before her admission she suffered a sudden severe syncope caused by another pacemaker malfunction. Chinese medicinals were administered immediately after admission.

The tongue body was pale, with a thick white coating; pulse was deep and fine.

Further results from diagnosis: pulse rate 42 beats per minute (bpm), blood pressure (BP) 100/70 mm/Hg.

Left heart was slightly enlarged, no sinus sound was detected. The lungs were normal, the liver and spleen not palpable. Plasma cholesterol levels were normal. X-ray showed an enlargement of the left heart edge beyond the left mid-clavicular line. An ECG showed arrhythmia in the atrio-ventricular border, ventricular extrasystoles and extensive myocardial ischemia.

Western medicine diagnosis: ischemic heart disease, sick sinus syndrome.

Chinese medicine diagnosis: weakness and collapse of Heart-*Yang*, *Qi* stagnation and Blood stasis.

Principle of treatment: tonify both *Yang* and *Qi*, invigorate Blood, remove Blood stasis.

Base formula[4]

Dang Shen 30 g Rx. Codonopsis	*Fu Pian* 15 g Rx. Aconiti
Huang Qi 30 g Rx. Astragali	*Gui Zhi* 12 g Rl. Cinnamomi
Chuan Xiong 12 g Rx. Ligustici	*San Qi* (powder) 9 g Rx. Notoginseng
Dan Shen 15 g Rx. Salviae	*Chi Shao Yao* 15 g Rx. Paeoniae Rubrae
Bai Mu Tong[5] 12 g Cs. Akebiae Mutong	

Auxiliary medicinals

1. With irritability and sleeplessness: *Fu Shen* 12 g, *Suan Zao Ren* 12 g, *Yuan Zhi* 12 g

---

[4] Traditionally, formulas were written horizontally, mostly in four rows, to better distinguish the four types of medicinals (emperor, minister, assistant, messenger). These days, many formulas that do not make these distinctions clear any more are written down vertically. I have decided to retain the original format in order not to change any information.
[5] Not to be confused with the discredited *Guan Mu Tong*, which contains aristolochic acid.

Case Study continues

2. With coughing and phlegm, nausea, vomiting: *Chen Pi* 12 g, *Fa Ban Xia* 12 g, *Fu Ling* (Poria) 12 g, *Zhu Ru* 12 g
3. With fullness and no appetite: *Hou Po* 20 g, *Bai Zhu* 14 g, *Zhi Ke* 12 g, *Sha Ren* 6 g, *Kou Ren* 6 g, *Sheng Jiang* 12 g
4. With atrio-ventricular conduction disturbances: *Sheng Mai Zhu She Ye* (pulse-generating injection, available in China, which is a preparation of *Sheng Mai Tang* pulse-generating decoction), twice daily, plus isopropyl-noradrenaline lozenges 10 mg, 1–3 times daily, until heart rate adjusts to 60–70 bpm, then discontinue.

Two weeks after treatment was started, frequency of palpitations was reduced and the pain became slighter. No more syncopes were observed. Heart rate levelled off at 65–68 bpm. ECG showed arrhythmia at the atrio-ventricular border and myocardial ischemia.

After 3 months of treatment the patient had no more complaints. She could stand up and perform normal activities. Another ECG revealed no presence of myocardial ischemia. The patient insisted on further prescriptions of Chinese medicinals and on regular examinations. Since then she has been in good health.

2. BLOOD STASIS DUE TO *QI* DEFICIENCY

Case Study 4.2   Exhaustion and atrophy after long illness

If Yuan-Qi *is so depleted that it cannot sufficiently supply the Blood vessels, then Blood will lack* Qi *that should propel its movement, thus it becomes stagnated and Blood stasis develops.*

> (Wang Qing-Ren ('Yi Lin Gai Cuo'))

Case study taken from the '*Yi Lin Gai Cuo*'.

In the beginning stages, the patient presented with heavy limbs and pain similar to muscle ache and gradual muscle atrophy. Thirst and appetite were decreased, complexion was yellowish-white, there was frothy cough, the patient was more nervous and irritable, and experienced afternoon fever and night sweat.

Physicians were consulted to correct this situation. At first, they prescribed *Yin*-tonifying, and later on *Yang*-strengthening medicinals, without success. Eventually it was concluded: 'This is a deficiency syndrome that is incapable of receiving tonification (*Xu Bu Shou Bu*). What's the reason behind this?'

In patients whose constitution gives rise to *Qi* and Blood deficiency originally, tonifying medicinals are prescribed to replenish the deficiency, and they will return to health. However, patients who are not in a state of deficiency become weak due to the protracted course of their condition. Thus, as soon as the disease is fought, *Yuan-Qi* will return by itself.

When searching for the disease, one will find neither superficial nor internal syndromes. All that can be observed are syndromes of Blood stasis. I often treat such cases. To restore health, nine prescriptions are given in easy cases. Eighteen prescriptions are given in severe ones.

Formula: Tong Qiao Huo Xue Tang (Orifices Opening, Blood Invigorating Decoction)

3 g	Radix Paeoniae Rubrae (*Chi Shao Yao*)
3 g	Radix Ligustici Wallichii (*Chuan Xiong*)
9 g	Semen Persicae (*Tao Ren*)
9 g	Flos Carthami (*Hong Hua*)
3 g	Herba Allii Fistulosum (*Lao Cong*)
5 g	Fructus Zizyphi Jujubae (*Da Zao*)
0.15 g	Moschus (*She Xiang*)
250 ml	Wine (*Huang Jiu*)

The decoction should be taken warm. To begin with, the first six medicinals are decocted and strained. Then add Moschus dissolved in warm wine.

If there is still substantial *Qi* deficiency after 3 prescriptions, add about 30 g Astragalus, taken in sips over the day. If there is no *Qi* deficiency, Astragalus can be omitted. Once the disease is removed, *Yuan-Qi* (Original *Qi*) will return by itself.

3. BLOOD STASIS DUE TO *YANG* DEFICIENCY COLD

Case Study 4.3   Scleroma

Physical overexertion, Cold, Summer-Heat and exhaustion can all damage Yang-Qi.

(Ye Tian-Shi)

Case study taken from Research Institute of Integrated Medicine for Skin Diseases, Tianjin, Chang Zhen Hospital for Skin Diseases. Patient Z. Male, 39-year-old worker, married admission 6.9.1978. Main complaints: hands and feet turning cold, and tightening and thickening of the skin affecting the face and limbs for 6 months.

History

In the winter of 1976 the patient's hands and feet started to turn cold. Upon exposure to cold, the skin changed to a chalk-whitish or cyanotic colour, accompanied by pain in the limbs. Gradually, facial skin and the skin of the limbs began to swell and to harden. As a result, movement of the hands became restricted. Also the skin on the neck, shoulders and breast hardened and swelled up, to a degree that deep inspiration became difficult. During the summer, the symptoms alleviated. There was no problem swallowing food or fluids. Appetite and general health were good.

The patient had previously been given 20 prescriptions of solely Blood invigoration herbs, but without success. There was no other relevant history. The patient smoked. He lived in Inner Mongolia, where winter temperatures can drop to about minus 10° Celsius.

The tongue body was pale, with a thin coating and the patient had a slippery pulse.

Results from examination showed normal constitution and diet. Facial skin was swollen, shiny and hardened, the nasolabial groove was absent, the tip of the nose was elevated and the lips were shrunken, therefore the patient experienced difficulties in opening the mouth.

Hands, feet, superior and anterior regions of the shoulders, lower leg and breast all presented as completely swollen and were shiny and hardened, with hands and anterior shoulders primarily affected. There was no pitting oedema, no pain, but restricted finger movements and difficulty in making a fist.

Heart and lungs were normal. The abdomen was soft upon palpation, the liver and spleen not enlarged. Blood: haemoglobin 13 g%, red blood count (RBC) 5.2 mio/mm^3, white blood count (WBC) 8000/mm^3, neutrophils 70%, lymphocytes 30%. Urine was normal. Erythrocyte sedimentation rate (ESR) was 7 mm/h. Chest X-ray, examination of upper gastrointestinal tract and gastric and intestinal mucosa were normal. ECG was normal.

Western medicine diagnosis: general thickening and tightening of the skin (systemic sclerodermatosis).

Chinese medicine diagnosis: Blood stasis due to Spleen- and Kidney-*Yang* deficiency.

Treatment principle: Strengthen and warm Spleen and Kidneys, invigorate Blood and remove stasis.

Formula (one bag per day)

Huang Qi 30 g Rx. Astragali	*Rou Gui* 10 g Cx. Cinnamomi
Gui Zhi 10 g Rl. Cinnamomi	*Fu Zi* 9 g Rx. Aconiti Praep.
Shou Wu 16 g Rx. Polygoni Multiflori	*Ji Xue Teng* 24 g Rx./Caulis Cs Jixueteng
Yuan Hu 12 g Rx. Corydalis	*Ru Xiang* 6 g Olibanum
Mo Yao 6 g Myrrha	*Ze Lan* 24 g Hb. Lycopi
Jin Yin Hua 24 g Fl. Lonicerae	*Dan Shen* 21 g Rx. Salviae
Xia Ku Chao 15 g Spica Prunellae vulg.	*Xuan Shen* 21 g Rx. Scrophulariae
Yu Jin 12 g Tu. Curcumae	

Mao Dong Qing (Ilex Pubescens) once daily 2 ml intramuscular.

Case Study continues

After only 2 weeks, the limbs felt warm to the touch and the Raynaud-like attacks subsided. The hard skin slowly became softer and slight perspiration was visible. After the treatment had continued for 6 months, the skin was basically normal and the patient was able to be discharged. Thereafter, the same formula was taken in a ready-made pill form for several months. Since then the disease has not reoccurred.

Discussion

Most patients with general thickening and tightening of the skin are sensitive to cold, present with a Raynaud's disease symptom, with hardened and swollen skin on the hands and feet etc. A slippery pulse and a swollen tongue body with little coating both belong to the syndrome of Spleen- and Kidney-*Yang* deficiency due to Blood stasis. Therefore, this formula can be used successfully in these cases.

The patient may still show signs of Heat syndromes, *Qi* and Blood deficiency syndromes, Spleen-*Qi* deficiency syndrome with Phlegm and Dampness and others. Consequently, treatment must always relate to syndrome differentiation.

4. BLOOD STASIS DUE TO EXOGENOUS PATHOGENIC COLD

Case Study 4.4   Acute pain

If harsh Cold is allowed to linger on, Blood coagulates and the vessels become impermeable. As a result the pulse becomes large and choppy, which indicates damage due to Cold.
(Huang Di Nei Jing, Su Wen)

Case study taken from Zhang Xi-Chun's 'Yi Xue Zhong Zhong Can Xi Lu' (*Essential notes about Chinese and Western Medicine*).

Mr G was about 50 years old, of slightly weak constitution. One day, he visited his friends in a neighbouring village, and people chatted and drank alcohol until late into the winter night. On his way home he was exposed to the cold temperature of the early morning. Then, halfway home, he suddenly experienced an unpleasant numb sensation in his legs and broke out in a sweat. He could not continue walking. He sat down to rest on the cold ground. When he arrived home, his legs hurt so much that he tried to warm them with hot bricks, which only aggravated the pain.

As he has some understanding of medicine, he self-prescribed some sweat-inducing formula; however, this further worsened his illness. As the medicinals were too hot, he vomited a few mouthfuls of blood, his stool was dry and hard. Eventually, he presented in my practice.

He lay on his back with his legs flexed, so I had to ask two assistants to support his legs. He expressed his pain by crying or screaming. He appeared to be in a very poor state. His pulse was wiry, fine and slightly accelerated.

In my view, the aggravated pain due to Heat is a sign of pathogenic Cold being driven further into the interior of the body. Sweat-inducing medicinals worsen the situation, because they can only expel Cold from the superficial parts, not from the bones and internal areas. Moreover, excessive perspiration diminishes *Qi* and Blood. Once this is the case, recovery will be even less likely.

Therefore I used *Huo Luo Xiao Ling Dan* (Wondrous Pill to Invigorate the Channels) plus 4 *Qian* dissolved *Jing Lu Jiao Jiao* (Gelatinum Cornu) and 2 *Qian Ming Tian Ma* (Gastrodia), taken together with the pills.

Once the patient took the medicine, the assistant holding the left leg felt a cold sensation in his hand, followed by immediate pain relief; however, the right leg did not improve. Suddenly, the following occurred to me: the human body pertains to *Yang* on the left and *Yin* on the right. *Jing Lu Jiao Jiao* (Gelatinum Cornu) is a strong *Yang* medicinal with greater effect on the left than on the right. Thus I prescribed the same medicine again, but simply replaced *Lu Jiao Jiao* (Gelatinum Cornu) with *Hu Gu Jiao* (Gelatinum Os Tigri). After that, the left leg recovered in the same way as the right leg.

5. BLOOD STASIS DUE TO EXOGENOUS PATHOGENIC HEAT

Case Study 4.5   Chronic aggressive hepatitis B

*If for seven, eight days of existing Heat...there
is still no defaecation, then there is Blood stasis.*
(Zhang Zhong-Jing)

*It appears to me that if a Heat syndrome has already
been present for 2 weeks without improvement,
then the disease no longer only affects the division
of the Qi. If the physical constitution is weak and
indicates deficiency, e.g. pale complexion, then it is
feared that the pathogenic factor may advance into
the Jue Yin channel (in this case, the Liver channel).*
(Ye Tian-Shi)

Case study taken from the medical records of the
302nd Hospital, Beijing, Dr Wang. Patient W, male,
15 year old student, single, admission 6.6.1984.
Main complaints: weakness and nausea for more
than a year, swelling of the lower limbs for 6 weeks.

History
In April 1983 nausea started, with loss of appetite,
aversion to fat, physical weakness, deep-yellow
urine. Laboratory examination revealed glutamate
pyruvate transaminase (GPT) 644 U/l, thymol turbidity
test (TTT) 13 U/l and stercobilin (STB) 4.4 mg/%.

After admission to hospital, *Yi Gang Ling* (a
Liver-strengthening medicine) and other remedies
were prescribed until there was no more jaundice
and laboratory values improved to TTT 9 U/l, GPT
628 U/l. As a result, the patient was discharged
and continued to take the prescriptions. Two
months later GPT 680 U/l, TTT 20 U/l, HBsAg (+)
and chronic aggressive hepatitis were detected, so
he was re-admitted. For 6 months he was treated
with bifendate (biphenyldicarboxylate), until values
dropped to GPT 180 U/l and TTT 18 U/l. The
medication was continued.

In April 1984, swelling of the legs was recorded,
in May STB was at 3.1 mg/%. Then, he was
admitted to our hospital.

TCM syndrome differentiation
On presentation the patient mentioned dizziness,
afternoon fever (around 38°C), a sensation of
swelling in the legs, distended abdominal wall
(medium-grade ascites) and furuncles on the skin
of the chest area.

The tongue body was slightly swollen, had a red
colour and showed tortoise-shell-like fissures, with
a thin white coating. The pulse was wiry.

Diagnosis on admission
BP 100/60 mm/Hg, mentally clear and cooperative,
no icteric skin colouration visible, but spider naevi
and typical palmar erythema, furunculosis,
petechiae all over the body, haemorrhagic bleeding
under the skin on the lower limbs, yellowish
sclerae. Heart and lungs normal, abdomen
distended, positive percussion with shifting
dullness, liver and spleen borders difficult to
evaluate, percussion pain in liver area.

Laboratory data: leukocytes 2800/mm³,
neutrophils 61%, leukocytes 36%, monocyte 2%,
eosinophils 1%, thrombocytes 42 000/mm³,
hematochrome 7 g/%, erythrocytes 1.79 mio/mm³,
erythrocyte sedimentation rate 16 mm/1/h, HBsAg
1:64, Anti-HBc inhibition rate 91%, Anti-HBcIgM
4.5, Anti-HBs negative, HBsAg positive, Hbe
negative; limulus lysate test (LLT) positive.

Western medicine diagnosis: chronic aggressive
hepatitis B, decompensated liver cirrhosis,
endotoxaemia.

Chinese medicine diagnosis: Blood stasis within
Blood deficiency syndrome and accumulation of
Heat toxins.

Treatment principle: cool and invigorate Blood,
clear Heat and toxins.

Prescription (twice daily, decoction)

Chi Shao 60 g	*Ge Gen* 30 g
Rx. Paeoniae Rubrae	Rx. Puerariae
Shuang Yin Hua 30 g	*Lian Qiao* 30 g
Fl. Lonicerae	Fr. Forsythiae
Bai Mao Gen 15 g	*Mu Dan Pi* 15 g
Rh. Imperatae	Cx. Moutan
Qian Cao 15 g	*Dang Gui* 15 g
Rx. Rubiae	Rx. Angelicae Sin

Case Study continues

Sheng Ma 6 g Rh. Cimicifugae	*Xian He Cao* 15 g Hb. Agrimoniae
Ze Xie 60 g Rh. Alismatis	*San Qi* (pulverised) 1.5 g Rx. Notoginseng
Shui Niu Jiao (pulverised) 1.5 g Cn. Bubali Cn = Cornu	

Accompanying therapy

Hydrochlorothiazide 25 mg/d, antisteron 20 mg/d, vitamin K1 10 mg/d, administered by infusion.

Blood transfusion 1000 ml, before and after albumin 380 g, prothrombin complex.

After admission there was a continuing fever with high peaks, occurring every 4–8 days, lasting for 2–3 days. This happened 10 times in total, to the effect that additionally 240 000 units of gentamicin were administered for 8 days, which failed to show any effect on the temperature. Eventually, by 13.11, the fever was gone.

Second diagnosis on 18.6.1984: Bilinibin (Bil) 9.3/3.9 mg/%, GPT 216 U/l, TTT 16 U/l, A/G 2.5/3.46 g%, prothrombin time/prothrombin agglutination (Pt/Pa) 33 sec/15% (lowest value 8.9%).

There was no more leg swelling, but thirst with taste of blood in the mouth was present. The tongue and pulse were the same as in the first consultation. The same prescription was issued, with the dosage of *Bai Mao Gen* increased from 15 g to 30 g.

Third diagnosis on 27.9.1984: Bil 5.5/2.2 mg%, GPT 334 U/l, GOT 304 U/l, Pt/Pa 23 sec/23.8%, albumin/glutamine (A/G) 2.38/3.16 g%, LLT (+), 30 min (+++), 24 hrs. (+++), endotoxin detection ≥10 ng%.

The patient had a wiry pulse and a red tongue body with tortoise-shell-like fissures, with a slightly yellowish coating. The formula was modified to the prescription given below, a decoction given twice daily.

Prescription

Chi Shao 80 g Rx. Paeoniae	*Pu Gong Ying* 15 g Hb. Taraxacum
San Leng 5 g Rh. Sparganii	*E Zhu* 15 g Rh. Curcumae Ezhu
Sheng Shan Zha 30 g Fr. Crategi	*Ku Shen* 15 g Rx. Sophorae
Ge Gen 30 g Rx. Puerariae	*Shuang Hua* 15 g Fl. Lonicerae

Lian Qiao 15 g Fr. Forsythiae	*Zhi Huang Qi* 15 g Rx. Astragali Praep.
Sheng Di Huang 15 g Rx. Rehmanniae	*Niu Xi* 15 g Rx. Achyrantis bid.
Gui Ban 15 g Plastrum testudnis	*Bie Jia* 15 g Carapax Amydae
Chuan Shan Jia 15 g Squama Manitis	*San Qi* (pulverised) 1.5 g Rx. Notoginseng
Shui Niu Jiao (pulverised) 1.5 g Cornu Bubalis	

Fourth diagnosis on 18.4.1985: Bil 2.3/1.0 mg/%, GPT 130 U/l (normal), GOT 112 U/l (normal), TTT 5 U/l, A/G 3.27/1.85 g%, Pt/Pa 24 sec/28.1%.

The patient had no further complaints, ascites were no longer present, the tongue body was pale red with fissures.

Modified formula

Chi Shao 30 g Rx. Paeoniae	*Ge Gen* 30 g Rx. Puerariae
Sheng Ma 30 g Rh. Cimicifugae	*E Zhu* 15 g Rh. Curcumae Ezhu
San Leng 15 g Rh. Sparganii	*Sheng Shan Zha* 30 g Fr. Crategi
Lian Qiao 15 g Fr. Forsythiae	*Zhi Huang Qi* 15 g Rx. Astragali Praep.
Niu Xi 15 g Rx. Achyrantis bid.	*Gui Ban* 15 g Plastrum testudnis
Chuan Shan Jia 15 g Squama Manitis	

Fifth diagnosis on 4.8.1985: Bil 2.5/1.4 mg/%, GPT, GOT, TTT all normal, A/G 3.38/2.55 g%, Pt/Pa 24 sec/28.1%, HBeAg negative, Anti HBc inhibition rate 99%, Anti-HBcIgM negative, hematochrome 10.5%.

After the patient was discharged, the last formula was continued until the end of 1985, when all biochemical laboratory values had fully returned to normal. After this the formula was changed from decoction to pills prepared with honey, which were taken for another year, then treatment was discontinued. Until this day, [sic] the beginning of the year 1988, the patient's state of health has remained in good condition without any further changes.

6. BLOOD STASIS DUE TO INJURY (CHRONIC BLOOD STASIS FOLLOWING ACUTE BLOOD STASIS)

Case Study 4.6   Chronic headache after concussion

After an injury from falling down, if the bad Blood does not recede from the interior,... then Qi and Blood are clotted and amassed.

(Huang Di Nei Jing Ling Shu, section 'Zei Feng' Thievish Wind)

Case study taken from the medical records of Chang Gui-Zhi and Chen Xing-Cai. Patient C, male 22 years old, presented for treatment on 5.6.1981.

Six months ago the patient was hit on the head by a large wooden beam due to lack of care. He then became unconscious, from which he recovered after 10 minutes.

After this event, the patient often complained of dizziness and headache, so he went to hospital for examination, where he was diagnosed with the aftermath of concussion (commotio cerebri). He was prescribed sedatives and analgesics without any improvement. He was ordered to have long-term rest.

The headache is described as tearing and localized in a fixed position. There is also unilateral tendency for dizziness and a feeling of pressure.

The patient has sensation of heat and restlessness, a bitter taste in the mouth and no appetite. He appears emaciated, has a dark complexion, and the tongue body is dark purple with Blood stasis spots on one side. He has a thin and yellowish tongue coating and a wiry and choppy pulse (*Xuan, Se*).

Syndrome differentiation: Blood stasis in the *Luo* channels of the brain, obstructed *Qi* movement. Treatment: invigorate Blood and remove stasis, remove obstructions from the channels and dispel pain.

Formula: modified Xue Fu Zhu Yu Tang (Anti-Stasis Chest Decoction) one bag per day, decoction

1.	Semen Persicae (*Tao Ren*)	10 g
2.	Flos Carthami (*Hong Hua*)	10 g
3.	Radix Rehmanniae (*Sheng Di Huang*)	15 g
4.	Radix Angelicae Sinensis (*Dang Gui*)	10 g
5.	Radix Paeoniae Rubrae (*Chi Shao Yao*)	10 g
6.	Radix Ligustici Wallichii (*Chuan Xiong*)	25 g
7.	Radix Glycyrrhizae (*Gan Cao*)	6 g
8.	Radix Bupleuri (*Chai Hu*)	10 g
9.	Fructus Citri Aurantii (*Zhi Ke*)	10 g
10.	Ram Cinnamomi (*Gui Zhi*)	6 g
11.	Radix Achyranthis Bidentatae (*Niu Xi*)	10 g
12.	Semen Vaccaria (*Wang Bu Liu Xing*)	10 g
13.	Vascularis Luffae (*Si Gua Luo*)	10 g
14.	Radix/Caulis Jixueteng (*Ji Xue Teng*)	30 g

After 40 days he had fully recovered. His body regained its strength, so he could return to work.

One year later he came for a routine examination, but there were no more complaints present.

Discussion

The ingredients *Tao Ren, Hong Hua, Chuan Xiong* and *Chi Shao* (1, 2, 6, 5) of *Xue Fu Zhu Yu Tang* (Anti-Stasis Chest Decoction) invigorate Blood and remove stasis. *Dang Gui* and *Sheng Di* (4, 3) invigorate and nourish Blood, *Chai Hu* (8) directs the effect of the medicinals upwards, *Gan Cao* (7) calms acute symptoms and works as an analgesic. *Wang Bu Liu Xing* (12) and *Ji Xue Teng* (14) were added to reinforce the effects of removing Blood stasis and obstructions from the channels, and to improve the pain-relieving properties. As a result the pain stopped and the syndrome was cleared.

7. BLOOD STASIS DUE TO BLOOD LOSS: BLOOD AND YIN DEFICIENCY

Case Study 4.7 Functional uterine bleeding, anaemia

Hundreds of diseases of the channels arise from Blood stagnation. The Blood governs in women. When the time has come the celestial cycles (Tian Gui) begin. If there is sufficient Kidney Qi, *then Blood will flow into the vessels. Thus every thirty days the menses occur, just like the waxing and waning of the moon.*

(Li Chan, 'Yi Xue Ru Men'
Introduction to Medicine)

Case study taken from Ha Li-Tian's *Fu Ke Yi An Yi Hua Xuan* (Selection of Case Records and Medical Lectures in Gynaecology). Patient Ms J, single, 23 years old, first consultation in April 1977. For the last 6 months her menstruation has been arriving earlier than usual and is prolonged.

Gynaecological examination, rectal: uterus relatively small, shifted horizontally etc.

Diagnosis: functional uterine bleeding, anaemic.

Previous hormone therapy for 3 months and treatment with medicinal plants failed to bring any substantial success.

Last menses started on 18th February and lasted for 40 days. Menstruation started 2 days prior to consultation with excessively heavy bleeding. Blood was of red colour with clots; the patient had slight pain in the abdomen, hip and back. She experienced a general feeling of weakness and lack of energy, dizziness and flickering in front of the eyes. Towards the evening she felt nausea and heat sensations; she had a dry mouth with a disinclination to drink a lot of fluids, no appetite and dry stool.

The patient had a fine and accelerated pulse, the tongue coating was thin and yellow.

TCM diagnosis: deficiency of *Yin* with Blood-Heat and Blood stasis.

Treatment principle: nourish *Yin*, cool Blood and disperse Blood stasis.

Formula
Three doses, decoction.

Nü Zhen Zi 9 g Se. Fruct. Ligustri	*Han Lian Cao* 9 g Hb. Ecliptae prostatae
Dang Gui Shen 12 g Corpus Rx. Angelicae Sin.	*Chuan Xu Duan* 9 g Rx. Dipsaci
Sang Ji Sheng 9 g Rl. Sangjisheng	*Dong Bai Wei* 12 g Rx. Cynanchi Baiwei
Chao Dan Pi 9 g Cx. Rx. Moutan	*Chao Huang Jing* 9 g Rh. Polygonati
Chao Di Yu 15 g Rx. Sanguisorbae Offic.	*Chuan Qian Chao* 9 g Rx. Cordifoliae
Chi Shao Yao 9 g Rx. Paeoniae Rubrae	*Liu Ji Nu* 15 g Hb. Artemisiae Anomalae
Xiang Fu Mi 9 g Rh. Cyperi	*Ling Xiao Hua* 4.5 g Fl. Campsis Grandiflora

Second consultation (21.4)
Volume of menstrual blood has reduced, but not ceased yet. No more evening nausea, mouth not dry any longer, back and hip pain improved, but still tiredness and lack of energy and dizziness. Pulse fine and soft, tongue body thin and white.

Explanation: Heat due to deficiency has improved, but there is still deficiency of *Qi* and Body Fluids.

Formula
Six doses of the previous formula plus *Qi*-tonifying medicinals.

Chuan Xu Duan 9 g Rx. Dipsaci	*Sang Ji Sheng* 9 g Rl. Sangjisheng
Chao Du Zhong 9 g Cx. Eucomniae	*Qing Dang Gui* 12 g Rx. Angelicae Sinensis Recens

Case Study continues

Shan Yu Rou 18 g
Fr. Corni off.

Wu Wei Zi 6 g
Se. Schisandrae

Tai Zi Shen 15 g
Rx. Pseudostellariae

Huang Qin Tan 6 g
Rx. Scutellariae Tostatae

Chuan Qian Cao 9 g
Rx. Cordifoliae

Chao Di Yu 15 g
Rx. Sanguisorbae

Zhong Lü Tan 9 g
Stipula Trachycarpi
Tostata

Hai Piao Qiao 9 g
Os sepiae seu sepiellae

Liu Ji Nu 12 g
Hb. Artemisiae anomalae

Third consultation (27.4)

After taking three doses of this formula the bleeding stopped. Menstruation lasted for 8 days. The patient was delighted as the menstruation was so short. She experienced no more dizziness, her appetite was improved, and her stool and urine normal. There was no sensation of heat, but some hip pain and tiredness remained.

Pulse and tongue had not changed. Thus another formula with *Qi*- and Blood-tonifying and digestion-improving medicinals was chosen to restore the function of Stomach and Spleen and Blood.

Five prescriptions of the following formula were given.

Sheng Huang Qi 15 g
Rx. Astragali

Tai Zi Shen 15 g
Rx. Pseudostellariae

Shan Yu Rou 9 g
Fr. Corni

Chuan Xu Duan 9 g
Rx. Dipsaci

Shang Ji Sheng 9 g
Rl. Sangjisheng

Chao Du Zhong 9 g
Cx. Eucomniae

Jin Gou Ji 9 g
Rh. Ciboti Barometz

Guan Chen Pi 6 g
Pc. Citri Reticulatae

Chao Shen Qu 12 g
Massa Fermentatae

Chao Huang Qin 4.5 g
Rx. Scutellariae

Sheng Ce Bai 9 g
Cacumen Biotae Orient.

Chuan Qian Cao 9 g
Rx. Cordifoliae

After taking five doses the patient fully recovered. I prescribed the patent remedies *Gui Pi Wan* once daily in the morning and *Liu Wei Di Huang Wan* once daily in the afternoon for 14 days. I also recommended the patient to eat a healthy diet and to avoid stress. In three subsequent check-ups duration of the menses and the volume of blood remained normal.

8. DRYNESS OF BLOOD IN CONNECTION WITH BLOOD STASIS

Case Study 4.8   Psoriasis

In the case of Blood stasis in the Zang-Fu organs and channels, heated Qi *thickens Blood stasis into dry Blood…When* Yin *is weak,* Yang *flares up and thus its hot-natured* Qi *combines with the Fire of the Heart, therefore the excess* Qi *can generate excess Fire.*

In essence, stagnated Blood is coagulated by blazing Qi *and thus Blood is too dry. For that reason, this syndrome entails febrile states of exhaustion, dry and rough skin and also scaling and lichenic skin. It is then termed 'Exhaustion due to Blood Dryness'* (Gan Xue Lao).

(Tang Zong-Hai, Xue Zheng Lun*)*

Case study taken from the medical records of Dr Zhou. Patient, Mrs M, 42 years old, worker, presented on 10.4.1987.

The patient has been suffering from psoriasis for 15 years, worsening during winter and becoming better during summer. Over the past 7 years many skin lesion have erupted. These skin changes were dark purple in colour and most predominant on the trunk, showing superficial, overlapping, white-greyish scallop-like scales. On the head, lesions were plaque-like and covered the upper part of the scalp. They were white, hard and extremely itchy, and underneath

Case Study continues

showed a small amount of bleeding when scratched.

Most hospital consultations diagnosed psoriasis. Despite many different prescriptions of both internal and external medicinals; there was no recovery; the condition even worsened over the years.

During menstruation she experienced pain, the bleeding was dark and there were clots. As soon as the clots were discharged the pain alleviated. Tongue diagnosis showed a tongue body that was dark red and slightly cyanotic, with stasis spots on the sides. The pulse was deep and choppy (*Chen, Se*).

TCM diagnosis: skin damage due to pathogenic factors and loss of balance of *Ying* and *Wei*, toxins invading the *Luo* vessels and Blood stasis due to long-term stagnation.

Treatment principle: transform Blood stasis, remove obstructions from the *Luo* vessels, invigorate Blood and expel pathogenic Wind. The formula used was a modification of the transforming blood stasis psoriasis decoction.[6]

E Zhu 20 g Rh. Curcumae Ezhu	*Ji Xue Teng* 50 g Rx./Cs. Jixueteng
Hong Hua 10 g Fl. Carthami	*Dan Shen* 15 g Rx. Salviae
Chuan Xiong 10 g Rx. Ligustici W.	*Wei Ling Xian* 15 g Rx. Clematidis
Chan Tui 10 g Ps. Cicadae	*Quan Xie* 10 g Buthus Martensi
Ci Ji Li 40 g Fr. Tribuli Terr.	*Bai Xian Pi* 30 g Cx. Dictamni Dasycarpi Radicis

---

[6] This formula is mainly used by Dr Zhou, which is why it is not included in the list of common Blood stasis formulas. The original formula contains *Dang Gui* 15 g, *Sheng Di* 30 g, *Shou Di* 20 g, *Ji Xue Teng* 50 g, *Xuan Shen* 20 g, *Dan Shen* 20 g, *Wei Ling Xian* 15 g, *Ci Ji Li* 20 g, *Fang Feng* 15 g, *Bai Xian Pi* 20 g and *Gan Cao* 10 g.

Twenty bags were prescribed. Thereafter, the itching decreased and the cornified skin lesions on the head became softer. The formula was continued with modifications, adding more Blood stasis transforming, hardness softening and Dryness moisturizing medicinals: *Wu Shao She* (Zaocys Dhumnades) 20 g, *Wu Gong* (Scolopendra Subspinipes) three pieces, *Mu Li* (Concha Ostrae) 30 g, as well as *Huang Jing* (Rhizoma Polygonati) 20 g.

After 24 doses of this combination the skin lesions were significantly reduced in amount and the pruritus had disappeared. However, general weakness and lack of energy with no appetite became noticeable. This was related to the chronic disease progress causing exhaustion, but also to the repeated consumption of attacking and dissolving formulas, which had led to syndromes of Spleen deficiency and *Qi* weakness. Consequently, the treatment principle of 'simultaneous attacking and tonifying' was indicated.

The following medicinals were removed from the previous formula: *Wei Ling Xian* (Radix Clematidis), *Bai Xian Pi* (Cortex Dictamni) and *Mu Li* (Concha Ostrae); the following were added instead: *Dang Shen* (Radix Codonopsitis) 25 g, *Huang Qi* (Radix Astragali) 20 g, *Bai Zhu* (Rhizoma Atractylodis Macrocephalae Praeparatae) 15 g and *Ji Nei Jin* (Endothel. Corneum Galli) 10 g.

Sixteen doses were prescribed. The appetite became normal, and an entire strengthening of the body was noticed as well. The skin lesions were healed for the most part. Thereafter, a modification in the form of medicinal pills of the Transforming Blood Stasis Psoriasis Decoction was prescribed for 2 months to help the patient to convalesce, adding *Huang Qi* (Radix Astragali) and *He Shou Wu* (Radix Polygoni Multiflori). One year later, a follow-up examination revealed a full recovery including a clinical confirmation. Since then, the illness has not reoccured.

9. PHLEGM COMBINING WITH BLOOD STASIS

Case Study 4.9   Chronic bronchial asthma

*Hemiplegia is caused by a combination of Qi
stagnation and Blood stasis. Alternatively,
Stomach-Heat produces Phlegm, which flows
into the channels and vessels and blocks their
passageways. Then, Qi and Blood cannot flow
either forward or backward.*

(Huang Di Nei Jing Su Wen)

Case study taken from Liu Shang-Gui's medical
records. Mrs L, 28 years old, admission date
28.12.1984.

When she was 2 years old, she had suffered
from a febrile cold with coughing and a wheezing
sound in her throat, which was treated with normal
pharmaceutical medicine. Over the past 5 years her
illness sometimes improved or sometimes deteriorated,
to the point where she had to be treated as an
inpatient. The diagnosis was bronchial asthma.

She was always treated with spasmolytic, anti-
infective drugs and different Chinese medicinals;
her condition would then improve and she was
able to be discharged.

One month ago, her situation deteriorated again
after a cold. She was admitted to the Occupational
Hospital and treatment began with theophylline
and antibiotics (kanamycin, amoxicillin), without
showing any marked result. When she presented to
us, apart from having a cough with thick, yellow-
green sputum, headache and sore limbs, she also
was noticeably exhausted, showed laboured
breathing with lifting of the shoulders, gasping for
air, mouth dryness, scant yellow urine and dry
stool. The tongue tip was red, the coating was thin
and yellow but also greasy (*Ni*), pulse was slippery
and accelerated.

Formula
The lung produced distinct wheezing sounds
bilaterally. There was an audible wet rhonchus (*Luo
Shen*) on the lung base. Leukocyte count was at
18 700, neutrophils at 87%. The diagnosis was
Phlegm-Heat in the Lung with asthma, therefore
the formula *Wei Jing Tang* originating from the
Sun Si-Miao's classic '*Qian Jin Fang*' was used.

Lu Gen 30 g Rh. Phragmitis	*Dong Gua Ren* 30 g Se. Benincasae Hisp.
Yi Yi Ren 20 g Se. Coicis Lachr.	*Tao Ren* 10 g Se. Persicae
Zhe Bei 10 g Bu. Fritillariae	*Fa Ban Xia* 10 g Rh. Pinelliae Tern.
Gua Lou 10 g Fr. Trichosanthis	*Xing Ren* 10 g Se. Pruni Armeniacae
Ge Gen 10 g Rx. Puerariae	*Ma Huang* 5 g Hb. Ephedrae
Zhi Gan Cao 3 g Rx. Glycyrrhizae Praep.	

After two prescriptions headache and sore limbs
disappeared and the asthmatic cough was
ameliorated. After another eight doses cough and
shortness of breath went away; only lack of
appetite, feeling weak and hip pain remained. As a
next step we removed *Ge Gen* and added *Dang
Shen* (Radix Codonopsis), *Bai Zhu* (Rhizoma
Atractylodis Macrocephalae), *Fu Ling* (Sclerotum
Poria), *Dang Gui* (Angelica Sinensis) and *Shou Di*
(Rehmannia Praeparata), and on 12.2.1985 the
patient was able to leave the clinic with no more
complaints. A routine examination 18 months later
revealed that the diseases had not re-occured.

Discussion
The patient was afflicted by an exogenous
pathogenic factor that reached the interior and
transformed into Heat, combined with the already
existing Phlegm and attacked the Lung. *Wei Jing
Tang* has the functions of cooling the Lung and
dissolving Phlegm, as well as removing Blood stasis
and expelling pus.

Because the disease had already been present
for more than 20 years, Spleen and Kidney had also
been affected. For this reason, Spleen and Kidney
tonifying medicinals were added in the second
prescription to strengthen the patient, in order to
achieve deep breathing and ease the asthma.

10. EXHAUSTION CAUSING BLOOD STASIS

Case Study 4.10

Regardless of food, drink or habitation, if the daily habits of life are out of proportion, this can all lead to failure of movement of Blood and Blood stasis. Hence poor Blood is responsible for a plethora of diseases.
(Wang Ken-Tang 'Zheng Zhi Zhun Sheng')

Case study taken from Zhang Xi-Chun's '*Yi Xue Zhong Zhong Can Xi Lun*' (*Essential notes about Chinese and Western Medicine*). Patient L, 25 years old, occupation tiler, suffered from Blood stasis and shortness of breath.

Aetiology
During repair works, while he was lifting heavy objects, he suddenly felt a pain in the costal arch, which improved after a few days. He was left with a feeling of having something stuck under the ribs, which disturbed his breathing.

General state
The patient's body used to be strong and well-built, but during the 6 months following his accident he steadily became weaker and often felt something stuck under the right rib cage that disturbed his breathing. When talking he often had to stop mid sentence and gasp for air, before he could continue. The condition got worse when he was angry.

His pulse was normal, just a little weak (*Ruo*).

Diagnosis
Blood stasis had developed due to overexertion, because Blood failed to flow back in the Liver channel and *Luo* vessels, which obstructed the passage of *Qi* which is ascending and descending during respiration. Due to the fortunate fact that the pulse, although weakened, remained palpable, *San Qi* (Radix Notoginseng) can be used on its own. It will gradually dissolve Blood stasis, so *Qi* can then regulate itself.

Prescription
San Qi 4 *liang* (~135 g) pulverized, take 1.5 *Qian* daily with 3 *Qian* wheat germ in a soup.

Effect
After 4 days a red-purple blood clot was discharged from the nose and breathing became a little easier. Once the whole prescription was finished, the patient fully recovered.

These ten case studies illustrate the various causes for Blood stasis. Twenty more case studies from both modern and ancient practice can be found in Section 3, Chapter 9.

SUMMARY

Both Blood and *Qi* should flow unobstructed through the body and mutually augment each other. But they can also exert a pathological influence on each other. If the flow of Blood or *Qi* slows down or becomes blocked, then Blood stasis will develop. If only one of them is disturbed, it will cause an imbalance that affects both. Stagnated Blood prevents fresh Blood from reaching the blocked site and from carrying out its nourishing and constructing functions. This causes impairment and weakening of many physiological functions, and the metabolic consequences of Blood stasis give rise to other disorders in turn, e.g. formation of Phlegm. Conversely, Blood stasis can commonly appear in combination with other syndromes that can cause Blood stasis. *Qi* stagnation, Blood and *Qi* deficiency, pathogenic factors such as Heat and Cold, and also any kind of Blood loss, exhaustion and incessant anger all belong to this category.

Chapter 5

Traditional diagnosis and syndrome differentiation of Blood stasis

Chinese diagnosis has four main components:

1. Visual diagnosis, including tongue diagnosis
2. Olfactory/auscultatory diagnosis (of less importance in Blood stasis)
3. Inquiry, and finally
4. Palpatory diagnosis, including pulse diagnosis.

Diagnosis for Blood stasis must be undertaken prior to syndrome differentiation. The most important elements are inquiring about the patient's personal history and inspection of the patient himself, particularly the tongue, skin, hair, lips etc.

Inspection and inquiry can be carried out according to the eight common principles (*Ba Gang*). This procedure will be used here, applying the *Zang Fu* organ classification. The *Zang Fu* organs are functional entities: they comprise the anatomical organ, its function and various other characteristics, hence they do not correspond exactly with the anatomical organ.

SPECIAL SYMPTOMS OF THE *ZANG FU* ORGANS

LIVER[1]

Of all the *Zang Fu* organs, the Liver is the most susceptible to Blood stasis. Typical signs of Blood

---

[1] As this book focuses on TCM, the word 'organs' usually indicates *Zang Fu* organs (functional entities). When anatomical organs in the sense of Western medicine are indicated, this is made clear.

stasis in relation to the Liver are: stabbing pain in the lower rib area, cyanotic nails and lips, dark complexion, painful menses with dark clots, purple-bluish sides of the tongue or dark Blood stasis spots on the side, and a wiry or tight pulse.

HEART

Signs of Blood stasis relating to the Heart include bluish or dark red lips, palpitations or tachycardia, stabbing pain and feeling tight in the chest. The tongue tip has a purple-bluish colour or these may be dark Blood stasis spots on the tip; the sublingual veins are dark or crooked and thick. The pulse is choppy or knotted.

LUNG

Blood stasis signs include a feeling of oppression or pain in the chest and coughing up dark, clotted blood. The tongue is bluish on the anterior parts (see colour plates) or shows black or dark marks that are typical for Blood stasis. The sublingual veins are dark or crooked and thick (sublingual varices).

MIDDLE BURNER

Epigastric pain, vomiting of blood or defecation with dark blood, and sometimes excessive hunger are all signs of Blood stasis relating to the Middle Burner. The typical Blood stasis signs can be seen in the centre of the tongue.

LOWER BURNER

The signs are abdominal pain or lower abdominal pain, abdominal masses and tongue signs in the posterior parts. In women, dysmenorrhoea, amenorrhoea, metrorrhagia, metrostaxis, premenstrual pain and dark, clotted blood indicate Blood stasis related to the Lower Burner.

In Blood stasis, inspection and observation of the above-mentioned signs can help in gathering the first important data. Smelling and listening are not so useful, but as there may be other accompanying syndromes present, such as Phlegm, one should not completely ignore this part of the traditional diagnosis. The most important

criterion for inspection is tongue diagnosis, which has a unique role in the diagnosis of Blood stasis.

TONGUE DIAGNOSIS

Although deficiency syndromes like Qi or Blood/Yin deficiency can also be implicated in Blood stasis, Blood stasis always involves an excess syndrome. The tongue body is a reliable indicator and should always be considered (see colour plate section).

A purple-bluish discolouration of the tongue body immediately alerts one to Blood stasis, but what exactly is the meaning of 'purple-bluish'? For the diagnostician who has not yet had the opportunity to observe thousands of tongue images it is not always easy to recognize this typical colouration. It should be made clear that this colouration, which can be found in both skin and tongue, is the result of poor blood circulation, resulting in a tendency for cyanosis. Chinese studies have shown that increased blood viscosity can lead to the development of this colouration, because the smaller blood vessels transport blood cells that are less oxygenated and thus more red-appearing. This increased blood viscosity has also been artificially recreated using injections of high molecular dextran solutions (molecular weight of 100 000–400 000 daltons.) It has also been shown that elevated blood lipids and a high proportion of immunoglobulins can slow down blood flow, which becomes particularly evident in the tongue capillaries due to lowered oxygenation saturation. Furthermore, chronic Blood stasis has also been linked with a reduction in capillaries.

To the expert eye, then, the difference is as striking as the difference between a piece of raw meat and a piece of raw liver displayed side by side on the meat counter. However, there is no substitute for experience when it comes to comparing tongue slides; the same goes for taking the pulse.

Dark blue or purple dots on the tongue with a purple shading of the tongue body generally indicates Blood stasis. The location of Blood stasis in the body can be determined from the region of the tongue affected, as taught in Chinese tongue diagnosis.

If dots or lines appear on one or both sides of the anterior tongue, then the Heart and Lung regions are affected, which hints at chest pain or chest *Bi* syndrome. Further back is the Liver and Gallbladder region, which can hint at syndromes such as Liver-*Qi* stagnation and other similar syndromes. If the spots are distributed on one side only instead of symmetrically, then only one side of the body is affected.

The different regions of the tongue are described in every good book on TCM.

The following section discusses the inspection of the bottom of the tongue in detail, as this is particularly relevant for the diagnosis of Blood stasis.

As well as their colour being an indication, sublingual veins that become engorged and crooked (sublingual varicosis) are unmistakable signs in tongue diagnosis: if they are dark blue or deep purple, or crooked and look 'angry' (as the Chinese say), then in most cases Blood stasis is present. These prominent veins then form a tortuous 'nest' on the bottom of the tongue. Small venules emerging from the ends of the veins are usually also a sign of Blood stasis. The number of stasis spots or dots, and the length and colour of the sublingual veins determine the degree of Blood stasis (see Figure 5.1).

As we can see in this figure, the bottom of the tongue can be divided into nine zones. Firstly, it is divided horizontally: above the upper end of the frenulum of the tongue (frenulum linguae) is the upper third, and below the frenulum linguae are the middle and lower thirds. Vertically there are three semicircle-like zones. The inner zone, which is well-defined anatomically, lies within the whitish margins (skin folds) that are present to the left and right of the sublingual veins.

This marks off the first segment. The middle and outer zones are both located outside this area and extend to the edge of the tongue. An imaginary dividing line halfway through this area separates the middle from the outer segment.

New vessel formations or enlargement of venules are assessed according to which segment they extend into. Whenever the sublingual veins pass over the midline at the end of the frenulum, this is regarded as sign for Blood stasis (see Figure 5.2).

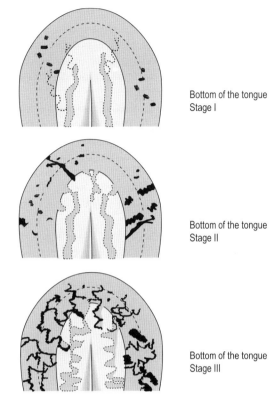

Bottom of the tongue
Stage I

Bottom of the tongue
Stage II

Bottom of the tongue
Stage III

Figure 5.1   Zones of the tongue showing stages of Bood stasis.

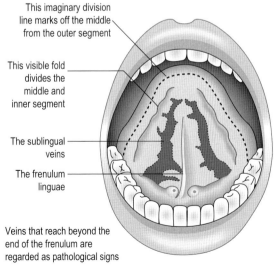

This imaginary division line marks off the middle from the outer segment

This visible fold divides the middle and inner segment

The sublingual veins

The frenulum linguae

Veins that reach beyond the end of the frenulum are regarded as pathological signs

Figure 5.2   Sign of Blood stasis: sublingual veins passing over the midline at the end of the frenulum.

The inspection of the bottom of the tongue is an indispensable tool in recognizing Blood stasis. I have often seen patients with a normal tongue surface but obvious stasis spots or other pointers on the bottom of the tongue; therefore all patients should have this examination.

It should be said that mixed tongue pictures occur quite frequently. In these cases, one must differentiate between Blood stasis and other pathogenic conditions. For example, in Blood stasis due to Cold, the purple-bluish tongue colour of the body is often covered by a thick white coating, so that only the colour on the sides of the tongue can be seen clearly.

Box 5.1 summarizes tongue diagnosis and includes a detailed differentiation of the sublingual veins as practised in many clinics in China today. This Box is based on the standard questionnaire of the Institute for Medical Research and Technology of the University for Traditional Chinese Medicine, Tianjin.

CONDITIONS FOR SUBLINGUAL DIAGNOSIS

Prior to sublingual diagnosis, the patient should not consume any food or drink and should avoid speaking (so this is best done before the oral history is taken). As in diagnosing the surface of the tongue, the face should be turned towards the brightest natural source of light. The angle of light should be chosen so that the floor of the tongue can be clearly seen. Unreflected daylight of at least 10 000 lux is suitable, or (for photographic recordings) a standard white light lamp of 4200° Kelvin and 10 000 lux or a D65 standard light source of 6500° Kelvin (in Europe). It is also possible to use a flash from a camera with white balance.

The patient should extend the tongue as far as possible towards the middle of the hard palate, keeping it relaxed to avoid a discolouration (a purple shading) resulting from backing up of blood. For the same reason, the inspection should

---

Box 5.1   Check-up list of tongue diagnosis

Tongue surface
- General appearance: normal; thick; stiff; teeth marks; cracks (shallow, medium, deep); tremor; deviated
- Tongue body colour: pale white; slightly pale; pale red; dark red; deep red; pale purple; purple; dark purple; deep purple; cyanotic; sides red; tip red
- Tongue body stasis spots: sides; middle; tip; sublingual;, dispersed
- Tongue coating appearance: thin; thin-sticky; sticky; thick-sticky; slippery; dry; like tofu; mirror tongue; geographical tongue; partially no coating; no coating
- Tongue coating colour: white; grey-white; white-yellow; yellow; dark yellow; yellow-brown; brown-grey; grey-black; black; burnt; discoloured other.

Bottom of tongue/sublingual veins
- Appearance at stem: no branching, double branched; multiple-branched; large area; crooked; enlarged; interrupted

- Length: passing over the tip of the frenulum yes/no?
- Shape: indistinct; enlarged at floor of the tongue – small towards the tip; enlarged and slightly crooked; evidently enlarged and crooked
- Colour: pale blue; pale red; red-purple; cyanotic-purple; black-purple.

Length of arteries and signs (degrees) of stasis
- 0: no veins, no elongated veins; no stasis dots or spots
- I: small veins reaching into outer zone; less than three stasis dots
- II: small veins enlarged and crooked, reaching into outer zone; less than 10 stasis dots/some stasis spots
- III: small veins evidently enlarged, crooked, rope-like, reaching into outer zone; dense accumulation of stasis dots/many stasis spots.

not exceed 3–5 seconds. A few seconds should pass before the tongue is shown for a second time, otherwise it may acquire a darker shading and the sublingual veins may protrude more visibly. It is best practice to demonstrate this procedure to the patient at the first consultation. It should be noted that some patients with very short frenulae can turn the tongue only slightly upwards.[2]

DETAILS OF SUBLINGUAL DIAGNOSIS

During sublingual diagnosis we need to evaluate:

- Colour and moisture of the tongue body
- Length and thickness, as well as shape of sublingual veins
- Length, distribution, location and colour of small venules and

---

[2] For photographic recording and storage, digital cameras with white balance (e.g. Nikon Coolpix 990) should be used to avoid film- and processing-induced shading.

Printing images of the tongue (slides, pictures) in books is restricted to the colours of a subtractive colour model (CYMK), whereas an additive colour model is available on the computer screen (RGB). This rather limits paper printing and makes it harder to display the different shadings of the tongue, and this can be observed in all printed samples. Finding the right setting of the colour mixture when processing pictures is also problematic, which is why digital cameras are preferred to normal mechanical ones: additive colour mixture as used on computer screens yields more exact picture quality, as pictures can be transmitted directly from the digital camera without undergoing any modifications during processing in a laboratory.

First, the computer screen settings need to be standardized: it is recommended that the brightness/contrast balance is adjusted to 2.2 gamma in PCs and 1.57 gamma in Apple Macintosh, according to IEC standard 61966 (Comission International de l'Eclairage). To my knowledge, currently the best available colour balance system for computer screens takes a picture of the colour spectrum and displays this on the screen (for example 'Monaco Sensor Colorimeter and Software Monaco EZ Color Profiling Software incl. IT-8 Template', 'Heidelberg View-Open ICC 2.0' or 'X-Rite Color DTP92 and Color Monitor Optimizer'). Afterwards, using a screen scanner, the image on the template and screen is scanned and the colour temperature of the screen is adjusted so both original and photographed image match.

- Size, colour and location of haemorrhagic signs of stasis (dots, spots, areas).

Colour

A purple colour on the bottom of the tongue differs from that of the surface of the tongue most clearly in cases of Blood stasis with Kidney-*Qi* and Heart-*Qi* deficiency. These two syndromes also generate most of the Blood stasis spots.

Moisture

Under normal conditions the bottom of the tongue is moister and paler than the surface (60% difference), but in older patients it becomes darker and less moist, and the mucous membrane becomes rougher.

During middle age, a relatively dry tongue signifies Body Fluid deficiency, caused for example by *Yin* deficiency, whereas, a tongue that is too moist on the bottom with a lot of saliva – especially if the mucous membrane is also thicker and the sublingual veins are obscured as if covered by fog – signifies Kidney- and Spleen-*Yang* deficiency with Dampness or water retention.

Sublingual veins

About three fifths of the length of the tongue and a thickness of approximately 2.5 mm are regarded as normal. The more the sublingual veins elongate towards the tip of the tongue, the more this points towards pathological changes. Such changes indicate the presence of Heat and infections.

Flaccid sublingual veins due to decreased vessel elasticity develop largely from chronic hyperviscosity of blood, caused for example by elevated blood lipids or a slow exsiccosis. The result is a widening of the vessel walls with the veins being distended, which causes them to visibly protrude. This sign suggests pain, tumour formation, dysmenorrhoea and amenorrhoea with *Qi* stagnation and Blood stasis. On the other hand, a flaccid widening of the veins, which makes them appear enlarged but indistinct from each other, suggests Blood stasis and Phlegm, as in arteriosclerosis.

Clear, pale blue, short and thin veins without any stasis dots point towards *Qi* deficiency or

Table 5.1 Signs and their causes

Sign	Cause
Diversified, red	Heat, high blood pressure, infections
Pale, purple, engorged	*Yin* deficiency with empty Heat or Blood-Heat, in headaches, migraine and late stages of *Wen Bing* diseases
Pale, clear	*Qi* deficiency and Blood stasis
Engorged like a hose, elongated and reaching up to the tip, dark red or pale purple	Severe Blood stasis, for example in apoplexies, angina pectoris, chronic asthma

Blood deficiency. Veins that are visibly filled up on one side only can occur congenitally. However, if they appear later on in life they can suggest aneurysms or circulatory problems of the carotid arteries. Black, dark veins point towards Cold or pain. Red veins indicate Heat, fever and infections.

Small vessels

Normally, the venules and branches of the main sublingual veins cannot be seen. However, the more they elongate, the more pronounced the Blood stasis. Elongated venules are classified into four degrees (0–III). (see Box 5.1).

Further signs are described in Table 5.1.

Stasis dots

There are three degrees of stasis dots: the smaller dots; stasis spots of the size of rice corns, which can be flat or raised; and converging stasis areas. Flat spots suggest *Qi* deficiency. The appearance of haemorrhagic stasis signs is classified into three degrees. Less than three dots indicates the first degree, less than ten indicates the second, and converging or more than ten dots indicates the third.

Although a few stasis dots, especially on the bottom of the tongue, are normal in elderly patients, in younger patients their appearance suggests digestive disorders, for example stomach ulcers due to the 'Liver attacks Spleen and Stomach syndrome'. In this case, the spots are visibly demarcated and mostly raised.

Dark red or dark purple stasis spots, particularly if they are raised and cannot be made to fade by pressing them with a cotton bud, suggest Blood stasis in high blood pressure, CHD, liver cirrhosis and asthma. Dark red or dark purple stasis areas, some of the size of a bean, that are clearly demarcated or hard suggest myocardial infarction or tumour formation due to loss of *Zheng-Qi* with Blood stasis. Typical diseases that become particularly visible in sublingual diagnosis are coronary heart diseases, high blood pressure, lung emphysema, cor pulmonale, chronic hepatitis and tumour formations.

The highest degree (III) of sublingual veins can be found mostly in CHD, and the lowest degree (I–II) in hepatitis. High blood pressure is characterized predominantly by the appearance of finely distributed vessels and several spots. In heart disease, the latter occur especially at the tip of the bottom of the tongue. In cor pulmonale the sublingual veins are heavily engorged due to the pressure in the pulmonary artery, and there are hard stasis spots that do not fade when pressed. Many tumours feature even larger hard stasis spots at the lower end of the bottom of the tongue. However, in hepatitis the venules become more evident and elongated and appear small and reddish, with spots on the sides only occurring occasionally.

The last part of traditional diagnosis is palpation. Also important at this stage is to palpate for painful, hard or palpable abdominal masses (resistances).[3] Local and persisting resistances,

---

[3] See Glossary.

and those that change location and are not always palpable, are differentiated. The former indicate Blood stasis, the latter *Qi* stagnation. Pulse diagnosis also belongs to this category.

PULSE DIAGNOSIS

The typical pulse for Blood stasis is choppy but powerful, which is caused by the low mobility of blood or by the lack of thin fluid substances within the blood. Li Shi-Zhen's Pulse Classic '*Ping Hu Mai Xue*' explains: 'Stagnated Blood accumulating in the interior gives rise to a tight and large pulse. However, if the pulse (in the presence of Blood stasis) is deep, small, choppy or weak, it is regarded as an unfavourable prognosis.'

Xu Da-Chun describes the *Se Mai* (choppy pulse) as follows:

The choppy pulse is stagnant and uneven, opposite to the slippery pulse, like a knife scraping bamboo, which cannot slide across smoothly and evenly. It feels slowed down, but not with regard to the amount of beats like the slow pulse, and is weak at the front and back like the short pulse. Both these and the choppy pulse indicate insufficient Qi within the pulse.

When palpated, the choppy pulse does not flow like a wave and leaves an unsatisfied sensation.[4] It is rough and stagnant, not harmonious, like a light knife that scrapes bamboo. It comes and goes reluctantly and feels like fine rain seeping away in the sand. Rain that falls on smooth jade runs smoothly off its surface; however, if it drops on sand it seeps away without any energy. The choppy pulse is neither very fine nor very soft nor like the fading pulse (Wei Mai). It feels as if it is about to fade and then it does not. The soggy pulse (Ru Mai) is superficial, soft and fine, the weak pulse (Ruo Mai) is deep, soft and fine. All three are similar to the choppy pulse. One must be able to distinguish them precisely and not confuse them.

A choppy and powerful pulse indicates Qi *stagnation or Blood stasis; one that is without power indicates deficiency syndromes and weakness. In order to determine the affected organ, the pulse positions should be used. The choppy pulse always suggests chronic or protracted diseases.*

So the choppy pulse is the 'ideal pulse' for Blood stasis. However, as Blood stasis usually occurs in combination with other syndromes, there may be a deep, wiry, tense or slow pulse, depending on the concomitant syndrome. In the case of *Qi* stagnation concurring, there are also often choppy, tight, wiry and knotted pulse qualities. Although not mentioned in the classics, an impalpable pulse that is due to vessel inflammation and vessel occlusion is also frequently encountered. In my experience, a 'purely' choppy pulse has become very rare in cases of Blood stasis in today's practice. More common is a pulse that feels like a knife scraping along a long piece of bamboo, which is deep, fine and flows up and down gradually without reaching a high pulse rate.

Due to the multitude of pulse combinations in Blood stasis and the existence of many concomitant syndromes, making a diagnosis based only on the pulse is not as straightforward as tongue diagnosis, inspection and taking a personal history. At this point I would like to emphasize that a choppy but powerful pulse indicates an excess syndrome, primarily Blood stasis, whereas as powerless choppy pulse indicates a deficiency syndrome, primarily deficiency of Blood. In the case of Blood stasis in combination with Blood deficiency, the dominating factor will determine the quality of the pulse.

SUMMARY

The following typical signs should be observed when Blood stasis is suspected:

- **Inspection:** Dry skin (cracked or scaly), petechiae, spider naevi, dark complexion, cyanotic nails and lips, dark or crooked and enlarged sublingual veins (sublingual varices) that branch out thinly over the border of the

---

[4] Xu surely means that the pulse is not sufficiently evident when it comes and goes. Only the peak is clearly palpable, thus it is just noticeable, but feels unsatisfactory when palpated.

area at the end of the frenulum. On the tongue, especially at the sides, there are dark Blood stasis spots or dots. The tongue is purple or slightly bluish.

- **Olfaction/auscultation:** There are no typical Blood stasis signs that could be sensed by the ear or nose. However, as Blood stasis frequently combines with other syndromes like Phlegm, this part of general diagnosis should not be neglected.
- **Inquiry:** General symptoms of Blood stasis include a chronic, fixed stabbing pain, aggravation of symptoms at night, bleeding or blood loss of any kind, and a numb and prickling sensation in the limbs. For example, with regard to the *Zang Fu* organs, there can be a sensation of pressure or pain in the chest, coughing of dark, clotted blood, painful menstruation with dark clots and many other gynaecological conditions. Mental symptoms often include forget-

fulness, irritability, depression and even psychosis.
- **Palpation:** Signs are abdominal resistances that are primarily fixed and hard, increased sensitivity to touch or warding off pain, and a powerful and choppy or a deep or fine pulse.

BLOOD STASIS IN COMBINATION WITH OTHER SYMPTOMS

Table 5.2 compares the typical signs and symptoms of Blood and *Qi* syndromes. These can also occur together, depending on the combination of Blood stasis with the other components. To give an example, Blood stasis and *Qi* deficiency may feature the following signs and symptoms: the patient feels generally weak and is quickly short of breath, with pale skin and face, dark purple tongue body with a little

Table 5.2 Differential diagnosis of various syndromes of Blood and *Qi*

Indicator	Blood stasis	*Qi* stagnation	Blood deficiency	*Qi* deficiency
Skin	Dry, cracked, petechiae, spider naevi	Normal	Sallow	Pale
Face/lips	Bluish, cyanotic	Normal	Grey-white, pale	Pale, white
Tongue	Bluish, purple with stasis dots	Normal, possibly slightly dark	Dry, little coating	Pale, swollen, teeth marks
Typical pulses	Choppy, deep, fine	Wiry	Fine, powerless	Weak
Mind/psyche	Forgetfulness, tends to mania	Tends to depression	Mental exhaustion	Lassitude, tiredness, no energy
Pain/sensation of pressure	Fixed location, sensitive to touch, worse at night	Strong, sudden	Numbness, cold limbs	Pain comes and goes, alleviated by pressure
Quality	Stabbing, pressing	Comes in bouts	Prickly	Dull
Location	Always same location	Often abdomen, breast, head	On extremities	Location varies
Menstruation	Clotted, dark blood, painful	Sensation of pressure in the breasts, often a prolonged cycle	Thin, light blood, prolonged cycle or amenorrhoea	Prolonged cycle, profuse menses, thin and light blood

Table 5.3   Blood stasis combined with other syndromes

Indicator	Blood stasis with Phlegm (excess)	Blood stasis with Heat (excess)	Blood stasis with Cold (excess)	Blood stasis with *Yang* deficiency	Blood stasis with *Yin* deficiency or Blood Dryness
Pain	Like Blood stasis or numb limbs, fullness	Like Blood stasis	Strong pain especially of the limbs and when moving	Pain alleviated by pressure or warmth	Like Blood stasis
Tongue	Thick white or thick greasy coating, dark purple body	Dry yellow coating, deep red or dark purple body with stasis spots	Thin white coating, dark purple body or stasis spots or dots	Slippery white coating, pale purple body, possibly with stasis spots	No or little coating, many cracks, dark red body with stasis spots
Pulse	Slippery, fine or wiry, fine	Accelerated, fine, possibly choppy	Fine, slow or wiry	Fine, weak or fine, deep	Weak, fine or weak, choppy
Skin/face	Swollen, partly greasy	Reddened, erythema	Partially pale or cyanotic	Cyanotic lips, oedema	Dry or scaly skin, lusterless skin
Digestion	Borborygmus, no appetite, nausea, scanty urine	Dry stool, dark urine, possibly blood (haemorrhagic diseases)	Thin and runny stool, partly with undigested food	Loose or runny stool, scanty urine without any pressure	Dry stool or constipation, scanty and dark urine
Other signs	Patient is often corpulent; many other symptoms possible	Irritability or apathy (during high fever)	Sensitive to cold or draught	Sensitive to cold, oedema especially of the legs	Dry mouth and brittle hair, skin diseases

white coating, loose stool or difficult defecation, and clear urine; he has consistent pain at a sensitive spot on the lower abdomen, etc. In this case, the combination of two syndromes needs to be considered, thus the treatment should involve both the 'branch' and the 'root'.

Table 5.3 compares different combinations of Blood stasis with other syndromes that are regularly seen in practice.

Apart from these, there are also other possible combinations, such as acute Blood stasis due to trauma in combination with chronic Blood stasis.

Finally, if Blood stasis is so common and mostly combines with other syndromes, how does the modern practitioner proceed in its treatment using the classical concept of Blood stasis? The following imaginary example (Box 5.2) will try to integrate both views (conventional medicine and TCM).

So far, we have learned about Blood stasis from the point of view of both conventional and Chinese medical systems and have looked at historical development, diagnosis, syndrome differentiation and its combination with other syndromes. Now we can proceed to the treatment of Blood stasis with TCM methods.

Box 5.2   Imaginary example

A 60-year-old glutton, who due to decreased thirst in old age takes in insufficient fluids, consumes many fatty and heavy meals instead. This generates both a lack of Body Fluids (*Yin* deficiency[5]) and endogenous formation of Heat or Phlegm. He has elevated blood lipids (pathogenic Phlegm) and the ratio of cells to plasma has been shifted in favour of the solid components of blood, the cells. Thus he has increased blood viscosity or 'thick blood'. The resulting poor capillary circulation generates a diminished supply of oxygen and nutrients to tissues, and an increased blood viscosity (Blood stasis). Over a long period of time, the most affected tissue will react by becoming acidic and showing functional disorders. Eventually, these will lead to organic disorders.

Now if, for example, another pathogenic factor is introduced, such as Wind in the form of an

infection, or Dryness as a climatic influence, the combination of endogenous and exogenous factors may now cause Blood stasis with Heat and manifest as a febrile disease, or cause Blood stasis with Dryness and manifest as psoriasis. In the latter case it becomes impossible to tell exactly to what extent endogenous *Yin* deficiency (root) or exogenous Dryness or Blood stasis (branch) caused the psoriasis. But it is not necessary to know, as the patient's condition itself is the basis of the diagnosis: the chief action of the formula is determined by which ever pathogenic factor prevails. Other factors are also incorporated into the treatment, because both endogenous root as well as branch and exogenous factors can be treated at the same time.

To obtain every detail of the aetiology may be of benefit to the therapist and contribute to his greater understanding. Yet, for the purpose of a successful treatment it is not absolutely necessary, as long as a precise diagnosis of the entire condition is carried out. Considering this, the above-mentioned pathological mechanisms must also be put into the right perspective.

---

[5] The terms in brackets stand for an overlap of both medical systems. This overlap is not always complete, because Blood stasis can manifest in other ways than hyperviscosity, and not every case of elevated blood lipids generates the typical symptoms of pathogenic Phlegm as defined in TCM.

SECTION **2**

Practical application

This part of the book is designed to link previous information with clinical application. First, basic treatment principles are presented and explained. After that, medicinals relevant to Blood stasis and their combinations with each other and with other medicinals are introduced. In addition, there is a list of the most commonly used formulas, which includes an analysis of their action, principles of action, contraindications and accompanying acupuncture therapy.

SECTION CONTENTS

Chapter 6

Examples of treatment principles for Blood stasis

Whilst Chinese medicine occasionally uses paradoxical treatment principles (e.g. warm diaphoretics for feverish states of Heat), the treatment principles for Blood stasis are based exclusively on an oppositional or allopathic model of prescription (e.g. Blood moving or cooling in case of Blood Heat, etc.).

The most common treatment principles deduced from syndrome differentiation are described below. They represent important building blocks in the treatment process. The treatment principle is the next step after diagnosis of the specific type of Blood stasis and analysis of its cause, and is the source of the right combination and modification of the formula.

Knowledge of the relevant medicinals and appropriate formulas is a prerequisite for the treatment principle, so the idea of the treatment principle is introduced before the medicinals themselves are mentioned, to enable the reader to follow the process in his mind.

There are certainly other principles, apart from the commonly occurring eleven principles introduced below. For example after birth, pathogenic Cold can manifest itself in the uterus, which would indicate *Sheng Hua Tang* (Generate Change Decoction); but pathogenic Cold could also manifest itself as rheumatic pain in the *Jing Luo* vessels. Then, *Shen Tong Zhu Yu Tang* (Anti-Stasis Pain Decoction) would be required. Or it could manifest itself as Cold in the chest presenting with heart pain and so on.

Table 6.1 with its examples does not replace syndrome differentiation and precise fine-tuning of the formula for each patient. A mere sympto-

Table 6.1 Treatment principles and formulas

Result of syndrome differentiation	Example of therapeutic principle	Example formula (Chinese /English)
Blood stasis with *Qi* stagnation	Invigorate Blood and move *Qi*	*Xue Fu Zhu Yu Tang*/Anti-Stasis Chest Decoction
Blood stasis with *Qi* deficiency	Invigorate Blood and tonify *Qi*	*Bu Yang Huan Wu Tang*/Five-Tenth Decoction[1]
Blood stasis with *Yin* deficiency	Invigorate Blood and nourish *Yin*	*Yang Yin Tong Bi Tang*/*Yin* Nourishing *Bi* Dissolving Decoction
Blood stasis with Blood deficiency	Invigorate Blood and nourish Blood	*Huo Luo Xiao Ling Tang*/Wondrous Pill to Invigorate the Channels
Blood stasis with pathogenic Cold	Invigorate Blood and dispel Cold	*Sheng Hua Tang*/Generate Change Decoction
Blood stasis with pathogenic Heat	Invigorate Blood and cool Heat	*Tao Ren Cheng Qi Tang*/*Qi* Rectifying Persica Decoction
Blood stasis with Phlegm	Invigorate Blood and transform Phlegm	*Xi Huang Wan*/Yellow Rhino Pills
Blood stasis with abdominal masses, Concretions, Conglomerations	Invigorate Blood and soften masses	*Da Huang Zhe Chong Wan*/Rheum Eupolyphaga Pill
Blood stasis with food stagnation	Invigorate Blood and purge	*Di Dang Tang*/Resistance Decoction
Blood stasis with bleeding	Invigorate Blood and stop bleeding	*San Qi Shi Xiao San*/Sudden Smile Powder with Notoginseng
Blood stasis with blockage of the *Luo Mai* (the collaterals)	Invigorate Blood and remove obstruction from the *Luo* channels	*Shen Tong Zhu Yu Tang*/Anti-Stasis Pain Decoction

matic treatment should be rejected. The same applies for acupuncture.

EXPLANATIONS OF THE PRINCIPLES IN DETAIL

1. BLOOD STASIS WITH *QI* STAGNATION: INVIGORATE BLOOD AND MOVE *QI*

Typical indications
Stabbing pain and feeling of oppression in the chest and hypochondrium, palpitations, depression, insomnia, frequent anger or other emotional factors. This is often caused by stagnation of Liver-*Qi*.

[1] Literally: Decoction to Tonify the *Yang* in Order to Restore the Five i.e. the hemi-phlegic half of the body: upper arm, lower arm, upper leg, lower leg and the paralized side of the head.

Related diseases
Liver and gallbladder diseases, coronary heart disease (CHD), nervous disorders.

Possible formulas
Xue Fu Zhu Yu Tang (Anti-Stasis Chest Decoction), *Ge Xia Zhu Yu Tang* (Anti-Stasis Abdomen Decoction), *Fu Yuan Huo Xue Tang* (Blood Invigorating Recovery Decoction), *Guan Xin Fang No. 2* (Coronary Decoction No. 2).

2. BLOOD STASIS WITH *QI* DEFICIENCY: INVIGORATE BLOOD AND TONIFY *QI*

Typical indications
Weakness, tiredness, shortness of breath, paralysis, chest pain especially under strain, lack of appetite.

Related diseases
Coronary heart disease (CHD), chronic hepatitis, stroke sequelae.

Possible formulas
Bu Yang Huan Wu Tang (Five-Tenth Decoction), *Huang Qi Si Wu Tang* (Astragalus Four Ingredients Decoction), *Ba Zhen Tang* (Eight Treasures Decoction).

3. BLOOD STASIS WITH YIN DEFICIENCY: INVIGORATE BLOOD AND NOURISH *YIN*

Typical indications
Sensation of heat in palms and soles, weight loss, night sweating, elevated temperature in the afternoon or evening, dizziness, dry eyes and skin, lustreless complexion.

Related diseases
Liver cirrhosis, leukaemia, tuberculosis, phlebitis, diabetes, low immunity.

Possible formulas
Xia Yu Xue Tang (Blood Stasis Purging Decoction), *Tao Hong Si Wu Tang* (Persica Carthamus Four Ingredients Decoction), *Liu Wei Di Huang Wan* (Rehmannia Six Pill),[2] *Qin Jiao San* (Gentiana Powder).

4. BLOOD STASIS WITH BLOOD DEFICIENCY: INVIGORATE BLOOD AND NOURISH BLOOD

Typical indications
Dizziness, insomnia, palpitations, pale complexion, pale lips and nails, dry stools, tinnitus.

Related diseases
Anaemia, loss of blood sequelae, neurasthenia, cardiac arrhythmias.

Possible formulas
Si Wu Tang (Four Ingredients Decoction),[3] *Huo Luo Xiao Ling Tang* (Wondrous Pill to Invigorate the Channels), *Tao Ren Shao Yao Tang* (Persica Paeonia Decoction).

---

[2] Literally: Radix Rehmannia Pill of the Six Medicinals.
[3] The formulas given here are listed at the back of the book, if they are Blood stasis formulas. Otherwise, they can be found in Bensky etc.

5. BLOOD STASIS WITH PATHOGENIC COLD: INVIGORATE BLOOD AND DISPEL COLD

Typical indications
1. Strong pain in a fixed location (e.g. chest area, costal area, abdomen), shortness of breath, heart pain, cold limbs.
2. Strong stabbing pain in the limbs, as if inflamed, but without reddening or heat, possibly stiff, numbness, lack of strength in arms and legs, cold climate worsens.
3. Pain in the lower abdomen after giving birth, feeling cold and weakness.

Related diseases
Postpartum infections, delayed uterine involution, no lactation, retention of placenta, infertility.

Possible formulas
Guan Xin Tang No. 2 (Coronary Decoction No. 2), *Zhi Shi Xie Bai Gui Zhi Tang* (Citrus Aurantium Allium Cinnamomum Decoction), *Shen Tong Zhu Yu Tang* (Anti-Stasis Pain Decoction), *Xiao Huo Luo Dan* (Small Channel Invigorating Pill).

6. BLOOD STASIS WITH PATHOGENIC HEAT: INVIGORATE BLOOD AND COOL DOWN HEAT

Typical indications
Burning pain in chest area and abdomen, irritability, nervousness, thirst, tendency to bleeding, feeling of heat, dry, hard stool, susceptibility to formation of furuncles.

Related diseases
Haemorrhagic diathesis (e.g. nose bleeding caused by Blood Heat), bronchioectasis, lung abscess, acute hepatitis B, septicaemia.

Possible formulas

Tao Hong Si Wu Tang (Persica Carthamus Four Ingredients Decoction), *Xi Jiao Di Huang Tang* (Rhino-Rehmannia Decoction), *Tao Ren Cheng Qi Tang* (Qi Rectifying Persica Decoction), *Xian Fang Huo Ming Yin* (Invigorating Drink of the Immortals), *Qing Re Xiao Du San* (Cooling Detoxifying Powder).

7. BLOOD STASIS WITH PHLEGM: INVIGORATE BLOOD AND TRANSFORM PHLEGM

Typical indications

Phlegm in its literal sense causing one to constantly clear one's throat due to the phlegm in the throat, coughing with phlegm; but also in its broad meaning, e.g. in certain types of paralysis or in *Bi*-syndrome of the chest.

Related diseases

Bronchitis, coronary heart disease, hyperlipi-daemia, hemiplegia, epilepsy and many kinds of 'strange' diseases that are out of the ordinary.

Possible formulas

Tao Hong Si Wu Tang (Persica Carthamus Four Ingredients Decoction), *Xi Huang Wan* (Yellow Rhino Pills).

8. BLOOD STASIS WITH ABDOMINAL MASSES: INVIGORATE BLOOD AND SOFTEN MASSES

Typical indications

Abdominal masses and gatherings, goitre and the like.

Related diseases

Myomas, ovarian cysts, lymph node swelling, tumours, especially of the vessels, prostatic hyper-trophy.

Possible formulas

Da Huang Zhe Chong Wan (Rheum Eupolyphaga Pill), *Gui Zhi Fu Ling Wan* (Cinnamon Poria Pill).

9. BLOOD STASIS WITH FOOD STAGNATION: INVIGORATE BLOOD AND PURGE

Typical indications
Food accumulation with stomach distension, feeling of distension and accumulation in the abdomen, digestive disorders with delayed diges-tion or cessation of digestion.

Related diseases
Pancreatitis, cholelithiasis, acute abdomen with cessation of digestion.

Possible formulas
Di Dang Tang (Resistance Decoction), *Tao Hong Cheng Qi Tang* (*Qi* Rectifying Persica Carthamus Decoction).

10. BLOOD STASIS WITH BLEEDING: INVIGORATE BLOOD AND STOP BLEEDING

Typical indications
Blood Heat syndromes, tendency to bleeding, poor blood coagulation, all types of haemor-rhages, including nose bleeding, bloody stool, excessive menstrual bleeding, excessive lochia or metrorrhagia etc.

Related diseases
All types of haemorrhages.

Possible formulas
San Qi Shi Xiao San (Notoginseng Sudden Smile Powder).

11. BLOOD STASIS WITH BLOCKAGE OF THE *LUO MAI* (COLLATERALS): INVIGORATE BLOOD AND REMOVE OBSTRUCTIONS FROM THE *LUO* CHANNELS

Typical indications
Limb pain with restriction of movement, worse at night.

Related diseases
Rheumatic *Bi*-syndrome (Arthritis), arthritis of the shoulder joint, lower back pain, lordosis of the neck.

Possible formulas
Huo Luo Xiao Ling Tang (Wondrous Pill to Invigo-rate the Channels), *Shen Tong Zhu Yu Tang* (Anti-Stasis Pain Decoction).

Composition and details of the listed formulas relevant to Blood stasis will be addressed in Chapter 7.

Chapter **7**

Blood stasis related medicinals, their application and combination

PART 1. BLOOD STASIS RELATED MEDICINALS

LISTING BLOOD STASIS RELATED MEDICINALS

Over 2000 years ago in the *Shen Nong Ben Cao Jing* (Divine Husbandman's Classic of the Materia Medica) 30 of the 365 listed medicinals were already being described as Blood invigorating, Blood transforming, Blood stasis breaking and dispelling. Even then, *Mu Dan Pi* (Moutan), *Niu Xi* (Achyranthis), *Chi Shao* (Paeonia Rubra), *Tao Ren* (Persica), *Shui Zhi* (Hirudo), *Meng Chong* (Tabanus), *Pu Huang* (Pollen) and many more had been recorded, which shows that Blood stasis was already being diagnosed and treated in China 2000 years ago. Today's list of medicinals that are linked with Blood stasis is of course much longer.

Although many medicinals were traditionally classified into different groups, I have listed below all medicinals directly related to Blood stasis according to the latest classification. As the characteristics of these drugs have already been discussed by Porkert, Paulus and Bensky, every drug is simply illustrated with a summary of its TCM actions. The main focus is on modern drug research, as that field was not accounted for by the authors mentioned above.

Scientific research in the most recent decades has confirmed that the concept of Blood stasis is closely linked to circulatory disorders. Moreover, relationships to metabolic disorders, immune functions and tissue changes such as neoplasms have been noted.

TCM traditionally employs Blood invigorating (*Huo Xue*) medicinals. This makes sense especially when we compare the most important general physiological changes in blood affected by Blood stasis with the actions of the medicinals:

1. Haemorheology: changes in blood are summarized as 'concentration, viscosity, clotting and clumping'. Concentration signifies a rise in blood lipids and albumin, as well as a raised haematocrit. Viscosity denotes a rise in blood and plasma viscosity, clotting is a rise in fibrinogen levels and increased blood clotting time. Clumping means raised thrombocyte aggregation.

2. Microcirculation: microcirculation is blood flow between the smallest arterioles and venules, i.e. blood flow in the capillaries. Here, blood stasis is characterized by a decrease in flow speed, partial obstruction of flow-through, raised pressure manifesting as changes in shape (crooking or formation of loops within the vessels) and leakage of blood through the vessel walls (haemorrhages).

3. Haemodynamics: here, Blood stasis presents as a circulatory disorder of a particular organ or tissue, caused by a narrowing or blocking of the vessels which decreases the amount of blood passing through.

Blood invigorating and Blood stasis breaking medicinals show their effect on these three precise areas; however, the effect is observed in different organs and in different mechanisms:

1. Action on blood viscosity: these medicinals work by improving blood flow in certain organs and peripheral vessels, for example by interfering in the coagulation process, by decreasing fibrinogen levels, by increasing the thrombus dissolving action of fibrinolysin (plasmin) and by making the formation of thrombocyte aggregation more difficult. Interestingly, this is achieved without causing an increased tendency towards bleeding, e.g. with *San Qi* (Notoginseng). Furthermore, blood lipid levels are lowered and immune function is increased.

2. Action on microcirculation: plasticity of erythrocytes as well as pathological small vessel diameters are both increased. In addition, vessel wall permeability is decreased, which prevents haemorrhages, and finally, blood flow velocity is increased.

3. General blood flow is enhanced by reducing vessel resistance, increasing flow rate, by vasodilation of peripheral and other vessels; and heart performance and arterial vessel function are improved. Every medicinal has specific sites of action, for example the cerebral vessels, coronary vessels and peripheral vessels. Due to the inhibitive action on inflammation inside the vessels, vascular inflammation is confined and thus thrombus and plaque formation is prevented. Furthermore, spastic vasoconstriction is inhibited by the analgesic action of the medicinals.

In addition, an antineoplastic action was noted in many medicinals of this class, which establishes the connection that was frequently recorded in ancient times: the link between Blood stasis and abdominal masses, a modern proof of the accuracy of traditional methods.

SIDE EFFECTS AND CONTRAINDICATIONS

According to Traditional Chinese Medicine, the use of Blood invigorating medicinals (especially groups 2 and 3, see below) can easily weaken *Qi* and especially Blood, particularly if taken over a longer period of time. Thus, *Qi*- and Blood-tonifying medicinals are often added to the prescription in order to protect the body from damage to *Qi* or Blood.

Even stopping bleeding can cause Blood stasis in the body. To prevent this from happening, Blood invigorating medicinals are sometimes added to a formula that stops bleeding. However, this does not apply to *San Qi* (Notoginseng), which is proven to invigorate Blood as well as to stop bleeding.

Furthermore, Blood invigorating formulas should only be used with great caution in pregnant women or in hypermenorrhoea (excessive menstrual bleeding) as these formulas have a blood dispelling effect. For all bleeding disorders, including haemophilia, most Blood invigorating medicinals are contraindicated.

As most Blood invigorating medicinals, especially those that move Blood (group 2 below) and break Blood stasis (group 3 below), actively influence blood coagulation and thrombolysis, simultaneous prescription of Western preparations that contain coumarin, heparin and hirudin should be avoided. Pharmaceutical hirudin, which is mostly employed in Japan, stems from the Chinese pharmacopoeia and is no less potent than older preparations. Nevertheless, many medicinals such as the above-mentioned *San Qi* (Notoginseng) also contain constituents that can stop bleeding. These constituents can prevent an overreaction in the body and therefore offer more safety in usage than conventional drugs. It is thus worth considering how to forego the simultaneous use of Blood invigorating/Blood stasis breaking medicinals and other 'blood thinning' drugs in clinical practice. This applies especially to the long-term use of certain drugs, e.g. all products containing acetylsalicylic acid (ASA).

In the following list, medicinals are given in alphabetical order according to the Chinese nomenclature, followed by a short Latin reference.

THE 46 MOST IMPORTANT BLOOD INVIGORATING AND BLOOD STASIS ELIMINATING MEDICINALS

The Chinese expression '*Huo Xue Hua Yu*', which describes these medicinals, translates literally as 'invigorate Blood transform Blood stasis', and thereby points to two different functions. However, in the latest pharmacological research, TCM makes a more precise differentiation, between three different groups of medicinals:

1. Blood harmonizing medicinals (group I)
2. Blood moving medicinals (group II)
3. Blood stasis breaking medicinals (group III).

In this context, Blood harmonizing medicinals (*He Xue Yao*) have a lesser Blood invigorating action but additionally nourish (*Dang Gui*) or cool (*Mu Dan Pi*) the Blood. Blood moving medicinals (*Huo Xue Hua Yu Yao*) are the 'classic' Blood

invigorating medicinals. They move Blood more strongly than the first group, transform Blood and therefore weaken it in the long term. They should always be combined with Blood nourishing medicinals (*Sheng Di, Dang Gui*). Typical Blood moving medicinals are Blood invigorating ones like *Hong Hua, Yu Jin,* and *Yi Mu Cao* (Leonurus). The third and most powerful group are Blood stasis breaking medicinals (*Po Xue, Qu Yu*), which are used in conditions of dry, long-standing stagnated Blood. Most of them can also remove obstructions from the vessels. They are the 'pipe-unblockers' for Blood stasis and should never be prescribed over a long period or without having balanced the formula with Blood nourishing medicinals, as they can otherwise easily weaken the Blood; in addition this group contains strong drugs, e.g. insect medicinals (*Chong Yao*). Typical representatives of this group are *Tu Bie Chong* (Eupolyphaga), *Mang Chong* (Tabanus), *Shui Zhi* (Hirudo), but also *Tao Ren* (Persica).

Further details concerning each medicinal can be found in Bensky's and Barolet: materia medica excellent work (see Appendix 7) which, as said before, does not yet incorporate modern scientific research [Translator's note: there is a new third edition 2004, which has been updated and revised]. I would encourage the reader to look up the extensively described traditional actions there. My short descriptions do not imply that they are less important; on the contrary, a good therapist will be flexible in his use of both kinds of knowledge and will apply both sides of the brain in the process of finding the right treatment principle.

GROUP I: 10 BLOOD HARMONIZING MEDICINALS

The medicinals in this group have a Blood forming and Blood harmonizing effect. They work in a milder way than the medicinals of the second or third group and additionally have a Blood cooling or nourishing action.

Chi Shao, Radix Paeoniae Rubrae

Taste: bitter
Dosage: 6–12 g
Temperature: slightly cold
Channel/Organ action: Liver

Traditionally used in China to eliminate stagnated Blood and pathogenic Heat in the Blood. Also used for the treatment of pain caused by Blood stasis, menorrhagia, amenorrhoea and acute inflammations with redness, swelling and pain.

New pharmacological research

Blood: prevents thrombosis formation and has an antisclerotic action.

Heart: has a heart muscle protective action, increases heart function, decreases pressure in the pulmonary artery.

Central nervous system (CNS): has a calming, analgetic and febrifugal action.

Further actions: antispasmodic on smooth musculature, antineoplastic, anti-inflammatory and antimycotic.

New clinical usage

Coronary heart disease, cor pulmonale, acute cerebral thrombosis, acute icteric hepatitis, mycotic dermatitis, acute traumatic sepsis and dermatitis.

Dan Shen, Radix Salviae Miltiorrhizae

Taste: bitter
Dosage: 6–18 g
Temperature: slightly cold
Channel/Organ action: Heart, Liver

Traditionally used in China to improve Blood circulation and to eliminate Blood stasis, especially in the treatment of dysmenorrhoea, amenorrhoea, abdominal masses caused by Blood stagnation, carbuncles and abscesses; it can also be used as a calming medicinal. Nowadays, it is often used in coronary heart disease.

New pharmacological research

Blood: improves microcirculation, has an antisclerotic effect and is used against thrombocyte aggregation.

Heart: increases heart function and coronary vessel circulation capacity.

Further actions: anti-inflammatory, antimycotic, anticarcinogenic, prevents liver damage, ischemic kidney damage, lung damage, anti-ulcerative, prevents endotoxin-induced shock, captures free radicals, has an oestrogenic action, protects from bronchial asthma and has a calming effect.

New clinical usage

Coronary heart disease, bacterial myocarditis in children, high blood viscosity, haemorrhoids, apoplexy, hepatitis, retinal vein thrombosis, whooping cough, nephritis, diabetes, haemorrhagic fever, malignant lymphomas and scleroderma.

Dang Gui, Radix Angelicae Sinensis

(traditionally in the Blood tonifying group)

Taste: sweet, pungent
Dosage: 6–15 g
Temperature: warm
Channel/Organ action: Lung, Heart, Spleen

It is used as:

1. A blood tonifying and circulation improving medicinal in menstrual disorders and
2. An emollient and laxative in chronic constipation in old age.

New pharmacological research

Blood: promotes haematopoiesis, especially erythropoiesis, has an antithrombotic action and prevents thrombocyte aggregation, lowers blood lipid concentration and increases microcirculation.

Heart: has an anti-ischemic and anti-arrhythmic action and lowers blood pressure.

Immune system: increases cellular and humoral immune function.

Further actions: has a relaxing action and alleviates pain in the smooth musculature of the uterus; has an antibacterial action on many different types of bacteria.

New clinical usage

Ischemic cerebral apoplexy, thrombophlebitis, cardiac arrhythmias, infantile pneumonia, menstrual disorders, uterus prolapse, chronic pelvic inflammation, cor pulmonale, hepatitis, herpes zoster.

Hong Jing Tian or Gao Shan Hong Jing Tian, Herba Rhodiolae Sachaliensis

(in most cases, this is traditionally categorised in the *Yang* tonic group)

Taste: sweet, astringent
Dosage: 9–15 g
Temperature: neutral
Channel/Organ action: Liver, Spleen

Traditionally used in China to invigorate and nourish the Blood and strongly tonify Kidney *Yang*. Used in old age weakness as well as in cardiac insufficiency, anaemia, dizziness due to low blood pressure and other weaknesses, where *Hong Jing Tian* has a strengthening and tonifying effect.

Less effective on the blood vessels, but more invigorating is the bitter and cold medicinal *Xia Ye Hong Jing Tian*, Radix et Rhizoma Rhodiolae Kirilowii, which is used more for ischemic heart disease. It acts on the Lung channel, cools Heat/toxins, has an analgetic effect in injuries and stops bleeding.

New pharmacological research
CNS: similar to Ginseng, *Hong Jing Tian* is a strong adaptogen, reduces stress, relaxes and counteracts the effects of tiredness.
Blood: blood pressure as well as blood sugar levels are regulated in both directions; it has an antioxidative effect on blood lipids.
Heart: strengthens heart contractility and reduces ischemic damage.
Immune system: *Hong Jing Tian* has anti-inflammatory, febrifugal and virostatic action.
Further actions: reduces the effects of radiation injuries and, depending on the dosage, has a contractile or relaxing effect on smooth musculature of the small intestine.

New clinical usage
Used in heart insufficiency in old age, reduced mental and physical capacity, anaemia, lung tuberculosis, diabetes, hypotension and in impaired mental activity.

Ji Xue Teng, Caulis Spatholobi

Taste: bitter
Dosage: 9–15 g
Temperature: slightly cold
Channel/Organ action: Liver, Kidney

Traditionally used in China to strengthen Blood circulation and remove obstructions from the channels and smaller vessels (*Luo* vessels). It is a Blood nourishing medicinal, especially for the treatment of abnormal menstruation caused by Blood deficiency and Blood stasis. Also used for inflammation of peripheral vessels, or thrombosis and numbness of the body and limbs. It is also effective in leukopenia caused by radiotherapy.

New pharmacological research
Blood: *Ji Xue Teng* promotes haematopoiesis (erythrocytes, thrombocytes, interleukin-2 and haemoglobin), counteracts blood clotting and lowers blood lipid levels.
Heart: reduces oxygen consumption of the heart muscle and increases heart rate.
Further actions: increases phosphate metabolism of the kidneys and uterus and has a calming action.

New clinical usage
Used in insufficiency of thrombocytes and in mammary gland hyperplasia.

Mu Dan Pi, Cortex Moutan Radicis

(traditionally in the group of cooling/Heat clearing medicinals)

Taste: bitter
Dosage: 6–12 g
Temperature: slightly cold
Channel/Organ action: Heart, Liver, Kidneys

It is used:

1. as a medicinal to cool Blood-Heat and for the treatment of bleeding together with fever, and
2. to improve circulation and eliminate Blood stasis in cases of appendicitis, furuncles, carbuncles and amenorrhoea.

New pharmacological research
Heart: lowers blood pressure, prevents arrhythmia and ischemia.
Blood: has an antisclerotic action and prevents thrombosis and haemorrhaging in the capillaries.
Further actions: has a spasmolytic effect in inflammation and is also calming, febrifugal, diuretic, antibacterial and contraceptive.

New clinical usage
Prevents bruising due to insufficient thrombocytes; used in urticaria, pruritus, fever due to
infections (appendicitis, cholecystitis pneumonia,
nephritis and many more), hypertension, allergic
rhinitis, amenorrhoea and dysmenorrhoea.

Shan Zha, Fructus Crataegi, Hawthorn Fruit

(traditionally in the group of digestion-improving
medicinals)

Taste: sour, sweet
Dosage: 9–15–30 g
Temperature: slightly warm
Channel/Organ action: Spleen, Stomach, Kidneys

Traditionally used in China to improve the digestion of fats and meats, it is often added to food. It
is also used to alleviate the feeling of fullness after
a heavy meal or to alleviate pain in the chest or
abdomen and invigorate the Blood, but mainly for
the treatment of stagnated food and digestive
problems, diarrhoea and pain in the chest and
abdomen.

New pharmacological research
Blood: significantly lowers blood lipids and blood
  pressure.
Heart: increases blood flow and amount of blood
  in the cardiac muscle and protects from the damaging effects of ischemia and hypoglycaemia.
Further actions: has an antioxidative effect, strengthens the immune system (t-lymphocytes) and
  is antibacterial.

New clinical usage
Hyperlipidaemia, hypertension, CHD, cardiac
arrhythmias, acute viral hepatitis, infectious
colitis, bacterial enteritis, digestive disorders,
inflammations in the kidneys and renal pelvis.

Sheng Di, Sheng Di Huang, Radix Rehmannia

(traditionally in the Blood cooling group)

Taste: bitter
Dosage: 6–30 g
Temperature: slightly cold
Channel/Organ action: Heart, Liver, Kidney

The fresh roots are used to treat thirst, exanthemas
and bleeding caused by pathogenic Heat. The dry
root (*Gan Di Huang*) has a similar effect and is also
used as a tonic in *Qi*-deficiency.

New pharmacological research
Blood: lowers blood sugar, stops bleeding and
  increases t-lymphocyte formation.
Heart: strengthens contractility.
Further actions: increases the plasma cAMP peak,
  anti-inflammatory, antibacterial, hepatoprotective (protects the liver from toxic damage), mild
  laxative and diuretic, increases resistance against
  lack of oxygen and alleviates radiation damage in
  the case of exposure to radioactive radiation.

New clinical usage
CHD, angina pectoris, myocarditis, hypertension
apoplexy, diabetes, anaphylactic shock, haemorrhages, hepatitis, neurodermatitis, measles, thickening of the oesophageal epithelium, retinary
phlebitis, acute otitis media, tonsillitis, externally
for all kinds of ulcers, protects from free radicals.

Wa Leng Zi, Concha Arcae

(traditionally also allocated to the Phlegm-
transforming medicinals)

Taste: salty, sweet
Dosage: 9–18 g
Temperature: neutral
Channel/Organ action: Liver, Spleen

Traditionally used in China to invigorate the
Blood, transform Phlegm and treat nodules and
abdominal masses (*Zheng* and *Jia*). Also for
stomach pain with sour regurgitation and chronic
epigastric pain.

New pharmacological research
This type and related bivalve molluscs produce
acetylcholine, active alkaline phosphatase and
other enzymes in the human body. Moreover, they
contain organic calcium amongst other minerals
and trace elements.

Stomach: *Wa Leng Zi* and its heat-processed form
  Duan Wa Leng Zi are used successfully in China
  together with *Gan Cao* (Glycyrrhiza) to treat

gastric and duodenal ulcers. Depending on the study, success rates lie between 86 and 92%.

Further actions: used in late stages of infestations with liver flukes (*Fasciola hepatica*) and other blood sucking parasites related to hepatomegaly or splenomegaly. Both organs regain their original size in 80–93% of studies conducted.

New clinical usage

In gastric and duodenal ulcers, liver and spleen enlargement caused by liver flukes and other parasites.

Yue Ji Hua, Flos Rosae Chinensis

Taste: sweet
Dosage: 6–12 g
Temperature: warm
Channel/Organ action: Liver

Traditionally used in China to invigorate the Blood, regulate the menses and reduce swelling. It is also helpful in Liver *Qi* stagnation of emotional cause, amenorrhoea, abdominal pain and feeling of pressure in the lower abdomen, ulcerative swellings and nodules before ulceration. The Chinese tea rose (*Yue Ji Hua*) is often replaced with the flower buds of the generic rose, although this contains completely different substances.

New pharmacological research
Heart: The essential oils of the tea rose, taken daily as a tea, improve and stabilize CHD and reduce the number of attacks.

New clinical usage
In CHD, liver cirrhosis and all types of menstrual disorders.

GROUP II: 27 BLOOD MOVING MEDICINALS

Medicinals in this group move and invigorate the Blood and eliminate Blood stasis. In comparison to the first group, the herbs of this group have a more concerted and stronger effect on Blood stasis.

Da Huang, Radix et Rhizoma Rhei

(traditionally in the purgative group)

Taste: bitter
Dosage: if cooked together with the decoction 6–12 g; 3–6 g if used as a purgative.
Temperature: slightly cold
Channel/Organ action: Spleen, Stomach, Large Intestine, Liver, Pericardium

It is used to purge, detoxify and cool pathogenic Heat, stagnant digestion and Blood stasis, in the treatment of fever, constipation and feeling of abdominal fullness, acute jaundice, acute appendicitis, amenorrhoea due to Blood stasis, haematemesis and epistaxis due to Heat in the Blood; used externally for burns, suppurative skin diseases, carbuncles and furuncles.

Da Huang is very versatile in modern medicine: it is used in many inflammatory, infectious, ulcerative and haemorrhagic illnesses of the digestive tract and other organs.

New pharmacological research
Digestive system: *Da Huang* (Rheum), briefly cooked, is a laxative due to its sennosides and 20 different, mostly heat-sensitive active ingredients. It increases peristalsis of the whole intestine and water absorption in the large intestine. Furthermore, it raises secretions of gastric acid, peptides, bile, and pancreatic enzymes throughout the digestive system.

Blood: *Da Huang* (Rheum) stops bleeding, lowers blood viscosity and blood lipids and increases microcirculation.

Heart: *Da Huang* (Rheum) increases force of contractions and lowers blood pressure.

Infections/Immune defence: *Da Huang* (Rheum) has anti-inflammatory, antiulcerative antibacterial and antibiotic as well as virostatic properties. Moreover, it inhibits the growth of certain cancer cells and lowers the temperature in fever.

Further actions: liver protective, diuretic and oestrogenic, it has been shown to lengthen the lifespan of laboratory animals by more than a quarter.

New clinical usage
Digestive system: oesophageal bleeding caused by liver cirrhosis, stomach ulcers of bacterial origin, acute stomach bleeding, chronic gastritis, acute pancreatitis, acute bleeding of the common bile

duct, constipation, ileus (blockage of the small or large bowel), toxic gut paralysis, intestinal typhoid, suppurative appendicitis, postoperative acute abdomen, rupture and sepsis of the colon/rectum caused by haemorrhoids.

Further uses: lipidaemia, kidney failure, haemorrhages of the urinary bladder and other organs, infectious haemorrhagic fever, suppurative tonsillitis, parotitis, chronic prostatitis, insecticide poisoning, amenorrhoea, cervical tumours and many more.

Chuan Xiong, Radix Ligustici Wallachii

Taste: pungent
Dosage: 6–12–15 g
Temperature: warm
Channel/Organ action: Liver, Gall-bladder, Pericardium

1. *Chuan Xiong*: Strengthens Blood circulation and promotes the flow of *Qi* in the treatment of abnormal menstruation, dysmenorrhoea, amenorrhoea.
2. Has analgesic action in the treatment of headaches and pain in the whole body due to Wind or Cold as well as headache due to concussion and pain after birth.
3. Has a drying effect in the treatment of pathogenic Dampness.

New pharmacological research
Heart: *Chuan Xiong* dilates peripheral and coronary vessels, lowers blood pressure and vessel resistance, increases the amount of blood in the heart and increases tolerance towards hypoxia, thereby unburdening the heart.
Blood: The medicinal increases microcirculation in general and blood circulation of the kidneys and the brain; it lowers the incidence of brain oedema, and prevents thrombocyte aggregation and thrombus formation.
Further actions: *Chuan Xiong* has antispasmodic action on the smooth musculature, calming action on the nervous system; moreover, it is antibacterial, and helps with radiation damage and lack of vitamin E.

New clinical usage
CHD, cardiac insufficiency, cardiac arrhythmia, angina pectoris, sudden cardiac arrest, cor pulmonale, cerebral ischemia, brain oedema, kidney failure, disseminated intravascular coagulation (DIC), thrombophlebitis, allergic shock (Arthus reaction), asthma, diabetes, stomach ulcers, dysmenorrhoea and psoriasis.

Chuan Shan Jia, Squama Manitis

Taste: salty, pungent
Dosage: 3–9 g
Temperature: slightly cold
Channel/Organ action: Liver, Stomach

Traditionally used in China:

1. as an emmenagogue and galactagogue, for the treatment of amenorrhoea, insufficient lactation and dysmenorrhoea;
2. for rheumatic *Bi*-syndrome caused by Wind and Dampness, to reduce inflammation and to dissolve pus in acute suppurative ulcers.

New pharmacological research
Blood: *Chuan Shan Jia* lowers blood viscosity and antagonizes blood clotting. It increases microcirculation and lowers blood vessel resistance.
Heart: it increases the blood flow and contraction force of the heart muscle and lowers oxygen consumption.
Further actions: *Chuan Shan Jia* is anti-inflammatory.

New clinical usage
Furuncles and other chronic ulcers that take a long time to heal, appendicitis, bladder stones, insufficient lactation.

Gui Jian Yu, Euonymus Alatus (Thunberg)

Dosage: 6–12 g

Traditionally used in women's disorders like Blood stasis with menstrual disorders, heavy lochia or metrorrhagia and pain after birth, as well as abdominal masses and heart pain.

New pharmacological research
Blood: it lowers blood viscosity as had been shown by the lowering of the shear rate, increases plasticity of erythrocytes, increases blood clotting time and flow speed in the capillaries, antago-

nizes thrombus formation (in vitro harvested thrombi were heavier and longer than normal) and also markedly lowers blood lipids.

Heart: *Gui Jian Yu* increases ejection fraction of the heart, lowers oxygen consumption and increases tolerance towards hypoxia and the contraction force.

Further actions: it increases tissue tolerance of ischemia and has a calming effect on the CNS.

New clinical usage

CHD, cardiac insufficiency, cardiac arrhythmias, angina pectoris, cor pulmonale as well as bleeding and pain after birth.

Hong Hua, Flos Carthami

Taste: pungent
Dosage: 9–15 g
Temperature: warm
Channel/Organ action: Liver, Heart

Traditionally used in China to improve Blood flow and relieve pain caused by Blood stasis, in the case of amenorrhoea, pains in chest and abdomen, painful swelling, hepatomegaly and splenomegaly; in addition it is used to treat pain due to traumatic wounds.

New pharmacological research

Heart: *Hong Hua* lowers blood pressure and blood lipids and increases contraction force of the heart muscle.

Blood: it has antithrombotic action, promotes the maturation of t- and b-lymphocytes and raises interleukin-2 production.

Further actions: anti-inflammatory, calming and analgetic.

New clinical usage

CHD, angina pectoris, arrhythmias (especially early systoles), ischemic and thrombotic apoplexies, arteriosclerosis of the cerebral arteries, thrombophlebitis, deafness after sudden sensorineural hearing loss, nasal polyps, menstruation disorders, traumata, haemorrhagic fever, short-sightedness in young people, duodenal ulcers and neurodermatitis, psoriasis, flat warts, solar dermatitis, erythema multiforme, lupus erythematosus and other skin diseases.

Similar medicinal in use: Fan Hong Hua, Zang Hong Hua, *Saffron, Stigma Krokus*

This medicinal consists of the dried stigmata of the saffron crocus, Crocus sativa (plant family iridaceae). It is traditionally used in China like *Hong Hua* (Carthamus) (see above), although the former has a stronger Blood invigorating action. Due to its high price it is rarely used.

Hu Zhang, Herba Polygonum Cuspidati

Taste: slightly bitter
Dosage: 9–18 g
Temperature: slightly cold
Channel/Organ action: Liver, Gallbladder, Lung

Traditionally used against Wind and Dampness pathogens, Blood stasis and pain with rheumatic *Bi*-syndrome, jaundice due to Heat-Damp, amenorrhoea, abdominal masses; also used against cough with Phlegm and traumata, especially burns.

New pharmacological research

Blood: *Hu Zhang* lowers blood pressure, blood sugar and blood lipids. Moreover, it improves microcirculation and raises the number of leukocytes and thrombocytes and decreases thrombocyte aggregation.

Further actions: antibacterial, virostatic, antitussive, antioxidative as well as useful against tumour formation and hook worms. It has a relaxing effect on the smooth musculature of the digestive tract, has a cholagogue action and is liver protective.

New clinical usage

Infantile pneumonia, acute viral hepatitis, jaundice in the newborn, hyperlipidaemia, leukopenia, haemorrhages of the digestive tract, cervical erosion, colpomycosis, toothache, stab wounds and burns.

Jiang Huang, Rhizoma Curcumae Longae

Taste: pungent, bitter
Dosage: 6–12 g
Temperature: warm
Channel/Organ action: Liver, Stomach

Traditionally used in China to relieve pain by regulating *Qi*-circulation as well as for pain in the chest area and abdomen, and dysmenorrhoea caused by *Qi*- and Blood stasis; also used for traumata and abdominal masses.

New pharmacological research

Blood: *Jiang Huang* lowers blood lipids and blood pressure, and is effective against arteriosclerosis and thrombocyte aggregation.

Further actions: liver protective, anti-inflammatory, antibacterial, virostatic, anticancer, abortive, contraceptive, antioxidative and captures free radicals.

New clinical usage

Dysmenorrhoea, chest pain, hyperlipidaemia, angina pectoris, inflammations (especially tooth or gum inflammations), applied externally for herpes zoster and herpes simplex infections (with curcuma tincture 30%).

Liu Ji Nu, Herba Siphonosteglae

Taste: pungent, bitter
Dosage: 6–12 g
Temperature: warm
Channel/Organ action: Urinary Bladder, Heart, Spleen

Traditionally used in China to relieve pain and remove stagnated Blood as well as for the treatment of abdominal pain due to Blood stasis and with painful swelling due to injury.

New pharmacological research

Lie Ji Nu increases tolerance of hypoxia and microcirculation and is antiseptic.

New clinical usage

Amenorrhoea, pain after birth, food stagnation with flatulence and pain, ulcerative colitis, old age anuria, abdominal and other traumata, burns.

Lu Lu Tong, Fructus Liquidambaris

(traditionally in the group of stopping bleeding medicinals)

Taste: bitter
Dosage: 6–12 g
Temperature: neutral
Channel/Organ action: Liver, Stomach

Traditionally used in China to stop bleeding and move Blood and *Qi*, remove obstructions from the vessels and relieve pain. It is mostly used in gynaecology, in Wind-Damp *Bi*-syndrome of the lower limbs and difficult urination with oedema.

New pharmacological research

Lu Lu Tong has antiallergenic action and used externally it has antiparasitic action.

Ma Bian Cao, Herba Verbenae

(traditionally in the antiparasitic group)

Taste: bitter
Dosage: 6–18 g
Temperature: cool
Channel/Organ action: Liver, Large Intestine

Traditionally used in China:

1. in the case of Blood stasis, to promote menstruation in amenorrhoea or dysmenorrhoea and in abdominal masses;
2. to treat malaria, and for the treatment of splenomegaly due to malaria; also for oedema;
3. as an antiparasite drug and to detoxify in conditions such as influenza and diphtheria.

New pharmacological research

Ma Bian Cao is effective against amoebas and other foreign microorganisms in the gut; it counteracts inflammation and pain, promotes blood clotting, stops cough and promotes lactation.

New clinical usage

Malaria, amoebic dysentery, bloody diarrhoea, schistosomiasis, filariasis and other worms, ulcerative colitis, infectious hepatitis, diphtheria, influenza, vaginal infections and acute and chronic pelvic inflammatory disease, oral and dental inflammations.

Mao Dong Qing, Radix Ilex Pubescens

Taste: pungent, bitter
Dosage: 24–60 g
Temperature: slightly cold
Channel/Organ action: Heart, Lung

Traditionally used in China:

1. to invigorate the Blood and remove obstructions from the channels and collaterals (*Luo*-vessels), in the treatment of Buerger's disease (presenile spontaneous gangrene), angina pectoris;
2. to lower fever, detoxify and as an anti-inflammatory in acute tonsillitis;
3. to stop coughing and promote expectoration in the case of acute bronchitis;
4. externally in burns and scalds.

New pharmacological research
Heart: *Mao Dong Qing* dilates the coronary arteries and increases the amount of blood flow to the heart.
Blood: prevents clotting.
Further actions: lowers blood pressure in the cerebral arteries, has anti-inflammatory and antibacterial action.

New clinical usage
CHD, ischemic apoplexy, thrombophlebitis of superficial veins, retinal changes, prostatitis, atrophic rhinitis, allergic rhinitis, haemorrhaging fever, wound infections, leprotic leg ulcers, aphthae.

Mo Yao, Myrrh, Resina Myrrhae

Taste: bitter
Dosage: 3–12 g
Temperature: neutral
Channel/Organ action: Liver

Traditionally used in China to alleviate pain caused by Blood stasis, for example all kinds of trauma-induced pain. *Mo Yao* (Myrrha) has a strong eliminating, Blood invigorating and Blood stasis dispersing action; furthermore, it reduces swelling.

New pharmacological research
Heart: *Mo Yao* increases the force of heart contractions and tolerance towards hypoxia.
Blood: lowers blood cholesterol levels.
Further actions: stimulates the respiratory centre and has an antimycotic action.

New clinical usage
Heart pain, high cholesterol levels, spinal and mammary tuberculosis, menstrual disorders, haemorrhages, ulcers and traumas.

Niu Xi, Huai Niu Xi, Radix Achyranthis Bidentatae

Taste: bitter, salty
Dosage: 9–18 g
Temperature: neutral
Channel/Organ action: Liver, Stomach

Traditionally used in China to improve Blood circulation and eliminate Blood stasis. It was also employed for illnesses or fractures of the joints, in amenorrhoea and haematuria.

New pharmacological research
Blood: *Niu Xi* has a dilating effect and lowers blood pressure.
Further actions: it promotes protein synthesis (wound healing) and has diuretic, anti-inflammatory, analgetic, antibacterial and abortive actions, and induces delivery by dilating the cervical canal.

New clinical usage
Epistaxis, infantile pneumonia, pain whilst urinating, toothache, functional uterine bleeding and chyluria (galactosuria).

Pu Huang, Pollen Typhae

(traditionally in the group of medicinals to stop bleeding)

Taste: sweet
Dosage: 6–12 g
Temperature: neutral
Channel/Organ action: Liver, Pericardium

Traditionally used in China to invigorate the Blood, stop bleeding, cool Blood and alleviate pain by eliminating Blood stasis. It was also used in the treatment of dysmenorrhoea, post partum abdominal pain and gastralgia. The charred medicinal is used as a haemostatic for all kinds of bleeding.

New pharmacological research
Heart: *Pu Huang* improves cardiac capacity and tolerance towards hypoxia and it protects the heart from the damaging effect of ischemia.
Blood: it lowers blood lipids (including cholesterol) and blood viscosity; it protects the endothelial cells of the blood vessels and regulates blood clotting; it lowers thrombocyte aggregation and has fibrinolytic action but it increases clotting speed and microcirculation; prevents arteriosclerosis.
Further actions: it regulates immune function in both directions, excites uterine musculature, relaxes bronchial vessels and increases intestinal peristalsis.

New clinical usage
CHD, hyperlipidaemia, ulcerative colitis, all kinds of haemorrhages, weeping eczema, to induce birth, leukorrhoea, insufficient post partum uterine involution, all kinds of menstrual disorders.

Qi Cao, Holotrichia Diomphalia

Taste: salty
Dosage: 0.5–2.0 g
Temperature: slightly warm
Channel/Organ action: Liver, Spleen

Traditionally used in the case of Blood stasis with *Qi* stagnation and pain, in amenorrhoea, epistaxis, feeling of fullness and oppression in the chest, fractures, insufficient lactation after delivery, herpes zoster, eye inflammations and mouth ulcers.

New pharmacological research
N/A

New clinical usage
Hepatitis B, tetanus, mycotic stomatitis.

Ru Xiang, Olibanum, Resina Olibani

Taste: pungent, bitter
Dosage: 3–12 g
Temperature: warm
Channel/Organ action: Heart, Liver, Spleen

Traditionally used in China to alleviate pain and reduce swelling. *Ru Xiang* is moistening and moves the *Qi* of the Blood, relaxes the sinews and invigorates the *Luo*-vessels. It is indicated for the treatment of pain due to Blood stasis, e.g. traumatic pain etc.

New pharmacological research
Blood: *Ru Xiang* (Olibanum) raises blood clotting speed but lowers thrombocyte aggregation; it also increases erythrocyte plasticity.
Further actions: it has anti-inflammatory and anti-bacterial action.

New clinical usage
Heart pain, intractable hiccups, appendicitis, traumas and rheumatic *Bi*-syndrome (arthritic diseases).

Rui Xiang, Flores/Folia Daphnae

Taste: pungent, sweet, salty
Dosage: 3–6 g
Temperature: warm
Channel/Organ action: Heart, Liver

Traditionally used in the treatment of all kinds of traumas and pain. It dispels pathogenic Wind and Dampness, alleviates pain and invigorates the Blood. Not to be confused with *Ru Xiang* (Olibanum), see above.

New pharmacological research
Rui Xiang protects the heart from the damaging effects of ischemia; it has a calming, anti-inflammatory, antithrombotic, antibacterial and a locally anaesthetic action; furthermore it inhibits intestinal peristalsis.

New clinical usage
CHD, severe pain, arthralgia, thrombophlebitis and as a local anaesthetic.

San Qi, Tian Qi, Radix Notoginseng, Radix Pseudoginseng (traditionally in the group of medicinals for stopping bleeding)

Taste: sweet, slightly bitter
Dosage: 1.5–9.0 g
Temperature: warm
Channel/Organ action: Liver, stomach

Is used as a styptic drug and painkiller, for the elimination of Blood stasis and to reduce swelling in the treatment of swelling and pain due to sprains, wounds and soft tissue injuries as well as all kinds of bleeding.

San Qi is a regulating medicinal, that can affect blood clotting, immunity and blood sugar levels in both directions.

New pharmacological research
Blood: San Qi (Notoginseng) promotes blood clotting and clotting speed as well as local vasoconstriction in the case of traumas. If no clotting is necessary, it counteracts thrombocyte aggregation, lowers fibrin and increases fibrinolysis time. In addition, it lowers blood lipid levels, increases erythrocyte and leukocyte count in the peripheral vessels, dilates peripheral blood vessels and thus lowers blood pressure.
Heart: San Qi (Notoginseng) increases heart muscle contractions, blood volume, oxygen saturation and microcirculation of the cardiac muscles; at the same time it lowers oxygen consumption and pulse rate and has an antiarrhythmic action.
Metabolism/Immune system: San Qi (Notoginseng) increases or decreases blood sugar levels and promotes DNA synthesis as well as protein synthesis of the kidneys and testes. It raises activity of natural killer (NK) lymphocytes and macrophages; concerning the latter functions, it also has an immune modulating effect in both directions.
Further actions: it protects brain cells from the damaging effects of ischemia and liver cells from toxic substances. It stimulates the smooth musculature of the uterus and protects the body from the effects of shock, radiation and cancer. Furthermore, it is virostatic, antimycotic, calming, analgetic and significantly increased the lifespan of laboratory animals.

New clinical usage
Angina pectoris, CHD, cardiac arrhythmias, hyperlipidaemia, hypertension, all kinds of apoplexies and cranial bleeding, internal and external traumas, all kinds of haemorrhaging, cancer, hepatitis, liver cirrhosis, acute nephritis, skin diseases and migraine.

Su Mu, Lignum Sappan

Taste: pungent
Dosage: 6–12 g
Temperature: neutral
Channel/Organ action: Liver

Traditionally used in China to alleviate pain and invigorate Blood; its main action is the treatment of bruises and other traumas, and of dysmenorrhoea and amenorrhoea accompanied by abdominal pain.

New pharmacological research
Heart/Blood: Su Mu increases the force of heart contractions, constricts the vessels and promotes blood clotting.
Further actions: Su Mu (Sappan) has a calming, antimycotic, and anti-inflammatory action. Moreover it is anticarcinogenic, used especially in the treatment of leukaemia.

New clinical usage
Tetanus, asthma, traumas, vitiligo.

Wang Bu Liu Xing, Semen Vaccariae

Taste: bitter
Dosage: 6–12 g
Temperature: neutral
Channel/Organ action: Liver, Stomach

Traditionally used as an emmenagogue and galactagogue in the treatment of menstrual disorders like amenorrhoea and insufficient lactation after birth. The raw seeds are used on ear acupuncture points instead of ear needles in acupressure; this makes the minor skin injuries of acupuncture unnecessary.

New pharmacological research
Wang Bu Liu Xing (Vaccaria) has a stimulating effect on the uterine musculature it also has

contraceptive action, lowers blood pressure, is analgetic and prevents tumour formation.

New clinical usage
Hypertension, rheumatic *Bi*-syndrome, herpes zoster, cough, insomnia, haemorrhoids, dysuria, intercostal neuralgia, dysmenorrhoea, amenorrhoea, promotes labour in the case of difficult delivery, acute mastitis and insufficient lactation after delivery.

The seeds are used in ear acupuncture in the treatment of juvenile short-sightedness.

Wu Ling Zhi, Faeces Trogopterori

Taste: sweet
Dosage: 6–12 g
Temperature: warm
Channel/Organ action: Liver

Traditionally used in China to alleviate pain and remove Blood stasis and *Qi*-stagnation, due to its function of moving *Qi*; it is mainly used in the treatment of gastric and abdominal pain due to smooth muscle cramps, and in dysmenorrhoea.

New pharmacological research
Blood: *Wu Ling Zhi* lowers blood viscosity and elevates an erythrocyte sedimentation rate that is too slow. It prevents thrombocyte aggregation and increases microcirculation.
Heart: it lowers oxygen consumption of the heart.
Further actions: it has a strong analgetic action and immune modulating (balancing) effect on the immune system. Moreover, *Wu Ling Zhi* (Trogopterus) has an antibacterial effect on a large amount of skin bacteria as well as tuberculosis bacteria.

New clinical usage
All acute states of pain (toothache, headache, sore limbs and so on), angina pectoris, snake bites, duodenal and gastric ulcers, chronic bronchitis, delayed uterine involution after delivery.

Yi Mu Cao, Kun Cao, Herba Leonuri

Taste: pungent, bitter
Dosage: 12–24–60 g
Temperature: slightly cold
Channel/Organ action: Pericardium, Liver

Traditionally used in China to strengthen circulation and to regulate the menstrual cycle, in abnormal menses or menstrual pain; it is also used as a diuretic in nephritic syndrome (oedema).

New pharmacological research
Heart: *Yi Mu Cao* increases circulation and microcirculation of the heart; it has a protective effect on cardiac muscle cells and lowers blood pressure.
Blood: it lowers blood viscosity, reduces clotting and thrombocyte aggregation, and by some other means prevents thrombus formation. It also inhibits agglomeration of antibodies among each other.
Further actions: it has contraceptive and anti-arteriosclerotic actions.

New clinical usage
CHD, angina pectoris, cor pulmonale, ischemic apoplexy, hypertension, menstrual disorders, incomplete uterine involution, acute nephritic syndrome, chronic glomerular nephritis, ascites due to liver cirrhosis, diabetes, prostatitis and urinary stones.

Yin Xing Ye, *Ginkgo leaves*, *Folia Ginkgo*

Taste: bitter, sweet, astringent
Dosage: 3–9 g
Temperature: neutral
Channel/Organ action: Lung, Heart

Traditionally used to treat pain and Blood stasis, but also cough, chest pain and shortness of breath.

New pharmacological research
Heart/blood: lowers the pulse rate, blood pressure, reduces plasma cholesterol and dilates the blood vessels.
Further actions: has a spasmolytic effect on the bronchi and smooth muscles, increases respiratory frequency.

New clinical usage
CHD, angina pectoris, high cholesterol levels, chronic bronchitis, Parkinson's disease, senile dementia.

Yu Jin, Radix Curcumae

Taste: pungent, bitter
Dosage: 6–12 g
Temperature: cold
Channel/Organ action: Heart, Liver, Lung

Traditionally used in China:

1. to alleviate pain and regulate stagnated *Qi*; treats chest pain, abdominal or pain in the hypochondrium due to *Qi*-stagnation and Blood stasis as well as pain in the liver area due to liver inflammation;
2. as a cholagogue in the treatment of jaundice due to liver disease.

New pharmacological research
Yu Jin raises cAMP levels in organ tissue and inhibits lymphocyte maturation. It has an anti-arteriosclerotic and antimycotic effect, protects from toxic liver damage and has an anti-arrhythmic action on the heart.

New clinical usage
Epilepsy, epistaxis, hepatitis due to cholecystopathy, heart pain, haematuria, hyperhidrosis and psoriasis.

Yuan Hu, Yan Hu Suo, Rhizoma Corydalis

Taste: pungent, bitter
Dosage: 4.5–12.0 g
Temperature: warm
Channel/Organ action: Heart, Liver, Spleen

Traditionally used in China to alleviate pain by invigorating the circulation of Blood and to regulate the circulation of *Qi*. It is frequently administered in the treatment of all kinds of pain in the chest and abdomen. Furthermore, this medicinal can raise the pain threshold and alleviate spastic pain; it also has a calming action.

New pharmacological research
Heart: *Yuan Hu* protects the heart from ischemic damage, lowers blood pressure and is anti-arrhythmic.
Blood: it lowers blood lipid levels, has an anti-arteriosclerotic action and improves circulation.

Further actions: it has a strong analgetic and locally anaesthetic effect, increases intestinal peristalsis and adrenal cortex secretion, it has an anti-ulcerative effect by reducing gastric secretions.

New clinical usage
Pain and neuralgias of all kind, insomnia, hypertension, CHD, cardiac arrhythmias, angina pectoris, myocardial infarction, gastritis, gastric and duodenal ulcers, acute pancreatitis, acute lower back pain and dysmenorrhoea; also used as a local anaesthetic.

Ze Lan, Herba Lycopi

Taste: pungent, bitter
Dosage: 6–12 g
Temperature: slightly warm
Channel/Organ action: Liver, Spleen

Traditionally used in China to strengthen circulation and to regulate the menstrual cycle, as well as for the treatment of abnormal menstruation and abdominal pain after delivery.

New pharmacological research
Ze Lan (Lycopus) inhibits clotting, fibrinogen and thrombocyte aggregation. It also increases plasticity of erythrocytes.

New clinical usage
CHD, cor pulmonale, lung emphysema, chronic bronchitis, jaundice due to liver disease, parotitis, haemorrhoids, postpartum pain, mastitis, female infertility.

Zi Ran Tong, Pyritum

Taste: pungent
Dosage: decoctions 3–15 g; powder 0.3–0.9 g
Temperature: neutral
Channel/Organ action: Liver

Traditionally used in China to treat fractures or to alleviate pain by dispelling stagnated Blood; also used for the treatment of traumatic injuries or fractures and pain due to Blood stasis.

New pharmacological research
N/A

New clinical usage
N/A

GROUP III: 9 MEDICINALS TO BREAK BLOOD STASIS

Medicinals in this group break and dissolve Blood stasis and attack hardenings due to Blood stasis. They have the most vigorous action.

E Zhu, Rhizoma Curcumae Ezhu, (previously known as Curcumae Zedoriae)

Taste: pungent, bitter
Dosage: 6–12 g
Temperature: warm
Channel/Organ action: Liver, Spleen

Traditionally used in China to alleviate pain and strengthen circulation, and for the treatment of pain in the chest and abdomen, abdominal masses, amenorrhoea etc. It is administered in serious cases of *Qi*-stagnation and Blood stasis as well as for combating cancer, especially cervical cancer.

New pharmacological research
Blood: *E Zhu* reduces thrombocyte agglutination time, lowers blood viscosity, improves microcirculation and increases glutamate pyruvate transaminase (GPT).
Cancer: *E Zhu* directly affects the DNA and RNA and prevents the formation of different types of cancer cells (sarcoma, lymphoma and others).
Infections: *E Zhu* has an antibacterial effect on a wide range of bacteria, virucidal effect on the respiratory syncytial (RS) virus and stops gastric inflammations and ulcerations.
Further actions: *E Zhu* has a contraceptive effect, increases the amount of blood flow through the femoral artery and stimulates gastric and intestinal smooth muscles.

New clinical usage
Cancer (especially cervical tumours), CHD, tonsillitis and pneumonia in children, consequences of high blood lipids, stomach ulcers, skin ulcers and neurodermatitis.

Gan Qi, Lacca Sinica Exsiccatae

Taste: pungent, bitter
Dosage: 0.05–0.10 g
Temperature: warm
Channel/Organ action: Stomach, Large Intestine, Small Intestine

Gan Qi is dried lacquer, which is extracted from the resin of Toxicodendron vernicifluum (Lacquer tree). Although it was mentioned in the *Shen Nong Ben Cao Jing* (Divine Husbandman's Materia Medica), it is rarely used nowadays. It treats Blood stasis, hip pain, cough, sensation of pressure and masses in the abdomen as well as ascariasis.

New pharmacological research
Gan Qi has a spasmolytic effect on smooth intestinal muscles, bronchi and uterus. It strengthens the contractile force of the cardiac muscles, constricts peripheral vessels and thus raises blood pressure.

New clinical usage
Worm infestations in children, abdominal pain, amenorrhoea and menstrual disorders.

Mang Chong, Meng Chong, Tabanus

Taste: bitter
Dosage: 1–3 g
Temperature: slightly cold
Channel/Organ action: Liver

Traditionally used to remove stagnated Blood and dispel swelling, so used in the treatment of serious cases of Blood stasis with pain as well as amenorrhoea and abdominal masses. *Meng Chong* is not in common use.

New pharmacological research
It dilates the blood vessels, increases tolerance towards hypoxia and activates the fibrinolytic system.

New clinical usage
Angina pectoris, cervical tumours, chronic hepatitis, bleeding internal haemorrhoids.

San Leng, Rhizoma Sparganii

Taste: bitter
Dosage: 6–12 g
Temperature: neutral
Channel/Organ action: Liver, Spleen

Traditionally used in China to remove stagnated Blood and for the treatment of pain and feeling of oppression of the chest, stagnated digestion with pain, abdominal masses, dysmenorrhoea and amenorrhoea.

New pharmacological research
Blood: *San Leng* prolongs clotting time, lowers blood viscosity, reduces thrombocyte aggregation and reduces time and gravity of a thrombus in vitro; it also increases blood flow and absorption rate of blood clots in the abdomen.
Further actions: in vitro, it stimulates and increases the contractile force of the smooth musculature of the uterus, dilates the vessels and is antineoplastic.

New clinical usage
Post-apoplexy hemiplegia, CHD, chronic pelvic inflammatory disease, extrauterine pregnancy, cervical tumours, renal stones.

Shui Zhi, Hirudo

Taste: pungent, salty
Dosage: 1.5–5.0 g
Temperature: neutral
Channel/Organ action: Liver

Traditionally used in China to remove stagnated Blood and to dispel swelling in pronounced cases of Blood stasis such as abdominal pain, amenorrhoea and masses in the abdomen, traumas, bruising etc.

New pharmacological research
Shui Zhi prevents thrombocyte aggregation, lowers blood lipids and lowers blood viscosity, thrombus absorption and flow speed.
Heart: it increases the Rb-86 assimilation of the heart muscle as well as blood volume and the entire microcirculation.

Further actions: it has an abortive effect in pregnancy.

New clinical usage
Ischemic and haemorrhagic apoplexies, cerebral thrombosis, angina pectoris, CHD, cor pulmonale, hyperlipidaemia, thrombophlebitis, liver cirrhosis, polycythaemia vera, eye diseases and oedema due to kidney function disorders.

Si Gua Lou, Fasiculus Vascularis Luffa

Taste: sweet
Dosage: 6–18 g
Temperature: neutral
Channel/Organ action: Lung, Stomach, Liver

This medicinal has only a mild Blood invigorating action; yet it is able to remove obstructions from the vessels.
Traditionally used in China:

1. to eliminate Wind- or Damp-*Bi* from the muscles and joints; to remove Blood stasis due to injury or hypochondriac pain;
2. in the treatment of breast abscesses;
3. in the case of viscous Phlegm in the Lung and cough with fever and chest pain due to Heat;
4. as a diuretic in cases of Summer Heat with fever and concentrated dark urine.

New pharmacological research
According to new (1998) research, Luffa stops coughing, has an antiasthmatic action and resolves Phlegm in the respiratory tract; it also has an anti-inflammatory action, alleviates pain, calms, and has antibacterial actions throughout the body. The antibacterial characteristics have already been established for *Staphylococcus aureus*, b-streptococci and other types of cocci, but especially for pneumococci.

New clinical usage
In the past as well as today, *Si Gua Lou* was administered for acute mastitis and in formulas for bronchial asthma. New applications are: treatment of herpes zoster as well as being the main ingredient in formulas for penile induration, chronic nephritis, anal fissures, epilepsy, thyroid nodules and uterine prolapse.

Tao Ren, Semen Persicae

Taste: bitter, sweet
Dosage: 6–9 g
Temperature: neutral
Channel/Organ action: Heart, Liver, Large Intestine

Traditionally used in China to:

1. remove Blood stasis in the treatment of amenorrhoea with abdominal pain, traumatic pain due to Blood stasis, pain in the hypochondrium area, as well as abdominal masses or pain;
2. treat constipation in the elderly or weak, or those with Blood deficiency syndrome.

New pharmacological research
Blood: *Tao Ren* increases blood flow in cerebral and peripheral vessels, is antithrombotic and prevents clotting by raising cAMP levels and lowering adenosine diphosphate (ADP) levels in thrombocytes.
Further actions: antitussive, antiphlogistic, antiallergic, antibacterial, analgetic, spasmolytic, counteracts fever, antioxidative; it promotes stool but can also treat diarrhoea by promoting diuresis; it stimulates the smooth muscles of the uterus; it is liver-protective; delays the aging process in vitro.

New clinical usage
Hepatitis, liver cirrhosis, CHD, cough, diabetes, skin diseases, trauma, menstrual pain, eye inflammations, chronic laryngitis and loss of voice, tonsillitis, epidemic haemorrhagic fever, acute kidney failure, chronic glomerulonephritis and pyelonephritis, gestational hypertension.

Tu Bie Chong, Zhe Chong, Bie Chong, Eupolyphaga

Taste: bitter
Dosage: 3–12 g
Temperature: slightly cold
Channel/Organ action: Liver

Traditionally used in China to alleviate pain due to Blood stasis as well as in the treatment of hepatomegaly and splenomegaly, lumbago and sprains. it is also used in the treatment of amenorrhoea, abdominal masses, contusions etc.

New pharmacological research
Blood: *Tu Bie Chong* inhibits blood clotting in different ways, and lowers blood lipids.
Heart: it improves heart function and increases tolerance of hypoxia.
Further actions: it has hepatoprotective action, absorbs free radicals and antagonizes cell mutations.

New clinical usage
CHD, tuberculosis of the lung and bone, fractures, hypertension, chest pain following overexertion, acute lower back pain and sciatica, external haemorrhoids, melanoma, nasal cancer, chronic hepatitis and sequelae of concussion.

Xue Jie, Sanguis Draconis

Taste: sweet, salty
Dosage: 0.5–2.0 g pulverized
Temperature: neutral
Channel/Organ action: Pericardium, Liver

It is used to remove Blood stasis, to alleviate pain and to promote wound healing in the treatment of trauma, wounds and bleeding.

New pharmacological research
Blood: *Xue Jie* lowers blood viscosity and thrombocyte aggregation.
Further actions: it has analgetic, anti-inflammatory, antibacterial and antimycotic action, increases plasma cAMP levels and lowers the plasma cGMP value, and increases the amount of blood in the coronary vessels.

New clinical usage
Internal and external bleeding (including cerebral and intestinal bleeding), traumas, chronic ulcers, coughing of blood, heavy menstrual bleeding, CHD, and angina pectoris.

PART 2. TABLES AND BOXES ON BLOOD INVIGORATING CHINESE MEDICINALS

The Tables and Boxes in Part 2 summarize and compare classical medicinals for removing Blood stasis.

Table 7.1   Classification of the medicinals according to their Blood invigorating group

Latin name	Chinese name	Group
Achyranthis Bidentatae, Radix	Niu Xi, Huai Niu Xi	(Group 2: Blood moving)
Artemisia Annua, Herba	Liu Ji Nu	(Group 2: Blood moving)
Angelicae Sinensis, Radix	Dang Gui	(Group 1: Blood harmonizing)
Carthamus, Flos	Hong Hua	(Group 2: Blood moving)
Corydalis, Rhizoma	Yuan Hu; Yan Hu Suo	(Group 2: Blood moving)
Crategus, Fructus	Shan Zha	(Group 1: Blood harmonizing)
Curcumae Longae, Rhizoma	Jiang Huang	(Group 2: Blood moving)
Curcumae, Radix	Yu Jin	(Group 2: Blood moving)
Curcumae Ezhu, Rhizoma	E Zhu	(Group 3: Blood stasis breaking)
Daphnae, Curcumae Ezhu Alatus	Gui Jian Yu	(Group 2: Blood moving)
Eupolyphaga	Tu Bie Chong, Zhe Chong, Bie Chong	(Group 3: Blood stasis breaking)
Ginkgo, Folia; ginkgo leaves	Yin Xing Ye	(Group 2: Blood moving)
Hirudo	Shui Zhi	(Group 3: Blood stasis breaking)
Holotrichia Diomphalia	Qi Cao	(Group 2: Blood moving)
Ilex Pubescens, Radix	Mao Dong Qing	(Group 2: Blood moving)
Lacca Sinica Exsiccatae	Gan Qi	(Group 3: Blood stasis breaking)
Leonuri, Herba	Yi Mu Cao; Kun Cao	(Group 2: Blood moving)
Ligustici Wallichii, Radix	Chuan Xiong	(Group 2: Blood moving)
Liquidambaris, Fructus	Lu Lu Tong	(Group 2: Blood moving)
Luffa, Fasiculus Vascularis	Si Gua Luo	(Group 3: mildly Blood stasis breaking)
Lycopus, Herba	Ze Lan	(Group 2: Blood moving)
Manitis, Squama	Chuan Shan Jia	(Group 2: Blood moving)
Moutan Radicis, Cortex	Mu Dan Pi, Dan Pi	(Group 1: Blood harmonizing)
Myrrhe; Resina Myrrhae	Mo Yao	(Group 2: Blood moving)
Notoginseng, Radix; Pseudoginseng, Radix	San Qi, Tian Qi	(Group 2: Blood moving)
Olibanum, Resina Olibani	Ru Xiang	(Group 2: Blood moving)
Paeoniae Rubrae, Radix	Chi Shao Yao	(Group 1: Blood harmonizing)
Persicae, Semen	Tao Ren	(Group 3: Blood stasis breaking)
Polygonum Cuspidati, Herba	Hu Zhang	(Group 2: Blood moving)
Pyritum	Zi Ran Tong	(Group 2: Blood moving)
Rehmanniae, Radix	Sheng Di; Sheng Di Huang	(Group 1: Blood harmonizing)
Rheum Palmatum, Radix et Rhizoma	Da Huang	(Group 2: Blood moving)
Saffron; Stigma Krokus	Fan Hong Hua, Zang Hong Hua	(Group 2: Blood moving)
Salviae Miltiorrhizae, Radix	Dan Shen	(Group 1: Blood harmonizing)
Sanguis Draconis	Xue Jie	(Group 3: Blood stasis breaking)
Sappan, Lignum	Su Mu	(Group 2: Blood moving)
Siphonosteglae, Herba, see Artemisia Annua Sparganii, Rhizoma	San Leng	(Group 3: Blood stasis breaking)
Spatholobi, Caulis	Ji Xue Teng	(Group 1: Blood harmonizing)
Tabanus	Meng Chong, Mang Chong	(Group 3: Blood stasis breaking)
Trogopterori, Faeces	Wu Ling Zhi	(Group 2: Blood moving)
Typhae, Pollen	Pu Huang	(Group 2: Blood moving)
Vaccariae, Semen	Wang Bu Liu Xing	(Group 2: Blood moving)
Verbenae, Herba	Ma Bian Cao	(Group 2: Blood moving)

Table 7.2 The pharmacological effects of Blood invigorating medicinals

Name of medicinal	Heart: increases amount of blood flow through coronary arteries	Blood vessels: vasodilating effect	Blood vessels: lowers blood pressure	Blood vessels: improves microcirculation	Blood: inhibits thrombocyte aggregation and thrombosis	Blood: lowers blood lipids	Gynaecology: uterus muscle	Gynaecology: other	Immune system: antiphlogistic or anti-ulcerative	Immune system: inhibits cancer growth	Nervous system: calming	Nervous system: alleviates pain	Other effects
Bie Chong					yes	yes							
Chi Shao (Paeonia rubra)	yes	yes		yes	yes		relaxes[a]		yes/yes		yes		increases heart capacity; relaxes smooth muscles of stomach and intestines
Chuan Shan Jia (Squama Manitis)	yes	yes		yes	yes								lowers heart oxygen consumption and blood viscosity
Chuan Xiong (Ligusticum)	yes	yes		yes	yes								promotes blood formation in the bone marrow
Da Huang (Rheum)	yes	yes	yes	yes	no	yes			yes		yes		stops bleeding, lowers viscosity, is also virostatic, antimycotic and antibacterial
Dan Shen (Salvia Miltiorrhiza)	yes	yes		yes	yes				yes		yes		antibacterial
Dang Gui (Angelica Sinensis)	yes	yes		yes	yes	yes					yes	yes	lowers heart oxygen consumption and antibody formation and increases macrophage phagocytosis

Table continues

[a] relaxes = a relaxing effect on the smooth muscles of the uterus

Table 7.2 The pharmacological effects of Blood invigorating medicinals (cont'd)

Name of medicinal	Heart: increases amount of blood flow through coronary arteries	Blood vessels: vasodilating effect	Blood vessels: lowers blood pressure	Blood vessels: improves microcirculation	Blood: inhibits thrombocyte aggregation and thrombosis	Blood: lowers blood lipids	Gynaecology: uterus muscle	Gynaecology: other	Immune system: antiphlogistic or anti-ulcerative	Immune system: inhibits cancer growth	Nervous system: calming	Nervous system: alleviates pain	Other effects
E Zhu (Curcuma Ezhu)	yes							c'ceptive[a]		yes			
Gan Qi (Lacca)	yes												spasmolytic effect on smooth muscles of intestines and bronchi
Gui Jian Yu (Euonymus)			no				relaxing[b]						lowers oxygen consumption and increases tolerance towards hypoxia and contractile force of the heart
Hong Hua (Carthamus)	yes	yes		yes	yes	yes	contractile[c]						blocks α-receptors
Hu Zhang (Polygonum Cuspidati)			yes	yes	yes	yes							lowers blood sugar and blood lipids, antibacterial, virostatic, counteracts coughing, antioxidative
Ji Xue Teng (Jixueteng)	yes	yes			yes	yes					yes		promotes blood formation, increases heart rate but lowers oxygen consumption
Jiang Huang (Curcuma Longa)	yes		yes		yes	yes	contractile	c'ceptive, abort.[d]		yes		yes	anti-arteriosclerotic, hepatoprotective, virostatic, antibacterial, antioxidative
Liu Ji Nu (Artemisia Anomalis)				yes									increases tolerance towards hypoxia, antiseptic

[a] c'ceptive = contraceptive effect
[b] relaxing = relaxing effect on smooth uterine muscles
[c] contractile = contractile effect on smooth uterine muscles
[d] abort. = abortive action

Table continues

Table 7.2 The pharmacological effects of Blood invigorating medicinals (cont'd)

Name of medicinal	Heart — increases amount of blood flow through coronary arteries	Blood vessels — vasodilating effect	Blood vessels — lowers blood pressure	Blood vessels — improves microcirculation	Blood — inhibits thrombocyte aggregation and thrombosis	Blood — lowers blood lipids	Gynaecology — uterus muscle	Gynaecology — other	Immune system — antiphlogistic or anti-ulcerative	Immune system — inhibits cancer growth	Nervous system — calming	Nervous system — alleviates pain	Other effects
Ma Bian Cao (Verbena)					no			lact.a	yes			yes	anti-amoebic, counteracts coughing, galactagogue increases tolerance towards hypoxia, activates fibrinolytic system
Mang Chong (Tabanus)		yes											
Mao Dong Qing (Ilex Pubescens)	yes	yes	only in cerebral arteries		yes				yes				antibacterial, lowers blood pressure in the cerebral arteries
Mo Yao (Myrrh)		yes	yes		yes				yes		yes	yes	
Mu Dan Pi (Moutan)							contractileb						prevents cardiac arrhythmias and ischemia, prevents capillary haemorrhaging, anticonvulsive, reduces fever, diuretic, antibacterial
Niu Xi (Achyranthis Bidentata)		yes						c'ceptive,c abort.d	yes			yes	promotes wound healing, diuretic, antibacterial, induces labour
Pu Huang (Typha)	yes	yes		yes	yes	yes	contractile					yes	

a lact. = has a galactagogue effect
b contractile = contractile effect on smooth uterine muscles
c c'ceptive = contraceptive effect
d abort. = abortive action

Table continues

Table 7.2 The pharmacological effects of Blood invigorating medicinals (cont'd)

Name of medicinal	Heart — increases amount of blood flow through coronary arteries	Blood vessels — vasodilating effect	Blood vessels — lowers blood pressure	Blood — improves microcirculation	Blood — inhibits thrombocyte aggregation and thrombosis	Blood — lowers blood lipids	Gynaecology — uterus muscle	Gynaecology — other	Immune system — antiphlogistic or anti-ulcerative	Immune system — inhibits cancer growth	Nervous system — calming	Nervous system — alleviates pain	Other effects
Ru Xiang (Olibanum)		yes							yes				increases erythrocyte plasticity
Rui Xiang (Daphna)		yes			yes								antibacterial, local anaesthetic
San Leng (Spargani)					yes					yes	yes		prolongs clotting time, lowers blood viscosity, increases absorption rate of blood clots in the abdomen
San Qi (Notoginseng)	yes	yes		esp. in the heart	yes								lowers heart oxygen consumption and pulse rate, anti-arrhythmic
Shan Zha (Crategus)	yes	yes				yes							strengthens the heart, promotes digestion, has anti-arrhythmic effect on the heart
Shui Zhi (Hirudo)				yes	yes, strongly	yes		abort.[a]	yes	yes			increases absorption of blood of the heart muscle
Su Mu (Sappan)	yes	no, constricts			yes				yes	yes	yes		antimycotic

[a] abort. = abortive action

Table continues

Table 7.2 The pharmacological effects of Blood invigorating medicinals (cont'd)

Name of medicinal	Heart: increases amount of blood flow through coronary arteries	Blood vessels: vasodilating effect	Blood vessels: lowers blood pressure	Blood vessels: improves microcirculation	Blood: inhibits thrombocyte aggregation and thrombosis	Blood: lowers blood lipids	Gynaecology: uterus muscle	Gynaecology: other	Immune system: antiphlogistic or anti-ulcerative	Immune system: inhibits cancer growth	Nervous system: calming	Nervous system: alleviates pain	Other effects
Tao Ren (Persica)							contractile[a]		yes				antiallergenic, counteracts coughing, promotes stool, counteracts diarrhoea
Wang Bu Liu Xing (Vaccaria)			yes				contractile[a]	c'ceptive[b]					
Wu Ling Zhi (Trogpterus)		yes			yes							yes	increases vascular permeability
Xue Ji (Sanguis Draconis)		yes								yes			
Yan Hu Suo (Corydalis)		yes		yes	yes				yes, yes		yes	yes	diuretic
Yi Mu Cao (Leonurus)	yes	yes	yes		yes		contractile					yes	lowers pulse and plasma cholesterol, increases respiration rate, has anticonvulsive effect on bronchi
Yin Xing Ye (Ginkgo)	yes	yes	yes									yes	
Yu Jin (curcuma)						yes							
Ze Lan (Lycopus)		yes			yes		contractile						inhibits fibrinogen, increases erythrocyte plasticity

[a] contractile = contractile effect on smooth uterine muscles

[b] c'ceptive = contraceptive effect

Box 7.1   Classification of the medicinals according to site of action (anatomical)

Mind
Dan Shen (Salvia Miltiorrhiza)
Chai Hu (Bupleurum)
Yuan Hu (Corydalis)
Su Mu (Sappan)
Rui Xiang (Daphna)
Hong Hua (Carthamus)
Chuan Xiong (Ligusticum Wallichii)

Epigastrium
Lu Lu Tong (Liquidambaris)
Wu Ling Zhi (Trogopterus)
Yan Hu Suo (Corydalis)

Kidney
Chuan Niu Xi (Cyathula)
Ji Xue Teng (Jixueteng)

Bladder
Yi Mu Cao (Leonurus)
Ze Lan (Lycopus)
Liu Ji Nu (Artemisia Anomalis)

Mammary gland, breast
Chuan Shan Jia (Squama Manitis)
Hong Hua (Carthamus)
Si Gua Luo (Luffa)
Wang Bu Liu Xing (Vaccaria)

Abdomen
San Leng (Spargani)
Tao Ren (Persica)
Tu Bie Chong (Eupolyphaga)
Yan Hu Suo (Corydalis)
Liu Ji Nu (Artemisia Anomalis)
Gan Qi (Lacca)

Uterus
Chi Shao (Paeonia Rubra)
Hong Hua (Carthamus)
San Leng (Spargani)
Su Mu (Sappan)
Tao Ren (Persica)
Tu Bie Chong (Eupolyphaga)
Wu Ling Zhi (Trogopterus)
Yan Hu Suo (Corydalis)
Yi Mu Cao (Leonurus), *Ze Lan* (Lycopus)
Liu Ji Nu (Artemisia Anomalis)

Box 7.2   Classification according to channel/organ action

Liver
Chuan Xiong (Ligusticum)
Dan Shen (Salvia Miltiorrhiza)
Yu Jin (Curcuma)
Jiang Huang (Curcuma Longa)
Tao Ren (Persica)
Hong Hua (Carthamus)
Niu Xi (Achyranthis Bidentata)
Ze Lan (Lycopus)
San Leng (Spargani)
E Zhu (Curcuma Ezhu)
Ru Xiang (Olibanum)
Mo Yao (Myrrha)
Wu Ling Zhi (Trogopterus)

Chuan Sha Jia (Squama Manitis)
Wang Bu Liu Xing (Vaccaria)
Yue Ji Hua (Rosa Chinensis)
Xue Jie (Sanguis Draconis)
Su Mu (Sappan)
Zi Ran Tong (Pyritum)
Shui Zhi (Hirudo)
Mang Chong (Tabanus)
Tu Bie Chong (Eupolyphaga)
Chi Shao (Paeonia Rubra)
Hu Zhang (Polygonum Cuspidati)
Qi Cao (Holotrichia)
Rui Xiang (Daphna)
Yuan Hu (Corydalis)

Box continues

Lung
Yu Jin (Curcuma)
Mao Dong Qing (Ilex Pubescens)
Hu Zhang (Polygonum Cuspidati)
Yin Xing Ye (Ginkgo)

Gallbladder
Chuan Xiong (Ligusticum)
Hu Zhang (Polygonum Cuspidati)

Heart
Chuan Xiong (Ligusticum)
Dan Shen (Salvia Miltiorrhiza)
Yu Jin (Curcuma)
Tao Ren (Persica)
Hong Hua (Carthamus)
Ru Xiang (Olibanum)
Mao Dong Qing (Ilex Pubescens)
Gui Jian Yu (Euonymus)
Liu Ji Nu (Artemisia Anomalis)
Rui Xiang (Daphna)
Yin Xing Ye (Ginkgo)
Yan Hu Suo (Corydalis)

Spleen
Jiang Huang (Curcuma Longa)
Ze Lan (Lycopus)

San Leng (Spargani)
Ru Xiang (Olibanum)
Liu Ji Nu (Artemisia Anomalis)
Qi Cao (Holotrichia)
Yan Hu Suo (Corydalis)

Large Intestine
Tao Ren (Persica)
Gan Qi (Lacca)

Kidney
Huai Niu Xi (Achyranthis Bidentata)

Stomach
Niu Xi (Achyranthis Bidentata)
Chuan Shan Jia (Squama Manitis)
Wang Bu Liu Xing (Vaccaria)
Gan Qi (Lacca)

Pericardium
Chuan Xiong (Ligusticum)
Yi Mu Cao (Leonurus)
Xue Jie (Sanguis Draconis)

Box 7.3   Classification according to temperature

Neutral
Tao Ren (Persica)
Niu Xi (Achyranthis Bidentata)
San Leng (Spargani)
Mo Yao (Myrrha)
Wang Bu Liu Xing (Vaccaria)
Xue Jie (Sanguis Draconis)
Su Mu (Sappan)
Zi Ran Tong (Pyritum)
Shui Zhi (Hirudo)
Yin Xing Ye (Ginkgo)
Hong Jing Tian (Rhodiola)

Cold medicinals
Yu Jin (Curcuma)
Jiang Huang (Curcuma Longa)
Mao Dong Qing (Ilex Pubescens)
Tu Bie Chong (Eupolyphaga)

Warm medicinals
Chuan Xiong (Ligusticum)
Hong Hua (Carthamus)
Ze Lan (Lycopus)
E Zhu (Curcuma Ezhu)
Ru Xiang (Olibanum)
Wu Ling Zhi (Trogopterus)
Yue Ji Hua (Rosa Chinensis)
Liu Ji Nu (Artemisia Anomalis)
Qi Cao (Holotrichia)
Rui Xiang (Daphna)
Yan Hu Suo (Corydalis)
Gan Qi (Lacca)

Cool medicinals
Dan Shen (Salvia Miltiorrhiza)
Yi Mu Cao (Leonurus)
Chuan Shan Jia (Squama Manitis)
Mang Chong (Tabanus)
Chi Shao (Paeonia Rubra)
Hu Zhang (Polygonum Cuspidati)

Box 7.4   Classification according to taste

Pungent
Chuan Xiong (Ligusticum)
Yu Jin (Curcuma)
Jiang Huang (Curcuma Longa)
Hong Hua (Carthamus)
Yi Mu Cao (Leonurus)
Ze Lan (Lycopus)
E Zhu (Curcuma Ezhu)
Ru Xiang (Olibanum)
Mao Dong Qing (Ilex Pubescens)
Su Mu (Sappan)
Zi Ran Tong (Pyritum)
Shui Zhi (Hirudo)
Tu Bie Chong (Eupolyphaga)
Liu Ji Nu (Artemisia Anomalis)
Rui Xiang (Daphna)
Yan Hu Suo (Corydalis)
Gan Qi (Lacca)

Sour/Astringent
Niu Xi (Achyranthis Bidentata)
Yin Xing Ye (Ginkgo)
Hong Jing Tian (Rhodiola)

Sweet
Tao Ren (Persica)
Wu Ling Zhi (Trogopterus)
Yue Ji Hua (Rosa Chinensis)
Xue Jie (Sanguis Draconis)
Rui Xiang (Daphna)
Yin Xing Ye (Ginkgo)
Hong Jing Tian (Rhodiola)

Bitter
Dan Shen (Salvia Miltiorrhiza)
Yu Jin (Curcuma)
Jiang Huang (Curcuma Longa)
Tao Ren (Persica)
Niu Xi (Achyranthis Bidentata)
Yi Mu Cao (Leonurus)
San Leng (Spargani)
E Zhu (Curcuma Ezhu)
Ru Xiang (Olibanum)
Mo Yao (Myrrha)
Wang Bu Liu Xing (Vaccaria)
Mao Dong Qing (Ilex Pubescens)
Mang Chong (Tabanus)
Chi Shao (Paeonia Rubra)
Hu Zhang (Polygonum Cuspidati)
Liu Ji Nu (Artemisia Anomalis)
Yin Xing Ye (Ginkgo)
Yan Hu Suo (Corydalis)
Gan Qi (Lacca)

Salty
Chuan Shan Jia (Squama Manitis)
Xue Jie (Sanguis Draconis)
Shui Zhi (Hirudo)
Tu Bie Chong (Eupolyphaga)
Qi Cao (Holotrichia)
Rui Xiang (Daphna)

PART 3. PEI YAO (COMBINING MEDICAL SUBSTANCES): THE MOST COMMON COMBINATIONS OF BLOOD INVIGORATING MEDICINALS

COMBINATIONS OF DIFFERENT BLOOD STASIS MEDICINALS

Many Blood invigorating medicinals are successfully combined to achieve an enhanced effect.

This chapter describes these combinations, and their underlying logic and main indications. Occasionally, one of these combinations already forms part of an established formula; in these cases, the formula's name is mentioned as well.

The combinations of medicinals listed in Box 7.5 and described below enhance the effect or increase the efficacy of the formula's action.

Box 7.5 Common combinations of Blood stasis medicinals

1. *Dang Gui–Chuan Xiong* (Radix Angelicae–Radix Ligustici)
2. *Tao Ren–Hong Hua* (Semen Persicae–Flos Carthami)
3. *Pu Huang–Wu Ling Zhi* (Pollen Typhae–Faeces Trogopteri)
4. *Ru Xiang–Mo Yao* (Olibanum–Myrrha)
5. *San Leng–E Zhu* (Rhizoma Sparganii–Rhizoma Curcumae Ezhu)
6. *Da Huang–Bie Chong* (Radix et Rhizoma Rhei–Eupolyphaga)
7. *San Qi–Bai Ji* (Radix Notoginseng–Rhizoma Bletillae)
8. *Dan Shen–Mu Dan Pi* (Radix Salviae Miltiorrhizae–Cortex Moutan Radicis)

Dang Gui–Chuan Xiong (Radix Angelicae Sinensis–Radix Ligustici)

Dang Gui is gentler in its nature, moistening, nourishing and invigorating Blood. It alleviates pain and swellings. *Chuan Xiong* is pungent, warm and aromatic, moving *Qi* and invigorating Blood; it also alleviates pain and dispels Wind pathogens. Together, they complement each other excellently: *Qi* and Blood are moved, Blood stasis is removed, the weakened Blood is nourished and pain is alleviated. In ancient times, this combination was called 'Buddha's Hands Powder' due to its marvellous effect.

Dosage
Dang Gui (Angelica) and *Chuan Xiong* (Ligusticum) 6–10 g of each.

Main indications
1. Menstrual disorders, especially with pain; difficult delivery; Blood stasis after birth with pain and bleeding.
2. Ulcers with swelling and pain.
3. Rheumatic-arthritic *Bi*-syndrome due to Wind and Dampness.

4. Headache due to Blood stasis or Blood deficiency, pain that is more apparent on the left side. Increase the dosage if there is severe pain: *Dang Gui* (Angelica) 10–20 g, *Chuan Xiong* (Ligusticum) 15–30 g.
5. Vomiting of Blood.

Tao Ren–Hong Hua (Semen Persicae–Flores Carthami)

Tao Ren (Persica) breaks Blood stasis, moistens Dryness and promotes stool. *Hong Hua* (Carthamus) is Blood invigorating, expels Blood stasis, removes obstructions from the vessels and alleviates pain. Together, they complement each other and make a Blood invigorating and obstruction removing medicinal, that can alleviate pain and swelling. The Blood invigorating effect and the name *Tao Hong Si Wu Tang* are based on this combination, which Wang Qing-Ren developed into *Xue Fu Zhu Yu Tang* (Anti-Stasis Chest Decoction).

Dosage
Tao Ren (Persica) and *Hong Hua* (Carthamus) 6–10 g of each.

Main indications
1. Blood stasis in the Heart, pain in the chest (including angina pectoris, coronary heart disease with pain and stomach pain).
2. Amenorrhoea, dysmenorrhoea.
3. Any kind of pain and swelling with Blood stasis (including trauma).

Pu Huang–Wu Ling Zhi (Pollen Typhae–Faeces Trogopterori)

Pu Huang (Typha) is pungent, aromatic and has a strong dispersing action. Its action is focused on the Blood, which it invigorates, stanches and cools. *Wu Ling Zhi* (Trogopterus) is sweet and warm and also acts principally on the Blood, invigorating Blood and expelling stasis; however, it also moves *Qi* and alleviates pain. These two medicinals are rarely used on their own, as they complement each other so well: obstructions are removed from the vessels, Blood is invigorated and stasis is dispelled, even severe pain is alleviated and swellings are reduced. This combination was called 'Shi Xiao San', which means 'Lost Smile Powder' as well as 'Sudden or Unexpected Smile Powder'. The first interpretation refers to the taste of *Wu Ling Zhi*; the latter suggests the unexpected abating of severe pain due to Blood stasis and the return to a happier state of mind.

Dosage
Pu Huang (Typhae) 6–10 g and *Wu Ling Zhi* (Trogopterus) 6–12 g.

Main indications

1. Heart or lower abdominal pain due to *Qi*-stagnation or Blood stasis (including angina pectoris and stomach pain).
2. Menstrual disorders, dysmenorrhoea (especially with lower abdominal pain), heavy metrorrhagia with pain and bleeding, incomplete involution of the uterus after birth.

Ru Xiang–Mo Yao (Olibanum–Myrrha)

Ru Xiang (Olibanum) has a pungent, aromatic and warm nature. It moistens and moves the *Qi* of the Blood, relaxes the sinews and invigorates the *Luo*-vessels. *Mo Yao* (Myrrha) is neutral, bitter, and has a strong draining action, which is enhanced when it is combined with *Ru Xiang* (Olibanum). Additionally, the two medicinals together invigorate Blood, and expel Blood stasis; the latter especially in the fields of traumatology and gynaecology. Wang Ken-Tang's *Ru Xiang Zhi Tong San* (Analgetic Olibanum Powder) contains this combination, which is also mentioned in the 'Yi Lin Gai Cuo'. Later, *Zhang Xi-Chun* extended it with *Dan Shen* (Salvia Miltiorrhiza) and *Dang Gui* (Angelica Sinensis) and in that way created his famous *Huo Luo Xiao Ling Dan* (Wondrous Pill to Invigorate the Channels), which is also noted in Case study 4.4 'Blood stasis due to exogenous pathogenic Cold' in Chapter 4, p. 28.

Dosage
3–10 g of each.

Main indications
1. Abdominal pain or lower abdominal pain due to *Qi* stagnation or Blood stasis, disorders of the menstrual cycle, menstrual pain or postpartum pain.
2. Trauma, painful, swollen abscesses, rheumatic *Bi*-syndrome due to Wind or Dampness.
3. Angina pectoris, extrauterine pregnancy.
4. Acute and subacute renal pelvic inflammation, also purulent, painful and swollen genitals and syndromes due to strong Fire toxins.

San Leng–E Zhu (Rhizoma Sparganii–Rhizoma Curcumae Ezhu/Zedoeriae)

San Leng (Spargani) is neutral, bitter, pungent and dispersing. It acts especially on the Blood, Liver and Spleen; apart from being one of the Blood stasis breaking medicinals, it also acts on the *Qi*. *E Zhu* is warm, bitter, pungent and acts especially well on the *Qi* of the Spleen and Liver. Among the *Qi* moving medicinals, it is one of those that also act on the Blood; it can also dissolve conglomerations. Together, they complement each other excellently, as they can move stagnated *Qi* as well as Blood. They can alleviate pain and dissolve gatherings.

Dosage
5–10 g of each.

Main indications
1. Amenorrhoea due to Blood stasis, dysmenorrhoea and pain after birth, abdominal masses of all kinds (concretions and conglomerations).
2. Hepatomegaly and splenomegaly.
3. Pain due to a blockage in the digestive system.
4. Swollen neoplasms (also malignant).

Da Huang–Tu Bie Chong (Radix et Rhizoma Rhei–Eupolyphaga)

Bitter *Da Huang* dissolves gatherings, purges stagnated food, by virtue of its cold nature drains Fire and cools the Blood, moves Blood stasis and removes obstructions from the vessels. *Bie Chong*, which is salty and cool, belongs to the *Chong*-medicinals,[1] which work powerfully to break Blood stasis. Like *Da Huang* (Rheum), it also acts

---

[1] See Glossary.

on the Liver and dissolves concretions and con-glomerations (*Zheng Jia*). If combined, the effect is amplified, with a strong dissolving effect on abscesses of all kind and Blood stasis.

This combination was first written down by Zhang Zhong-Jing as *Da Huang Bie Chong Wan* (Rheum Eupolyphaga Pill) in the '*Jin Kui Yao Lüe*'.

When the herbs are being boiled, *Da Huang* should only be added during the last few minutes if its purging action is to be emphasized. Boiling it from the beginning will emphasize its Blood invigorating but not its purging action.

Dosage
Da Huang (Rheum) 3–10 g, *Tu Bie Chong* (Eupolyphaga) 3–6 g.

Main indications
1. Amenorrhoea due to Blood stasis, abdominal masses and digestive disorders.
2. Dry, cracked or scaly skin, afternoon fever.
3. Pain and swelling with bruises due to traumata.

San Qi–Bai Ji (Radix Notoginseng–Rhizoma Bletillae)

San Qi (Notoginseng) has a sweet, slightly bitter nature. It is characterized by its simultaneous Blood invigorating and stopping bleeding actions. Furthermore, it reduces swelling and has an analgetic action. *Bai Ji* has a bitter, sweet and astringent nature. It can also stop bleeding and promote wound healing. In addition, it has a toni-fying effect on the Lung. TCM holds that: '*San Qi* moves, but doesn't collect, *Bai Ji* collects, but doesn't move'. Here, collecting indicates contract-ing the wound and moving indicates the moving of the Blood, e.g. in a haematoma. This com-bination is especially suitable for bleeding and thrombosis.

Dosage
3–10 g of each.

Main indications
1. Injuries of the lung with bleeding, for example as in tuberculosis, emphysema etc.

2. All kinds of haemorrhaging such as hae-matemesis, haematuria, haematochezia, epis-taxis etc.

Dan Shen–Mu Dan Pi (Radix Salviae Miltiorrhizae–Cortex Moutan Radicis)

Dan Shen (Salvia Miltiorrhiza) invigorates and nourishes Blood and transforms Blood stasis. It also reduces swelling and has an analgetic and calming action. *Dan Pi* (Moutan) cools Blood and Heat, invigorates Blood and dispels stasis. In addi-tion, it cools the Liver and lowers blood pressure, so it can also be administered in feverish Heat syndromes and residual Heat in the body. Together these two have a Blood cooling and invigorating action, dispelling stasis and pro-moting wound healing as well as cool pathogenic Heat, due to their slightly cool nature.

Dosage
Dan Pi (Moutan) 6–10 g and *Dan Shen* (Salvia Miltiorrhiza) 10–15 g.

Main indications
1. To treat Wind-Heat pathogens that have pene-trated into the Blood, and thus Heat-toxins with skin eruptions, all kinds of haemorrhag-ing, measles and other kinds of infectious dis-eases with fever and skin phenomena.
2. Blood stasis with Heat syndrome, menstrual disorders, abdominal masses, lower abdomi-nal pain, heavy metrorrhagia and so on.
3. *Yin* deficiency syndromes with false Heat (gen-erated by *Yin* deficiency), idiopathic low-grade fever of continuing duration.
4. Rheumatic Heat *Bi*-syndrome, typical joint inflammations (calor, rubor, dolor).

OTHER MEDICINALS OFTEN COMBINED WITH BLOOD STASIS REMOVING MEDICINALS

- In the case of Blood stasis with pathogenic factors in exterior conditions, but also in the case of Wind and Wind-*Bi*, **exterior relieving medicinals** are prescribed.

In the case of Blood stasis due to Phlegm and hardenings, either **Phlegm resolving** or **purging medicinals** are prescribed. Amongst those are *Ban Xia, Jie Geng, Sang Bai Pi* and *Mang Xiao.*

In the case of Blood stasis due to pathogenic Cold or *Yang* deficiency, **warming medicinals** are prescribed. Herbs that are often combined with Blood stasis medicinals are *Gui Zhi, Gui Rou, Sheng Jiang, Gan Jiang* and *Fu Zi.* They are often used in gynaecological and rheumatic diseases.

In the case of Blood stasis due to *Qi* deficiency and stagnation, *Qi* **tonifying** or *Qi* **moving medicinals** are often prescribed in combination with Blood stasis removing medicinals: *Xiang Fu, Wu Yao, Chuan Lian Zi, Qing Pi, Chen Pi* etc. are *Qi* moving medicinals; *Huang Qi, Dang Shen, Gan Cao, Bai Zhu* etc. strengthen the *Qi* and are used in *Qi* deficiency. When the *Qi* is moving, then Blood will move as well.

In the case of Blood stasis with pathogenic Heat in the Blood and a tendency to bleeding, **cooling medicinals** or **medicinals that stop bleeding** are administered. For example, *Ce Bai Ye, Xi Cao, Gui Hua, Di Yu, San Qi* and *Sheng Di Huang* are used.

In the case of Blood stasis due to internal Heat with Heat Toxins, **Blood cooling medicinals** like *Pu Gong Yin, Ding Cao, Hong Teng, Ye Ju Hua* etc. are prescribed. They aim at treating internal and external abscesses and inflammations.

1. EXTERIOR RELIEVING MEDICINALS

Sheng Jiang, Rhizoma Zingiberis Recens

This belongs to the pungent, warm and exterior relieving medicinals. It is used:

1. as a diaphoretic in illnesses due to Wind and Cold;
2. as an antiemetic.

New pharmacological research and new clinical usage
Fresh ginger is febrifugal, alleviates pain and inhibits inflammations; is calming, strengthens the heart and lowers blood pressure; has an antiemetic and antiulcerative action, promotes stomach and intestinal motility, stimulates pepsin and gastric acid secretion and is liver protective; it also has cholecystokinetic, antioxidative, antibacterial and antimycotic, anticoagulative and antimutagenic actions.

Apart from traditional usages (see above), nowadays this herb is used in chronic gastritis and ulcerations, diarrhoea, enteritis, rheumatic pain, burns and worm infestations.

It is an ingredient of the following Blood stasis removing formula: *Wen Jing Tang* (Menses Warming Decoction). It is readily used in Blood stasis due to Cold.

Fang Feng, Radix Ledebouriellae, new name: Radix Saposhnikoviae

It belongs to the pungent, warm, exterior relieving medicinals. It is used:

1. as a diaphoretic in illnesses due to Wind and Cold and rheumatic pain;
2. as a spasmolytic in tetanus.

New pharmacological research and new clinical usage
Fang Feng lowers fever, has analgetic, antiphlogistic and antimicrobial actions, reduces thrombocyte aggregation, counteracts shock and is calming.

Apart from traditional usages (see above), this herb is nowadays used in skin diseases such as acne rosacea, urticaria, psoriasis, alopecia, vitiligo, warts and furuncles as well as in rheumatic pain, toothache and alopecia.

It is an ingredient of the following Blood stasis removing formulas: *Shu Jing Huo Xue Tang* (Relaxing the Vessels Decoction), and *Huang Qi Fang Feng Tang* (Astragalus Ledebouriella Decoction). It is used especially in Blood stasis with rheumatic pain.

Qiang Huo, Rhizoma/Radix Notopterygii

Qiang Huo belongs to the pungent, warm, exterior relieving medicinals. It is used:

1. as an exterior relieving medicinal in Wind and Cold with headache;
2. as an exterior relieving medicinal in Wind and Dampness; as a herb with antirheumatic and

analgetic actions it is employed in the treatment of rheumatic pain especially in the upper half of the body.

New pharmacological research and new clinical usage

Qiang Huo has analgetic, antiphlogistic and antibacterial actions and lowers fever. These characteristics correspond to its classical usage for which it is still used nowadays in cases of infections. In addition, it has antiallergenic and antiepileptic actions. It also has an anti-arrhythmic effect on the heart, so it is used nowadays as an anti-arrhythmic medicine. Another modern application is its use in the treatment of conjunctivitis.

It is an ingredient of the following Blood stasis removing formulas: *Shen Tong Zhu Yu Tang* (Anti-Stasis Pain Decoction) and *Shu Jing Huo Xue Tang* (Relaxing the Vessels Decoction). It is readily used in Blood stasis due to Cold.

Chai Hu, Radix Bupleuri

This belongs to the pungent, cool, exterior relieving medicinals. It is used:

1. as an antipyretic or in intermittent fever, e.g. malaria;
2. to remove Liver *Qi* stagnation with pain in the sides and chest;
3. to tonify Spleen *Qi* in visceroptosis and connective tissue weakness.

New pharmacological research and new clinical usage

It is effective against microorganisms, has anti-inflammatory and febrifugal actions, is calming, alleviates pain, has antitussive, hepatoprotective, antineoplastic and antioxidative actions, and prevents mutations and radiation injuries. It strongly influences the following body systems: immune system, digestive system, metabolism of fat, protein and sugar, as well as kidney and heart function.

New clinical applications for its use are, apart from infections, the treatment of liver and gall bladder diseases, arteriosclerosis, acute nephritis, hypothyroidism, diseases of the skin, kidney, heart and blood vessels.

It is an ingredient of the following Blood stasis removing formulas: *Xue Fu Zhu Yu Tang* (Anti-Stasis Chest Decoction), and *Fu Yuan Huo Xue Tang* (Blood Invigorating Recovery Decoction). It is used for treating Blood stasis in association with Liver-*Qi* stagnation.

Ge Gen, Radix Puerariae

Ge Gen belongs to the pungent, cool, exterior relieving medicinals. It is traditionally used:

1. as a diaphoretic to treat fever accompanied by pain in the neck and back;
2. to quench thirst in fever;
3. in headaches related to hypertension and coronary heart disease;
4. to promote eruptions of measles.

New pharmacological research and new clinical usage

It relaxes smooth muscles and dilates coronary vessels, protects the heart from ischemic damage and arrhythmia, and lowers heart rate, blood pressure, blood sugar, blood lipids and body temperature. It increases peripheral circulation by lowering peripheral vessel resistance, it inhibits adrenergic β-receptors and thrombocyte aggregation.

It is used nowadays in conditions such as migraine, hypertension, hyperlipidaemia, acute deafness, coronary heart disease (CHD), angina pectoris and cardiac arrhythmias as well as in various skin diseases.

It is an ingredient of the following Blood stasis removing formulas: *Jie Du Huo Xue Tang* (Detoxifying, Blood Invigorating Decoction), and a modified version of *Wen Jing Tang* (Menses Warming Decoction) and in modern preparations against hepatitis (see Case study 4.5 in Chapter 4).

Sheng Ma, Rhizoma Cimicifugae

It belongs to the pungent, cool, exterior relieving medicinals. It is traditionally used:

1. to promote circulation in the treatment of measles;
2. to detoxify in sore throat and stomatitis;
3. to re-establish the normal position of the organ in splanchnoptosis.

New pharmacological research and new clinical usage

Sheng Ma lowers fever; it has antiphlogistic, antibacterial and analgetic actions; it has an inhibitory function on the CNS, stimulates and removes cramps from smooth muscles, and lowers blood pressure and heart rate.

For these reasons it is used in uterus prolapse and gastroptosis, heavy metrorrhagia, skin diseases, haematochezia, infectious diseases and acute sinusitis.

It is an ingredient of the following Blood stasis removing formulas: *Yu Long Gao* (Jade Dragon Paste, also called *Shen Yu Gao*), and in modern preparations that treat hepatitis (see Case study 4.5 in Chapter 4).

Lian Qiao, Herba Forsythia

This belongs to the pungent, cool, exterior relieving medicinals. It is traditionally used:

1. in colds and infectious diseases with fever (invasion of febrile infectious factors into the *Ying* level (Nutritive energy));
2. in the treatment of purulent ulcers, furuncles, carbuncles, exanthema and erythema;
3. in anuria and painful urination (*Lin* syndrome).

New pharmacological research and new clinical usage

Lian Qiao has an antiseptic effect on a vast array of microorganisms, lowers fever and is antiphlogistic, which relates to its classical usage. Furthermore, it has antiemetic, hepatoprotective and blood pressure lowering actions; except in states of shock, it increases heart function and capillary circulation.

Today, it is predominantly applied in the area of acute febrile infectious diseases. Apart from respiratory infections, its indications were extended to include acute hepatitis and nephritis as well as purulent skin infections. It is also used as an antiemetic medicine.

It is an ingredient of the following Blood stasis removing formulas: *Yu Long Gao* (Jade Dragon Paste, also called *Shen Yu Gao*), *Jie Du Huo Xue Tang*

(Detoxifying, Blood Invigorating Decoction) and *Tong Jing Zhu Yu Tang* (Anti-Stasis Exanthema Decoction).

2. PHLEGM TRANSFORMING MEDICINALS

Ban Xia, Rhizoma Pinelliae

Ban Xia belongs to the Phlegm resolving, cough stopping medicinals. It is traditionally used:

1. as an expectorant in the treatment of coughing with profuse thin Phlegm;
2. as an antiemetic in nausea, vomiting and vomiting during pregnancy.

New pharmacological research and new clinical usage

New research in the main bears out its classical applications: *Ban Xia* helps to resolve Phlegm and has expectorant, antitussive and antiemetic effects, and inhibits fibrosis of the Lung.

Apart from its classical fields of use, it is nowadays prescribed in gastrointestinal disorders, vomiting in pregnancy, globus sensation in the throat, CHD, dizziness, psychoneuroses, round worms and skin diseases.

It is an ingredient of the following Blood stasis removing formulas: *Wen Jing Tang* (Menses Warming Decoction) and *Dian Kuang Meng Xing Tang* (Psychosis Decoction).

Jie Geng, Radix Platycodi

Jie Geng belongs to the Phlegm resolving, cough stopping medicinals. It is traditionally used:

1. as an expectorant and to dissolve pus;
2. in coughing due to respiratory infections or lung abscess;
3. in the treatment of sore throat.

New pharmacological research and new clinical usage

Jie Geng has mucolytic, antitussive, antiphlogistic, antiulcerative, analgetic and immune stimulating actions. It alleviates pain, lowers fever and is calming. Furthermore, it lowers heart rate, cholesterol levels, blood sugar levels and blood pressure.

It counteracts tumour formation and relaxes the smooth muscles of the gut.

Today, as in ancient times, it is used in the treatment of respiratory diseases such as pneumonia, chronic bronchitis, asthmatic bronchitis, emphysema, acute tonsillitis and laryngitis as well as sinusitis. Apart from that, it is also prescribed in enteritis and haemorrhagic fever.

It is an ingredient of the following Blood stasis removing formulas: *Xue Fu Zhu Yu Tang, Ge Xia Zhu Yu Tang, Hui Yan Zhu Yu Tang* (Anti-Stasis Chest Decoction, Anti-Stasis Abdomen Decoction, Anti-Stasis Epiglottis Decoction).

Sang Bai Pi, Cortex Mori

This belongs to the Phlegm resolving, cough stopping medicinals. It is classically used:

1. as an antitussive in the treatment of coughing due to Lung Heat;
2. as a diuretic in oedema and anuria.

New pharmacological research and new clinical usage
Sang Bai Pi has antibacterial, febrifugal and diuretic actions, which are confirmed by its classical application. Furthermore, it has a calming and analgetic effect, increases contractility of the heart and gut motility, and by peripheral vasoconstriction helps to prevent shock.

Nowadays, it is used in pleuritis, oedema and excessive salivation in infants.

It is an ingredient of the following Blood stasis removing formula: *Dian Kuang Meng Xing Tang* (Psychosis Decoction).

3. INTERIOR WARMING MEDICINALS

Rou Gui, Cortex Cinnamomi

It is classically used:

1. to warm *Yang Qi* of the Kidney in the treatment of chronic diarrhoea accompanied by cold limbs, oliguria and oedema due to kidney hypofunction;
2. against lower abdominal pain due to Cold and in the treatment of gastrointestinal disorders due to Cold.

New pharmacological research and new clinical usage
Rou Gui (not to be confused with *Gui Zhi*, Ramulus Cinnamomi) has antibacterial, antiulcerative, analgetic and febrifugal actions and increases gut motility; this largely corresponds to its classical application. Furthermore, it has an indirect anabolic building effect due to its inhibitory action on the catabolic glucocorticoids. It increases leukocyte production and radiation tolerance; it prevents ischemic damage to the heart muscle to a large degree, and thrombocyte aggregation.

Apart from its classical usage, it is nowadays also used in bronchial asthma and acute colitis.

It is an ingredient of the following Blood stasis removing formulas: *Shao Fu Zhu Yu Tang, Ai Fu Nuan Gong Wan* (Anti-Stasis Lower Abdomen Decoction and Artemisia Cyperus Pill).

Gan Jiang, Rhizoma Zingiberis

It is used:

1. to warm Stomach and Spleen in the treatment of nausea, vomiting, abdominal pain and diarrhoea;
2. to warm the Lung in the treatment of chronic bronchitis with thin and frothy white Phlegm.

New pharmacological research and new clinical usage
Gan Jiang is dried ginger and not to be confused with fresh *Sheng Jiang*, Rhizoma Zingiberis Recens.

Dried ginger as well as fresh ginger alleviates pain and has febrifugal, anti-inflammatory, antibacterial, antiemetic and antiulcerative actions. It also increases gut motility and gastric secretion. It can affect blood pressure in both directions. Furthermore, it has a cholagogue action, inhibits thrombosis and thrombocyte aggregation and reduces the amount of worms and intestinal parasites.

It still fulfils its classic role as a medicinal for intestinal diseases, such as duodenal ulcers, worm infestation and acute bacterial enteritis, but recently it has also been used successfully in treating rheumatic pain and hip or leg pain.

It is an ingredient of the following Blood stasis removing formulas: *Shao Fu Zhu Yu Tang* (Anti-Stasis Lower Abdomen Decoction) and *Sheng Hua Tang* (Generate Change Decoction).

Xiao Hui Xiang, Fructus Foeniculi

It is traditionally used to dispel Cold and regulate the smooth flow of *Qi*, and it alleviates pain in the treatment of Cold and pain in the lower abdomen as well as in bloatedness and pain in the testicles.

New pharmacological research and new clinical usage

Fennel seeds have antiulcerative, analgetic, antiphlogistic, antibacterial, antineoplastic and antiasthmatic actions, resolve phlegm and have a cholagogue effect. Furthermore, they can relax the bronchi, stimulate the CNS, increase intestinal motility and bronchial secretions, inhibit blood clotting and have an oestrogen-like effect in the endocrine system (including a galactagogue effect).

Modern applications include: intestinal obstruction, abdominal pain of differing origin in infants and duodenal ulcers etc.

It is an ingredient of the following Blood stasis removing formulas: *Shao Fu Zhu Yu Tang* (Anti-Stasis Lower Abdomen Decoction) and *Xiao Hui Xiang Ju* (Fennel Tincture).

Ai Ye, Folia Artemisia Argyi

It belongs to the interior warming medicinals and to the group of medicinals that stop bleeding. It is used to warm the uterus and stop bleeding in the treatment of functional bleeding of the uterus, sterility and dysmenorrhoea.

New pharmacological research and new clinical usage

Apart from the proven effect that it can stop bleeding (if given as a decoction) and the disinfecting properties of its smoke (Moxa), which both correspond to its traditional applications, *Ai Ye* has many other effects: it suppresses cough, has mucolytic, antibacterial, antiasthmatic and antiallergic effects, and its smoke was successfully used in treating breathing problems due to tuberculosis of the lung. Furthermore, it increases phagocytosis in macrophages, has a cholagogue effect on liver and gallbladder, strengthens the heart and stimulates uterine muscles.

Its modern applications have therefore been extended to include: chronic bronchitis and hepatitis, acute bacterial hepatitis, allergies, candidiasis and all kinds of haemorrhaging.

It is an ingredient of the following Blood stasis removing formula: *Ai Fu Nuan Gong Wan* (Artemisia Cyperus Pill).

4. *QI* MOVING MEDICINALS

Chen Pi, Pericarpium Citri Reticulatae

It is traditionally used:

1. as a carminative and stomachic to regulate the transportation function of the Spleen;
2. to regulate *Qi* in the treatment of a gastrointestinal feeling of fullness, vomiting and hiccup;
3. as an expectorant in coughing with profuse amounts of Phlegm.

New pharmacological research and new clinical usage

Chen Pi increases blood pressure and counteracts shock. In addition, it relaxes stomach and gut muscles, has virustatic, antioxidative, antiasthmatic and mucolytic actions and resolves gall stones. Therefore, apart from its classical indications, it is also used in shock, ulcers and gall stones.

It is an ingredient of the following Blood stasis removing formulas: *Dian Kuang Meng Xing Tang* (Psychosis Decoction) and *Shu Jing Huo Xue Tang* (Relaxing the Vessels Decoction).

Zhi Qiao/Zhi Ke, Fructus Citrus Aurantium

It is not to be confused with the much stronger *Zhi Shi*, Fructus Immaturus Citrus Aurantii. Its traditional usage is similar to it: as a carminative to move stagnated *Qi* and stagnated food in the gastrointestinal tract in the treatment of dyspepsia, constipation and fullness after eating due to food stagnation. Due to its milder action, it is more suitable for elderly, weak or very young patients, equally in *Qi* stagnation with constipation.

New pharmacological research and new clinical usage

Zhi Ke has a spasmolytic effect on intestinal muscle cramps and raises blood pressure. Similar to *Zhi Shi*, it is used according to classic criteria. New indications include different types of connective tissue weaknesses, such as umbilical, inguinal and scrotal hernias, gastroptosis, uterus prolapse and other types of splanchnoptosis.

It is an ingredient of the following Blood stasis removing formulas: *Xue Fu Zhu Yu Tang, Ge Xia Zhu Yu Tang, Jie Du Huo Xue Tang* (Anti-Stasis Chest Decoction, Anti-Stasis Abdomen Decoction and Detoxifying, Blood Invigorating Decoction).

Xiang Fu, Rhizoma Cyperi

It is used:

1. as a carminative, spasmolytic and analgesic in the treatment of feelings of oppression and pain in the chest, especially in a disorder of Liver-*Qi*.
2. in the treatment of abdominal pain due to dysmenorrhoea and menstrual disorders.

New pharmacological research and new clinical usage

Xiang Fu has an oestrogen-like effect, inhibits the CNS, strengthens heart function and resolves bronchial spasms. It has antibacterial, analgetic, antiphlogistic and febrifugal actions. Apart from its classic applications, it is nowadays also used in hip pain and externally in the treatment of flat warts.

It is an ingredient of the following Blood stasis removing formulas: *Ge Xia Zhu Yu Tang* (Anti-Stasis Abdomen Decoction), *Tong Qi San* (*Qi* Passage Powder), *Dian Kuang Meng Xing Tang* (Psychosis Decoction) and *Shen Tong Zhu Yu Tang* (Anti-Stasis Pain Decoction).

5. *QI* STRENGTHENING MEDICINALS

Ren Shen, Radix Panax Ginseng and *Dang Shen*, Radix Codonopsis Pilosulae (today often used as an affordable substitute for ginseng)

Whilst Ginseng strengthens the *Qi* of the whole body, *Dang Shen* acts only on the *Qi* of the Middle (Spleen, Stomach). Nevertheless, palpitations, weak limbs, lack of appetite and thin stools are all indications for *Dang Shen*.

Of course there are many books[2] available on studies concerning ginseng; no other medicinal is as well-researched. As this book covers mainly Blood regulating medicinals, I will not go into too much detail on ginseng.

New pharmacological research and new clinical usage

Ginseng promotes memorization and memory, capacity, improves heart function, nucleic acid formation in the cells and protein metabolism, and stimulates the adrenal cortex endocrine system and haematopoiesis. It reduces thrombocyte aggregation and cancer cell growth and can regulate the CNS, blood pressure, blood sugar and immune system (cellular and humoral) in both directions. It protects heart muscle cells and other cells from anoxia damage and shock. Furthermore, ginseng contains oestrogen-like substances, lowers prostaglandin E (PGE) and F (PGF) levels and decreases the ratio of PGE to PGF, and increases incretion of tri-iodothyronine and therefore also T4 plasma levels and cAMP plasma levels. Moreover, it has hepatoprotective and environment-adaptation-promoting actions, increases performance and has antioxidative, antineoplastic and antimutagenic actions; it can delay the aging process and prolong life in laboratory animals etc.

Ginseng is prescribed in the following conditions:

- Heart: cardiac arrhythmias, sinus arrhythmia in old age, CHD, acute myocardial infarction and endotoxic myocarditis;
- Circulation/blood: shock, hypo- and hypertension, hypercholesterolemia, hyperlipidaemia, increased coagulation tendency, leukocyte and erythrocyte anaemia;

---

[2] For example Steven Fulders *The Tao of Medicine* (new title: *Book of Ginseng*) is dedicated exclusively to ginseng research. Although its studies are mostly from the 1970s, it is one of the most complete works. A more modern, but less comprehensive book is *Recent Advances in Chinese Herbal Drugs*, published in 1991 by Beijing Science Press and SATAS, Belgium. The research in this work dates from the 1980s. The most recently published material is unfortunately only available in Chinese at the moment. Because of limited space, this material can only be touched on in this book.

- Digestion/metabolism: acute and chronic hepatitis, digestive disturbances, anal prolapse and diabetes;
- Further conditions: sexual disorders, all kinds of functional disorders, neurasthenia, carcinoma, allergic rhinitis and rheumatoid arthritis.

Dang Shen has haematopoietic, adaptogenic and calming actions and increases stress tolerance; it is antibacterial, antiphlogistic and analgetic. It increases cellular immune defence, plasma cortisone levels and blood sugar levels. It protects tissue from the damaging effects of ischemia.

Today, its applications include: anaemia, CHD, acute altitude sickness, gastric ulcers, nephritis, digestive weakness, psoriasis, purulent ulcers and neuroses etc.

Wang Qing-Ren frequently used *Dang Shen* in his formulas: he included it in *Ji Qiu Hui Yang Tang* (Emergency *Yang* Recovery Decoction), *Zhi Xie Tiao Zhong Tang* (Anti-Diarrhoea Centre Regulating Decoction), *Zhu Wei He Rong Tang* (*Wei* and *Ying* Strengthening Decoction) and *Ke Bao Li Su Tang* (Guaranteed Resuscitation Decoction).

Huang Qi, Radix Astragali Membranacea

It is used:

1. to tonify the *Qi* and as an antihidrotic in the treatment of spontaneous sweating, night sweating, uterine and anal prolapse;
2. to resolve pus and to promote wound healing in the treatment of chronic ulcers;
3. as a diuretic in chronic nephritis accompanied by oedema and proteinuria.

New pharmacological research and new clinical usage

Huang Qi markedly stimulates the whole immune system; it has diuretic and antiphlogistic actions, largely corresponding to its classical indications. Furthermore, it lowers blood pressure in the treatment of essential hypertension, has a positive inotrope effect on the heart and increases tolerance towards anoxia, skin collagen content and erythrocyte plasticity.

It is used today, in addition to its classical applications, in the treatment of hepatitis and ulcers of the digestive tract.

As Blood stasis often goes together with *Qi* deficiency, *Huang Qi* is one of the herbs that are most commonly combined with Blood stasis removing medicinals. It is found in: *Huang Qi Fang Feng Tang* (Astragalus Ledebouriella Decoction), *Ai Fu Nuan Gong Wan* (Artemisia Cyperus Pill), *Bu Yang Huan Wu Tang* (Five-Tenth Decoction), *Huang Qi Tao Hong Tang* (Astragalus Persica Carthamus Decoction), *Huang Qi Chi Feng Tang* (Astragalus Red Wind Decoction), *Huang Qi Gan Cao Tang* (Astragalus Liquorice Decoction), *Ke Bao Li Su Tang* (Guaranteed Resuscitation Decoction), *Zhu Yang Zhi Yang Tang* (Anti-Itching Yang Tonifying Decoction), *Zhu Wei He Rong Tang* (*Wei* and *Ying* Strengthening Decoction), *Bao Yuan Hua Chi Tang* (Origin Protecting Anti-Dysentery Decoction) and *Zhi Xie Tiao Zhong Tang* (Anti-Diarrhoea Centre Regulating Decoction).

Gan Cao, Radix Glycyrrhizae Uralensis

It is used:

1. to increase Heart and Spleen function in the treatment of *Qi* deficiency syndromes in these organs;
2. as a spasmolytic and antitussive for coughing and for peptic ulcers;
3. as an antiphlogistic for sore throat, furuncles and carbuncles;
4. for detoxification in drug poisoning or overdose.

New pharmacological research and new clinical usage

Gan Cao has an antiallergic, corticoid-like effect on the body, yet also has antiulcerative and antineoplastic actions. It lowers blood lipids and has a virustatic effect on different lentiviruses and other viruses such as herpes simplex, herpes zoster and the HIV virus.

Its modern applications therefore comprise endocrine diseases such as Addison's disease, Duchenne's disease, viral hepatitis, AIDS, ulcers, and otitis and rhinitis of various origins.

It is an ingredient of the following Blood stasis removing formulas: as Glycyrrhiza (*Gan Cao*) is generally used as a harmonizing ingredient in all formulas, it is often to be found in Blood stasis removing formulas, for example in *Xue Fu Zhu Yu*

Tang (Anti-Stasis Chest Decoction), *Ge Xia Zhu Yu Tang* (Anti-Stasis Abdomen Decoction), *Tao Hong Cheng Qi Tang* (*Qi* Rectifying Persica Carthamus Decoction), *Da Huang Zhe Chong Wan* (Rheum Eupolyphaga Pill), *Shu Jing Huo Xue Tang* (Relaxing the Vessels Decoction), *Sheng Hua Tang* (Generate Change Decoction), *Wen Jing Tang* (Menses Warming Decoction), *Fu Yuan Huo Xue Tang* (Blood Invigorating Recovery Decoction).

6. *YIN* OR *YANG* TONIFYING MEDICINALS

Bai Shao, Radix Paeonia Lactiflorae

This belongs to the group of *Yin* tonifying medicinals. It is used:

1. to nourish Blood and to regulate menstrual flow in the treatment of menstrual disorders;
2. as a spasmolytic and analgetic in headaches, abdominal pain, spasms of the leg muscles etc.

New pharmacological research and new clinical usage
Modern research was able to demonstrate that *Bai Shao* is one of the medicinals with the broadest effects on the immune system. On the one hand, it can stimulate the immune response in people with low immunity; on the other hand, it has an inhibiting effect on autoimmune reactions and allergies. In addition, it has antiphlogistic, analgetic, antibacterial, febrifugal and calming actions. It increases tissue tolerance towards hypoxia, protects liver cells from toxic damage and lowers blood pressure by dilating peripheral vessels.

Its modern applications therefore comprise all kinds of immune disorders, hepatitis B, acute pancreatitis and trigeminal neuralgia.

It is an ingredient of the following Blood stasis removing formulas: *Da Huang Zhe Chong Wan* (Rheum Eupolyphaga Pill), *Shu Jing Huo Xue Tang* (Relaxing the Vessels Decoction), *Ai Fu Nuan Gong Wan* (Artemisia Cyperus Pill), *Wen Jing Tang* (Menses Warming Decoction), *Ke Bao Li Su Tang* (Guaranteed Resuscitation Decoction), *Zhi Xie Tiao Zhong Tang* (Anti-Diarrhoea Centre Regulating Decoction), *Zhu Wei He Rong Tang* (*Wei* and *Ying* Strengthening Decoction).

Wu Zhu Yu, Shan Zhu Yu, Shan Yu Rou, Fructus Evodia

It belongs to the group of *Yang* tonifying medicinals. It is used:

1. to warm the Centre, dispel Cold pathogens, e.g. diarrhoea due to deficiency of Spleen or Kidney *Yang*;
2. to normalize smooth flow of *Qi* in ascending *Qi* of the Stomach, or Liver *Qi* disorders such as vomiting, sour regurgitation, stomach pain, stabbing hypochondriac pain, a wiry or weak pulse;
3. in the treatment of hernias such as inguinal or scrotal hernias;
4. in the flaring-up of Fire as in aphthae or oral ulcers.

New pharmacological research and new clinical usage
Wu Zhu Yu slightly raises body temperature and promotes intestinal motility. Furthermore, it has antiulcerative and hepatoprotective actions and alleviates pain; it has an antibiotic effect on bacteria, viruses and endoparasites (also: vibrio cholera, ascarides). All these correspond to the classical usage of the medicinal. Apart from that, it markedly lowers blood pressure, stimulates the CNS and uterine muscles and has an antiparasitic effect on ectoparasites such as dermatomycoses.

Its modern applications therefore comprise classical indications such as a variety of intestinal disorders (vomiting, diarrhoea, enteritis etc.) and oral ulcers, as well as new indications such as uterine bleeding, hypertension, irritable bowel disease and skin conditions such as eczema, neurodermatitis and dermatomycoses.

It is an ingredient of the Blood stasis removing formula *Ke Bao Li Su Tang* (Guaranteed Resuscitation Decoction) as well as being used in modern formulas like the one in Case study 4.7 'Blood stasis due to loss of Blood' (Blood and *Yin* deficiency) in Chapter 4.

7. HEAT COOLING MEDICINALS

Sheng Di Huang, Radix Rehmanniae

It is used:

1. to cool down Heat and especially Blood Heat, for example in infectious diseases with Heat pathogens in the Blood level (haemorrhages, exanthema);
2. to nourish the *Yin* and generate body fluids, for example in *Yin* deficiency or continuous low fever, constipation, dry mouth and 'bone-steaming fever' or in the case of damaged body fluids and diabetic states;
3. to cool down Heart Fire blazing causing aphthae, irritability, insomnia, afternoon fever and so on.

New pharmacological research and new clinical usage

Due to its different way of preparation from *Shou Di* (Rehmannia Preparata), *Sheng Di Huang* (Rehmannia) contains different ingredients and therefore has different actions and indications. It lowers glucocorticoid levels and influences the whole adrenocorticoid system, regulates the cAMP β-adrenoreceptor relationship and coronary circulation as well as blood pressure in both directions. Furthermore, it inhibits leukaemia and tissue aging by binding free radicals; it also has antibacterial properties and stops bleeding.

Today, apart from its classical applications, it is used in rheumatoid arthritis and skin diseases such as neurodermatitis and urticaria.

It is an ingredient of the following Blood stasis removing formulas: *Xue Fu Zhu Yu Tang* (Anti-Stasis Chest Decoction), *Ai Fu Nuan Gong Wan* (Artemisia Cyperus Pill), *Die Da Wan* (Trauma Pill), *Jie Du Huo Xue Tang* (Detoxifying, Blood Invigorating Decoction), *Hui Yan Zhu Yu Tang* (Anti-Stasis Epiglottis Decoction), *Shu Jing Huo Xue Tang* (Relaxing the Vessels Decoction), *Tao Hong Si Wu Tang* (Persica Carthamus Four Ingredients Decoction) and *Yang Yin Tong Bi Tang* (Yin Nourishing *Bi* Dissolving Decoction).

Pu Gong Yin, Herba Taraxacum

It is used:

1. in Heat and Fire-toxins (e.g. sore throat) or Fire Dampness pathogens in the Liver (jaundice, red, swollen eyes and so on);
2. in Heat disorders of other organs (emphysema, *Lin* syndrome with painful urination);

3. in Heat-toxins of the skin, such as furuncles, carbuncles, abscesses, lymphadenitis;
4. in insufficient lactation or breast abscess with Heat syndromes.

New pharmacological research and new clinical usage

Pu Gong Yin is one of the most potent anti-inflammatory medicinals and has an antiseptic effect on a vast number of microorganisms. It stimulates the immune system and has antiulcerative, cholagogue and hepatoprotective actions.

It is used in many acute infections, e.g. respiratory infections, parotitis, tonsillitis, gastritis, retinitis, mastitis, old age prostatitis, appendicitis, nephritis, purulent dermatitis and other inflammations like gastric ulcer, haemorrhoids and anal fissures.

It is an ingredient of modern formulas such as the one in Case study 4.5 'Blood stasis due to exogenous pathogenic Heat' in Chapter 4.

Qian Cao, Radix Rubiae Cordifoliae

Qian Cao belongs to the group of Blood cooling and stopping bleeding medicinals. It is used:

1. to treat all kinds of bleeding due to Heat in the Blood, e.g. uterine bleeding, coughing of blood, bloody stools etc.
2. in pain due to Blood stasis, as it is Blood invigorating and able to dispel stasis, especially in injuries, chest pain and lower abdominal pain.

New pharmacological research and new clinical usage

The root has bacteriostatic action against streptococci and staphylococci as well as against several kinds of viruses (influenza). Furthermore, it has a relaxing effect on smooth muscles. It is antitussive and promotes expectoration.

In North China, gynaecologists like prescribing it together with Blood invigorating medicinals (e.g. in uterine bleeding and amenorrhoea). In dermatology, it is combined with other Blood cooling medicinals in the treatment of skin diseases and carbuncles. Moreover, it is used together with medicinals that stop bleeding to treat ulcerative colitis, epistaxis and haemoptysis.

MEDICINALS OF OTHER GROUPS WHICH ARE FREQUENTLY COMBINED WITH BLOOD INVIGORATING MEDICINALS

She Xiang, Moschus

It belongs to the orifices opening medicinals. It is used:

1. as a central nervous system stimulant in the treatment of unconsciousness due to high fever, acute infections and apoplexy;
2. to improve circulation and reduce inflammation in the treatment of painful swellings due to abscesses, carbuncles, furuncles and Buerger's disease (presenile spontaneous gangrene).

New pharmacological research and new clinical usage

In small amounts, *She Xiang* has a stimulating effect on the CNS, whilst in larger amounts, it has an inhibitory effect. In addition, it has an androsterone effect on the body and is abortive in early pregnancies. It stimulates adrenergic β-receptors and increases heart muscle contractility, memory function and immunity. It has analgetic, antiphlogistic and antiulcerative actions, and is effective in the smallest amounts (less than 1 g).

Its modern applications are: CHD, migraine, chronic hepatitis, early stage liver cirrhosis; it is also used in the external treatment of rheumatic pain and abscesses.

It is an ingredient of the following Blood stasis removing formulas: *Tong Qiao Huo Xue Tang* (Orifices Opening, Blood Invigorating Decoction), *Qi Li San* (Seven *Li* Powder), *Yu Long Gao* (Jade Dragon Paste, also called *Shen Yu Gao*) and *Tong Jing Zhu Yu Tang* (Anti-Stasis Exanthema Decoction).

Di Long, Lumbricus

It belongs to the group of Liver-Wind extinguishing medicinals. It is used:

1. to cool down Heat, in convulsions and cramps with high fever;
2. to remove obstructions from the vessels; used in asthma and in the treatment of rheumatoid pain and after apoplexies, particularly if there is hemiplegia;
3. externally in leg ulcers, eczema, erysipelas and burns.

New pharmacological research and new clinical usage

Di Long has febrifugal, calming, antiasthmatic, anti-arrhythmic (in vitro) and spermicidal actions, and lowers blood pressure. In addition, it counteracts shock and has antihistamine effects. It stimulates the smooth muscles of the uterus and inhibits blood clotting, thrombosis formation and tumour growth.

Its modern applications comprise chronic bronchial asthma, chronic bronchitis, whooping cough, hypertension, thrombosis, epidemic parotitis, sequelae of meningitis and herpes zoster.

It is an ingredient of the following Blood stasis removing formulas: *Bu Yang Huan Wu Tang* (Five-Tenth Decoction), *Shen Tong Zhu Yu Tang* (Anti-Stasis Pain Decoction) and *Tong Jing Zhu Yu Tang* (Anti-Stasis Exanthema Decoction).

Mang Xiao, Mirabilitum

This belongs to the group of purging medicinals. It is used as a purgative in the treatment of constipation and externally for acute mastitis. Although purgatives are rarely combined with Blood invigorating medicinals, *Da Huang* (Rheum) and *Mang Xiao* (Mirabilitum) are occasionally considered for the treatment of abscesses and digestive stagnation with Blood stasis. A review of the usage of *Da Huang* can be found in Part 1 of this chapter under the heading 'Group II: 26 Blood moving medicinals' (p. 59) and in Part 3 under 'Combinations of different Blood stasis medicinals' (p. 79).

New pharmacological research and new clinical usage

Mang Xiao has purgative, diuretic and antiphlogistic actions. Apart from its function of clearing the intestines, it is also administered for gallbladder-related pain, chronic renal failure, purulent abdominal infections, swellings after fractures, appendicitis, mastitis, fallopian tube blockage, thrombophlebitis, painful and swollen haemorrhoids, manic-depressive states, hordeolum sty and constipation.

Mang Xiao is part of the following Blood stasis removing formulas: *Tao Hong Cheng Qi Tang* (Qi Rectifying Persica Carthamus Decoction), and *Zhi*

Tong Mo Yao San (Analgesic Myrrh Powder With Additions).

SUMMARY

Blood invigorating medicinals can nowadays be divided into three categories: Blood harmonizing medicinals (*He Xue Yao*), Blood moving medicinals (*Huo Xue Yao*) and Blood stasis breaking medicinals (*Po Xue, Qu Xue*). They can be distinguished according to their strength and their other qualities, for example nourishing, cooling, stopping bleeding and many more.

According to the most recent pharmacological research, Blood invigorating medicinals can be successfully employed in the following illnesses:

1. Heart diseases: CHD, angina pectoris and myocardial infarction are typical Blood stasis diseases. Blood invigorating medicinals increase heart function and heart muscle blood and oxygen supply. Typical representatives of this group are, for example, *Chuan Xiong* (Ligusticum), *Dan Shen* (Salvia Miltiorrhiza) and *Chi Shao* (Paeonia Rubra).
   a. In addition, Blood invigorating medicinals lower blood viscosity, which is blood flow resistance. This increases tissue circulation and prevents blood fluid losses through the capillary walls.
   b. Most Blood invigorating medicinals relax and dilate peripheral vessels, arterioles and venules of the lung and thus reduce pressure on the heart, lower blood pressure in the pulmonary artery and in this way decrease cardiac preload.

2. Cerebral diseases: Blood invigorating medicinals significantly improve circulation of blood through the brain in patients with infarctions and multiple infarctions. Moreover, Blood invigorating medicinals can reduce thrombocyte aggregation and surface activity of erythrocytes, thrombocytes and coagulation factor VIII. In addition, the activity of fibrinolysin (plasmin) is increased. They have also shown excellent results in epidemic encephalitis with acute diffuse intravascular coagulation.

3. Respiratory diseases: Blood invigorating medicinals relax spasms even in the smallest vessels and reduce vesicular damage to the alveolar tissue of the lung. They protect capillary walls and decrease thrombosis and thrombocyte aggregation. Lung function in general and lung microcirculation are improved and the dangers of inflammatory changes are reduced. In this way, oxygen supply is increased.
   a. The most marked effect of Blood invigorating medicinals is observed in lung diseases in infantile pulmonary adenovirus infections, tuberculosis of the lung, chronic obstructive lung disease and cor pulmonale.

4. Kidney diseases: in illnesses such as nephrotic syndrome, chronic glomerular nephritis and kidney failure, there is always a high tendency towards clotting. In this case, it is immaterial whether this high tendency towards clotting only affects kidney function or contributes to the development of the above named diseases. It poses an immediate danger which can be easily reduced by prescribing Blood invigorating medicinals. Not only do these medicinals improve microcirculation and lower blood viscosity, they also increase blood flow and control thrombocyte aggregation.
   a. In addition, *Mu Dan Pi* (Moutan), *Tao Ren* (Persica) etc. prevent organ rejection in kidney transplantation and prolong survival time.

5. Hepatitis: a pathologic product that always arises in hepatitis is Blood stasis and this can equally lead to typical consequences of hepatitis (e.g. lassitude). By administering Blood invigorating medicinals, causative factors of hepatitis can be removed, symptoms can be alleviated and normal function can be restored.

   The use of Blood invigorating medicinals has proven to be of great value in severe hepatitis, chronic aggressive hepatitis, ascites due to liver cirrhosis and acute viral hepatitis. In addition, recovery from jaundice can be accelerated and the symptoms of icteric hepatitis can be alleviated.

6. Intestinal diseases: repeated enemas with Blood invigorating medicinals were able to successfully treat ulcerative colitis in China. Oral administration of Blood invigorating, cooling and detoxifying medicinals proved to be very effective in postoperative intestinal adhesion. Peristalsis as well as the absorption rate of infectious fluid in the abdominal cavity was increased, thus enabling the adhesions to be dissolved and normalization to be attained. Oral administration of San Qi (Notoginseng) both in Crohn's disease and in ulcerative colitis showed a significant reduction of volume of blood in the stool.

7. Diabetes: clinical studies were able to demonstrate that diabetics generally have a highly elevated blood viscosity, decelerated erythrocyte electrophoresis, a marked rise in thrombocytes and disturbances in microcirculation. In this case, Blood invigorating medicinals not only improve blood viscosity, but also reduce the dangers of diabetic sequelae such as heart disease and cerebrovascular disease.

8. Gynaecology: Blood invigorating medicinals such as Yi Mu Cao (Leonurus), Hong Hua (Carthamus) etc. not only regulate all kinds of menstrual disorders, but also take care of postpartum uterine bleeding and incomplete uterine involution. Moreover, Blood invigorating medicinals are used in chronic pelvic inflammations, Polycystic Ovarian Syndrome (PCOS), also known as Stein-Leventhal Syndrome, extra-uterine pregnancies and many other conditions. Additionally, these medicinals show a marked effect in postmenopausal syndromes and the elimination of side effects of long-term oestrogen administration.

9. Dermatology and immune system: San Leng (Spargani), E Zhu (Curcuma Ezhu), Dan Shen (Salvia Miltiorrhiza), Ru Xiang (Olibanum), Mo Yao (Myrrha) and many other medicinals have great effect in treating psoriasis. Blood invigorating medicinals, which also remove obstructions from the vessels, are used in sar-coidosis of the lower limbs, scleroderma, lupus erythematosus and rubella infections. Furthermore, Blood invigorating medicinals can improve microcirculation disorders due to disturbed immune reactions and can increase oxygen supply in Cold-induced erythematous dermatitis (see also Case study 4.4 'Blood stasis due to exogenous pathogenic Cold' in Chapter 4 (p. 28).

10. Mind and nervous system: clinical examinations of the last years have shown a clear relationship between Blood stasis and the mind. For example, patients suffering from insomnia, schizophrenia and neuroses showed deviations from normal values of microcirculation upon examination of their nail beds. This normalized after administration of Blood invigorating medicinals.

    Schizophrenia, panic attacks, psychoses and other mental diseases are treated with Tao Ren (Persica), Yu Jin (Curcuma), Chi Shao (Paeonia Rubra), Dan Shen (Salvia Miltiorrhiza), E Zhu (Curcuma Ezhu) and many other medicinals. As they do not have any side effects, they have proven themselves over antipsychotic drugs.

11. Sense organs: Blood invigorating medicinals are vasodilative and have an anticonvulsive effect on retinal arterioles. In this way, they improve circulation and prevent ischemia of the eye. They are used to treat atrophy of the optic nerve, reduce arterial and venous pressure and to stop haemorrhaging in the eye. Additionally, they increase the absorption of blood clots.
    a. Research over the past years has shown that in chronic glaucoma, blood viscosity is significantly raised; thus, Blood invigorating medicinals are indicated. They are effective in tinnitus, hardness of hearing, chronic blocked nose, nasal polyps, epistaxis, rosacea nose, vocal cord nodules and many other conditions.

12. Oncology: Blood invigorating medicinals and anti-cancer drugs are a successful combination for acute leukaemia and nasal cancer. This increases the success rate and reduces

side effects. At the same time, the danger of metastasis is reduced.

a. *E Zhu* (Curcuma Ezhu), administered on its own, demonstrated excellent results in the treatment of early-stage cervical tumours.

Common combinations amongst Blood invigorating medicinals are given in Box 7.5 on p. 80 of this chapter.

Generally, it can be noted that a combination of Blood invigorating medicinals with other Blood invigorating medicinals, amongst which are medicinals of a cooling, warming, *Qi* tonifying, *Qi* moving, Phlegm transforming, dispersing or purging nature, increases the total effect. Therefore, integrating such combinations into formulas is the treatment of choice in Blood stasis and its related illnesses.

Chapter **8**

Blood stasis in the practice of TCM – formulas and acupuncture

Although it has the smaller part within the treatment plan, acupuncture will be considered first, for the following three reasons:

1. Acupuncture works at the *Qi* level and can only reach the Blood via the *Qi*. Herbal treatment, however, can have a direct effect on the Blood level, which is necessary in Blood stasis.

2. In the classical works on acupuncture there were never any indications given with regard to syndromes, rather they related directly to specific symptoms. In modern Chinese literature point combinations are composed according to experience of Western diseases, not according to traditional syndromes.

3. Blood stasis is a syndrome that manifests in various parts of the body, but it is still of a universal nature: this means that Blood flow is disturbed everywhere in the body. Only a drug that reaches everywhere can tackle such a general disturbance. Acupuncture works better in cases of local Blood stasis, so there may exist point combinations for CHD, apoplexy, psoriasis, dysmenorrhoea and so on, but no combinations for the whole body.

The interested practitioner will find countless point combinations for conditions with Blood stasis listed under the respective disease in the relevant literature (e.g. Maciocia). To every formula I have also added a few points and combinations, which of course should be modified – as well as the formula – according to each patient. The following paragraphs deal mainly with the general treatment of Blood stasis.

ACUPUNCTURE IN THE CASE OF BLOOD STASIS

How to treat impure Blood: the pathogen invades the collaterals and from there also the channels. Eventually, it accumulates in the blood vessels. Its hot or cold nature has not developed yet, it behaves like the breaking waves: sometimes they come and sometimes they depart. Therefore, the symptoms are not always present. The treatment must seize and stop the pathogen. After it has been stopped it will accumulate in one place and then needs to be discharged together with the impure (static) Blood. If it stays in the channels for a longer period of time, blockage with Bi *syndrome will develop.*

(Taken from the *'Zhen Fang Jiu Li'* (*Six Chapters on Acupuncture Methods*) by Wu Kun (1551–1620)).

The successful treatment of Blood stasis in TCM is usually achieved by means of the prescription of herbs (by using Blood invigorating medicinals etc.). Acupuncture can also contribute significantly towards increasing the flow of blood, removing obstruction from the vessels and moving *Qi* and Blood. Furthermore, many diseases that were caused by Blood stasis present with pain, which can be effectively treated with acupuncture.

San Yin Jiao (SP 6) is usually selected for general disorders of Blood. Another important point is the *Hui*-Meeting point of Blood, *Ge Shu* (BL 17). The literature always mentions *Lie Que* (LU 7) for blood diseases, and the bleeding technique on *Wei Zhong* (BL 40) using the three-edged needle (*San Ling Zhen*) is also often noted.

To stop bleeding the appropriate points are LIV 1 and SP 1 with SP 10.

To treat Blood stasis due to emotions (e.g. Liver-*Qi* stagnation) the appropriate points are HR 7, P 7 and DU 26.

The general points that are effective for Blood stasis include LIV 2, LIV3, SP 6, L.I. 11, P 5 and BL 60.

The methods described below are now frequently employed in China to invigorate Blood in case of Blood stasis.

1. Blood invigorating manipulation of the *Luo* vessels (collaterals)

In the chapter 'Twelve sources of the nine needles' of the '*Ling Shu*', it is stated: 'Whenever acupuncture is used, . . . accumulated and old Blood should be removed.' In the chapter 'Explanation of the needles' in the '*Su Wen*' it is stated: 'in order to remove accumulated and old Blood, one must allow the Blood to come out.' In the '*Ling Shu*' chapter 'Concerning needles', '*Luo* vessel pricking' is mentioned which is supposed to mean bloody needling (bloodletting using a three-edged needle). Modern research has shown that this method is efficient in clinical routine. It is used especially for headache (*Tai Yang*, extra point M-HN 9 – Deadman nomenclature) and hip pain (puncture *Wei Zhong*, BL 40, in the popliteal fossa) due to Blood stasis.

2. Method for invigorating Blood and moving *Qi*

In the chapter 'Ascending pain' of the '*Su Wen*' it is stated: 'When pathogenic Cold invades the channels, accumulates and coagulates, Blood will leave the blood vessels and flow outwards, thus Blood is deficient and *Qi* cannot flow through the blood vessels and is blocked, so a sudden pain arises.' The same chapter continues: 'Internal damage due to depression and gloominess makes the *Qi* rebellious and it flows upwards, whereby the six *Shu* points become obstructed and the moisturizing *Qi* cannot move freely, so Blood accumulates and fails to disperse, Body Fluids become concentrated.' If left untreated, this will lead to all sorts of gatherings (abdominal masses).

This suggests that exterior pathogens and disturbed emotions can lead to internal damage, which in turn results in *Qi* stagnation and Blood stasis. As *Qi* is the commander of Blood, according to the '*Nei Jing*', moving *Qi* in case of Blood stasis due to *Qi* stagnation can also invigorate the Blood. The following points are appropriate for this: *Qi* moving points such as *Tan Zhong* (in the middle of the breast, *Hui*-Meeting point of the *Qi*, REN 17) for the Upper Burner, *Zhong Wan* (on the midline of the abdomen, *Hui*-Meeting point of the *Fu* organs, REN 12) for the Middle Burner and *Qi Hai* (on the midline of the lower abdomen, Sea of *Qi*, REN 6) for the Lower Burner. Blood invigorating points like *Ge Shu* (*Hui*-Meeting point of the Blood, BL 17) combined with *Xue Hai* (this name means: 'Sea of Blood', SP 10) are the main points for the whole body; *Nei Guan* (P 6) is an important point for the treatment of heart and vessel diseases; *Zu San Li* (ST 36) together with *Cheng Shan* (BL 57) are important points in the treatment of gastrointestinal diseases with Blood stasis; *Wei Zhong* (BL 40) is an important point for back and hip pain that is caused by Blood stasis.

3. Method for invigorating Blood and warming the channels

As the '*Nei Jing*' says: 'When there is a constitutional internal deficient Cold condition (due to deficiency of the warming nature of *Yang*), the channels and blood vessels are blocked and impenetrable.' This means that for interior and exterior Cold, which 'froze' the Blood and so led to Blood stasis, the principle of warming the channels is appropriate. For this effect one should first puncture *Da Zhui* (DU 14) and *Qu Chi* (L.I. 11) with warm needles (needles with moxa on the tip) to expel Cold from the exterior. Subsequently, one should use warm needling and moxibustion on the back *Shu* points (including *Ashi* points), followed by a *Ba-Guan* (Chinese cupping method) treatment.

4. Method for invigorating the Blood and moisturizing *Yin*

Internal Heat can be caused by *Yin* deficiency as well, resulting in a deficient Fire syndrome, which concentrates and coagulates the Blood. Blood stasis is therefore the result of a protracted *Yin* deficiency. The root treatment focuses on using a Blood invigorating and *Yin* moisturizing method: the essential *Mu* and *Shu* points of the *Yin* channels are selected, such as *San Yin Jiao* (SP 6), *Yin Ling Quan* (SP 9), *Tai Xi* (KID 3), *Shen Shu* (BL 23), *Gan Shu* (BL 18), *Pi Shu* (BL 20), *Guan Yuan*

(REN 4), *Qi Hai* (REN 6) and so on. At every session only 2–3 points should be chosen to avoid furthering the deficiency by using too many needles.

As a matter of principle, acupuncture is a method that consumes *Qi* despite the fact that 'tonifying' is commonly mentioned. As the body does not receive any new energy (except when moxibustion is used), the energy present in the body is merely either accumulated, or guided to one point (i.e. tonification). A genuine supplementation can only be accomplished by using moxa, herbal prescriptions, diet and external *Qi* in *Qi Gong*. For this reason, if conditions of long-term deficiency present, medicinals should be prescribed in addition. In this way, acupuncture and herbal treatment can complement each other excellently.

According to modern research, the application of Blood invigorating acupuncture proved very efficient for the following diseases: autoimmune diseases, ischemic apoplexy, schizophrenia, sclerodermatitis, protruding of the eyes related to hyperthyroidism and arthritic diseases of the rheumatic sphere. The underlying principle of Blood invigorating acupuncture is assumed to be primarily related to regulatory mechanisms of the immune system and metabolism. A disturbed immune reaction is one of the aetiological pathogenic influences of Blood stasis, which I was able to prove in my experimental studies in China.[1]

There is also the possibility of removing stagnation from the channels by needle pricking with the three-edged needle (*San Ling Zhen*) followed by cupping; this method also applies in the case of Heat, pain and swelling, provided an excess syndrome is evident. Treatment examples are especially acute erysipelas, rheumatoid arthritis, stiffness of the fingers (for which the 4 extra channel points *Si Feng* can be used) and acute Blood stasis due to traumata.

[1] GR Neeb: 'Experimental generation in animal models of the chronic Blood stasis syndrome and investigation of its pathological consequences' published at the 1998 Annual Congress of the Society for Integrated Chinese and Western Medicine, Tianjin, as well as in various journals. Excerpts available in the *Zeitschrift für TCM* Jan 1999, p. 48 ff.

As mentioned before, one should not forget that only syndrome differentiation can provide a precise treatment plan. For this reason, this information is to be understood as a guideline only. More detailed specifications concerning the treatment of the individual syndromes with acupuncture are provided together with the formulas and should be equally as open to modification as the prescriptions.

The method often used in Taiwan according to Master Tong (*Dong Shi Zhen Jiu*) also promises good results when treating diseases related to Blood stasis. However, non-conventional points are predominantly selected for this method, so no specifications can be made here. One of the special characteristics is needle pricking all the points on the back, i.e. they may be needled using a sterile lancet, which is far easier than the three-edged needle used in orthodox acupuncture. This method has proven very successful in practice and is therefore very popular amongst orthodox acupuncturists in Taiwan.

In the '*Nei Jing*', acute Blood stasis due to injuries accounted for a quarter of all causes of Blood stasis, these causes being traumata, coagulations due to Cold, emotional causes and protracted consumptive diseases. There, it is stated: 'Injury resulting from a fall generates poor Blood in the interior, which will not resolve.' (Chapter 58 '*Ling Shu*', 'Thievish Wind'). This quotation refers to acute Blood stasis accompanied by bruises, which in ancient times as well as nowadays responds well to needle pricking.

Professor Unschuld (Munich) holds the opinion that in China's antiquity at the time of the '*Nei Jing*', acupuncture points were predominantly used in this way,[2] because fine needle acupuncture had yet to become more prevalent; this happened at a later stage. This could be another indication of the great age of Master Tong's method.

FURTHER REFERENCES FROM ACUPUNCTURE CLASSICS

'*Zhen Jiu Zi Shang Jing*' (Experiences with Acu-Moxa therapy, 1220) by Wang Zhi-Zhong:

Shi Men (REN 5) treats postpartum flow of Blood, accumulations of Blood and metrorrhagia.
Tian Shu (ST 25) and *Zhong Ji* (REN 3) treat accumulations of Blood and blood clots.
Lou Gu (SP 7) and *Qu Quan* (LIV 8) treat Blood stasis and abdominal masses (*Jia*).
Qiu Xu (GB 40) and *Zhong Fu* (LU 1) treat Blood stasis in the interior.

'*Yi Xue Ru Men*' (Elementary Medicine, 1575) by Li Chan:

In the case of Blood stasis in the chest and abdomen select *Zu San Li* (ST 36).
In the case of Blood stasis in the chest select *Ju Gu* (L.I. 16).

'*Zhen Jiu Da Cheng*' (Great Compendium of Acupuncture, 1601) by Yang Ji-Zhou:

If Blood becomes concentrated select *Xuan Zhong* (GB 39).
Concentrated Blood, accumulated in the chest and abdomen, treat with *Shen Shu* (BL 23).

ESSENTIAL FORMULAS AND ACUPUNCTURE IN THE TREATMENT OF BLOOD STASIS

Blood regulating prescriptions consist of regulating and other medicinals and are designed to activate Blood and its flow, to stimulate Blood circulation or to stop bleeding. They are generally used in the treatment of haemorrhaging and Blood stasis. All Blood syndromes are first differentiated on the basis of Cold/Heat and deficiency/excess.

Blood regulating prescriptions can be classified further into formulas that invigorate Blood and stop bleeding. This book will mainly focus on Blood invigorating formulas.

During the diagnosis one should also be aware how urgent the condition is: if the syndrome is acute and there are severe symptoms (e.g. heavy bleeding or pain due to stasis), one should first concentrate on the symptoms and then on the cause.

If the syndrome is of a chronic nature and symptoms are mild, one should concentrate on the treatment of the causes. The use of Blood invigor-

---

[2] Unschuld, *Medicine in China: A History of Ideas*, p. 96, middle paragraph (see Appendix 7).

ating medicinals may easily weaken *Qi* and Blood, especially if prescribed for a longer period of time. For this reason, *Qi* and Blood tonifying medicinals are usually added. This will protect the body from damage to *Qi* and Blood. On the other hand, stopping bleeding may easily lead to Blood stasis in the interior, so Blood activating medicinals are sometimes added to prevent Blood stasis from forming inside the body. In contrast, *San Qi* (Radix Notoginseng) has been shown to be able to both invigorate Blood and stop bleeding.

Furthermore, Blood invigorating prescriptions should be used with care during pregnancy or in women with excessive menstruation (hypermenorrhoea), as these prescriptions have a Blood stasis dispelling character.

They are often used in the treatment of, for example, traumata accompanied by swelling and pain, abdominal pain due to Blood stasis or hemiplegia due to stagnation of Blood in the channels and collaterals. The formulas may also be used in the initial stages of ulcerative diseases, amenorrhoea and dysmenorrhoea, but also for continuous postpartum haemorrhaging.

One word of caution to all inexperienced practitioners of Chinese herbal medicine: the prescription of individual or several medicinals that are aimed at the same pathology, which is commonly practised here in the West, is rather the exception in China. It is often the case that medicinals not targeting the main symptoms are prescribed in order to reduce side effects or to prevent potential consequences of the disease.

The experience and knowledge of such combinations have been used successfully for many centuries, and these are now being verified in terms of pharmacological research. Experiments with protein-induced arthritis in laboratory rats showed that monotherapy with decocted *Chou Wu Tong* (Clerodendrum trichotomum) or *Xi Xian Cao* (Herba Siegesbeckia orientalis) had no effect on arthritis, whereas the combined prescription in a ratio of 2 : 1 led to a significant reduction.[3] Because of this, (especially in the study of prescribing med-

icinals in TCM) the indication of certain traditional combinations should not be ignored simply because there might be no apparent and direct relationship with the main syndromes treated by the formula.

In China it is the custom to modify the formula according to the situation; however, here in the West this should only be practised by those familiar with the action of the medicinals and those who have gained sufficient experience. Experimenting at the expense of the patient should be avoided at all costs.

For the advanced practitioner the flexible use of prescriptions is the desired aim of phytotherapy, which according to the World Health Organization (WHO) is the suggested object of medicine in the twenty first century. I would go as far as to argue that all standard prescriptions should only act as reference material and there is no need to learn them by heart, provided the practitioner is totally familiar with the medicinals and is able to use them flexibly to compose individualized prescriptions. How were the first formulas conceived, if not in this way?

In the next part of the chapter, the 32 essential formulas for the treatment of Blood stasis are categorized as follows:

1. Acute local Blood stasis due to traumata and infections that modify the vessels' permeability.
2. Chronic generalized Blood stasis characterized by pain or other symptoms.
3. Chronic local Blood stasis in distinct areas of the body, such as the head, chest, abdomen, lower abdomen.
4. Chronic local Blood stasis conditions with mainly gynaecological indications.[4]

It should be noted that many formulas by virtue of their wide range of indications may belong to two groups at the same time. For example, **Tao Hong Si Wu Tang** (Persica Carthamus Four Ingredients Decoction) would belong to both the second and the fourth group, as it can be used for

---

[3] Ou Ming: *Chinese-English Manual of Common Used Prescriptions on Traditional Chinese Medicine*, Hong Kong, 1989 (see Appendix 7).

[4] For further details on the pathological and diagnostic differentiation of these four groups the reader is referred to the author's dissertation (see Appendix 9).

all kinds of menstrual disorders as well as for a range of diseases that were either the cause or result of Blood stasis. However, as there are far more specific formulas available for menstrual disorders, I chose to include this formula in the second group.

At times, the demarcations are blurred and the practitioner should be flexible enough in his syndrome differentiation to recognize that some of the prescriptions listed in the gynaecological group may also be suitable for male patients.

Furthermore, practitioners should understand that standard prescriptions from the classics often reflect the simplified experience of having treated many patients, whose indications have been reduced to a 'common denominator'. Nevertheless, the indispensable principle of syndrome differentiation (*Bian Zheng Lun Zhi*) strongly suggests an individualized modification of the base formula for every patient. Due to the large Chinese pharmacopoeia there are, of course, many possibilities of combining similar medicinals and thus even more standard prescriptions; however, as modern examples from China demonstrate (see Chapter 4), formulas are *always* modified to consider the exact pathological situation of the individual case.

This structure should, above all, be a guideline, not a dogma.

Boxes 8.1–8.4 show the groupings of essential formulas for Blood stasis.

Box 8.2   Group II: Generalized chronic Blood stasis (emphasis is on the syndrome)

Shen Tong Zhu Yu Tang	(Anti-Stasis Pain Decoction)
Bu Yang Huan Wu Tang	(*Yang* Tonifying Five-Tenth Decoction)
Dan Shen Yin	(Salvia Drink)
Shi Xiao San	(Sudden Smile Powder)
Shou Nian San	(Hand-made Pill)
Huo Luo Xiao Ling Dan	(Wondrous Pill to Invigorate the Channels)
Shu Jing Huo Xue Tang	(Relaxing the Vessels Decoction)
Da Huang Zhe Chong Wan	(Rheum Eupolyphaga Pill)
Di Dang Tang	(Resistance Decoction)
Tao Hong Si Wu Tang	(Persica Carthamus Four Ingredients Decoction)
Yang Yin Tong Bi Tang	(*Yin* Nourishing *Bi* Dissolving Decoction)
Dian Kuang Meng Xing Tang	(Psychosis Decoction)

Box 8.3   Group III A: Specific chronic Blood stasis (emphasis is on the location)

Tao Hong Cheng Qi Tang	(*Qi* Rectifying Persica Carthamus Decoction)
Xue Fu Zhu Yu Tang	(Anti-Stasis Chest Decoction)
Tong Qiao Huo Xue Tang	(Orifices Opening, Blood Invigorating Decoction)
Ge Xia Zhu Yu Tang	(Anti-Stasis Abdomen Decoction)
Guan Xin Er Hao Fang	(Coronary Decoction No. 2)

Box 8.1   Group I: Acute localized Blood stasis (in traumas and acute infections)

Fu Yuan Huo Xue Tang	(Blood Invigorating Recovery Decoction)
Qi Li San	(Seven *Li* Powder)
Die Da Wan	(Trauma Pill)
Jie Du Huo Xue Tang	(Detoxifying, Blood Invigorating Decoction)
Tong Jing Zhu Yu Tang	(Anti-Stasis Exanthema Decoction)
Hui Yan Zhu Yu Tang	(Anti-Stasis Epiglottis Decoction)

Box 8.4   Group III B: Specific chronic Blood stasis (commonly used formulas from gynaecology)

Shao Fu Zhu Yu Tang	(Anti-Stasis Lower Abdomen Decoction)
Gong Wai Huai Yun Fang	(Extra Uterine Pregnancy Formula)
Wen Jing Tang	(Menses Warming Decoction)
Ai Fu Nuan Gong Wan	(Artemisia Cyperus Pill)
Sheng Hua Tang	(Generate Change Decoction)
Gui Zhi Fu Ling Wan	(Cinnamon and Poria Pills)
Xia Yu XueTang	(Blood Stasis Purging Decoction)
Yong Quan San	(Gushing Spring Powder)
Xi Huang Wan	(Yellow Rhino Pills)

GROUP I: *ACUTE LOCALIZED BLOOD STASIS* (IN TRAUMAS AND ACUTE INFECTIONS)

1. *Fu Yuan Huo Xue Tang* (Blood Invigorating Recovery Decoction)

This formula is administered in the treatment of stabbing, almost unbearable pain, mostly caused by traumas. It is effective for Blood stasis in the costal area, calms the Liver and removes obstructions from the *Luo* vessels.

Ingredients

1. Rhizoma et Radix Rhei (Da Huang)	30 g
2. Radix Bupleuri (Chai Hu)	15 g
3. Radix Angelicae Sinensis (Dang Gui)	9 g
4. Semen Persicae (Tao Ren)	9 g
5. Flos Carthami (Hong Hua)	6 g
6. Squama Manitis (Chuan Shan Jia)	6 g
7. Radix Trichosanthis (Tian Hua Fen)	9 g
8. Radix Glycyrrhizae (Gan Cao)	6 g

Application

This formula is taken as a warm decoction. It can be used in all severe pain conditions due to trauma or in Liver *Qi* stagnation with Blood stasis and hypochondriac pain.

Action

1. Removes Blood stasis and invigorates Blood.
2. Calms the Liver and removes obstructions from the *Luo* vessels.

Explanation

This formula employs Rhizoma et Radix Rhei (*Da Huang*) to quickly disperse Blood stasis in the costal area and by virtue of its cold nature to cool down Heat. Radix Bupleuri (*Chai Hu*) is used to smooth the flow of stagnated Liver *Qi* and thus alleviate pain. Radix Angelicae Sinensis (*Dang Gui*) nourishes the Blood and prevents exhaustion due to Blood regulating medicinals. Semen Persicae (*Tao Ren*) and Flos Carthami (*Hong Hua*) move the Blood and dispel Blood stasis. Squama Manitis (*Chuan Shan Jia*) breaks up Blood stasis and promotes flow of *Qi* in the *Luo* vessels. Radix Trichosanthis (*Tian Hua Fen*) acts in the Blood level, drawing the action of the other medicinals to that area. At the same time, it cools down Heat and alleviates swellings. Radix Glycyrrhizae (*Gan Cao*) helps to alleviate an acute state and harmonizes the other medicinals. This formula consists mainly of Blood invigorating medicinals.

To increase the *Qi* moving effect, other medicinals like *Chuan Xiong* (Ligusticum), *Yu Jin* (Curcuma), *Ru Xiang* (Olibanum), *Mo Yao* (Myrrha), *Tu Bie Chong* (Eupolyphaga) and *Yan Hu Suo* (Corydalis) can be added.

In clinical practice, this formula is often used in painful traumas of all kinds, as it has a strong analgesic and antithrombotic effect and reduces swelling.

Suggested acupuncture treatment

The points BL 17, SP 10, LIV 14 and GB 34 can be used, with a reducing manipulation. BL 17 and SP 10 activate Blood flow and remove Blood stasis. LIV 14 regulates Liver *Qi*. GB 34 is the *He*-Sea point of the Gall-Bladder meridian and can relieve hypochondriac pain.

2. *Qi Li San* (Seven *Li* Powder)

The Chinese *Li* is a measuring unit and corresponds to 0.031 grams. Seven *Li* Powder means that the maxiumum dosage of this formula is seven *Li*, that is approximately 2.2 grams.

It activates Blood circulation, dispels Blood stasis, stops bleeding and alleviates pain. It is used externally in injuries, for example sprained ankles or fractures with Blood stasis. Clinical symptoms are, for example, local swelling, burns, bleeding due to cuts or stab wounds and similar injuries. The formula can be used internally as well as externally.

Ingredients

1. Sanguis Draconis (Xue Jie)   30 g
2. Flos Carthami (Hong Hua)   5 g
3. Resina Olibani (Ru Xiang)   5 g
4. Myrrha (Mo Yao)   5 g
5. Moschus (She Xiang)   0.4 g
6. Borneolum (Bing Pian)   0.4 g
7. Catechu (Er Cha)   7.5 g
8. Cinnabaris (Zhu Sha)   4 g
    (is no longer used)

Application
The ground powder is to be kept airtight, as it contains many volatile substances. The prescription is 0.22–2.20 g, to be taken with wine or warm water. It can also be mixed with alcohol and applied externally. Available in ready-made form.

Action
1. Activates circulation and dispels Blood stasis.
2. Alleviates pain and stops bleeding.

Indicated in injuries and traumas of all kind: Blood stasis and swelling due to bruises, spraining or fracture; bleeding due to cuts or stab wounds and similar injuries.

Explanation
The formula is a frequently used remedy for an array of symptoms caused by traumatic injuries with Blood stasis. It causes movement of Blood and *Qi*, dispels Blood stasis and stops bleeeeding and pain.

Sanguis Draconis (*Xue Jie*) is the main ingredient of this formula, and it can dispel stasis and alleviate pain and stop bleeding. Flos Carthami (*Hong Hua*) equally dispels Blood stasis and activates Blood circulation. Resina Olibani (*Ru Xiang*) and Myrrha (*Mo Yao*) activate the *Qi* and break up stasis, in order to reduce pain and swelling. Aromatic musk (*She Xiang*) and Borneolum (*Bing Pian*) activate the *Qi* and the circulation of Blood and open the meridians and *Luo* vessels. Cooling Catechu (*Er Cha*) clears Heat and improves the body's ability to retain fluids. Therefore, together with Sanguis Draconis (*Xue Jie*) it has the effect of stopping bleeding. Cinnabaris (*Zhu Sha*) calms the mind, which is also often impaired after traumatic injuries.

Suggested acupuncture treatment
In the treatment of traumas like fractures or ruptured tendons, the focus should lie predominantly on herbal treatment.

3. *Die Da Wan* (Trauma Pill)

This formula treats exhaustion, traumas of the musculoskeletal system, for example with hip joint pain, all kinds of external abcesses, and also arthritis due to pathogenic factors.

Ingredients

1. Rhizoma Rhei (*Jiu Jun*) cooked in wine
2. Rhizoma Cyperi (*Jiu Xiang Fu*) cooked in wine
3. Radix Notoginseng (*San Qi*)
4. Flos Carthami (*Hong Hua*)
5. Eupolyphaga (*Tu Bie Chong*)
6. Pyritum (*Zi Ran Tong*)
7. Radix Angelicae (*Jiu Dang Gui*) cooked in wine
8. Radix Paeoniae Rubrae (*Chi Shao*)
9. Lignum Sappan (*Su Mu*)
10. Radix Rehmanniae (*Sheng Di Huang*)

Application

Grind the ingredients in equal parts and form into balls of roughly 3 g each using honey. Take one pill twice daily with alcohol or warm water.

Action

1. Removes acute Blood stasis due to trauma or operations.
2. Alleviates pain and reduces swelling.

Typical indications are exhaustion, traumas or pain of the musculoskeletal system (fractures, tendon injuries, hip pain and many more), furuncles and all kinds of external abcesses as well as arthritic joint pain due to Wind or Dampness.

Explanation

Amongst Blood invigorating medicinals, *San Qi* and *Su Mu* work especially well in cases of pain. *Chi Shao*, *Zi Ran Tong* and the preparation *Da Huang* (*Jiu Jun*) remove Blood stasis and, together with *Sheng Di*, cool the heated Blood. At the same time, *Sheng Di* and *Dang Gui* harmonize it, as this formula contains strong Blood stasis breaking medicinals such as *Tu Bie Chong*, which concurrently reduces swellings. Simultaneously, *Xiang Fu* moves the *Qi*, so that Blood can flow better. This is also to prevent stagnated Liver *Qi* from impairing the recovery process. Altogether, the formula acts against the stasis, swellings, pain and anger that accompany a trauma.

This formula is, in different variations, available in ready-made form.

Suggested acupuncture treatment

In the treatment of traumas of the musculoskeletal system, the focus should lie predominantly on herbal treatment.

Acupuncture has proven useful as an additional therapy against the concomitant pain of traumas. Choice of points is based on local *A-Shi* (painful) points and distant points to activate *Qi* and Blood, for example SP 10 and ST 36.

4. *Jie Du Huo Xue Tang* (Detoxifying, Blood Invigorating Decoction)

This formula invigorates and cools Blood in the case of diarrhoea with vomiting and fever due to the exsiccosis induced by Blood stasis.

Ingredients	
1. Fructus Forsythiae (*Lian Qiao*)	8 g
2. Radix Puerariae (*Ge Gen*)	8 g
3. Radix Bupleuri (*Chai Hu*)	12 g
4. Radix Angelicae Sinensis (*Dang Gui*)	8 g
5. Radix Rehmanniae (*Sheng Di Huang*)	20 g
6. Radix Paeoniae Rubrae (*Chi Shao*)	12 g
7. Semen Persicae (*Tao Ren*)	32 g
8. Flos Carthami (*Hong Hua*)	20 g
9. Fructus Citri Aurantii (*Zhi Ke*)	4 g
10. Radix Glycyrrhizae (*Gan Cao*)	8 g

Application

This formula is taken as a warm decoction.

Action

1. Cools down Heat Toxins in the Blood in early-stage febrile infectious diseases (*Wen Bing*).
2. Moves the heated and dried-out Blood.

Typical indications are feverish diarrhoea with vomiting and severe loss of fluids, a tendency towards cramps due to exsiccosis, signs of dehydration such as sunken eyes etc., cold limbs, severe sweating. It should be admininstered in the early stage of febrile infectious diseases (*Wen Bing*) such as measles, meningitis, post-encephalitic syndrome and the sequelae of poliomyelitis.

Explanation

This clinically tested formula acts by cooling down Heat with *Lian Qiao*, *Chai Hu*, *Ge Gen* and *Gan Cao*. It also cools the Blood with *Sheng Di* and *Chi Shao*, amplified by the Blood invigorating medicinals *Dang Gui*, *Tao Ren* and *Hong Hua*. As *Qi* is the 'leader of Blood', a small amount of *Zhi Ke* is added to support moving the Blood. As *Dang Gui* harmonizes the Blood, it prevents exhaustion caused by the Blood moving and Blood stasis breaking medicinals. Additionally, *Gan Cao* harmonizes the effect of the medicinals.

Suggested acupuncture treatment

To accompany his formula, Wang Qing-Ren suggests needle-pricking (*Ci Lou*) the point LU 5 with a three-edged needle or a lancet.

5. *Tong Jing Zhu Yu Tang* (Anti–Stasis Exanthema Decoction)

This formula is effective in dark or purple exanthema, pustules, blotchy rash (exanthema) or in fluid filled vesicles due to acute infections.

Ingredients	
1. Semen Persicae (*Tao Ren*)	32 g
2. Flos Carthami (*Hong Hua*)	16 g
3. Radix Paeoniae Rubrae (*Chi Shao*)	12 g
4. Squama Manitis (*Shan Chuan Jia*)	16 g
5. Spina Gleditsiae Sinensis (*Zao Jiao Ci*)	24 g
6. Fructus Forsythiae (*Lian Qiao*)	12 g
7. Lumbricus (*Di Long*)	12 g
8. Radix Bupleuri (*Chai Hu*)	4 g
9. Moschus (*She Xiang*)	0.3 g

Application
This formula is taken as a warm decoction. Musk, however, is not boiled, but drunk together with the decoction.

Action
1. Strongly moves Blood and *Qi*.
2. Cools Blood Heat in febrile infectious diseases (*Wen Bing*) with exanthema.
3. Opens the orifices.

This formula acts on febrile diseases (*Wen Bing*) as well, like the aforementioned *Jie Du Huo Xue Tang*; however, it is more effective on those diseases where toxins have already come out as an exanthema and Blood stasis is more distinct. Therefore, typical indications are dark, purple exanthema of all kinds accompanied by an urge to retch, irritability and insomnia during the day and night. Recently, this formula has been used in skin diseases with Blood stasis, even if they were not related to *Wen-Bing* diseases.

Explanation
Tao Ren, *Hong Hua* and *Chi Shao* constitute three of the five pillars of herbal treatment of Wang Qing-Ren (the other two are Angelica (*Dang Gui*) and

Ligusticum (*Chuan Xiong*)). *Shan Chuan Jia* is salty, it dissolves masses and can break Blood stasis. *Chai Hu* lifts the *Qi* and *She Xiang* relieves the fever-dulled senses. *Zi Jiao Ci* invigorates the Blood, reduces swellings and brings out pus whilst *Di Long* guides the herbs into the vessels and together with *Lian Qiao* lowers the heated *Yang*.

Additions: if the stool is very dry, 8 g of Rhizoma Rhei (*Da Huang*) should be added during the last 2–5 minutes of cooking.

If, after a few days, vesicles filled with white or clear secretions start to appear, musk (*She Xiang*) should be left out and replaced with 20 g of Astagalus (*Huang Qi*). At the same time, the amounts of Squama Manitis (*Shan Jia*) and Spina Gleditsiae (*Zao Jiao Ci*) should be halved.

Eventually, after about 7–8 days, the amounts of Semen Persicae (*Tao Ren*) and Flos Carthami (*Hong Hua*) should be halved as well and Astagalus (*Huang Qi*) can be increased to 32 g.

This formula can be used for a closely disseminated smallpox rash, regardless of whether it is still covered or erupting. Alternatively, it can be administered to treat small pointed pustules that are developing into macules all over the body, or to treat pustules that have a measles-like or blotchy rash in between, or fluid-filled vesicles. The colour can be either purple, dark or black; the accompanying symptoms may feature retching, irritability, insomnia during the day and night, as well as other unfavourable signs and symptoms.

All these symptoms demonstrate that there is an obstruction of Blood in the vessels due to Blood stasis. Medicinals in this formula are neither too hot nor too cold, neither too attacking nor too purging; it truly is a well balanced formula.

6. *Hui Yan Zhu Yu Tang* (Anti–Stasis Epiglottis Decoction)

Already during the times of Wang, this formula was used to treat frequent choking when drinking liquids in patients who had had smallpox for 5 or 6 days. Nowadays, it is used for different problems of the throat and vocal cords.

Ingredients

1. Semen Persicae (*Tao Ren*)	15 g
2. Flos Carthami (*Hong Hua*)	15 g
3. Radix Glycyrrhizae (*Gan Cao*)	9 g
4. Radix Platycodi (*Jie Geng*)	12 g
5. Rhizoma Rehmanniae (*Sheng Di*)	12 g
6. Radix Angelicae (*Dang Gui*)	6 g
7. Radix Scrophulariae (*Xuan Shen*)	3 g
8. Radix Bupleuri (*Chai Hu*)	3 g
9. Pericarpium Citri Aurantii (*Zhi Ke*)	6 g
10. Radix Paeoniae Rubrae (*Chi Shao*)	6 g

Application

This formula is taken as a warm decoction.

Action

Removes Blood stasis, relieves the throat, moves *Qi* and resolves Phlegm.

This formula is indicated for choking when drinking, sore throat, vocal cord inflammation with throaty voice or loss of voice.

Suggested acupuncture treatment

To treat sore throat with Heat, needle-prick the source points of the fingers, especially SJ 1 and LU 10 and 11 and the ten extra points on the fingertips (*Shi Xuan*).

To treat loss of voice, a point combination called *Shi Yin* (Loss of Voice No. 88.32) from the Dong family tradition (*Dong Shi Zhenjiu*), used mainly in Taiwan, has proven very beneficial. The first of the two points is located with the patient sitting down and his knees bent. It is on the inner (medial) side of the knee joint, in line with BL 54 behind the head of the tibia. The second point is to be found 2 *cun* (body inches) below.

GROUP II: GENERALIZED CHRONIC BLOOD STASIS (EMPHASIS IS ON THE SYNDROME)

7. Shen Tong Zhu Yu Tang (Anti-Stasis Pain Decoction)

This formula is especially suited to treating Blood stasis with severe pain due to arthritis and rheumatoid conditions (*Bi* syndrome). There is often a blockage in the meridians and *Luo* vessels, which shows in a stiffness of the limbs.

Ingredients

1. Radix Gentianae Qinjiao (*Qin Jiao*)	3 g
2. Radix Ligustici Wallichii (*Chuan Xiong*)	6 g
3. Semen Persicae (*Tao Ren*)	9 g
4. Flos Carthami (*Hong Hua*)	9 g
5. Radix Glycyrrhizae (*Gan Cao*)	6 g
6. Rhizoma Seu Radix Notopterygii (*Qiang Huo*)	3 g
7. Myrrha (*Mo Yao*)	6 g
8. Radix Angelicae Sinensis (*Dang Gui*)	9 g
9. Faeces Trogopterori (*Wu Ling Zhi*)	6 g
10. Rhizoma Cyperi (*Xiang Fu*)	3 g
11. Radix Achyranthis Bidentatae (*Niu Xi*)	9 g
12. Lumbricus (*Di Long*)	6 g

Application

This formula is taken as a warm decoction.

The main effect of this formula is based on removing the *Bi* syndrome and removing obstructions from the vessels with *Qin Jiao* (Gentiana Qinjiao), *Qiang Huo* (Notopterygium) and *Di Long* (Lumbricus). They all move *Qi* and Blood and remove pain. In clinical practice, it is administered for shoulder pain, elbow pain, hip, leg and knee pain or generalized pain.

If there is evidence of a slight Heat syndrome, add *Cang Zhu* (Rhizoma Atractylodes Lanceae) and *Huang Bai* (Cortex Phellodendri). With deficiency and weakness, a large amount of *Haung Qi* (Astragalus) must be added, approximately 40–80 g.

Suggested acupuncture treatment

The following points can be used to treat Blood stasis and pain due to *Bi* syndrome: BL 15, BL 17, SP 10, BL 18, BL 12, BL 20, GB 34 and local painful points.

8. *Bu Yang Huan Wu Tang* (*Yang* Tonifying Five-Tenth Decoction)

This formula tonifies the *Qi* and promotes circulation; in addition, it promotes the function of the (*Qi*) vessels and removes obstructions from them. Wang Qing-Ren specially devised this formula to treat hemiplegia after apoplexy (paralysis after stroke).

Ingredients	
1. Radix Astragali (*Huang Qi*)	20 g
2. Radix Angelicae Sinensis (*Dang Gui Wei*)	6 g
3. Radix Ligustici Wallichii (*Chuan Xiong*)	3 g
4. Radix Paeoniae Rubrae (*Chi Shao Yao*)	6 g
5. Semen Persicae (*Tao Ren*)	3 g
6. Flos Carthami (*Hong Hua*)	3 g
7. Lumbricus (*Di Long*)	3 g

Application

This formula is taken as a warm decoction. It is used for the sequelae of apoplexy, e.g. facial paralysis with paralysis of the mouth and eye, difficult speech and dysphagia, uncontrollable drooling, paralysis of the limbs, dry and hard stool, urinary incontinence or polyuria and muscular atrophy. Typical signs are a slow pulse and white tongue coating.

Action

1. Tonifies *Qi*.
2. Activates circulation and removes Blood stasis.
3. Promotes the functions of the meridians and *Luo* vessels, removes obstructions.

Explanation

This formula treats the frequently occuring Blood stasis, *Qi* stagnation and paralysis of the meridians and *Luo* vessels after a stroke.

Huang Qi is used in large amounts to tonify the *Yang* and *Qi*, which indirectly promotes Blood circulation, which, additionally, is specially stimulated by *Dang Gui* (Angelicae Sinensis). Radix Ligustici Wallichii (*Chuan Xiong*), Radix Paeoniae

Rubrae (*Chi Shao Yao*), Semen Persicae (*Tao Ren*) and Flos Carthami (*Hong Hua*) also invigorate the Blood. The Blood invigorating medicinals are only used sparingly, as the focus of the formula is to tonify *Qi* and remove obstructions from the vessels. Lumbricus (*Di Long*) has a strong effect in that direction.

Modern Chinese medicine administers this formula not only for strokes, but also for paralyses of different origin.

Caution

In order to be able to employ this formula correctly, the patient has to be conscious; otherwise, an orifices opening formula such as *An Gong Niu Huang Wan* (Calm the Palace Calculus Bovis Pill) or similar is indicated. Furthermore, the patient's body temperature has to be normal and, in case the stroke was caused by a ruptured vessel, the bleeding has to have stopped. Ideally, the pulse should be weak and soft.

The formula is contraindicated in *Yin* deficiency with Heat in the Blood. However, high blood pressure is not a contraindication.

Suggested acupuncture treatment

The points L.I. 15, 11 and 4, SI 5, GB 30 and 34, ST 36 and 41, BL 60, and further points according to the individual situation, are indicated, with a reinforcing manipulation.

As the *Yang* is weakened after a Wind-stroke, main points on *Yang* meridians have to be tonified. Since the *Yang Ming* vessel is closest to *Qi* and Blood, it should receive special focus.

Points have to be chosen according to syndrome differentiation, for example Wind stroke of the meridians or of the *Zang Fu* organs, spastic or atrophic paralysis and so on. Because of this, acupuncture in the treatment of stroke and its sequelae is a large field, which cannot be discussed here in every detail. I refer readers to the works of Maciocia and others, or to one of my next books *China's Secret Acupuncture Techniques*, which will deal with this topic extensively.

9. *Dan Shen Yin* (Salvia Drink)

This formula activates circulation of Blood, removes Blood stasis, activates the movement of

Qi and alleviates pain. It is specially suited for the treatment of Heart or Stomach pain due to *Qi* stagnation and Blood stasis.

Ingredients	
1. Radix Salviae Miltiorrhizae (*Dan Shen*)	30 g
2. Lignum Santali Albi (*Tan Xiang*)	5 g
3. Fructus Amomi (*Sha Ren*)	5 g

Application
This formula is taken as a cold (cooled-down) decoction.

Action
1. Activates the Blood and removes Blood stasis.
2. Activates the flow of *Qi* and alleviates pain.

Explanation
This formula treats Heart or Stomach pain due to *Qi* stagnation and Blood stasis. The large dosage of Radix Salviae Miltiorrhizae (*Dan Shen*) is intended to activate the Blood and remove Blood stasis. Lignum Santali Albi (*Tan Xiang*) and Fructus Amomi (*Sha Ren*) activate *Qi* circulation and alleviate pain.

It is a relatively safe formula in so far as its relation of *Yin* and *Yang* is almost neutral and there is only a very slight tendency towards Cold. Therefore, we often administer this formula in cases of stable angina pectoris, as Radix Salviae Miltiorrhizae (*Dan Shen*) also has a mild vasodilating effect. Moreover, it improves circulation in the coronary vessels as well as heart function and microcirculation, is antiarteriosclerotic and prevents thrombocyte aggregation.

Suggested acupuncture treatment
The following points can be used, with a reducing manipulation: BL 17, SP 10, REN 12, ST 36, P 6.

BL 17 and SP 10 activate circulation and help remove Blood stasis. REN 12 is the front *Mu* point of the Stomach meridian. ST 36 is its *He*-Sea Point. Together with P 6, they can regulate the flow of Stomach-*Qi* and eliminate stomach pain.

10. Shi Xiao San (Sudden Smile Powder)

This formula promotes blood flow and dispels Blood stasis. It also dispels abscesses and alleviates pain. It is commonly used for different kinds of pain in the chest and abdomen related to stasis.

Ingredients
1. Faeces Trogopteri (*Wu Ling Zhi*)
2. Pollen Typhae (*Pu Huang*)

Application
To be mixed in equal parts and pulverized. About 6 g are taken with wine or vinegar water. It can also be prepared as a warm decoction, but it has an unpleasant taste.

Typical symptoms are, for example, continuous bleeding or retention of the placenta after birth, pain with irregular menstruation and stabbing pain in the lower abdomen.

Action
1. Activates circulation of Blood and removes Blood stasis.
2. Removes abscesses and stops pain.

Explanation
Often a part of larger formulas, it treats different kinds of Blood stasis accompanied by pain. It is specially suited for Blood stasis in the Liver.

Faeces Trogopteri (*Wu Ling Zhi*) and Pollen Typhae (*Pu Huang*) are combined to activate circulation of Blood, remove Blood stasis and stop bleedings and pain. Vinegar and wine can amplify this effect. As this formula puts a Blood invigorating and stasis-dispelling action first, it is not strong enough to activate the *Qi*. For this reason, other *Qi* active medicinals are added, for example a combination of this formula with *Jin Ling Zi San* (Meliae Toosendan Powder) or the addition of Astragalus (*Huang Qi*).

Other combinations with this formula are Tang Zong-Hai's *Gui Xiong Shi Xiao San* (Angelica and Ligusticum Sudden Smile Powder) with Ligusticum Chuanxiong and Angelica Sinensis. These herbs augment the Blood stasis breaking action with a nourishing effect.[5] In heavy bleeding due to trauma, use *San Qi Shi Xiao San* (Notoginseng Sudden Smile Powder) which contains a larger dose of Radix Notoginseng.

Suggested acupuncture treatment
Use points BL 17 and SP 10, with a reducing manipulation.

BL 17 is one of the eight *Hui*-Meeting points which influence the Blood. Therefore, it can be used in different illnesses related to the Blood. In this case, it is needled to activate the Blood. SP 10, the sea of Blood, can activate Blood circulation and dispel Blood stasis.

11. Shou Nian San (Hand-made Pill)

The name *Shou* (hand) and *Nian* (to knead) refers to the kneading of the pill by hand. It is used in epigastric and abdominal pain due to *Qi* stagnation and Blood stasis.

Ingredients	
1. Rhizoma Corydalis (*Yan Hu Suo*)	6 g
2. Faeces Trogopteri (*Wu Ling Zhi*)	6 g
3. Fructus Tsaoko (*Cao Guo*)	6 g
4. Myrrha (*Mo Yao*)	6 g

Application
This formula is taken as a warm decoction.

Explanation
The main action of this formula is similar to *Shi Xiao San*, but it has a stronger warming effect and therefore is specially suited for Cold with Blood stasis. Apart from that, it also promotes Blood circulation, removes Blood stasis and alleviates pain.

Suggested acupuncture treatment
Use the points BL 17, SP 10 and SP 8 with reducing and moxibustion manipulation.

---

[5] More on this can be found in the third part in the translation of the classics (Chapter 11): 6. Excerpts from Tang Zong Hai's '*Xue Zherg Lun*' (Treatise on Blood syndromes).

12. *Huo Luo Xiao Ling Dan* (Wondrous Pill to Invigorate the Channels)

This formula is a general remedy with many possible modifications for all kinds of pain du to *Qi* stagnation and Blood stasis. It invigorates the Blood, removes stasis and alleviates pain.

Ingredients	
1. Radix Angelicae Sinensis (*Dang Gui*)	15 g
2. Radix Salviae Miltiorrhizae (*Dan Shen*)	15 g
3. Resina Olibani (*Ru Xiang*)	15 g
4. Myrrha (*Mo Yao*)	15 g

Application
This formula is taken as a warm decoction. Typical indications are Heart and abdominal pain, neck, leg and elbow pain, swellings and bruises due to trauma, carbuncles, furuncles, multiple abcesses, lymph node swelling and abdominal masses as well as ulcers.

Action
1. Invigorates Blood and removes Blood stasis.
2. Removes obstructions from the *Luo* vessels and alleviates pain.

Explanation
This formula treats many kinds of pain resulting from *Qi* stagnation and Blood stasis. It acts on external injuries as well as on Blood stasis of the internal organs. Radix Angelicae Sinensis (*Dang Gui*) nourishes the Blood and at the same time activates Blood circulation. Radix Salviae Miltiorrhizae (*Dan Shen*) helps Radix Angelicae Sinensis (*Dang Gui*) and further intensifies the removal of Blood stasis. Resina Olibani (*Ru Xiang*) and Myrrha (*Mo Yao*) invigorate *Qi* and dispel Blood stasis. In addition, they have an analgetic effect.

Suggested acupuncture treatment
Use points BL 17, SP 10 and the points described below. Manipulation should be even method (neither reinforcing nor reducing) or reducing.

BL 17 and SP 10 generally activate circulation and thus work against Blood stasis. Depending on the location of the pain, the following points can be added: BL 15, REN 14, HE 6 and REN 17 for chest pain; REN 12, ST 36, SP 15 and SP 14 for abdominal pain. As pain acupuncture is such a big area, not all points can be listed here. However, the guideline to incorporate painful (*A-Shi*) points into treatment is always valid.

13. *Shu Jing Huo Xue Tang* (Relaxing the Vessels Decoction)

This formula removes obstructions from meridians and *Luo* vessels, invigorates Blood and expels Dampness. It is administered for a weak or deficient patient with pain due to an attack of exogenous factors like Wind or Dampness.

Ingredients	
1. Radix Angelicae Sinensis (*Dang Gui*)	5 g
2. Radix Paeoniae Lactiflorae (*Bai Shao*)	4 g
3 Radix Rehmanniae (*Sheng Di Huang*)	4 g
4. Radix Ligustici Wallichii (*Chuan Xiong*)	3 g
5. Semen Persicae (*Tao Ren*)	4 g
6. Poria Cocos (*Fu Ling*)	3 g
7. Rhizoma Atractylodis (*Cang Zhu*)	4 g
8. Pericarpium Citri Reticulatae (*Chen Pi*)	4 g
9. Rhizoma et Radix Notopterygii (*Qiang Huo*)	3 g
10. Radix Angelicae Dahuricae (*Bai Zhi*)	3 g
11. Radix Clematidis (*Wei Ling Xian*)	4 g
12. Radix Stephaniae Tetrandrae (*Fang Ji*)	3 g
13. Radix Ledebouriellae (*Fang Feng*)	3 g
14. Radix Gentianae (*Long Dan Cao*)	3 g
15. Radix Achyranthis Bidentatae (*Niu Xi*)	4 g
16. Radix Glycyrrhizae (*Gan Cao*)	2 g

Application
This formula is taken as a warm decoction on an empty stomach. The ingredients are cooked together with three big pieces of fresh ginger (*Sheng Jiang*).

Typical indications are deficiency pain due to exogenous pathogenic factors transformed into excessive pain, for example sore muscles and limbs, numbness of the legs or pain radiating down the legs as well as rheumatic pain in the extremities.

Action
1. Removing obstructions from the meridians and *Luo* vessels.
2. Removal of Blood stasis.
3. Expelling pathogenic Dampness.

Explanation
The typical course of disease of patients for whom this formula is suitable is characterized by an excessive consumption of alcohol, sexual over-indulgence or internal injuries leading to a general weak state. This is followed by an intrusion of pathogenic factors like Wind, Cold, Heat or Dampness into the meridians and *Luo* vessels generating painful *Bi* syndrome.

In response, Radix Angelicae Sinensis (*Dang Gui*), Radix Paeoniae Lactiflorae (*Bai Shao*), Radix Rehmanniae (*Sheng Di Huang*) and Radix Ligustici Wallichii (*Chuan Xiong*) are used to nourish the Blood and activate Blood circulation. Semen Persicae (*Tao Ren*) acts against Blood stasis. Poria Cocos (*Fu Ling*) expels Dampness via diuresis. Rhizoma Atractylodis (*Cang Zhu*) dries pathogenic Dampness. Pericarpium Citri Reticulatae (*Chen Pi*) regulates flow of *Qi* and dries as well. Rhizoma et Radix Notopterygii (*Qiang Huo*), Radix Angelicae Dahuricae (*Bai Zhi*), Radix Clematidis (*Wei Ling Xian*), Radix Stephaniae Tetrandrae (*Fang Ji*) and Radix Ledebouriellae (*Fang Feng*) move the stagnated *Qi*, dispel Wind and Dampness and have an analgetic effect. Radix Gentianae (*Long Dan Cao*) expels pathogenic Heat and Dampness and Radix Achyranthis Bidentatae (*Niu Xi*) activates the Blood and tonifies the body via Kidney and Liver. Radix Glycyrrhizae (*Gan Cao*) harmonizes the medicinals.

Suggested acupuncture treatment
Use the points BL 15, 18, 21, 20, 12; REN 4, SP 9, BL 17, LIV 5 and local *A Shi* points. Use reinforcing manipulation; reducing should be avoided.

The Heart controls the Blood and the Liver stores the Blood, therefore BL 15 (Back *Shu* point of the Heart) and BL 18 (Back *Shu* point of the Liver) are used to tonify the Blood. BL 20 (Back *Shu* point of the Spleen) and BL 21 (Back *Shu* point of the Stomach) are used to strengthen the Middle

Burner and thus indirectly to increase production of *Qi* and Blood. BL 12, REN 4 and SP 9 expel pathogenic Wind, Cold and Dampness. BL 17 activates Blood circulation and LIV 5 activates *Qi* circulation. In addition, *A Shi* local points are needled to reduce pain.

14. *Da Huang Zhe Chong Wan* (Rheum Eupolyphaga Pill)

This formula is most suitable for removing Blood stasis and generating new tissue.

Ingredients	
1. Rhizoma et Radix Rhei (*Da Huang*)	400 g
2. Radix Scutellaria (*Huang Qin*)	80 g
3. Radix Glyzhyrriza (*Gan Cao*)	120 g
4. Semen Persicae (*Tao Ren*)	80 g
5. Semen Pruni Armeniacae (*Xing Ren*)	80 g
6. Radix Paeoniae Lactiflorae (*Bai Shao Yao*)	160 g
7. Radix Polygonatum (*Shou Di Huang*)	400 g
8. Lacca Exsiccatae (*Gan Qi*)	40 g
9. Tabanus (*Mang Chong*)	80 g
10. Hirudo (*Shui Zhi*)	80 g
11. Holotrichia (*Qi Cao*)	80 g
12. Eupolyphaga (*Tu Bie Chong*)	40 g

Application
The twelve medicinals are mixed and pulverized, then formed into balls of 3 g each using honey. Take 3 × 5 pills daily with alcohol or warm water.

Typical indications are Blood stasis due to overexertion, exhaustion and weakness syndrome with emaciation or swollen abdomen with inability to eat or drink, dry scaly skin and dark eyes and dark eye circles, abdominal pain, abdominal masses, menstrual disorders, amenorrhoea and afternoon fever.

Action
1. Dispels Blood stasis.
2. Promotes formation of Blood.
3. Removes obstructions from the meridians and dissolves fixed abdominal masses (*Zheng* Blood clots).

Explanation
This formula treats Blood stasis due to exhaustion, also called *Gan* exhaustion. Due to the weakness, there is also *Qi* and *Yin* deficiency. Rheum, Persica and Lacca act against Blood stasis with dry Blood clots in the abdomen. They also remove obstructions from the vessels. The *Chong* (insect) medicinals Tabanus, Hirudo, Holotrichia and Eupolyphaga break and dissolve Blood stasis. To promote haematopoiesis and regulate the Middle, *Shu Di Huang, Bai Shao* and *Gan Cao* (strengthens Spleen) are added. Scutellaria and Pruni Armenica invigorate Lung *Qi* and resolve stagnant Heat due to Blood stasis.

Caution/contraindications
This formula is contraindicated in pregnancy due to the drastic potential of its insect ingredients (Eupolyphaga etc.).

Suggested acupuncture treatment
To move Blood stasis in general, points such as LIV 2, LIV 3, SP 6, SP 8, L.I. 11, P 5 and BL 60 can be used. Severe *Qi* deficiency and general weakness cannot be eliminated by acupuncture, as acupuncture cannot add energy but works with the energy already present.

On the contrary, every acupuncture treatment, even when reinforcing methods are applied, is a process that consumes energy for the patient. For this reaon, acupuncture is contraindicated when the patient is very weak. New energy can then only be supplied from outside, with medicinals.

15. *Di Dang Tang* (Resistance Decoction)

This formula first treats the so-called *Xu Xue* syndrome (from the *Shang Han Lun*) with Blood Heat due to Blood stasis, which it breaks and purges.

Ingredients	
1. Hirudo (*Shui Zhi*)	30 pc (pieces)
2. Tabanus (*Meng Chong*)	30 pc
3. Semen Persicae (*Tao Ren*)	20 pc
4. Rhizoma et Radix Rhei (*Da Huang*)	48 g

Application

The ingredients are boiled together, and the decoction is taken after it has cooled down.

Typical indications for this formula are Blood Heat due to Blood stasis with symptoms such as forgetfulness, feeling of fullness in the chest, dry mouth, thirst with aversion to swallowing the fluid, feeling of abdominal fullness with abdominal distension, dark, hard stool but normal urine, irritability, menstrual disorders, deep and irregular pulse (knotted or intermittent), sometimes with large pulse waves.

16. *Tao Hong Si Wu Tang* (Persica Carthamus Four Ingredients Decoction)

This formula is effective for all kinds of menstrual disorders due to Blood stasis and for a whole range of diseases linked with Blood stasis as a cause or effect.

Ingredients	
1. Radix Angelicae (*Dang Gui*)	9 g
2. Semen Persicae (*Tao Ren*)	9 g
3. Radix Paeoniae Rubrae (*Chi Shao*)	9 g
4. Radix Ligustici Wallichii (*Chuan Xiong*)	6 g
5. Flos Carthami (*Hong Hua*)	6 g
6. Radix Rehmannia (*Sheng Di Huang*)	15 g

Application

The ingredients are boiled together, and the decoction is taken after it has cooled down.

Typical indications for this formula are amenorrhoea, dysmenorrhoea, menstruation that is too heavy or too weak, too frequent or too irregular, bleeding with dark, clotted Blood that takes a long time to stop.

Action

General invigoration of Blood and regulation of menstruation.

Explanation

This formula is based on the Blood forming and Blood invigorating formula *Si Wu Tang*

(Four Ingredients Decoction), with the addition of Semen Persicae (*Tao Ren*) and Flos Carthami (*Hong Hua*). The original Paeonia Lactiflora (*Bai Shao*) was replaced with Paeonia Rubra (*Chi Shao*) in order to achieve a Blood invigorating effect instead of a *Yin* nourishing effect.

The *Yin* moistening preparation Radix Rehmanniae (*Shu Di*) was replaced with the non-heated *Sheng Di*. Instead of moistening and nourishing Blood and *Yin*, the desired effect was to cool and invigorate Blood. By adding the medicinals Persica and Carthamus which both dispel Blood stasis, a balanced Blood stasis dispelling formula was created.

Nowadays, in addition to the above named menstrual disorders, it is used in chronic pelvic inflammation, after apoplexies due to the rupture of a vessel with hemiplegia, nervous headaches, and in trauma of the head such as concussion. Additionally, it is administered in psoriasis, extrauterine pregnancy or various forms of neuritis.

Suggested acupuncture treatment

It is not possible to give acupuncture prescriptions for this formula due to the broad range of its action. Details can be found under the respective diseases or syndromes.

17. *Yang Yin Tong Bi Tang* (*Yin* Nourishing *Bi* Dissolving Decoction)

This formula is effective for *Yin* and *Qi* deficiency of Kidney and Liver with Blood stasis.

Ingredients	
1. Semen Persicae (*Tao Ren*)	9 g
2. Flos Carthami (*Hong Hua*)	9 g
3. Radix Rehmannia (*Sheng Di Huang*)	12 g
4. Semen Ligustri (*Nü Zhen Zi*)	15 g
5. Semen Trichosanthes (*Gua Lou*)	30 g
6. Radix Codonopsitis (*Dang Shen*)	9 g
7. Rhizoma Cyperi (*Xiang Fu*)	9 g
8. Tuber Ophiopogones (*Mai Men Dong*)	9 g
9. Rhizoma Corydalis (*Yuan Hu*)	9 g

Application

This formula is taken as a warm decoction.

Typical indications are chest and Heart pain, dizziness and tinnitus, dry mouth, light flashes in the eye and insomnia due to *Yin* or Blood deficiency in relation to Blood stasis.

Action

1. Nourishes and invigorates Blood and *Yin*.
2. Removes obstructions from the vessels.

Explanation

This formula treats causes and consequences at the same time as it nourishes a weak *Yin* and Blood of Kidney and Liver with *Sheng Di Huang* (Rehmannia), *Nü Zhen Zi* (Ligustrum) and *Mai Men Dong* (Ophiopogonis) and thus prevents flaring-up of Liver *Yang*. Whilst *Dang Shen* (Salvia) tonifies *Qi*, *Xiang Fu* (Cyperus), *Yuan Hu* (Cory-dalis) and *Gua Lou* (Trichosanthes) move the stagnated *Qi* in the chest and alleviate pain. *Tao Ren* (Persica) and *Hong Hua* (Carthamus) remove Blood stasis due to Blood deficiency.

Nowadays, this formula is also used in Heart disease and for the consequences of hypertension.

18. *Dian Kuang Meng Xing Tang* (Psychosis Decoction)

This formula is effective for cases of manic depressive psychoses with Blood stasis and *Qi* stagnation.

Ingredients	
1. Semen Persicae (*Tao Ren*)	32 g
2. Radix Bupleuri (*Chai Hu*)	12 g
3. Rhizoma Cyperi (*Xiang Fu*)	8 g
4. Caulis Akebiae Mutong (*Mu Tong*)	12 g
5. Radix Paeoniae Rubrae (*Chi Shao*)	12 g
6. Rhizoma Pinelliae (*Ban Xia*)	8 g
7. Pericarpium Arecae (*Da Fu Pi*)	8 g
8. Pericarpium Citri Reticulatae (*Qing Pi*)	8 g
9. Pericarpium Citri Reticulatae Viride (*Chen Pi*)	12 g
10. Cortex Mori Albae (*Sang Bai Pi*)	12 g
11. Fructus Perilla (*Su Zi*)	16 g
12. Radix Glycyrrhizae Uralensis (*Gan Cao*)	20 g

Application

This formula is taken as a warm decoction. If a large amount of Phlegm is present, it is combined with *Wen Dan Tang* (Gall-Bladder Warming Decoction).

Action

Dispels Blood stasis, moves stagnated Liver-*Qi* and transforms Phlegm.

Explanation

Here, the main Blood stasis removing medicinals are the large amounts of Semen Persicae (*Tao Ren*) and Radix Paeoniae Rubrae (*Chi Shao*), which also cools the Blood. Rhizoma Cyperi (*Xiang Fu*), Pericarpium Arecae (*Da Fu Pi*), Pericarpium Citri Reticulatae (*Qing Pi*) and Pericarpium Citri Reticulatae Viride (*Chen Pi*) prevent *Qi* stagnation, which in this case manifests predominantly in the Liver. This also explains the ingredient Radix Bupleuri (*Chai Hu*), as it is a medicinal especially suited to smooth Liver-*Qi* and cool down Heat. Another cooling medicinal is Cortex Mori Albae (*Sang Bai Pi*) which is added for its calming function. Further medicinals against Dampness and Phlegm are the Heart Fire cooling Caulis Akebiae Mutong (*Mu Tong*), as well as Rhizoma Pinelliae (*Ban Xia*), which together with the stool-promoting Fructus Perilla (*Su Zi*) direct *Qi* downwards.

Radix Glycyrrhizae Uralensis (*Gan Cao*) is detoxifying and harmonizes the other medicinals.

In this case, three causes of psychological disorders are tackled: Blood stasis, Heat (often together with constipation) and Phlegm. Under these conditions, there is often *Qi* stagnation. This stagnation is moved as well.

In order to increase the anti-stasis effect and cool down Heat, the following medicinals can be employed: Angelica (*Dang Gui*), Carthamus (*Hong Hua*), Ligusticum (*Chuan Xiong*), Rehmannia (*Sheng Di*) and Moutan (*Mu Dan Pi*).

Clinical signs

Typical indications are abnormal states of mind such as constant crying, laughing, singing and swearing no matter who is present; dreamlike confusion, aggression such as throwing of objects etc.

Further signs are insomnia, lack of appetite, dark complexion, dark or purple tongue with protruding sublingual veins and a deep, rough pulse.

Although this formula had fallen into oblivion, it is now used successfully again in cases of manic-depressive psychosis and schizophrenia. As Blood stasis has an effect on the mind, for example in cases of forgetfulness or confusion due to Blood stasis, these severe conditions can also be caused by a severe chronic Blood stasis. For the treatment to be successful, there has to be a valid diagnosis of Blood stasis. Furthermore, it should be differentiated as to whether the Blood stasis is mostly in the Heart or Liver. In the latter case, there is usually more aggression.

Caution
Due to the cooling and *Qi* moving nature of its ingredients, the formula should not be given over a prolonged amount of time. In case of patients with *Qi* deficiency, the formula should only be administered with caution and with the addition of *Qi* tonifying medicinals (e.g. Radix Astragali).

Suggested acupuncture treatment
Use points P 6 and 7, SP 6, HE 7, BL 17 and LIV 3 (both reducing); in marked Blood stasis in the Heart add BL 14 and 15, REN 14 and BL 44; in marked Blood stasis in the Liver add LIV 14, GB 13, DU 24 and BL 18.

With regard to manipulation, apart from reducing needling on BL 17 and LIV 3, neither a reinforcing nor a reducing technique should be applied.

P 6 and P 7 as well as SP 6 move the Blood and calm the mind. BL 17 tonifies the Blood, HE 7 calms and LIV 3 moves stagnating Liver Blood.

BL 14 and 15 are the *Shu* points of Heart and Pericardium and REN 14 is the front *Mu* point of the Heart. These, together with BL 44, all calm down the mind and the first three also have a Blood moving action.

The points LIV 14 and BL 18, needled for Blood stasis of the Liver, are *Mu* and *Shu* points and invigorate stagnating Liver-Blood. GB 13 and DU 24 are used for treating aggression in Liver syndromes.

GROUP III A: SPECIFIC CHRONIC BLOOD STASIS (EMPHASIS IS ON THE LOCATION)

19. Tao Hong Cheng Qi Tang (Qi Rectifying Persica Carthamus Decoction)

Tao Hong Cheng Qi Tang cools Heat and removes Blood stasis. This formula is particularly effective for Blood stasis and Heat in the Lower Burner, manifesting as acute lower abdominal pain, delirium, irritability, thirst, nocturnal fever, but with normal urination. It is also applied in severe cases of manic psychoses.

Ingredients	
1. Semen Persicae (*Tao Ren*)	12 g
2. Rhizoma et Radix Rhei (*Da Huang*)	12 g
3. Ramulus Cinnamomi (*Gui Zhi*)	6 g
4. Mirabilitum Depuratum (*Mang Xiao*)	6 g
5. Radix Glycyrrhizae Praeparatae (*Zhi Gan Cao*)	6 g

Application
This formula is taken as a warm decoction.

Action
Tao Hong Cheng Qi Tang is cooling and dispels Blood stasis.

Clinical symptoms
Accumulation of Blood in the Lower *Jiao* (Burner): acute lower abdominal pain, normal urination, delirium, irritability, thirst, nocturnal fever or mania in severe cases.

Explanation
This formula consists of *Tiao Wei Cheng Qi Tang* (Rheum and Mirabilitum Combination) plus

Semen Persicae (*Tao Ren*) and Ramulus Cinnamomi (*Gui Zhi*). As stated in the '*Jin Kui Yao Lüe*', it treats Blood stasis in the Lower *Jiao*. If a person is affected by a *Tai Yang* syndrome and the exterior pathogens are not removed, the factors will descend further into the channels; once they reach the interior, they transform into Heat, which accumulates and coagulates Blood in the Lower Burner, which eventually results in Blood stasis.

As the water passages have not been affected, urination remains normal. Acute lower abdominal pain is the result of Blood stasis in the Lower Burner. Delirium, irritability, thirst, nocturnal fever and mania also suggest the presence of Heat in the Blood. In this formula, Semen Persicae (*Tao Ren*) dispels Blood stasis. Rhizoma et Radix Rhei (*Da Huang*) dispels Heat and stagnation. These two are the emperor medicinals of this formula, dispelling Blood stasis and cool Heat.

Ramulus Cinnamomi (*Gui Zhi*) activates the circulation of Blood and assists Semen Persicae (*Tao Ren*) in dispelling Blood stasis. Mirabilitum Depuratum (*Mang Xiao*) disperses Heat and mildly dispels Blood stasis. It is often combined with Rhizoma et Radix Rhei (*Da Huang*) to clear internal Heat. Radix Glycyrrhizae Praeparatae (*Zhi Gan Cao*) supplements *Qi* and regulates the Middle Burner. Moreover, by supplementing *Qi* it prevents *Qi* from suffering any damage due to the harsh actions of the other medicinals.

The range of clinical applications of this formula has been expanded since ancient times; now it may also be used for:

1. Sports injuries, bruises, difficult evacuation or urination.
2. Headache, a feeling of pressure in the head, red eyes or toothache due to excessive Fire.
3. Epistaxis and vomiting of dark blood due to Blood-Heat.
4. Blood stasis in women, amenorrhoea, continued bleeding after delivery, lower abdominal distension and pain, shortness of breath.

The action of this formula should always be remembered; as it is able to break Blood stasis and clear Heat, a thorough diagnosis should always be made before such harsh measures are taken. Qin Bo-Wei, one of the most famous physicians of modern times (1901–1970), remarked concerning this in the '*Qian Zhai Yi Xue Jiang Cao*': 'Wang Qing-Ren had a good method for breaking Blood stasis; he also employed Blood invigorating medicinals. However, it is unwarranted to resort to Blood stasis breaking methods at the smallest hint of Blood stasis.'

Caution/contraindications
This formula should be used when Wind-Cold is no longer in the exterior. If there are still exterior symptoms, one should first use diaphoretic medicinals before this formula is prescribed. Not to be used during pregnancy.

Suggested acupuncture treatment
Use points L.I. 11, L.I. 4, BL 40, SP10, BL 17, KID 6, LU 7, ST 37, ST 36. L.I. 11 and L.I. 4 cool Heat in the internal *Yang Ming* channel. BL 40 cools Heat in the Blood level. SP 10 and BL 17 activate the circulation of Blood and dispel Blood stasis. KID 6 nourishes Water and restrains Fire. LU 7, the *Luo*-Connection point of the Lung channel, can penetrate to the Large Intestine and thus cool Heat in the Lower Burner. ST 37, the lower *He*-Sea point of the Large Intestine channel, can soothe the flow of *Qi* inside the channel. ST 36 nourishes Middle Burner *Qi* and prevents the Stomach from being damaged due to the strong activation of Blood within the body.

20. *Xue Fu Zhu Yu Tang* (Anti–Stasis Chest Decoction)

This formula is used for chronic stabbing pain that usually occurs in the chest and always at the same location, which is caused by *Qi* stagnation and Blood stasis. Thus this formula activates *Qi* and Blood in the 'residence of Blood', i.e. in the space above the diaphragm.

Further clinical manifestations are headache, pain below the costal arch, persistent hiccup, a retching sensation without vomiting, palpitations, insomnia, a sensation of Heat, irritability, anger and nervousness. There are often other signs such as a dark tongue body with stasis spots or dots, dark lips and a wiry and slow or choppy and fine pulse.

Ingredients	
1. Semen Persicae (*Tao Ren*)	12 g
2. Flos Carthami (*Hong Hua*)	9 g
3. Radix Rehmanniae (*Sheng Di Huang*)	9 g
4. Radix Angelicae Sinensis (*Dang Gui*)	9 g
5. Radix Paeoniae Rubrae (*Chi Shao Yao*)	6 g
6. Radix Ligustici Wallichii (*Chuan Xiong*)	5 g
7. Radix Glycyrrhizae (*Gan Cao*)	3 g
8. Radix Bupleuri (*Chai Hu*)	3 g
9. Fructus Citri Aurantii (*Zhi Ke*)	6 g
10. Radix Platycodi (*Jie Geng*)	5 g
11. Radix Achyranthis Bidentatae (*Niu Xi*)	9 g

Application
This formula is taken as a warm decoction.

Action
1. Activates the circulation of Blood and removes Blood stasis.
2. Activates the circulation of *Qi* and removes pain.

Clinical symptoms
Blood stasis in the chest: persistent and stabbing pain in the chest and head, pain in the lower costal arch, persistent hiccup, dry retching, palpitations, insomnia, restlessness at night, nervousness, irritability, sensation of Heat and fever, dark red tongue with petechiae, dark lips, yellowish sclera and a wiry and slow or choppy and fine pulse.

Explanation
This formula treats various clinical manifestations of Blood stasis in the chest and Upper Burner. Blood stasis in the chest generates stabbing chest pain and headaches, which occur quite frequently and are in a fixed location. Commonly, Blood stasis also generates Heat in the body, which may affect the Stomach by causing *Qi* to ascend, and thus retching and hiccup develop.

Other symptoms such as palpitations, insomnia, restlessness at night, nervousness, irritability and afternoon fever arise from Blood stasis in the chest and Liver-*Qi* stagnation.

A dark red tongue with petechiae suggests Blood stasis. A wiry and slow or choppy and fine pulse suggest Blood stasis and pain. Semen Persicae (*Tao Ren*) and Flos Carthami (*Hong Hua*) are used for breaking stasis and activating the circulation of Blood. Radix Rehmanniae (*Sheng Di Huang*), Radix Angelicae Sinensis (*Dang Gui*), Radix Paeoniae Rubrae (*Chi Shao Yao*) and Radix Ligustici Wallichii (*Chuan Xiong*) nourish Blood, activate the circulation of Blood and remove Heat. Radix Glycyrrhizae (*Gan Cao*) and Radix Bupleuri (*Chai Hu*) are used for soothing Liver-*Qi*, thus *Qi* is brought back into flow and the chest pain will stop. Fructus Citri Aurantii (*Zhi Ke*) has the effect of breaking stasis and activating the circulation of *Qi*. Radix Platycodi (*Jie Geng*) guides the action of the herbs upwards to treat Blood stasis in the chest. Radix Achyranthis Bidentatae (*Niu Xi*) guides Blood downwards to assist in dispelling stagnated Blood.

In modern practice, this formula is also used in the treatment of arteriosclerotic heart diseases, coronary heart diseases (CHD), the sequelae of concussion, but also insomnia with memory disorders, senile dementia and similar conditions.

It is also applied in gynaecology to treat amenorrhoea and dysmenorrhoea by omitting *Jie Geng* (Platycodon) and adding *Xiang Fu* (Cyperus), *Yi Mu Cao* (Leonurus), *Ze Lan* (Lycopus) and other medicinals.

Suggested acupuncture treatment
Use points BL 21, ST 36, SP 6, BL 15, BL 17, SP10, P 6, SP 4, SI 4, LIV 2. Use reinforcing and reducing manipulation.

BL 21, ST 36, SP 6, BL 15, BL 17 and SP10 activate the flow of *Qi*, dispel Blood stasis and nourish both *Qi* and Blood. P 6 and SP 4 can dispel stagnation in the chest. SI 4 regulates the flow of *Shao Yang Qi*. LIV 2 regulates the flow of Liver-*Qi*. When combined, these points help to remove pain and Blood stasis in the chest.

21. *Tong Qiao Huo Xue Tang* (Orifices Opening, Blood Invigorating Decoction)

This formula is employed for Blood stasis in the head and limbs accompanied by pain and the consequences of stasis such as hair loss, tinnitus and hardness of hearing, eye and gum inflammation, *Gan* deficiency syndrome, diseases that are characterized by cyclical attacks, fatigue, tuberculosis, amenorrhoea, bad breath and skin blemishes.

Ingredients		
1. Radix Paeoniae Rubrae (*Chi Shao Yao*)	3 g	
2. Radix Ligustici Wallichii (*Chuan Xiong*)	3 g	
3. Semen Persicae (*Tao Ren*)	9 g	
4. Flos Carthami (*Hong Hua*)	9 g	
5. Herba Allii Fistulosum (*Lao Cong*)	3 g	
6. Fructus Zizyphi Jujubae	5 g	
(*Da Zao*)	(approx. 2–3 pc.)	
7. Moschus (*She Xiang*)	0.15 g	
8. Wine (*Huang Jiu*)	250 ml	

Application

This filtered decoction of the first six ingredients is taken warm with *She Xiang* and white wine. It is used in all cases of Blood stasis in the head and the face, but also for amenorrhoea. The addition of Moschus and spring onions achieves a greater opening effect of the orifices.

In my personal experience, this formula is highly effective as long as the (unfortunately expensive) Moschus is employed. It is very effective in treating difficult diseases that have failed to respond to other therapies, such as chronic tinnitus, alopecia, skin diseases etc.

Today, Moschus is no longer harvested by killing the Musk deer, but is scraped out of the musk gland, which grows again every year. This should address the concerns of animal welfare activists.

Suggested acupuncture treatment

The following points may be selected for removing Blood stasis from the head: BL 15, BL 17, SP 10, DU 23, *Yin Tang* (extra) and L.I. 4.

22. *Ge Xia Zhu Yu Tang* (Anti-stasis Abdomen Decoction)

This formula is used for Blood stasis in the abdomen and hypochondrium area, characterized by fixed pain, swellings and lumps in the abdomen, abdominal masses (especially in chil-

dren), a sensation of heaviness in the abdomen, and chronic diarrhoea that may also be due to Kidney deficiency.

Ingredients		
1. Faeces Trogopteri (*Wu Ling Zhi*)	9 g	
2. Radix Angelicae Sinensis (*Dang Gui*)	9 g	
3. Radix Ligustici Wallichii (*Chuan Xiong*)	6 g	
4. Semen Persicae (*Tao Ren*)	9 g	
5. Cortex Moutan Radicis (*Mu Dan Pi*)	6 g	
6. Radix Paeoniae Rubrae (*Chi Shao Yao*)	6 g	
7. Radix Linderae (*Wu Yao*)	6 g	
8. Rhizoma Corydalis (*Yan Hu Suo*)	3 g	
9. Radix Glycyrrhizae (*Gan Cao*)	6 g	
10. Rhizoma Cyperi (*Xiang Fu*)	3 g	
11. Flos Carthami (*Hong Hua*)	9 g	
12. Fructus Citri Aurantii (*Zhi Ke*)	5 g	

Application

This formula is taken as a warm decoction. It aims at moving Blood and *Qi* below the diaphragm, particularly if abdominal masses have already formed and a fixed stabbing pain or a persistently uncomfortable sensation of pressure or fullness is evident.

In terms of action, it is related to *Shao Fu Zhu Yu Tang* (Anti-Stasis Lower Abdomen Decoction); however, its main effect focuses on the treatment of Blood stasis with Heat, whereas *Shao Fu Zhu Yu Tang* is more suitable for Blood stasis with Cold.

One should exercise caution when prescribing this formula over a longer period of time, as it contains several medicinals for breaking Blood stasis, which may deplete *Qi* and Blood.

Suggested acupuncture treatment

The following points may be selected for removing Blood stasis from the abdomen: BL 15, BL 17, SP 10, LIV 3, GB 34 and LIV 14.

23. *Guan Xin Er Hao Fang* (Coronary Decoction No. 2)

Since its first application in 1978, this formula has been used successfully in the treatment of various heart diseases, primarily for the long-term management of angina pectoris and coronary heart disease.

Ingredients	
1. Radix Ligustici Wallichii (*Chuan Xiong*)	15 g
2. Radix Paeoniae Rubrae (*Chi Shao*)	15 g
3. Radix Salviae Miltiorrhizae (*Dan Shen*)	30 g
4. Flos Carthami (*Hong Hua*)	15 g
5. Lignum Dalbergiae Odiferae (*Jiang Xiang*)	15 g

Application

This formula is taken as a warm decoction. In terms of TCM, it has the action of removing stasis and pain, activating stagnated *Qi* and removing obstructions from the vessels.

Explanation

Chuan Xiong (Ligusticum) assumes the role of the emperor herb by invigorating *Qi* and Blood, removing stasis and stopping pain, supported by double the amount of *Dan Shen* (Salvia Miltiorrhiza), which also invigorates Blood, dispels stasis and at the same time nourishes the Heart and Blood. *Hong Hua* (Carthamus) and *Chi Shao* (Paeonia Rubra) are the two 'minister herbs' that further amplify the main effect. Finally, *Jiang Xiang* (Dalbergia) is added for moving *Qi* and stopping pain, and today this is commonly combined with *Dan Shen* (Salvia Miltiorrhiza) for formulas that are effective for heart disorders.

Apart from CHD and angina pectoris, this formula is also applied successfully in cases of acute thrombotic stroke.

Suggested acupuncture treatment

For acute pain in the chest, traditional acupuncture selects the paints REN 17, HT 6, P 6 and *Hua Tuo* extra points 4 to 6 (next to the spinal column). In the case of deficiency or Cold, moxibustion may also be applied.

In modern scalp acupuncture, the points on the first lateral line on both sides of the vertex (*E pang xian* 1) are selected.

In terms of manipulation, for acute attack of angina pectoris P 6 and HT 6 are needled obliquely towards the body and may be slightly reinforced or manipulated with strong stimulation using the 'sparrow pecking' method (*Que Zhuo Fa*) until the sensation of *Qi* has reached the site of pain; retain for 30 minutes.

In China, the combination of two points by threading the needle under the skin is often employed. Provided the Western patient's consent is given (it sounds worse than it actually is), the needle may be threaded from *Tanzhong* (REN 17) down to *Jiuwei* (REN 15). The *Huatuo Jiaji* points should also be needled $1/2$ to 1 *cun* directed towards the spinal column, so that the sensation of *Qi* can spread to the chest area.

In scalp acupuncture (more appropriate for long-term effect), two needles per line are employed, which are stimulated every 1–5 minutes and then retained for 2 hours. During manipulation, the patient should perform slow deep breathing (this is absolutely vital in an acute attack!).

GROUP III B: SPECIFIC CHRONIC BLOOD STASIS (COMMONLY USED FORMULAS FROM GYNAECOLOGY)

24. *Shao Fu Zhu Yu Tang* (Anti-Stasis Lower Abdomen Decoction)

This formula is used particularly in gynaecology for Blood stasis accompanied by masses and gatherings in the lower abdomen, regardless of whether there is pain or not. It is also effective for lower abdominal pain without abdominal masses and for lower abdominal distension and fullness. It is also used for dysmenorrhoea that begins with back pain and a distended lower abdomen.

Moreover, it can be employed in the treatment of polymenorrhoea (several periods per month in close succession), where there are blood clots which are dark or purple. The formula is also used for uterine bleeding accompanied by lower abdominal pain or for bright bleeding with leukorrhoea, and for infertility.

Ingredients	
1. Fructus Foeniculi (*Hui Xiang*)	1.5 g
2. Rhizoma Zingiberis (*Gan Jiang*)	3 g
3. Rhizoma Corydalis (*Yan Hu Suo*)	3 g
4. Radix Angelicae Sinensis (*Dang Gui*)	9 g
5. Radix Ligustici Wallichii (*Chuan Xiong*)	3 g
6. Cortex Cinnamomi (*Rou Gui*)	3 g
7. Radix Paeoniae Rubrae (*Chi Shao*)	6 g
8. Pollen Typhae (*Pu Huang*)	9 g
9. Faeces Trogopteri (*Wu Ling Zhi*)	6 g

Application
This formula is taken as a warm decoction.

The main effect of this formula is based on removing stasis in the lower abdomen, regulating menstruation and eliminating pain. Due to its contents of fennel seeds, cinnamon, ginger and the remaining predominantly warm ingredients, this formula has a warm property and is therefore particularly suitable for treating Blood stasis due to Cold or with a concomitant Cold syndrome.

Suggested acupuncture treatment
The following points may be selected for treating Blood stasis in the lower abdomen: BL 15, BL 17, SP 10, REN 3, ST 25, SP 8.

25. *Gong Wai Huai Yun Fang* (Extra Uterine Pregnancy Formula)

This formula is effective for extrauterine pregnancy with threatened abortion.

Ingredients	
1. Radix Salviae Miltiorrhizae (*Dan Shen*)	15 g
2. Radix Paeoniae Rubrae (*Chi Shao*)	9 g
3. Semen Persicae (*Tao Ren*)	9 g
4. Resinum Olibani (*Ru Xiang*)	9 g
5. Myrrha (*Mo Yao*)	9 g

Application
This formula is taken as a warm decoction. It is indicated for hard lower abdominal distension that quickly increases in size, and a slight dark purple-red bloody discharge that increases in amount. In the case of extreme pain, the limbs may be icy cold, there may be dizziness, light flashes in the eye and perspiration. Depending on the case, the patient may also faint. The pulse is hidden (*Fu Mai*).

Explanation
The main effect of this formula is to break Blood stasis and invigorate Blood. Therefore, a high dosage of *Dan Shen* (Radix Salvia) is prescribed in combination with *Chi Shao* (Paeonia Rubra) and *Tao Ren* (Persica) to amplify the Blood invigorating effect. *Ru Xiang* (Olibanum) and *Mo Yao* (Myrrha) are particularly indicated for pain due to stasis. Together these medicinals can invigorate Blood, dispel stasis, reduce swelling and stop pain.

Note: extrauterine pregnancy is usually one of three types: extrauterine pregnancy with shock, miscarriage with a clotted discharged mass and unstable extrauterine pregnancy. The present formula is indicated for the last type.

In the case of low or unstable blood pressure due to loss of blood accompanied by a deficiency syndrome, the formula may be supplemented with ginseng; also in the case of cold extremities with aconite, in the case of inflammation and Heat with *Mu Dan Pi* (Moutan), *Bie Jia* (Amyda), *Zhi Ke* (Pericarpium Citri Aurantii) and *Chuan Shan Jia* (Squama Manitis), and in the case of Cold with *Cang Zhu* (Atractylodes), *Hou Po* (Magnolia) and *Ai Ye* (Artemisia).

Suggested acupuncture treatment
Knowledge of the abortive, i.e. delivery inducing points, is vital, and these should be avoided in the case of threatened abortion, e.g. L.I. 4, KID 7, BL 67, *Duyin* (extra 11).

26. *Wen Jing Tang* (Menses Warming Decoction)

In China, *Wen Jing Tang* is often used in gynaecology in the treatment of Blood stasis due to deficiency Cold in the *Ren Mai* and *Chong Mai*. In these channels, *Wen Jing Tang* warms and scatters Cold, invigorates and nourishes Blood and dispels stasis.

Ingredients

1. Fructus Evodiae (*Wu Zhu Yu*)		9 g
2. Ramulus Cinnamomi (*Gui Zhi*)		6 g
3. Radix Angelicae Sinensis (*Dang Gui*)		9 g
4. Radix Ligustici Wallichii (*Chuan Xiong*)		6 g
5. Radix Paeoniae Lactiflorae (*Bai Shao*)		6 g
6. Cortex Moutan Radicis (*Mu Dan Pi*)		6 g
7. Colla Corii Asini (*E Jiao*)		9 g
8. Tuber Ophiopogonis (*Mai Men Dong*)		9 g
9. Radix Ginseng or Codonopsitis (*Ren Shen* or *Dang Shen*)		6 g
10. Rhizoma Pinelliae (*Ban Xia*)		6 g
11. Radix Glycyrrhizae (*Gan Cao*)		6 g
12. Rhizoma Zingiberis Recens (*Sheng Jiang*)		6 g

Application

This formula is taken as a warm decoction. Typical indications are irregular menstruation, raised temperature in the afternoon, irritability, hot palms and soles, dry mouth and lips, fullness and abdominal pain, excessive bleeding after delivery and infertility.

Action

1. Warms the vessels and scatters Cold.
2. Nourishes Blood and removes Blood stasis.

Explanation

This formula was designed especially for Blood stasis due to Cold and deficiency of the *Ren Mai* and *Chong Mai*, which have a close relationship to pregnancy (*Ren*) and menstruation (*Chong*), and may both lead to a Cold syndrome in the case of deficiency. This in turn leads to Blood stasis and *Qi* stagnation, and may occasionally manifest as deficient Heat (false Heat syndrome). Thus this formula treats the cause and the consequences by warming and supplementing both channels, by nourishing Blood and strengthening the weakened *Qi*.

Fructus Evodiae (*Wu Zhu Yu*) and Ramulus Cinnamomi (*Gui Zhi*) warm the channels, scatter Cold and activate stagnated Blood. Radix Angelicae Sinensis (*Dang Gui*), Radix Ligustici Wallichii (*Chuan Xiong*) and Radix Paeoniae Lactiflorae (*Shao Yao*) regulate menstruation, stimulate the cir-

culation of Blood and nourish Blood. Cortex Moutan Radicis (*Mu Dan Pi*) also stimulates the circulation of blood and removes deficient Heat symptoms such as afternoon fever and hot palms and soles. Colla Corii Asini (*E Jiao*) and Radix Ophiopogonis (*Mai Men Dong*) nourish the *Yin* and by doing so clear deficient Heat. Radix Ginseng (*Ren Shen*) and Radix Glycyrrhizae (*Gan Cao*) tonify *Qi* and strengthen the Spleen to promote the movement of Blood, because it is the Spleen's function to 'hold' the Blood inside the blood vessels. Rhizoma Pinelliae (*Ban Xia*) disperses masses in the body and assists in removing Blood stasis. Rhizoma Zingiberis (*Sheng Jiang*) warms, stimulates the Stomach to improve digestion and absorption, and harmonizes the other medicinals.

Suggested acupuncture treatment

Use the points REN 6, KID 13, SP 6, DU 4, KID 3, BL 17, SP 10, BL 20, ST 36 with moxibustion and reinforcing manipulation.

REN 6 works on the uterus. KID 13 is the Meeting point of the Kidney channel and the *Chong Mai*. The combination of these points regulates both the *Ren Mai* and *Chong Mai*. SP 6 nourishes Blood and *Yin*. DU 4 and KID 3 warm and nourish the Kidney to scatter Cold. BL 17 and SP 10 stimulate the circulation of Blood and remove Blood stasis. ST 36 and BL 20 tonify the Spleen and strengthen Middle *Qi*.

27. Ai Fu Nuan Gong Wan (Artemisia Cyprus Pill)

In comparison to *Wen Jing Tang*, this formula does not act as strongly on Blood stasis; however, it is stronger for nourishing Blood and for warming, especially the uterus. For this reason it is used for Cold and deficiency affecting the uterus and concurrent Blood deficiency.

Ingredients

1. Folium Artemisiae Argyi (*Ai Ye*)		90 g
2. Rhizoma Cyperi (*Xiang Fu*)		180 g
3. Fructus Evodiae (*Wu Zhu Yu*)		90 g
4. Radix Ligustici Wallichii (*Chuan Xiong*)		90 g

Ingredients continues

Ingredients (cont'd)	
5. Radix Paeoniae Lactiflorae (*Bai Shao*)	90 g
6. Radix Astragali (*Huang Qi*)	90 g
7. Radix Dipsaci (*Xu Duan*)	45 g
8. Radix Rehmanniae (*Sheng Di Huang*)	30 g
9. Cortex Cinnamomi (*Rou Gui*)	15 g
10. Radix Angelicae Sinensis (*Dang Gui*)	90 g

Application

The ingredients are ground and processed with vinegar and flour into pills, of which 12–15 g are taken as one dose.

Typical indications are leukorrhoea, menstrual disorders, abdominal pain, infertility, a sallow yellowish complexion, cold limbs, tiredness, lethargy and no appetite.

Action

1. Warms the uterus and nourishes Blood.
2. Invigorates Blood.

Explanation

As this formula has stronger Blood nourishing and warming actions than *Wen Jing Tang*, but a less strong effect on Blood stasis, it is especially suitable for patients with Blood-Cold in the Uterus and Blood deficiency.

Ai Ye (Artemisia) is one of the gynaecological medicinals that warm and stop bleeding. It is combined with *Ruo Gui* (Cortex Cinnamomi) and *Wu Zhu Yu* (Evodia) to amplify the warming nature of the formula. *Dang Gui* (Angelica Sinensis), *Bai Shao* (Paeonia) and *Shou Di* (Rehmannia Praeparata) nourish Blood, *Chuan Xiong* (Ligusticum) invigorates Blood. *Huang Qi* (Astragalus) strongly supplements *Qi* whilst *Xiang Fu* (Cyperus) moves *Qi* and regulates the menses. *Xu Duan* (Dipsacum) consolidates the *Chong Mai* and *Ren Mai* and removes obstructions from the vessels. Vinegar has a general stabilizing effect on losses of fluids and Blood.

Suggested acupuncture treatment

Use the points REN 6, KID 13, SP 6, DU 4, KID 3, SP 10, BL 20, ST 36 with moxibustion and a reinforcing manipulation.

28. *Sheng Hua Tang* (Generate Change Decoction)

This formula nourishes the Blood and promotes the formation of Blood, but also invigorates Blood and transforms stasis, as is implied by its name *Sheng Hua* 'generate and change' (i.e. changing (transforming) stasis of the old Blood and generating new Blood). It is also worth mentioning that *Sheng* can also mean delivery, which is why this formula is commonly used following a delivery.

It invigorates Blood, removes stasis, warms the channels and stops pain. The associated syndrome is postpartum Blood stasis with Cold and Blood deficiency.

Ingredients	
1. Radix Angelicae Sinensis (*Dang Gui*)	25 g
2. Radix Ligustici Wallichii (*Chuan Xiong*)	9 g
3. Semen Persicae (*Tao Ren*)	6 g
4. Rhizoma Zingiberis (*Gan Jiang*)	2 g
5. Radix Glycyrrhizae Praeparatae (*Zhi Gan Cao*)	2 g

Application

This formula is taken as a warm decoction. Typical indications are continued bleeding (metrorrhagia), for example due to retention of the placenta, a sensation of cold and pain in the lower abdomen, a dark purple tongue body and a deep, knotted pulse.

Action

1. Invigorates Blood and removes Blood stasis.
2. Warms the channels and stops pain.

Explanation

After delivery, the mother's Blood is usually affected by deficiency and is therefore more susceptible to pathogenic Cold, which then leads to Blood stasis. For this reason, this formula uses Radix Angelicae Sinensis (*Dang Gui*) to nourish and activate Blood. Radix Ligustici Wallichii (*Chuan Xiong*) and Semen Persicae (*Tao Ren*) invigorate the Blood, whilst the latter also dispels Blood stasis. Rhizoma Zingiberis (*Gan Jiang*) warms the body, scatters Cold and stops pain. Radix Glycyrrhizae Praeparatae (*Zhi Gan Cao*) harmonizes all the ingredients.

In the case of Cold due to chilled food accompanied by abdominal binding and pain, *Rou Gui* (Cortex Cinnamomi) may be added. If blood clots are not yet dissolved, one should definitely not prescribe *Qi* tonifying medicinals such as Astragalus or Ginseng, otherwise the pain will not stop. Recently, this formula has also been used successfully for treating insufficient lactation.

Caution
This formula is not suitable for patients with Blood stasis and internal Heat, as most of its ingredients are of a warming nature.

Suggested acupuncture treatment
The points REN 3, ST 30, SP 8 and REN 4 should be used with moxibustion and a reinforcing and reducing manipulation.

REN 3 acts on the uterus. ST 30 is the Meeting point of the Stomach and *Chong Mai* channels, thus the combination of these two points can regulate the *Chong Mai* and *Ren Mai*. SP 8 is the *Xi*-Cleft point of the Spleen channel; it can stimulate the circulation of Blood and stop pain. Moxibustion on REN 4 can scatter Cold and remove pain.

29. *Gui Zhi Fu Ling Wan* (Cinnamon and Poria Pills)

This is a very balanced formula that is suitable for invigorating Blood, removing Blood stasis and gently dissolving abdominal masses (*Zheng* concretions).

In China, it is commonly used for Blood stasis in the Uterus with restless foetus, continued bleeding with dark blood and lower abdominal pain that is aggravated by pressure.

Ingredients	
1. Ramulus Cinnamomi (*Gui Zhi*)	9 g
2. Poria Cocos (*Fu Ling*)	9 g
3. Cortex Moutan Radicis (*Mu Dan Pi*)	9 g
4. Semen Persicae (*Tao Ren*)	9 g
5. Radix Paeoniae Rubrae (*Chi Shao*)	9 g

Application
This formula is taken as a warm decoction or processed with honey into pills, of which 3–5 g are taken per day.

Typical indications are preceding Blood stasis in the Uterus or present Blood stasis with restless foetus, bleeding presenting with dark blood and accompanied by lower abdominal pain that is aggravated on pressure.

Action
1. Activates circulation of Blood and dispels Blood stasis.
2. Dissolves abdominal masses.

Explanation
This is a well balanced and mild formula, as it is designed to treat Blood stasis and loss of Blood without damaging the foetus or the mother. Ramulus Cinnamomi (*Gui Zhi*) is employed to warm and activate Blood. Poria Cocos (*Fu Ling*) drains Heat by virtue of its diuretic effect and thus calms the foetus. It also nourishes the Heart and Spleen. As chronic Blood stasis often entails Heat syndromes with all kinds of bleeding, Cortex Moutan Radicis (*Mu Dan Pi*) and Radix Paeoniae Rubrae (*Chi Shao*) are employed to invigorate as well as cool the Blood.

When prescribed as a honeyed bolus, the formula has an even milder action, and this is ideal in the later stages of pregnancy.

Furthermore, it can be used for irregular menstruation or post-menstrual abdominal pain as well as for prolonged lochia or metrorrhagia with dark blood.

Caution
This formula is not suitable for Blood stasis with Heat, and should not be used if Blood stasis is not present.

Suggested acupuncture treatment
It is safer to avoid acupuncture in the case of a restless foetus.

30. *Xia Yu XueTang* (Blood Stasis Purging Decoction)

This formula is used for amenorrhoea or postpartum pain and concretions (*Zheng*) in the lower abdomen due to Blood stasis.

Ingredients	
1. Rhizoma et Radix Rhei (*Da Huang*)	9 g
2. Semen Persicae (*Tao Ren*)	9 g
3. Eupolyphaga (*Bie Chong*)	9 g

Application

This formula is taken as a warm decoction, or ground and mixed with honey into pills and taken together with alcohol.

Typical indications are similar to those mentioned for *Tao Hong Cheng Qi Tang* (*Qi* Rectifying Persica Carthamus Decoction), the difference being that the latter formula treats Heat and stasis binding in the lower abdomen that also affects the Mind. The present formula treats Blood stasis with dry Blood stagnating in the umbilical area, which is palpable, but without pain or mental changes.

31. *Yong Quan San* (Gushing Spring Powder)

This formula is indicated for postpartum insufficient lactation due to *Qi* stagnation and Blood stasis.

Ingredients	
1. Semen Vaccaria (*Wang Bu Liu Xing*)	9 g
2. Semen Trichosanthis (*Tian Hua Fen*)	4.5 g
3. Radix Glyzyrrhizae (*Gan Cao*)	9 g
4. Radix Angelicae (*Dang Gui*)	4.5 g
5. Squama Manitis (*Chuan Shan Jia*)	9 g

Application

The ingredients are ground and taken together with pig's trotters soup. The typical indication is postpartum insufficient lactation due to Liver-*Qi* stagnation or Blood stasis caused by Blood deficiency.

Action

1. Nourishes and invigorates the Blood and soothes Liver-*Qi*.
2. Removes obstructions from the *Luo* vessels and generates milk.

Suggested acupuncture treatment

Use the points REN 17 and ST 18 with the needle directed towards the nipple. In the case of Liver-*Qi* stagnation add SI 1, P 6 and LIV 3; in the case of Blood deficiency add BL 20 and ST 36. Use reinforcing manipulation, except P 6 and LIV 3 which should be reduced.

REN 17 regulates *Qi* of the chest and ST 18 promotes lactation by regulating the *Qi* of the *Yang Ming* channel. BL 20 and ST 36 tonify the Spleen and Stomach, thus promoting the formation of *Qi* and Blood. SI 1 promotes lactation in general, P 6 and LIV 3 bring stagnated Liver-*Qi* back into flow.

32. *Xi Huang Wan* (Yellow Rhino Pills)

Although the name of this formula mentions the word '*Xi*' (rhinoceros), there are no parts of the rhinoceros contained in it. It is used for hardenings and lumps in the breasts and lymph glands.

Ingredients	
1. Calculus Bovis (*Niu Huang*)	1 g
2. Moschus (*She Xiang*)	4.5 g
3. Olibanum (*Ru Xiang*)	30 g
4. Myrrh (*Mo Yao*)	30 g
5. Millet (*Huang Mi*)	30 g

Application

The first four ingredients are mixed and ground. Then they are mixed with the pulverized millet, rolled into small balls and slowly dried (do not heat as there are volatile compounds). Three to six of these balls are taken with alcohol or warm water twice daily.

Typical indications are hardenings and lumps in the breasts and lymph glands. The latter are hard but movable and painless and feel like pearls under the skin. The colour of the skin is unchanged.

Action

1. Invigorates blood and stops pain.
2. Detoxifies and dissolves hardenings.

Explanation

Calculus Bovis (*Niu Huang*) has a cooling, detoxifying and Phlegm transforming effect in this formula. Moschus (*She Xiang*) removes obstructions from all vessels and removes swellings and lumps. Olibanum (*Ru Xiang*) and Myrrh (*Mo Yao*) invigorate Blood and dispel Blood stasis. Finally, millet harmonizes the Spleen and strengthens the Stomach.

In China, this formula is mostly available as a patent remedy and is used for benign breast lumps, lymphadenitis and idiopathic swollen lymph nodes.

Caution

This formula is contraindicated for pregnant women and patients with *Yin* deficiency and a false Heat syndrome. Long-term application is not recommended as this will injure Stomach *Qi*.

SUMMARY

Table 8.1 gives a short overview comparing these formulas.

IMPORTANT PATENT REMEDIES RELEVANT TO BLOOD STASIS

At this point a few important patent remedies that are relevant to Blood stasis are presented. Due to the different names used for these in various provinces in China, several related patents will be summarized into one category. In each case, the composition is valid for the first patent name. Due to the variety of names and the multitude of patent remedies only a small selection can be presented here, the efficacy of which I was able to test for myself in clinical practice.

Paralysis, post–apoplectic hemiplegia and *Bi* syndrome

Da Huo Luo Wan (Beijing and Tianjin)
Ren Shen (Ginseng)
Niu Huang (Calculus Bovis)
She Xiang (Moschus)
Shui Niu Jiao (Cornu Bovis)
Bing Pian (Borneolum)

Huang Lian (Coptidis)
Dang Gui (Angelica Sinensis)
Quan Xie (Buthus)
Tian Ma (Gastrodia)
Wu Shao She (Zaocys)

- Actions: removes obstructions from the vessels, moves Blood and expels Wind-Dampness from the channels.
- Indications: used in post-apoplectic hemiplegia, paralysis, *Bi*-syndrome, arthralgia.
- Contraindications: pregnancy (as Moschus induces labour).

Tianma Wan (Chongqing), **Tianma Pian** (Guangdong), **Tianma Qufeng Bu Pian** (Nanjing)
Tian Ma (Gastrodia)
Dang Gui (Angelica Sinensis)
Sheng Di Huang (Rehmannia)
Huai Niu Xi (Achyranthis Bidentata)
Du Zhong (Eucomnia)
Qiang Huo (Notopterygium)
Fu Zi (Aconitum Praeparata)
Bi Xie (Dioscorea Hypoglauca)
Xuan Shen (Scrophularia)

- Actions: expels Wind-Dampness, moves *Qi* and Blood, stops pain.
- Indications: paralysis and numbness in the limbs, gait problems, stroke sequelae and rheumatic arthritis.
- Contraindication: use with caution during pregnancy.

Hui Tian Zaizao Wan (Liaoning), **Yinao Fujian Wan** (Jinan), **Sanqi Pian** (Yunnan), **Nao Xueshuan Pian** (Tianjin)
Ren Shen (Ginseng)
Niu Huang (Calculus Bovis)
She Xiang (Moschus)
Shui Niu Jiao (Cornu Bovis)
Bao Gu (Os Leopardis)
Tian Ma (Gastrodia)
Xue Jie (Sanguis Draconis)
Yang Xue (Sanguis Naemorhedi)

- Actions: moves Blood, extinguishes Wind, transforms Phlegm.
- Indications: facial paralysis and hemiplegia.
- Contraindication: none, but *Nao Xueshuan Pian* is only used for thrombotic apoplexy as it contains Hirudo.

Table 8.1 Comparison of formulas

Group	Formula	Site of action	Symptom/syndrome	Concomitant factor of Blood stasis
I	*Fu Yuan Huo Xue Tang* (Blood Invigorating Recovery Decoction)	Rib area	Extreme pain	Trauma
	Qi Li San (Seven *Li* Powder)	Localized trauma	Pain	Trauma
	Die Da Wan (Trauma Pill)	Musculoskeletal system, skin	Pain	Exhaustion/trauma/ Cold/Wind
	Jie Du Huo Xue Tang (Detoxifying, Blood Invigorating Decoction)	Entire body	Exsiccosis due to diarrhoea with vomiting	Deficiency of Body Fluids
	Tong Jing Zhu Yu Tang (Anti-Stasis Exanthema Decoction)	Skin	Skin reactions and changes	Heat
	Hui Yan Zhu Yu Tang (Anti-Stasis Epiglottis Decoction)	Neck and throat	Problems of the vocal cords and throat	Phlegm
II	*Shen Tong Zhu Yu Tang* (Anti-Stasis Pain Decoction)	Musculoskeletal system, especially joints	Severe pain	Depending on the type of *Bi* syndrome: Heat/Wind/Cold
	Bu Yang Huan Wu Tang (*Yang* Tonifying Five-Tenth Decoction)	Brain, paralysed side of the body	Hemiplegia	*Qi* deficiency
	Dan Shen Yin (Salvia Drink)	Heart and stomach	Pain	*Qi* stagnation
	Shi Xiao San (Sudden Smile Powder)	Chest, abdomen	Pain, abdominal masses (*Zheng* concretions)	Only Blood stasis
	Shou Nian San (Hand-made Pill)	Epigastrium, abdomen	Pain	*Qi* stagnation, Cold
	Huo Luo Xiao Ling Dan (Wondrous Pill to Invigorate the Channels)	Entire body	Pain	*Qi* stagnation and also traumas
	Shu Jing Huo Xue Tang (Relaxing the Vessels Decoction)	Muscles, limbs	Pain, numbness	Dampness or *Bi* syndrome with exhaustion or weakness
	Da Huang Zhe Chong Wan (Rheum Eupolyphaga Pill)	Abdomen, vessels	Exhaustion, abdominal masses	*Qi* and *Yin* deficiency, Heat
	Di Dang Tang (Resistance Decoction)	Entire body, colon	Dark and hard stools and other typical symptoms	Heat in the Blood area
	Tao Hong Si Wu Tang (Persica Carthamus Four Ingredients Decoction)	Entire body, menstruation, skin	Menstrual disorders, typical symptoms	Blood and *Yin* deficiency
	Yang Yin Tong Bi Tang (*Yin* Nourishing *Bi* Dissolving Decoction)	Chest, heart, Kidney and Liver (TCM organs)	Heart *Bi*, pain, *Yin* deficiency syndrome	*Yin* deficiency and *Qi* or Blood deficiency, *Qi* stagnation
	Dian Kuang Meng Xing Tang (Psychosis Decoction)	Psyche, mind	Confusion, manic-depressive psychosis	Phlegm, Heat, Liver-*Qi* stagnation

Table continues

Table 8.1   Comparison of formulas (cont'd)

Group	Formula	Site of action	Symptom/syndrome	Concomitant factor of Blood stasis
III A	Tao Hong Cheng Qi Tang (Qi Rectifying Persica Carthamus Decoction)	Lower Burner, head, Blood division	Typical signs of Heat syndrome	Heat
	Xue Fu Zhu Yu Tang (Anti-Stasis Chest Decoction)	Chest, mind	Typical signs of Blood stasis	Qi stagnation
	Tong Qiao Huo Xue Tang (Orifices Opening, Blood Invigorating Decoction)	Head and skin	Typical signs of Blood stasis and blockage of the orifices	None
	Ge Xia Zhu Yu Tang (Anti-Stasis Abdomen Decoction)	Abdomen, hypochondrium area	Pain, abdominal masses, fullness	Qi stagnation
	Guan Xin Er Hao Fang (Coronary Decoction No. 2)	Chest, heart	Pain, crushing pain, shortness of breath	Q stagnation
III B	Shao Fu Zhu Yu Tang (Anti-Stasis Lower Abdomen Decoction)	Lower abdomen	All gynaecological indications, pain	Cold
	Gong Wai Huai Yun Fang (Extra Uterine Pregnancy Formula)	Abdominal cavity	Pain, extrauterine pregnancy	None
	Wen Jing Tang (Menses Warming Decoction)	Ren Mai and Chong Mai	Deficiency Heat syndrome, menstrual disorders	Cold, Qi deficiency of the Ren and Chong Mai
	Ai Fu Nuan Gong Wan (Artemisia Cyperus Pill)	Uterus	Menstrual disorders, abdominal pain	Qi deficiency, Blood deficiency, Cold in the Uterus
	Sheng Hua Tang (Generate Change Decoction)	Blood, the breast in females	Pain, prolonged postpartum haemorrhaging	Cold and Blood deficiency after blood loss
	Gui Zhi Fu Ling Wan (Cinnamon and Poria Pills)	Lower abdomen, foetus, abdomen	Pain, restless foetus, prolonged haemorrhaging, conglomerations	Heat
	Xia Yu Xue Tang (Blood Stasis Purging Decoction)	Periumbilical area	Abdominal masses (Zheng)	None
	Yong Quan San (Gushing Spring Powder)	Female breast glands	Insufficient lactation	Liver-Qi stagnation or Blood deficiency
	Xi Huang Wan (Yellow Rhino Pills)	Female breast, lymph glands	Lumps, hardenings, lymphoma	Phlegm, probably Heat

Coronary heart diseases

Acute angina pectoris

Guan Xin Su HeWan (Styrax Coronary Pill), **Su Xiao Tong Xin Wan** (Tianjin), **Guan Xin Su He Wan** (Shandong), **Huo Xin Wan** (Guangdong), **Xin Bao** (Guangdong)

Su He Xiang 80 g (Styrax)
Bing Pian 150 g (Borneol)
Ru Xiang 150 g (Olibanum)
Tan Xiang 300 g (Santalum)
Mu Xiang 300 g (Aucklandia Lappa)

This formula is processed using a low temperature into approximately 1000 pills weighing 1 g each. Allow one pill per intake to dissolve under the tongue or administer the dissolved pill via an endotracheal tube. 1–3 pills daily or in an acute attack.

- Actions: opens the orifices by virtue of its content of essential oils, moves *Qi* and stops pain.
- Indication: angina pectoris due to CHD, sensation of pressure or fullness in the chest, partly with shortness of breath in the case of (according to TCM) *Qi* stagnation in the chest due to turbid Phlegm.
- Contraindication: *Qi* deficiency syndrome.

Chronic coronary heart disease

Fu Fang Dan Shen Pian (Wuxi, Shengxian, Tianjin and Shanghai), **Fu Fang Danshen Gao** (Jining), **Huang Qi Dan Shen Pian** (Tianjin), **Fu Fang Dan Shen Pian** (Zhejiang), **Fu Fang Dan Shen Di Wan** (Guangdong), **Huo Xue Tong Mai Pian** (Beijing)

Fu Fang Dan Shen Pian was approved by the American Food and Drug Administration (FDA) for the treatment of CHD in 1998.

Dan Shen (Salvia), *San Qi* (Notoginseng) and *Bing Pian* (Borneol) are used in a ratio of 6 : 3 : 1. A few similar patents also contain a *Qi* tonic such as Astragalus or Ginseng.

- Actions: invigorates the Blood, opens the orifices by virtue of its content of essential oils, moves *Qi* and stops pain.
- Indications: angina pectoris due to CHD, sensation of pressure or fullness in the chest, partly with shortness of breath in the case of (according to TCM) *Qi* stagnation in the chest due to Blood stasis and *Qi* stagnation.

- Contraindication: *Qi* deficiency syndrome (except *Huo Xue Tong Mai Pian* and *Huang Qi Dan Shen Pian*).

Rheumatic diseases

An Luo Tong Pian (Shanghai), **Xiao Luo Tong Pian** (Shandong)

Ingredients: mainly 1–2 medicinals such as *Yan Hu Suo* (Corydalis), *Gui Mao Zhen*, *Yuan Hua* etc.

- Actions: expels Blood stasis and Wind, stops pain.
- Indications: arthralgia and rheumatic pain.
- Contraindications: varies according to each remedy, but mostly none.

Shenjindan Jiaonang (Wehai, Shandong)

Di Long (Lumbricus)
Ma Qian Zi (Semen Strychni)
Hong Hua (Carthamus)
Ru Xiang (Olibanum)
Mo Yao (Myrrha)
Fang Ji (Stephania Tetrandra)
Gu Sui Bu (Drynaria)

- Actions: breaks Blood stasis and moves Blood and *Qi*, removes obstructions from the channels and collaterals, stops pain and reduces swelling.
- Indications: periarthritis of the shoulder, cervical spondylosis, sciatica, arthritic pain in the extremities and neck due to fractures.
- Contraindications: not during pregnancy and breastfeeding due to its content of *Ma Qian Zi*.

Baogujiu (Taoyuan), **Hugu Yaojiu** (Beijing), **Hugu Jiu** (Beijing)

Bao Gu (Os Leopardis)
Yi Yi Ren (Coix)
Bi Xie (Dioscorea Hypoglauca)
Yin Yang Huo (Epimedii)
Shou Di (Rehmannia Praeparata)
Chen Pi (Citrus Reticulata)
Yu Zhu (Polygonatum Odoratum)
Niu Xi (Achyranthis Bidentata)
Xiang Jia Pi (Periploca Radix)
Dang Gui (Angelica Sinensis)

- Actions: the medicinal wines mentioned here are all suitable for expelling Wind and Wind-

Dampness, for removing obstructions from the vessels and for invigorating the Blood.

- Indications: Cold-*Bi* and Damp-*Bi* characterized by arthralgia and numbness in the limbs, muscle pain and weak legs and back.
- Contraindications: pregnancy and patients with Fire syndromes due to *Yin* deficiency and high blood pressure.

Gynaecological diseases

Fukang Ning Pian (Tianjin), *Danggui Jingao Pian* (Lanzhou), *Fuke Shi Wei Pian* (Sichuan), *Jin Ji Chongji* (Guangdong), *Nü Bao* (Jilin), *Yi Mu Cao Gao* (Tianjin)

Dang Gui (Angelica Sinensis)
San Qi (Notoginseng)
Bai Shao (Paeonia)
Yi Mu Cao (Leonurus)
Xiang Fu (Cyperus)

- Actions: removes Blood stasis and *Qi* stagnation, stops pain.
- Indications: dysmenorrhoea, amenorrhoea, metrorrhagia, postpartum lochias, pain etc. *Jin Ji Chongji* is especially suitable for endometriosis and all pelvic inflammations. It contains medicinals from the local province.
- Contraindications: pregnancy; no restrictions for *Jin Ji Chongji*.

Pain and injuries

Yuanhu Zhitong Jiaonang (Shanxi), *Yuanhu Zhitong Pian* (Shandong)

Contains *Yuan Hu* (Corydalis) and *Bai Zhi* (Angelica Dahurica).

- Indications: *Yuanhu Zhitong Jiaonang* is used particularly for headache, stomach pain, hepatic pain and dysmenorrhoea.
- Contraindication: use with caution during pregnancy.

Qili San (Beijing), *Jiufen San* (Beijing)

For the composition of *Qili San*, see *Qi Li San* in Appendix 5.

- Actions: breaks stasis, invigorates Blood, promotes circulation, stops pain and reduces swelling.
- Indications: all kinds of traumatic pain, hypochondriac pain due to hepatitis.

- Contraindications: pregnancy; *Jiufen San* is also contraindicated in high blood pressure, heart and kidney diseases.

Yunnan Baiyao (Kunming)

This patent remedy stems from the family tradition of the *Yi* minority in Yunnan, who sold the formula to the government during the 1950s. Its unpatented predecessor was used successfully for gunshot wounds in the Sino-Japanese War of Resistance. The ingredients are top secret; apart from local herbs of the *Yi* minority it certainly contains *San Qi* (Notoginseng) and *Huo Xiang* (Patchouli).

- Actions: *Yunnan Baiyao*, like *San Qi*, has a universal application as it not only stops pain but also stops bleeding and moves Blood.
- Indications: These include all kinds of injuries, both internal and external, swellings, abscesses, circulation problems as in thrombophlebitis, and menstrual disorders such as dysmenorrhoea and irregular menstruation, where the remedy should be taken with some wine. The powder can be applied externally on abscesses and wounds and will immediately stop bleeding. Every bottle of *Yunnan Baiyao* also contains one small red pill, which is an especially strong dose of the medicine. This can be used in the case of severe injuries, and especially in transient ischaemic attack (TIA, temporary disorder of cerebral circulation) and in the acute stage of stroke (ischemic and thrombotic). Never take more than one pill per day. Since 1998 *Yunnan Baiyao* has also been available as a spray.
- Contraindications: pregnancy; on the first day of intake no fish or sour and cold food should be consumed to avoid indigestion. The red emergency pill should not be taken for minor injuries.

RESEARCH REPORTS ON THE 10 MOST COMMON TREATMENT METHODS FOR BLOOD STASIS, CLASSIFIED ACCORDING TO WESTERN DISEASE DEFINITIONS

Having discussed the pharmacological effects and the application of Blood invigorating medicinals in the earlier part of the chapter, we go on now to outline the actual combinations of medicinals used by individual physicians and hospitals.

However, the inexperienced TCM practitioner is advised that the prescriptions must be used flexibly and modified according to the individual condition of the patient. Hardly any CHD patient in China would be prescribed an unmodified prescription of 'Coronary Decoction No. 2' (*Guan Xin Er Hao*). It is one of the studied aims of TCM to avoid both cookery book acupuncture and standard prescriptions. This may make studying TCM more difficult, but it is actually one of its best features as there will be greater and more precisely directed efficacy in treatment. The prescriptions listed for each disease are to be understood as a starting point and not as a dogma.

1. Heart and vascular diseases

Coronary heart disease (CHD)

'Chest *Bi* disease', *Xiong Bi* in Chinese as described in the '*Jin Kui Yao Lüe*', is characterized primarily by a sensation of pressure or tension in the chest, and also by pain but to a lesser degree. Within the clinical picture of CHD, this would correspond to its mild initial stages as well as to an unusual condition such as painless attacks of angina pectoris or silent myocardial ischemia and infarcts. Severe disease and conditions characterized by greater pain are usually related more to the syndromes of 'heart pain', *Xin Tong*, as described in the '*Nei Jing*' (pain in the middle of the chest reaching under the ribs, pain in the shoulder that radiates to the back). Another possibility is that such severe pain would relate to 'crushing pain', *Jue Xin Tong*, mentioned in the '*Ling Shu*' (pain as if stabbed in the heart, accompanied by cold hands and feet, cold sweating and weakness). Both these types coincide more usually with unstable angina pectoris or acute myocardial infarction.

Even worse is the 'absolute (literally: true) heart pain' – *Zhen Xin Tong* – which in its pathology coincides exactly with acute infarction. It was also described in the '*Ling Shu*': 'Cyanosis of the hands and feet as far as the joints, extreme pain, starting in the morning it will lead to death at night, and starting in the evening it will lead to death in the morning . . .'. The disease names mentioned in the classics are thus classified by Dr Gu according to their degree: chest-*Bi*, heart pain, crushing pain and eventually absolute heart pain.

Following a review of 333 cases of CHD in a clinical study of angina pectoris, infarction, heart insufficiency and arrhythmia, Dr Gu from Zhejiang concluded that CHD would predominantly present itself as fundamentally an illness of deficiency, but would manifest symptoms of excess. These deficiency syndromes include in particular a combined pattern of *Qi* and *Yin* deficiency, followed by *Qi* deficiency and *Yin* deficiency, *Yang* deficiency and finally a combined pattern of *Yin* and *Yang* deficiency.

Using *Zang Fu* differentiation, most of the *Qi* deficiency syndromes were Heart-*Qi* deficiency (66.5%), most of the *Yang* deficiency syndromes were Heart-*Yang* deficiency (60.5%) and most of the *Yin* deficiency syndromes were patients suffering from Liver-*Yin* deficiency (75.1%).

Amongst the excess syndromes, the primary syndrome was a combined pattern of *Qi* stagnation and Blood stasis, which appeared either in isolation or in combination with deficiency syndromes (98.19%).

Dr Wang Bao-He, from the Second University Hospital for TCM, used *Hongjingtian* capsules in the treatment of 100 cases of chest-*Bi* syndrome with angina pectoris. (*Hongjingtian*, Rhodiola Rosea L, is a native plant from traditional Tibetan medicine and has Blood invigorating and stasis dispelling properties.) The rate of efficacy was 53% with 37 cases of complete recovery and 48 cases of significant improvement after an average of 4.77 ± 2.52 days.

Heart insufficiency

When the *Kangxinshuai* formula (*Dang Shen, Fu Zi, Wu Jia Pi, Chi Shao, Chuan Xiong, Ji Xue Teng, Yi Mu Cao, Ze Lan, Mai Men Dong*) was used for congestive left heart failure in a study of the TCM Research Institute Chongqing, a positive effect was shown in 96.5% of the cases. Of these 70% showed a significant improvement, so that digitalis treatment could be discontinued after 3–7 days. Dr Xu employed an equally successful formula called *Xinshuai Heji*, which contains *Huang Qi, Tai Zi Shen, Ze Xie, Ting Li Zi, Sang Bai Pi, Zi Dan Shen, Wu Wei Zi, Che Qian Zi* and *Dang Gui*.

High blood pressure

The Second Hospital of Taian City in Shandong province used the principle of 'invigorating Blood and strengthening the Kidney' in its formula *Xue Ping* in the treatment of high blood pressure. The formula contained *Huang-Jing* extract, *Sang Ji Sheng*, *Mao Dong Qing*, *Xia Ku Cao*, *Huai Mi*, *Niu Xi*, *Gu Jing Cao*, *Guo Teng*, *Sheng Ma* and other medicinals. In a study of 200 elderly patients with Kidney deficiency and Blood stasis, blood pressure was significantly lowered.

Arrhythmia

The Xiyuan Research Hospital, Beijing, employed classical formulas according to the principle of 'Wenyang fumai' (warming *Yang* and recovering the pulse), e.g. *You Gui Yin* (Kidney *Yang* Drink), *Zhen Wu Tang* (True Warrior Decoction), *Bao Yuan Tang* (Origin Preserving Decoction), *Er Chen Tang* (Two Old Decoction) etc. The average heart rate was raised from 46.65 to 58.18 beats per minute (bpm). The department of Heart Pathology Research of the Shandong TCM Hospital treated 60 patients successfully using its own formula *Jianxin Fumai Ling*, which contains *Huang Qi*, *Dan Shen*, *Gan Song*, *Chuan Xiong* and *Gui Zhi*. The average heart rate was raised from 53.2 to 61.1 bpm, resulting in a rate of efficacy of 83.3%.

Peripheral vascular diseases

Dr Fan Jian-Zhong's formula *Tong Mai Fang*, containing *Fu Zi*, *Huang Qi*, *Dou Zhi*, *She Xiang*, *Gan Jiang*, *Gui Zhi*, *Hu Zhang* and *Gan Cao*, managed to fully break up thrombi in 46 out of 53 patients with thrombotic vasculitis, and in 4 patients it reduced the thrombi. After 2 months, 15 patients were cured and 33 had significantly improved.

Over a period of 23 years (1968–1991), Dr Wei achieved a total curative rate of 92% using a medicated wine 'Tongbi Huoxue Jiu'. The formula is based on a modification of *Huang Qi Gui Zhi Wu Wu Tang* (Astragalus and Cinnamon Five Ingredients Decoction) and contains *Dan Shen* (Salvia Miltiorrhiza), *Huang Qi* (Astragalus), *Dang Gui* (Angelica Sinensis), *Zang Hong Hua* (Saffron), *Ma Huang* (Ephedra), *Chang Pu* (Acorus), *Shui Zhi* (Hirudo), *She Xiang* (Moschus), *Rou Gui* (Cortex Cinnamomi), *Gan Jiang* (Zingiberis) and *Chen Pi* (Citrus Reticulata), all preserved in rice wine.

Using his formula *Mai Yan Ling* (Vasculitis Preparation), and without adding any further drugs such as antiphlogistics, Dr Chen from the Yinan Research Institute for Vascular Diseases, Henan province, achieved a treatment efficacy of 97.3%, compared to the control group treated with orthodox drugs reaching an efficacy of 87.1%. In subsequent follow-ups, it was recorded that relapse in the latter group was 21.77%, whilst it was only 11.45% in the experimental group treated with *Mai Yan Ling*.

Thrombophlebitis

Dr Tang Yhu-Xuan from Shanghai employed his formula *Qingre Tongyu Tang* in 43 cases of inflammatory venous thrombosis for 2 weeks. A full recovery was achieved in 26 patients, a significant improvement in 10, an improvement of symptoms in 5 and no effect in 2 patients. The total efficacy rate was 95.23%. His formula consisted of *Cang Zhu* (Atractylodes) 15 g, *Huang Bai* (Phellodendron) 15 g, *Dang Gui* (Angelica Sinensis) 30 g, *Shui Zhi* (Hirudo) 30 g, *Yi Yi Ren* (Coix) 30 g, *Xuan Shen* (Scrophularia) 45 g, *Yin Hua* (Lonicera) 45 g, *Huang Qi* (Astragalus) 15 g, *Quan Xie* (Buthus) 10 g, *Wu Gong* (Scolopendra Subspinipes) 3 pieces and *Gan Cao* (Glycyrrhiza) 5 g.

2. Diseases of the liver and metabolism

Hepatitis

In the Yunnan Provincial Hospital, Professor Su Lian treats hepatitis B and C patients with modifications of his Spleen-*Qi* strengthening, Liver calming and Blood invigorating prescriptions 1 to 4. The base formula contains *Chai Hu* (Bupleurum) 10 g, *Bai Shao* and *Chi Shao* (Paeonia Lactiflora and Rubra) 15 g each, *Fu Ling* (Poria) 9 g, *Chao Bai Zhu* (Atractylodes Macrocephala Praeparata) 12 g, *Dan Shen* (Salvia Miltiorrhiza) 15 g, *Yi Yi Ren* (Coix) 20 g, *Jian Shan Zha* (Crategus Tosta) 15 g, *Huang Qi* (Astragalus) 30 g, *Chong Lou* (also known as *Zao Xiu*) 10 g, *Zao Ren* (Ziziphus Spinosa) 20 g, *Ye Jiao Teng* (Caulis Polygoni Multifloris) 30 g, *Zi Hua Di Ding* (Viola Yedoensitis) 20 g, *Sang Ji Sheng* (Ramulus Loranthi) 30 g, *Sheng Gan Cao* (Glycyrrhiza Recens) 4 g. He explains that after taking these medicinals for 2–3 months patients would have no further complaints and the clinical findings would also be negative. Pharmacologically, his formula combines virustatic herbs such as *Zi Hua Di Ding*, immune strengthening herbs such as *Huang Qi*, Blood invigorating herbs such as *Dan Shen* and hepato-protective herbs such as *Chai Hu*. All these medicinals confine the hepatitis and prevent its sequelae. At the same time, herbs for promoting digestion such as *Shan Zha* and relaxing herbs such as *Suan Zao Ren* are prescribed to remove the concomitant symptoms of hepatitis.

Liver cirrhosis

In a study of 105 patients suffering from cirrhosis due to chronic hepatitis, Dr Yu Hui-Yin used his formula *Huang Qi Dan Shen Huang Jing Tang* (Astragalus Salvia Polygonatum Decoction) and achieved a full recovery in 42.9%, a significant improvement in 29.5% and a measurable effect in 18.1%. The total efficacy rate was 90.5%. The formula contains *Huang Qi* (Astragalus), *Dan Shen* (Salvia), *Huang Jing* (Polygonatum), *Ji Nei Jin* (Endothelium Galli), *Ban Lan Gen* (Istadis), *Lian Qiao* (Forsythia), *Jiang Cao* (Patrinia), *Bai Zhu* (Atractylodes Macrocephala), *Fu Ling* (Poria), *Yu Jin* (Curcuma), *Dang Gui* (Angelica), *Nü Zhen Zi* (Ligustrum) and *Zi He Che* (Placenta).

Diabetes

Dr Guo from Beijing used his formula *Xian Zhen Pian* (Epimedium Lucidum Tablets) in 34 cases of type II diabetes. After 2 months he had not only achieved a lowering of blood sugar levels by 61.8% and a reduction in levels of lipid peroxides (LPO), but also an increase in levels of superoxide dismutase (SOD) and high density lipoprotein-cholesterol (HDL-C). His formula contains *Yin Yang Huo*, *Nü Zhen Zi*, *Huang Qi*, *Dan Shen*, *He Shou Wu*, *Tu Si Zi*, *Gou Qi Zi*, *Huang Jin* and *Shan Zha*.

Circulation disorders that are common in diabetics can be treated very successfully with Blood invigorating medicinals. Dr Li from the Kaifeng TCM Hospital, Henan province, successfully treated 51 patients suffering from pathological changes of the retina with his formula *Bushen Huoxue Fang*. The formula contained *He Shou Wu* (Radix Polygoni Multiflori), *Huang Jing* (Polygo-

natum), *Shi Hu* (Herba Dendrobii), *Yin Yang Huo* (Epimedii), *Ge Gen* (Radix Puerariae), *Chi Shao* (Paeonia Rubra), *Chuan Niu Xi* (Cyathula), *San Qi* (Notoginseng) and other medicinals.

3. Cerebral diseases

Apoplexy

Wang Qing-Ren's *Bu Yang Huan Wu Tang* (Yang Tonifying Five Tenth Decoction) is still used with modifications in the treatment of apoplexy. The First Hospital of Harbin City prescribed a modified version of this formula to 19 patients with acute embolic apoplexy over a period of 25 days. There were 14 cases with significant improvement, 4 cases with mild improvement and one case with no improvement. The formula contained *Chuan Xiong* (Ligusticum), *Tao Ren* (Persica), *Di Long* (Lumbricus), *Chi Shao* (Paeonia Rubra), *Huang Qi* (Astragalus), *Dang Gui* (Angelica Sinensis) and in addition *Chuan Shan Jia* (Squama Manilis), *Dan Shen* (Salvia Miltiorrhiza) and *Ge Gen* (Pueraria).

A certain Dr Lü reported an efficacy rate of 97.3% in a study of 37 patients: 25 were cured and 11 showed a significant improvement. His modification contained *Chuan Xiong* (Ligusticum), *Tao Ren* (Persica), *Hong Hua* (Carthamus), *Di Long* (Lumbricus), *Chi Shao* (Paeonia Rubra), *Huang Qi* (Astragalus), *Dang Gui* (Angelica Sinensis) and also *Dan Shen* (Salvia Miltiorrhiza), *Ge Gen* (Pueraria), *Gui Zhi* (Ramulus Cinnamomi), *Sang Zhi* (Morus A), *Chuan Niu Xi* (Cyathula), *Ji Xue Teng* (ibid) and *Tong Bian* (Infantis Urina).

Dr Zhang Ji-Fen from the Tianjin Dongli TCM Hospital reported the treatment of 32 cerebrovascular accidents with *Angong Niuhuang Wan* (Calm the Palace Calculus Bovis Pill), which resulted in an improved action of invigorating Blood, removing obstructions from the vessels and opening the orifices. The formula was prepared as an injection: 40–60 ml with 5% glucose per 500 ml were administered once daily. One course of treatment lasted for 30 days. According to the criteria of the 2nd National Cerebrovascular Accident Conference, the curative rate was 65.63%, the efficacy rate was 34.37% and the average recovery time was 27.36 days.

Dr Wang Wenbo from the Tianjin Hexi TCM Hospital reported the treatment of 35 patients with ischemic apoplexy, who were prescribed a combination of *Huazhuo-Quyu* Decoction and infusions of *Huang Qi* (Astragalus). The *Huazhuo-Quyu* Decoction contains *Chuan Xiong* (Ligusticum), *Dan Shen* (Salvia Miltiorrhiza), *Tao Ren* (Persica), *Dang Gui* (Angelica Sinensis), *Di Long* (Lumbricus), *Yu Jin* (Curcuma), *Shi Chang Pu* (Acorus), *Tian Zhu Huang* (Concretio Silicea Bambusae), *Ji Xue Teng* (Jixueteng), *Wu Shao She* (Zaocys Dhumnades), *Chen Pi* (Pericarpium Citri Reticulatae), *Pei Lan* (Herba Eupatorii Fortunei) and *Fu Ling* (Sclerotium Poriae Cocos). After patients were admitted to hospital, the decoction was administered twice daily, along with 20 ml of *Huang Qi* infusion together with 200–500 ml of glucose once daily. The longest course of treatment was 3 months, the shortest 16 days. In total, 13 patients were cured, 10 experienced a significant improvement, 9 a mild improvement, and 3 showed no effect.

Senile dementia (including multi infarct dementia (MID) and Alzheimer's disease)

Blood invigorating medicinals have a particular effect on patients with MID. When used for this purpose they are commonly combined with Phlegm transforming or Kidney strengthening medicinals. The patent remedy *Yi Zhi Ling* was used in 51 cases of senile dementia in the Shandong TCM University Hospital. A full recovery was achieved in 18 patients, a significant improvement in 13, an improvement in 16 and no improvement in 4 patients. The total efficacy rate was 92%. *Yi Zhi Ling* is based on the treatment principle 'strengthen the Kidney, invigorate Blood, remove Phlegm and stasis'.

Parkinson's disease

The most common established formulas used by the Shanghai TCM University are *Xi Feng Tang* (Wind Allaying Decoction) and *Rou Gan Huo Xue Tang*. The former contains *Tian Ma* (Gastrodia), *Quan Xie* (Buthus), *Gou Teng* (Ramulus Uncariae Cum Uncis), *Wu Gong* (Scolopendra Subspinipes) and *Yang Jin Hua* (Flos Daturae), and was prescribed for Liver-Wind (96.5% total efficacy rate in 58 patients). The latter formula contains *Shou Di* (Rehmannia Praeparata), *Huai Niu Xi* (Achyranthis Bidentata), *Dang Gui* (Angelica Sinensis),

Gou Qi Zi (Lycium), *Shou Wu* (Radix Polygoni Multiflori), *Bai Shao* (Paeonia Lactiflora), *Dan Shen* (Salvia Miltiorrhiza), *Mu Gua* (Fructus Chaenomelis) and *Ji Xue Teng* (Jixueteng), which was used for Liver and Kidney deficiency with Blood stasis in the collaterals. Modifications of this formula were used in the treatment of 48 cases of Parkinson's disease and achieved an efficacy rate of 60.7%.

4. Gynaecological diseases

Female infertility

According to an investigation carried out by the Shanghai Long Hua Hospital in 1987, the highest incidence in 257 cases of female infertility was due to Blood stasis (29.57%), followed by Kidney-*Yang* deficiency (27.63%). All other syndromes had a minor incidence (2–12%). The formulas most commonly used for infertility due to Blood stasis are Wang Qing-Ren's *Shao Fu Zhu Yu Tang* (Anti-Stasis Lower Abdomen Decoction), *Ge Xia Zhu Yu Tang* (Anti-Stasis Abdomen Decoction) and their modifications. *Wu Jin Wan* (Black Gold Pill), a patent remedy, is frequently used as well. In the treatment of ovarian cysts, Blood invigorating medicinals are combined with Kidney-*Yang* tonics. Another patent formula frequently used here is *Gui Zhi Fu Lin Wan* (Cinnamon and Poria Pills).

In the East-West Clinic in Shipai, the Taiwanese Professor Chang Chung-Kwo from Taipei treated 108 cases of infertility, which were partly due to tubal adhesions, and had been given up on by conventional gynaecologists. He prescribed decoctions containing *Wang Bu Liu Xing* (Vaccaria), *Yu Jin* (Curcuma), *Dan Shen* (Salvia Miltiorrhiza) and other medicinals, which after a treatment course of 2–6 months resulted in the patients becoming pregnant.

Menstrual disorders

Blood invigorating medicinals are prescribed in nearly all menstrual disorders, especially lower abdominal pain during menstruation, pain all over the body and in the chest, and headache (migraine). Further conditions treated with Blood invigorating medicinals and formulas, depending on the case, include intermenstrual bleeding, prolonged menstruation, heavy excessive bleeding and scanty bleeding.

Dr Tian from Shanghai employed a modification of Wang Qing-Ren's *Xue Fu Zhu Yu Tang* (Anti-Stasis Chest Decoction) in 70 cases of dysmenorrhoea. This resulted in 34 cases of full recovery, 31 of significant improvement and 5 cases of no recovery.

For complaints related to the menopause, *Ge Xia Zhu Yu Tang* (Anti-Stasis Abdomen Decoction) and *Wen Jing Tang* (Menses Warming Decoction) are often used in China, as emphasized by Maciocia in his book[6] on gynaecology.

Pregnancy

Most Blood stasis medicinals are contraindicated during pregnancy. Exceptions are *Chi Shao* (Paeonia Rubra), *Si Gua Luo* (Luffa), *Ji Xue Teng* (Jixueteng), *Dan Shen* (Salvia Miltiorrhiza) and *Dang Gui* (Angelica Sinensis), which are used, for example, as part of a special formula called *Gong Wai Yun* Formula No. 2 (Extra Uterine Pregnancy Formula No. 2) in cases of extrauterine pregnancy. In cases of threatened habitual abortion due to Blood stasis, Wang Qing-Ren's *Shao Fu Zhu Yu Tang* (Anti-Stasis Lower Abdomen Decoction) is used.

Delivery

Due to the potential danger of abortion, other Blood invigorating medicinals are not used during pregnancy. However, they are often used during and shortly after delivery. In cases of difficult delivery or labour, a special formula called *Cui Sheng Yin* (Labour-Inducing Drink) is used. In the case of breech delivery, *Bao Chan Wu You San* (Delivery Protecting Carefree Powder) is used, which was originally used by the famous gynaecologist Fu Qing-Zhu.

Other gynaecological disorders

One hundred and fifteen cases of chronic pelvic inflammation were treated by Dr Huang, Shanghai, using a modification of *Shao Fu Zhu Yu Tang* (Anti-Stasis Lower Abdomen Decoction). After three treatment courses he recorded a full recovery in 33 patients (no further abdominal pain, no clinical findings, and in a case of previous infertil-

ity the patient was able to become pregnant) and a significant improvement in 51 patients (mostly absent symptoms, no clinical findings, adnexitis no longer detectable, and in a case of previous infertility the patient was able to become pregnant). There was an improvement in 28 patients (reduced symptoms, guarding pain reduced as well, palpable masses had been softened, adnexitis swelling had gone down) and no improvement in 6 patients (i.e. no improvement of symptoms, clinical examination remained positive). Thus, the total efficacy rate was 94.9%.

5. Skin diseases

Dermatology includes various diseases that are difficult to treat in Chinese Medicine. This is partly due to the fact that many of today's skin diseases, e.g. neurodermatitis and allergies to various new substances and environmental toxins, were unknown in ancient times, therefore new strategies have to be developed. Still, in some diseases TCM gets better results than Western medicine. In addition to the predominant treatment principles of cooling Heat-Toxins, expelling Wind and Dampness and supplementing deficiency, invigorating Blood and breaking stasis are also used.

Skin diseases that respond well to these medicinals are categorized as follows:

1. Skin diseases with a fixed pain, e.g. herpes zoster, painful erythemas etc.
2. Skin diseases with lichenification, e.g. erythema nodosum, erythema induratum, various warts and tuberculid lesions.
3. Skin diseases characterized by a rough, dry skin such as sclerotic skin lesions, psoriasis, neurodermatitis, chronic eczema, lichen planus etc.
4. Skin diseases due to vascular changes, e.g. scleroderma, generalized lupus erythematosus, dermatitis, polymyalgia rheumatica, rheumatic fever, rheumatoid arthritis and tuberculous polyarteriitis etc.

One example will be presented from each category.

Herpes zoster

Dr Hu Jian-Hua treated 132 cases of herpes zoster accompanied by severe pain using Blood invigor-

---

[6] G. Maciocia: *Obstetrics and Gynaecology in Chinese Medicine* (see Appendix F).

ating, pain stopping and Heat-toxins cooling medicinals. Symptoms receded in between 2 (earliest) and 17 days (latest), giving an average of 7.5 days. The earliest time the pain receded was on the third day, the latest time was on the thirtieth day (average: 10.6 days).

Verrucae

Dr Zhao Wu from Shanghai treated 67 cases of molluscum contagiosum with three courses of 10 days each using a modification of *Tao Hong Si Wu Tang* (Persica Carthamus Four Ingredients Decoction). After 30 days, 49 cases were cured, 12 were significantly improved, 5 were improved and 2 cases showed no effect. This resulted in a total efficacy rate of 97%. The formula mainly contained *Tao Ren* (Persica), *Hong Hua* (Carthamus), *Dang Gui* (Angelica Sinensis), *Chi Shao* (Paeonia Rubra), *Sheng Di* (Rehmannia), *Chuan Xiong* (Ligusticum), *Ma Qian Zi* (Semen Strychni), *Zi Cao* (Lithispermum), *Bai Jiang Cao* (Patrinia), *Xia Ku Cao* (Prunella), *Ban Lan Gen* (Isatis), *Yi Yi Ren* (Coix) and other medicinals.

Psoriasis

Dr Li Zheng-Yin from Shanghai treated 126 cases of psoriasis for 45–60 days using a modification of *Huang Qi Tang* (Astragalus Decoction). Seventy-eight patients (61.9%) experienced a full recovery, 34 patients (27%) had a basic recovery, and in 7 patients (5.6%) symptoms improved, resulting in a total efficacy rate of 97.5%. The formula consisted of *Huang Qi* (high dosage), *Dang Gui* (Angelica Sinensis), *Dan Shen* (Salvia Miltiorrhiza), *Hong Hua* (Carthamus), *Ji Xue Teng* (ibid), *Sheng Di Huang* (Rehmannia), *Bi Xie* (Dioskorea Hypoglauca) and *Ci Ji Li* (Tribuli). In the case of pronounced symptoms of Blood-Heat he added *Sheng Gui Hua* (Osmanthus) and *Bai Mao Gen* (Imperatus); in the case of respiratory or tonsillar infections he added *Jin Yin Hua* (Lonicera) and *Ban Lan Gen* (Isatis); in the case of Blood-Dryness he added *Tian Men Dong* (Asparagus), *Mai Men Dong* (Ophiopogonis) and *Lu Feng Fang* (Nidus Vespae).

Purpura-like, lichenoid dermatitis

Dr Xu Li-Ying treated 20 cases of this kind of dermatitis with three courses each of 4 weeks duration. His prescription was discontinued for a few days during menstruation. He achieved a full recovery in 8 patients (40%), a significant improvement in 6 and an improvement in 5 patients. His formula contained *Shui Niu Jiao*, *Sheng Di Huang* (Rehmannia), *Chi Shao* (Paeonia Rubra), *Mu Dan Pi* (Moutan), *Zi Cao* (Lithispermum), *Tao Ren* (Persica), *Hong Hua* (Carthamus), *Dang Gui* (Angelica Sinensis) and *Yi Mu Cao* (Leonurus). An improvement set in on average between the first and second week.

His colleague Dr Zhu Guang-Dou used a similar formula in 279 cases of purpura and achieved a full recovery in 47.3%, a significant improvement in 21.5%, an improvement in 18.3% and no effect in 13.3% of all patients. In total, the efficacy rate was 86.7%.

6. Oncological diseases

The 'Huang Di Nei Jing' had already attributed abdominal masses and all kinds of tissue hardening to stagnation of *Qi* or Blood stasis, as for example with 'Ji and Ju', 'Zheng and Jia'. Those gatherings that move around and are not fixed are ascribed to *Qi*, whilst those that are fixed and hard come into the category of Blood diseases, that is Blood stasis. This category includes benign as well as malignant tumours, hence Blood invigorating medicinals play an important role in oncology. Many anticarcinogenic, mutation-inhibiting and immune-stimulating medicinals are to be found in the section on the pharmacological action of Chinese herbs, including a large number of Blood invigorating medicinals. In addition, my own research has shown that Blood stasis itself may constitute a carcinogenic factor. In China it is now common practice to treat cancer by prescribing Blood invigorating medicinals in combination with cancer-inhibiting drugs; if the patient receives chemotherapy at the same time, other medicinals may be added to reduce or neutralize its side effects.

Blood stasis medicinals are most commonly combined with herbs having the following actions: moving *Qi*, cooling Heat-toxins, softening and dissolving masses, removing obstructions from the collaterals, and tonifying (*Fu Zheng*). They may also be combined with drugs used in chemotherapy. A few examples from clinical investigations are presented below.

Dr Wang Chuang-Cai from Shanghai treated 44 cases of terminal oesophageal cancer using Blood invigorating and Phlegm transforming medicinals; patients experienced an average further life span of 11 months after treatment (up to 15 months in 50% of the cases). Symptoms were removed in 24 patients, partly alleviated in 16, slightly alleviated in 3, and remained unchanged in 1 patient. The base formula, which was modified for every case, contained 30 g each of *Tian Nan Xing* (Arisematis), *Ban Xia* (Pinellia) and *Gua Lou* (Trichosanthis), 15 g each of *Zhi Ke* (Pericarpium Citri Aurantii) and *Shan Zha* (Crataegus), and 10 g each of *Huang Yao Zi* (Dioscorea Bulbifera), *Chen Pi* (Pericarpium Citri Reticulatae), *Ji Xing Zi* (Impatiens Balsamica), *Wang Bu Liu Xing* (Vaccaria), *E Zhu* (Curcuma Ezhu), *Tu Bie Chong* (Eupolyphaga), *Chuan Shan Jia* (Squama Manitis) and *Chan Pi* (Bufo).

In cases of *Qi* deficiency he added *Huang Qi*, *Dang Shen*, *Xi Yang Shen*, *Bai Zhu*, *Fu Ling*; in cases of Blood deficiency he added *Tian Men Dong*, *Mai Men Dong*, *Sheng Di Huang*, *Huang Jing* and *Gui Ban*; in cases of Spleen deficiency he added *Bai Zhu*, *Fu Ling*, *Bian Dou*, *Ji Nei Jin*, *Shan Zha Qu* (Massa Fermentata Con Crataegi) and *Gu Mai Ya*; in cases of ascending Stomach-*Qi* he added *Ding Xiang*, *Hong Xiang Teng* (Dalbergia Hancei), *Fu Xuan Hua* and *Dai Zhe Shi*; in cases of oedema he added *Zhu Ling*, *Fu Ling*, *Bai Zhu* and *Che Qian Zi*.

Cytotoxic agents that act against tumour cells are *Mo Yao* (Myrrha), *Mu Dan Pi* (Moutan), *Chi Shao* (Paeonia Rubra), *Da Huang* (Rheum), *Yue Ji Hua* (Rosa Chinensis), *E Zhu* (Curcuma Ezhu), *Tu Bie Chong* (Eupolyphaga), *Wu Gong* (Scolopendra Subspinipes), *Mang Chong* (Tabanus), *Quan Xie* (Buthus), *Dan Shen* (Salvia Miltiorrhiza) and the patent remedy *Yunnan Baiyao*. *Da Huang Zhe Chong Wan* (Rheum Eupolyphaga Pills), *Bie Jia Jian Wan* etc. are used especially for liver cancer. In the treatment of cervical tumours, *E Zhu* (Curcuma Ezhu) has shown good results. The National *E Zhu* Research Foundation investigated 173 cases of cervical cancer and achieved a recovery rate of 28.9% after a short treatment period, resulting in a total efficacy rate of 71.1%.

Comparing radiotherapy to concomitant TCM treatment and radiotherapy, there were significant differences evident. Dr Cai Wei-Min from Shanghai treated nearly 200 patients suffering from nasopharyngeal carcinoma, of whom 105 were only treated with radiotherapy and 92 received TCM herbs and radiotherapy. After 1, 3 and 5 years the survival rates in the radiotherapy group were 80%, 33.3% and 24%; in the combined treatment group, survival rates were 91.2%, 67.4% and 52.5%. (P < 0.05–0.01).[7] These figures speak for themselves.

7. Urogenital diseases

Chronic nephritis
Dr Wang from Beijing treated 47 patients using a combination of Spleen- and Kidney-*Yang* warming medicinals (*Ba Ji Tian*, *Yin Yang Huo*, *Fu Zi Pian*, *Rou Gui*, *Huang Qi*, *Dang Shen*, *Bai Zhu*) and Blood invigorating and stasis transforming medicinals (*Dang Gui* (Angelica Sinensis), *Chuan Xiong* (Ligusticum), *Hong Hua* (Carthamus), *Chi Shao* (Paeonia Rubra), *Dan Shen* (Salvia Miltiorrhiza) and *Yi Mu Cao* (Leonurus)). His results were complete recovery in 36 cases, significant improvement in 6, an improvement in 3 and no improvement in 2 cases.

Chronic renal failure (CRF)
The treatment of chronic renal failure subsumes several treatment principles. Professor Zhang Da-Ning of the Tianjin TCM Municipal Hospital used Kidney strengthening and Blood invigorating medicinals in 128 cases of CRF, achieving a significant improvement in 84.4% of cases and a total efficacy rate of 51.5%. His own formulas were *Huo Xue Tang* (Blood Invigorating Decoction) containing *Chi Shao* (Paeonia Rubra), *Dan Shen* (Salvia Miltiorrhiza), *Ze Lan* (Lycopus), *San Leng* (Spargani), *E Zhu* (Curcuma Ezhu), *Tao Ren* (Persica) and others, as well as *Huoxue Huayu* Capsules (Blood Invigorating Stasis Transforming Capsules) containing *Wu Gong*, *Tian Xian Zi* and others, *Zi Bu Shen Gan Tang* (Kidney Liver Nourishing Decoction) containing *Nü Zhen Zi*, *Han Lian Cao*, *Shan Zhu Yu*, *Gui Ban*, *Dang Gui*, *Bai Shao* and others, *Shen Shuai Guanzhongye* (Kidney Insuffi-

---

[7] Cai Wei-Min in *Zhong Yi Za Zhi* 1983(3):36.

ciency Decoction) containing *Da Huang, Chi Shao, Da Huang Yan, Huang Qi, Fu Zi, Qing Dai* and others, one cooling formula and one for strengthening the Middle.

Prostatitis and prostatic enlargement

Dr Wang Shao-Jin from Tianjin use modified versions of *Fu Fang Di Hu Tang* (Earth Dragon – Tiger Decoction) containing *Di Long* (Lumbricus), *Hu Zhang* (Polygonum Cuspidati), *Mu Tong* (Akebia), *Che Qian Zi* (Plantago), *Lai Fu Zi* (Rhaphanus), *Huang Qi* (Astragalus), *Chuan Shan Jia* (Squama Manitis) and *Gan Cao* (Glycyrrhiza). In the case of *Yang* deficiency he added *Wu Zi Yan Zong Wan*, the Five Seeds Procreation Pill, containing *Wu Wei Zi* (Schisandra), *Tu Si Zi* (Cuscuta), *Gou Qi Zi* (Lycium), *Fu Pen Zi* (Rubus) and *Che Qian Zi* (Plantago). In cases of Blood-*Jing* deficiency he added *Sheng Di Huang* (Rehmannia), *Bai Mao Gen* (Imperatus), and in cases of narrowing of the prostate he added *E Zhu* (Curcuma Ezhu) and *Lei Wan* (Omphalia).

Dr Li also achieved good results with his formula *Qian Lie Xian Pian* (Prostate Tablets), containing *Yu Xing Cao* (Herba Houttuyniae), *Feng Wei Cao* (Herba Pteris Multifida Poir.), *Tu Fu Ling* (Smilax), *Che Qian Cao* (Herba Plantaginis), *Dan Shen* (Salvia Miltiorrhiza), *Yi Mu Cao* (Leonurus), *Bi Xie* (Diocorea Hypoglauca), *Chuan Lian Zi* (Semen Melia Toosendan), *E Zhu* (Curcuma Ezhu), *Rou Cong Rong* (Cistanches), *Lu Lu Tong* (Liqidambaris), *Dan Pi* (Moutan), *Nü Zhen Zi* (Ligustrum), *Mai Men Dong* (Ophiopogonis) and *Sheng Gan Cao* (Glycyrrhiza Recens).

In the case of prostate enlargement in elderly men, Dr Chen's *Yiyuan Kaichan Tang* (Source Nourishing and Opening Decoction) is commonly used, containing *Ba Ji Tian* (Morinda), *Shou Di* (Rehmannia Praeparata), *Wu Yao* (Lindera), *Tao Ren* (Persica), *Hong Hua* (Carthamus), *Shan Yao* (Dioscorea), *Bai Shao* (Paeonia), *Huang Qi* (Astragalus), *Rou Gui* (Cortex Cinnamomi) and *Ju He* (Epicarpium Citrus). Dr Yang's formula *Shen Ling Liu Huang Tang* (Codonopsis Poria Five Yellows Decoction) is also regarded as highly efficient, containing *Dang Shen* (Codonopsis), *Fu Ling* (Poria), *Sheng Di* (Rehmannia), *Huang Qi* (Astragalus), *Huang Lian* (Coptis), *Huang Bai* (Phellodendron), *Huang Jing* (Polygonatum), *Pu Huang* (Typha), *Niu Xi* (Achyranthis Bidentata) and *Che Qian Zi* (Plantago).

Anuria

Dr Zhou's *Long-Bi San* (Anuria Powder) with *Chuan Shan Jia* (Squama Manitis) and *Rou Gui* (Cortex Cinnamomi) in a ratio of 6 : 4 and Dr Li Wen-Biao's modification of *Shengma-Huangqi-Tang* with *Huang Qi* (Astragalus), *Dang Gui* (Angelica Sinensis), *Hua Shi* (Talcum), *Sheng Ma* (Cimicifuga), *Chai Hu* (Bupleurum), *Gan Cao* (Glycyrrhiza), *Shi Chang Pu* (Acorus) and *Zhu Ye* (Bambusa) both prove to be highly effective in everyday clinical practice.

8. Chronic haematopoietic disorders

In 121 cases of chronic haematopoietic disorders, Dr Chen Qiu-Shi used a modification of *Liu Wei Di Huang Wan* (Rehmannia Six Pill) with Blood moving medicinals and achieved an efficacy rate of 83.3%. Apart from the ingredients of *Liu Wei Di Huang Wan*, the formula also included *Ji Xue Teng* (Jixueteng), *Dang Gui* (Angelica Sinensis), *Bai Shao* (Paeonia), *Dan Shen* (Salvia Miltiorrhiza) and other Blood invigorating medicinals. Dr Chen Yun-Qi used a similar formula in 4 cases with haematopoietic disorders. His formula, which was equally effective clinically, contained *Sheng Di Huang* (Rehmannia), *Nü Zhen Zi* (Ligustrum), *Han Lian Cao* (Eclipta), *Gou Qi Zi* (Lycium), *Zhi Shou Wu* (Polygoni Multiflori Praeparata), *Tu Si Zi* (Cuscuta), *Huang Qi* (Astragalus), *Dang Shen* (Codonopsis), *Bai Zhu* (Atractylodes Macrocephala), *Huang Jing* (Polygonatum), *Dan Shen* (Salvia Miltiorrhiza), *Ji Xue Teng* (Jixueteng), *Dang Gui* (Angelica Sinensis), *Chuan Xiong* (Ligusticum), *Tao Ren* (Persica) and *Zhi Ma Zi* (Sesamum).

9. Lung emphysema

Jiangong Hospital in Beijing treated many patients with emphysema that became aggravated during winter. When these patients were treated for a course of 3 months prior to the aggravation of the disease, it did not reoccur. The formula was called *Fei Qi Zhong Wan* (Emphysema Pill) and contained *Dan Shen* (Salvia Miltiorrhiza), *Chi Shao* (Paeonia

Rubra), *Shi Hu* (Herba Dendrobii), *Hong Hua* (Carthamus), *Xing Ren* (Pruni Armeniaca), *Wang Bu Liu Xing* (Vaccaria), *Huang Qi* (Astragalus), *Gou Qi Zi* (Lycium), *Pu Gong Ying* (Herba Taraxacum) and *Dong Chong Xia Cao* (Cordyceps Sinensis) as a medicated bolus.

10. Effect on symptoms of old age

In the treatment of lipofuscin pigments Dr Mo from Sichuan compiled his own formula called *Yishen Huayu Tang* (Kidney Strengthening Stasis Transforming Decoction), which consisted of *Shou Di* (Rehmannia Praeparata), *Shan Yao* (Diocorea), *Shan Zhu Yu* (Cornum), *Dan Shen* (Salvia Miltiorrhiza), *Tu Si Zi* (Cuscuta), *Rou Cong Rong* (Cistanches), *Fu Ling* (Poria), *Mu Dan Pi* (Moutan), *Jiang Can* (Bombyx), *Hong Hua* (Carthamus), *Ze Xie* (Alismatis) and others.

Out of 34 patients, in 14 the marks completely disappeared, in 10 they were significantly reduced, in 7 they were slightly reduced and in 3 patients the marks remained unchanged. This resulted in a total efficacy rate of 91.8%, in comparison with the control group (64%), which had been treated with vitamin E and C as well as external applications.

Professor Zhang Da-Ning from the Tianjin TCM Municipal Hospital treated 400 patients suffering from ten significant signs of old age, according to his statistics: skin folds, loss of hair, reduction of mental and physical strength etc. After a few months of treatment, in 142 patients there was a pronounced improvement, in 247 there was a visible improvement and in 11 patients no improvement was noted.

COMMENTARY

I am aware that this list of biomedically-defined diseases, which includes the actual research results of treatment applications, may be very tempting, especially for beginners in TCM, but I would strongly advise against acquiring such a 'cookery book' treatment style, for the following reasons:

1. One of the great strengths of TCM is its flexibility in approaching the individual condition of the patient. Whoever foregoes this in favour of a 'quick fix' has failed to grasp the essence of TCM and should instead practise a less complex therapy such as kinesiology (touch for health) or something similar, because it applies fewer parameters in treatment.[8]

2. All the examples listed above are generalized from innumerable cases. In fact, virtually every formula varies a little (except for patent remedies), in order to cater for the individual symptoms of each patient.

3. To gain maximum efficacy in treatment, i.e. to achieve the best possible treatment results, TCM *must* be applied according to its rules. If TCM is carried out with an allopathic mindset (in the case of disease A prescribe medication B), it will not only prolong the patient's suffering but also damage the practitioner's reputation, because a longer treatment will entail more costs, and in the long run patients will stop coming back.

4. The study and thorough analysis of clinical research, and of the case studies in the next chapter, can help improve one's own understanding and practical skills in the application of Chinese medicine. This is why clinical research and case studies are presented and discussed here.

---

[8] This is not supposed to mean that I consider these methods as poor but rather as comparatively simple. Applied kinesiology only applies two parameters during testing, namely 'good' or 'not good' (similar to a principle of black and white, like *Yin* and *Yang*). However, it does not qualify or combine its information, which is not only possible but essential in Chinese medicine.

Chapter **9**

Practical cases: 20 further case studies from the ancient and modern practice of famous TCM physicians

Qin Bo-Wei, the great TCM doctor of the twentieth century, stresses the importance of analysing cases studies, which is the last step of studying TCM. It should become the life-long habit of every TCM doctor. By doing so, every newcomer can retrace the thoughts of 'master doctors', everyone at an advanced stage can learn from his colleagues and every 'master doctor' can see that there is more than one way of treating patients successfully.

The examples contained herein – like those cases presented in the first section of this book – come from classical and modern works, so a wide variety of case histories is ensured.

CLASSICAL CASE STUDIES

These stem predominantly from the Ming and Qing dynasties, where it first became the custom to draw up case records and to pass them on to other people for study. I have attached a short analysis to every case.

The first three cases were handed down by Ye Tian-Shi (1667–1746), one of the fathers of the febrile disease theory (*Wen Bing*). The work '*Ling Zheng Zhi Nan Yi An*' is not from him, but from the records of his students.

Ye was convinced that in long-term disease or enduring pain conditions the *Luo* vessels had to be treated as well, as it is stated in the '*Nei Jing*': 'Long-term disease enters the *Luo* vessels.' His conclusion was that repeated damage to the *Luo* vessels leads to *Qi* stagnation and Blood stasis, so he developed a 'Luo freeing method' (*Tong Luo Fa*).

For mild cases, this method employs laxatives with a pungent flavour, like Zhang Zhong-Jing's *Xuan Fu Hua Tang* (Inula Decoction), combined with Blood invigorating medicinals. For severe cases insects (*Chong*) are used as medicinals to break Blood stasis, as in Zhang's *Da Huang Zhe Chong Wan* (Rheum Eupolyphaga Pill), along with Lumbricus, Buthus and so on.

Ye coined this phrase: 'Blood stasis disorders also affect the *Qi* and in *Qi* disorders Phlegm is certain to accumulate.' This is clearly reflected in his treatment style.

Case 4 stems from Xu Da-Chun (1693–1772), the 'Leonardo' of Qing dynasty China, who was a brilliant physician, scientist and artist. Many case studies are to be found in the extensive works he left behind.

Case 5 was written by the famous physician Wu Ju-Tong (1758–1836), alongside Ye Tian-Shi another protagonist of the febrile disease theory (*Wen Bing*), who elegantly brought together the works of his predecessors and combined them with his own experiences.

Case 6 stems from Ding Gan-Ren (1866–1926), who assisted in creating modern TCM with his research and teaching in Shanghai. Here, he discusses the same syndrome as Ye Tian-Shi. While Ye describes the syndrome in the first case from the point of view of the febrile disease school (*Wen Bing*) and uses the so-called *Shi-Fang* (modern prescriptions), Ding presents the point of view of the *Jing-Fang* school (*Shang Han / Jing Kui* prescriptions).

Case 7 stems from Zhang Zhong-Hua from the middle of the Qing dynasty (approximately 1790). He devised plain and logical treatment principles but was also willing to strike new paths. He was also very concerned with gynaecology, as seen in this case of infertility.

Case 8 stems from the records of Zhang Xi-Chun (1860–1933), who stood at the borderline of classic (imperial) and modern TCM. He tried to integrate Western medical knowledge with TCM.

Case 9 stems from Zhao Wen-Kui (1870–1933), who still treated the imperial family at their court at the end of the Qing dynasty, and remained active as a doctor in the first days of the Republic. He was a specialist in pulse diagnosis, about which he published a book called the '*Wen Kui Mai Xue*' (*Wen-Kui's Pulse Diagnosis*). Unfortunately, nothing is mentioned about the pulse in this case study. It is interesting to compare this case to case 5, as Zhao also supported the *Wen Bing* school, and represents here the opinion of his time faced with the same syndrome.

Case 10 was penned by Cao Ren-Bai (1767–1834) of the Qing dynasty, whose case records – like those of Zhang Zhong-Hua – were collected by Qin Bo-Wei (1901–1970), the 'great TCM doctor of modern times', and thus remained preserved for our time. He set high standards for himself and others, as shown by his remark: 'When a physician devotes all his abilities to treatment, there is no disease under the sun he could not cure. If a disease is not cured, in my opinion this is due to the physician not having devoted all his abilities to the treatment.'

Compared with modern case studies, the ancient case records may often appear very short, reduced to the essentials; it was assumed that the reader already had good medical knowledge. For example, indications of the dosage or the pulse rate were often left out. Nevertheless, these cases still provide a fund of information with regard to the genuine, classic thinking of the ancients.

Case Study 9.1   Blood accumulation: Heat invading the room of Blood (*Re Ru Xue Shi*) (from Ye Tian-Zhi's '*Ling Zheng Zhi Nan Yi An*')

Patient Wu, Heat disease for 70 days, right pulse long, left pulse deep, tongue appears shrunken. Patient asks for cold drinks, there is restlessness and irritability. The Mind is sometimes clouded, sometimes clear.

The disease started on the third day of the menses. When the Heat-*Qi* sank downwards, Blood had just become deficient in the interior. This should be dealt with as Blood stasis with internal Heat, but as the disease has already

Case Study continues

progressed to a dangerous point, it must be treated (as described in the '*Jin Kui*') as a case of Blood accumulation, with mental symptoms (as if one had gone mad). Literally: '. . . the patient behaves as if mad, as the Heat has accumulated in the Lower Burner' (i.e. there is no water accumulation in the abdomen, but rather Blood stasis).

Prescription: *Sheng Di* (Rehmannia), *Mu Dan Pi* (Moutan), processed *Da Huang* (Rheum), *Tao Ren* (Persica), *Ze Lan* (Lycopus) and *Ren Zhong Bai* (Hominis Urinae Sedimentum).

Author's commentary

As is the case in many classics, Ye Tian-Shi gives no dosages as this knowledge is assumed in the medically educated reader. His diagnosis is succinct: with respect to the pathology he knows that during menstruation a febrile disease is more likely directly to attack the division of the Blood, which is empty due to the menses. The long pulse on the right confirms this: a long pulse indicates toxic Heat in the Blood or in the *Yang Ming*. A shrunken tongue suggests *Yin* deficiency, as the tongue obtains its full size from Body Fluids (*Yin*). A thirst for cold drinks and nervous irritability are also signs for Heat and deficiency of Body Fluids. Clouding of consciousness suggests that the Pericardium is affected by Heat in the Blood.

Surprisingly, the formula contains only substances with Blood invigorating actions: *Sheng Di Huang* and *Mu Dan Pi* also cool the Blood, *Ze Lan* drains urine, *Da Huang* promotes stool (not added at the end here, therefore the effect is focused on moving Blood). *Tao Ren* also promotes stool, but moisturizes it as well. Finally, the formula contains *Ren Zhong Bai*, also known as *Niao Bai Ning*, urine sediment

(Hominis Urinae Sedimentum), which collects on the walls of latrines, and is then dried and heated. Li Shi-Zhen describes it in the '*Ben Cao Gang Mu*': '. . . its effect is based on diuresis, it clears stasis in the Liver and Kidneys, Triple Burner, Lung, abdomen and lower abdomen. It is able to excrete pathogenic fluids and dispels Blood stasis.'

The reader may be surprised to hear that although today this 'revolting excremental drug' no longer belongs to the list of common medicinals, the urine of the working class masses is collected in each of the major cities of China in order to reclaim hormones which are excreted in trace amounts along with the urine. Hormones are active even in the smallest amounts; one should be careful not to deny this somewhat strange drug its effect. Today it is understood that the normally sterile urine contains urokinase and hormones such as 17-ketosteroids, oestrogen, 17-oxycorticosterone and gonadotrophins, as well as vitamins (B_1, B_2, B_6 and C) and essential minerals.

Case study 9.6 relates to the same syndrome, but is resolved in another way.

Case Study 9.2   Stomach pain: long–term disease invades the Blood (*Jiu Re Ru Xue*) (from Ye Tian-Zhi's '*Ling Zheng Zhi Nan Yi An*')

Patient Qin has been suffering from stomach pain for a long time. The illness got worse due to heavy work and overexertion, and eventually led to Blood stasis in the collaterals. Furthermore, rebellious *Qi* and nausea suggest obstruction of the local vessels and collaterals. Exterior- and interior-attacking medicinals were prescribed before, but this brought about no change for the patient. In this case, a quick-acting treatment is not suitable, because the patient is already emaciated and thin, therefore a gradual dispersal of Blood stasis should be employed.

Case Study continues

Dr[1] Ye writes in another paragraph concerning such diseases: 'This treatment is suitable when the patient presents with a fixed pain in the stomach,

a purple and dark tongue, a choppy pulse and a dark and dull complexion.'

Prescription: *Qing Lang Chong* (Catharsius Molossus), *Tu Bie Chong* (Eupolyphaga), *Wu Ling Zhi* (Trogopterus), *Tao Ren* (Persica), *Gui Zhi* (Ramulus Cinnamomi), *Chuan Niu Xi* (Cyathula), the juice of one stored *Xie Bai* (Allium root, called *Bai Niu Zhi Fa Wan*).

[1] At the imperial court, there was an equivalent of a doctorate; however, Ye Tian-Shi and most other physicians at that time and today did and do not hold a doctorate. However, I will keep to the tradition of using the title 'Dr' for every Chinese whose occupation is that of physician.

Author's commentary

It was Ye Tian-Shi who developed the theory that chronic diseases can disturb the Blood and that treatment should proceed slowly using non-drastic medicinals. In this case, there are two causes for the Blood stasis: long-term disease and exhaustion. Probably at the same time the *Qi* of the Liver, which stores Blood, was stagnated, so it attacked the Spleen, which in turn failed to process food as usual: as a result, the patient is emaciated, and the weakened *Qi* of the Stomach attacks upwards.

Thus, Doctor Ye prescribed onion juice and cinnamon to warm the Yang of the Middle and to treat the pain. These two medicinals remove obstructions from the *Luo* vessels (collaterals) and expel Cold – one of the three causes of the pain – at the same time.

Qing Lang Chong is cold, salty and goes into the Liver. Its action is to break stasis, dissolve hardness, calm and purge. New reports suggest it has anticarcinogenic effects. *Tu Bie Chong* also belongs

to the medicinals that break up stasis and dissolve hardness. *Wu Ling Zhi* stops pain and works on the Liver, but also on the Spleen, like the two previous medicinals. It is also used for a sensation of distension and heaviness (*Pi*) in the stomach. *Chuan Niu Xi* invigorates the Blood, like *Huai Niu Xi*; however, it does not guide the action of the formula downwards but rather concentrates on the middle area. *Tao Ren* breaks up stasis and also treats abdominal pain and promotes stool. The whole effect of the formula is directed towards breaking up Blood stasis, stopping pain and warming the Middle. From today's point of view, the formula may appear a little unbalanced, thus for long-term prescription one would have to add harmonizing medicinals such as *Da Zao*, *Fo Shou* or – provided the patient has no high blood pressure – *Gan Cao*, as the *Chong*-medicinals are not always very well tolerated by the stomach.

Case Study 9.3 Headache: persistent Blood stasis in the *Luo* vessels (*Jiu Re Ru Luo*) (from Ye Tian-Zhi's '*Ling Zheng Zhi Nan Yi An*')

Here the Yang-*Qi* is blocked by pathogens and cannot disperse in the orifices. In the classic text 'Zhou Li',[2] toxic[3] medicinals were used to cure

[2] Also called 'Li Jing', *Classic of the Rites* from the Zhou dynasty.
[3] Toxic in the sense of being derived from poisonous animals like wasps, scorpions, snakes etc.

diseases. This text mentions that *Chong*-drugs are used for dispelling stasis in the Blood, attacking accumulated pathogens and for removing obstructions. This is a classical method that has been forgotten by physicians. As the pain floods the brain, nausea and a feeling of vomiting arise in the epigastrium; and so – if there is a concomitant Liver syndrome – a deficiency syndrome develops,

Case Study continues

with a long-term disease present. While the pathogen is attacked (which depletes *Qi* and Blood), the healthy (Blood) needs to be nourished at the same time.

Prescription: *Chuan Xiong* (Ligusticum), *Dang Gui* (Radix Angelicae), *Ban Xia* (Rhizoma Pinelliae), *Zhi Quan Xie* (Scorpio Praeparata), *Jiang Zhi* (Sap Zingiberis Recens), *Feng Fang* (wasp's nest).

Author's commentary

In this third case study, which is similar to the second, Dr Ye uses the classical method of removing obstructions from the *Luo* vessels with *Chong*-drugs (wasp's nest and scorpion), which in this respect prove more efficient than herbal drugs. He also considered *Qi* stagnation, caused by Phlegm and Blood stasis, which develops during chronic disease, and this is treated by Pinellia and Chuanxiong.

Ginger juice prevents nausea and warms the *Yang*. Angelica root invigorates and nourishes the Blood. As we can see, Dr Ye frequently used insect drugs, which used to be common in ancient times but had nearly been forgotten in his time. Most of these medicinals that remove obstructions from the collaterals or extinguish Wind also have a Blood invigorating effect.

Case Study 9.4   Pain: generalized Blood stasis in the channels and *Luo* vessels (from Xu Da-Chun)

A patient called Xiu-Dong in the town of Wu had a strange disease: he suffered from pain that started in his back and then travelled to his chest and ribs. During the daytime, everything was normal, including his food and drink intake, but in the evening his pain would start and cause him to scream with pain all night long, which also disturbed the entire neighbourhood. After 5 years of ineffective treatments by physicians, the family's money was all used up and Xiu-Dong was ready to put an end to it all. However, his mother told him: 'You already have children, a daughter and a son for whom you must care. Instead, let me die, then I will not have to listen to all the mourning.' Because he wanted to drown himself, the relatives took pity on him and got a doctor (i.e. Dr Xu).

I said: 'This is a case of Blood stasis blocking the channels and *Luo* vessels.' I said to my son Xi:

'This is an unusual disease. A wide variety of therapies needs to be tried to help this patient. We can learn a lot here.'

As he was treated at home, and nothing was lading, I used acupuncture, moxibustion, applied heat and all sorts of medicinal preparations. Gradually, the pain was alleviated and was lasting for shorter periods of time. Eventually, after a month, he recovered and couldn't stop thanking me. But I replied: 'It's me who should thank you. Usually when I'm treating seriously ill patients I have to use all my knowledge to achieve success. These days, however, patients want to see immediate results after just one prescription. If they still haven't recovered after three prescriptions, they just go to another physician. But you believed in me all the way through, and eventually I learnt to understand your disease. How could I not be indebted to you?'

Author's commentary

Judging from the context, in spite of the fact that the patient's family hardly had any money, the physician adopted all available means to increase his own therapeutic knowledge. Although this case does not describe the treatments in detail, and Dr Xu merely explains that he employed all known methods, we can take a leaf out of his book as regards his ethics even today.

Case Study 9.5   Blood stasis due to Liver depression (*Gan Zhuo*; also known by wiseman as Liver fixity: translator's note) (from Wu Ju-Tong – Zi-name Wu Tang)

Liver depression presenting with painful areas in the hypochondrium, called *Gan Zhuo* (Liver-Blood *Qi* stagnation),[4] is often encountered in gynaecology. Many physicians fail to notice the presence of Heat and the aversion to Cold. Thus they falsely put this down to Wind-Cold and prescribe medicinals to treat Wind.

The Liver belongs to Wind (according to the Five Phases), so the use of Wind expelling (and warm) medicinals will increase Wind.

The Liver controls the sinews and ligaments. The presence of Cold contracts the sinews and ligaments in the entire body (Liver-Wind convulsions).

The Liver opens into the eyes (orifice). When Cold is present, the eyes cannot close during night or day, and there is insomnia lasting for over a week. Moreover, the Liver regulates the smooth flow of *Qi*. In the case of a Liver condition (and when exterior relieving medicinals have been wrongly prescribed) *Qi* flows upwards but fails to descend, stagnation is generated and this results in constipation. Urine can be passed but it has a (dark) reddish colour. If the physician treats this with the wrong method once again, assuming a gastrointestinal disease, and prescribes *Da Huang* (Rheum) for purgation, or *Huo Ma Ren* (Semen Cannabis) for promoting the stool, the following symptoms will result: 'no food, no appetite, no stool, no sleep'.

The pulse is unmistakably big and arrives in waves (*Hong, Da Mai*), the body is hot and restless and the patient cannot lie down flat to sleep; there are persistent urges to vomit, nervousness and irritability. The deterioration is doubled due to the two wrong treatments. As it is stated in the '*Jin Kui Yao Lüe*': 'One wrong treatment can just be tolerated; however, two of them may lead to a life-threatening situation.' Even someone who is not a sage will realize that such a case cannot turn out all right. . . .

When the disease manifests initially with pain in the costal arch and an incorrect tonifying method is employed, Blood stasis will accumulate further, and exhaustion (*Lao*) develops due to long-standing cough. This weakens the bones to such a degree that the patient will no longer be able to get up from bed. This is a sign of Blood stasis and stagnation. If the sputum smells foul, then abscesses have already developed from the *Gan Zhuo* (Liver-Blood *Qi* stagnation). If the pulse was hollow, big and choppy (*Kou, Da, Se Mai* = Blood deficiency) the day before yesterday, then big and with clear signs of Blood stasis yesterday, and today the Blood is in overwhelming motion, what else could it be other than Blood stasis?

If tonifying medicinals are given, the disease will reoccur after a short interruption; however, if the obstructions are removed from the vessels at the same time, it will work every time. This is my humble opinion. . . .

Prescription: *Jiang Zhen Xiang* (Lignum Acronychiae), *Su Zi* (Perilla), *Dang Gui* (Angelica Sinensis), *Tao Ren* (Persica), *Xuan Fu Hua* (Inula), *Chen Xiang* (Aquilaria), *Chuan Lian Pi* (Rhizoma Melia Toosendan), *Huang Lian* (Rhizoma Coptidis), *Yu Jin* (Tuber Curcuma).

---

[4] This is a form of Blood stasis and *Qi* stagnation of the Liver mentioned in the '*Jin Kui Yao Lüe*', where the patient perceives both hot drinks and pressure on the diseased area to have an alleviating or comforting effect.

Author's commentary

After describing various wrong treatments of Blood stasis and their consequences, which mostly lead to conditions of Heat, Dr Ye finally explains how the excess syndrome of Blood stasis can worsen and stagnate further following false tonification. This results in Blood-Heat (consequence: coughing of blood) and eventually in a deficiency condition (branch) alongside the Blood stasis (root). Tonifying may be appropriate but will only yield short-term results, because the excess condition of Blood stasis remains present. Therefore, one must prescribe a combination of Blood moving and *Qi* moving medicinals to remove obstructions from the vessels, as seen in Dr Ye's formula.

Jiang Zhen Xiang is related directly to the Liver, causes *Qi* to descend, removes stasis and impure Blood, and stops pain in the chest. Regarding *Su Zi*, it is unclear whether there might be a fault in his notes as this is predominantly used for cough with phlegm. More probably, *Su Geng* (Ramulus Perilla) is meant, which relieves tightness of the chest.

Dang Gui (in this case the lower part of the root) has a stronger effect on invigorating the Blood than the head of the root, which is better for nourishing the Blood, and is often used in gynaecology. *Tao*

Ren and *Yu Jin* also belong to the Blood invigorating medicinals of this formula; *Yu Jin* also moves stagnant Liver-*Qi*.

Chen Xiang is its counterpart: whilst *Yu Jin* primarily invigorates Blood and also moves *Qi*, *Chen Xiang* moves *Qi* but also invigorates the Blood, stops pain and regulates abdominal distension. *Chuan Lian Zi*, in this case the rhizome, also moves *Qi* and is predominantly used for pain due to Liver stagnation attacking the Stomach. *Xuan Fu Hua* causes *Qi* to descend and transforms Phlegm, like *Su Geng* and *Jiang Zhen Xiang*.

Although *Yu Jin* cools the Blood and *Chuan Lian Zi* clears Heat, *Huang Lian* is still the single exclusively cooling medicinal. Presumably it is used to cool Heart-Fire that was caused by Phlegm and stagnation. While the history does not exactly describe insomnia or irritability, it can be assumed that the patient did have these symptoms in addition to a sensation of heat.

In summary, this formula regulates Liver-*Qi*, moves the Blood, transforms Phlegm and stops pain. This case should be compared with Case study 9.9, which features similar symptoms.

Case Study 9.6 Heat generates Blood stasis in the lower abdomen (*Re Ru Xue Shi*) (from Ding Gan-Ren)

Menstruation set in during an infection (*Shang Han*) so that pathogenic Heat went all the way down to the Chamber of Blood (uterus) and led to a mixture of Blood stasis and Heat. Thus the pathogen could neither reach the exterior nor the lower part. All this led to a sensation of febrile heat sometimes with chills, as well as a clouded mind and incoherent speech, as if seeing ghosts. The area of the chest and ribs was painful, the coating of the tongue was yellowish, and the patient had a bitter taste in her mouth. The lower abdomen was painful and sensitive to touch, the *Qi* in this region was not moving (stagnation). The pulse was wiry and rapid, the disease appeared severe and dangerous. It was feared that the

disease might proceed to the *Jue Yin* stage (Liver and Pericardium channels).

Hoping for success I chose *Xiao Chai Hu Tang* (Small Bupleurum Decoction) and added medicinals to cool Heat and remove stasis. This would on the one hand loosen the pathogen by harmonizing the Middle, and on the other hand remove the pathogen by draining Heat and stasis. Prescription: *Chai Hu* (Bupleurum), *Huang Qin* (Scutellaria), *Ling Yang Jiao* (Antelopis), *Zang Hong Hua* (Saffron), *Tao Ren* porridge (Persica), *Qing Pi* (Fraxinus), *Tong Cao* (Tetrapanacus), *Chi Shao* (Paeonia Rubra), *Qing Ding Wan* (Cold Arresting Pill) and *Sheng Pu Huang* (Pollen Typhae Recens).

Author's commentary

It is interesting to compare this case with Case study 9.1 by Ye Tian-Shi, who presented the same syndrome. While Ye based his diagnosis 'Heat invades the Blood division directly' on his own theory of the Four Levels *Wei, Qi, Ying, Xue* (for his formula, see above), Ding Gan-Ren proceeds according to the Six Stages model of the '*Shang Han Lun*'; his prescription is composed solely according to the *Jing-Fang* (prescriptions of Zhang Zhong-Jing). He selected *Chai Hu* and *Huang Qin* from *Xiao Chai Hu Tang* (Small Bupleurum Decoction) to loosen the pathogen by harmonizing the *Shao Yang* and added *Ling Yang Jiao* and *Qing Pi*, which focus on cooling Liver-Fire. Furthermore, he added *Qing Ding Wan* (Cold Arresting Pill) and *Tong Cao* to cool and drain Heat by diuresis. For removing stasis, he added *Zang Hong Hua* (Saffron), *Tao Ren* (Persica), *Chi Shao* (Paeonia Rubra), and *Pu Huang* (Pollen Typhae).

In contrast to the first case, there is an additional involvement of the Pericardium already underway, caused by Heat, leading to incoherent speech and clouding of consciousness, which was obviously more advanced in this case. Be that as it may, both relate to the quote in the '*Jin Kui*' on *Xu Xue* (Blood accumulation): '. . . the patient acts as if mad due to stagnation of Heat in the Lower Burner.' Ding tries to eliminate the Heat via the urine, whilst Ye tries to cool the Blood and eliminate Heat via the stool. Both methods have their own logic. The only question is, which one is better?

Case Study 9.7   Chronic Blood stasis (infertility and PMS) (from Zhang Zhong-Hua)

Painful menstruation for many years, infertility, pain begins three days before menstruation, there are palpable hardenings in the lower abdomen, similar to concretions and conglomerations (*Zheng Jia*). No appetite and poor digestion with weight loss and lassitude.

There are so many methods to regulate menstruation, why were they not applied for so long by the physicians? And once they had been used continuously for many years, why was there no effect? After I had learnt that she had not been ill in her youth, but rather that the disease had started after her marriage (which means after the first time she had intercourse), the cause of the pain became clear to me. This syndrome is not described in the classics. According to the method and formula described in the '*Ji Yin Gan Mu*' (*Systematic Description of Gynaecological Diseases*, written by the famous gynaecologist Wu Zhi-Wang of the Ming dynasty), the name of which we will not yet reveal, the formula must not be taken at the usual times, only when the premenstrual pain sets in; once the menses start it is discontinued until the onset of the next premenstrual pain.

Prescription: *San Leng* (Spargani), *E Zhu* (Curcuma Ezhu), *Yuan Hu* (Corydalis), *Xiang Fu* (Cyperus), *Zhi Jun* (processed *Da Huang*), *Gui Shen* (end-root of *Dang Gui*), *Mu Dan Pi* (Moutan), *Chuan Xiong* (Ligusticum), *Tao Ren* (Persica) and *Zhi Shi* (Fructus Immaturus Citrus Aurantii).

After the patient had taken three daily prescriptions before her second menstruation, a large amount of dark purple, clotted blood was discharged; amongst this was one lump that looked like an embryo but in fact was not. The following menstruation was regular and without pain. This syndrome belongs to the group gatherings in the uterus. After this lump had eventually loosened, there were no further doubts.

Author's commentary

Dr Zhang's formula makes use of the commonly combined duo that invigorate Blood stasis, *San Leng* and *E Zhu* (see also Chapter 7), which are often used nowadays in oncology in the treatment of uterine carcinoma and so on. *Mu Dan Pi* and *Dang Gui* have a Blood harmonizing effect, whereas *Mu Dan Pi* is better for cooling Blood and *Dang Gui* for invigorating Blood. *Dang Gui* and *Chuan Xiong* also constitutes a popular pair, a combination called 'Buddha Hands Powder'. *Tao Ren* and processed *Da Huang* are also used to invigorate Blood, but in addition they can eliminate the clotted Blood via

the stool. Regarding *Qi*, *Zhi Shi* moves the *Qi* of the Middle whilst *Xiang Fu* focuses on Liver-*Qi*, where they are supported by *Yuan Hu Suo* and *Chuan Xiong*, both of which can move *Qi* as well as Blood.

This formula is a very neat combination of medicinals to move *Qi* and Blood, transform stasis and cool Blood-Heat. It demonstrates how a balanced and harmonious formula consisting of only 10 ingredients can be put together. In composition, it is somewhat similar to *Ge Xia Zhu Yu Tang* (Anti-Stasis Abdomen Decoction) by Wang Qing-Ren.

Case Study 9.8   Ulcerative colitis: Blood stasis and Heat in the Lower Jiao (from Zhang Xi-Chun)

Patient Huai, 30 years old. Initially, there was white-red (mucus and blood) diarrhoea, which eventually turned into red diarrhoea with a foul smell. There were shreds of mucus within the discharged bloody water, which looked like singed tissue. This was always combined with a stabbing pain in the middle of the abdomen. There was a nervous irritability and inability to eat or drink. The pulse was wiry and slightly rapid (*Xuan*, *Shuo*), approximately five beats per breath. The pulse was strong in the deep layer, thus the presence of internal Heat was clear. . . . The Heat moved down to the intestine and manifested as colitis. Due to the prolonged diarrhoea the intestinal tissue was affected, so ulcerated bits of tissue were also discharged.

Because of this, medicinals to treat ulcerations and intestinal inflammation were recommended, used in combination to cool Heat, loosen toxins, transform Blood stasis and generate new tissue.

Prescription: *Jie Du Sheng Hua Dan* (Antitoxic Transformation Pill): *Jin Yin Hua* 30 g, *Bai Shao* (Paeonia) 18 g, *Gan Cao* (Glycyrrhiza) 9 g, *San Qi* (Notoginseng) 9 g, *Ya Dan Zi* 60 pc.

Preparation: to begin with, half of the *San Qi* and half of the *Ya Dan Zi* was swallowed down with sugared water. Then, the remaining three ingredients were decocted and sieved. After that, what was left of the first two medicinals was swallowed in the same way and then the decoction was drunk.

After just one prescription the pain abated and the pulse became more harmonious and slower. The subsequent stool had a fairly normal colour and became less red. Finally, I used *Bai Tou Weng Tang* (Pulsatilla Decoction); after two prescriptions the patient recovered fully.

Prescription: *Bai Tou Weng Tang* (from '*Shang Han Lun*'): *Bai Tou Weng* (Pulsatilla) 9 g, *Huang Bai* (Phellodendron) 12 g, *Huang Lian* (Coptis) 12 g, *Qin Pi* (Fraxinus) 12 g; or *Bai Tou Weng Tang* (from Sun Si-Miao's '*Qian Jin Yi Fang*'): 6 g each of *Bai Tou Weng* (Pulsatilla), *Huang Bai* (Phellodendron), *Huang Lian* (Coptis), *Qin Pi* (Fraxinus), *Shao Yao* (Diocorea), *E Jiao* (Asinus), *Hou Po* (Magnolia), *Fu Zi* (Aconitum Praeparata) and *Fu Ling* (Poria), 9 g each of *Dang Gui* (Angelica Sinensis), *Gan Cao* (Glycyrrhiza), *Gan Jiang* (Zingiberis), *Long Gu* (Os Draconis), *Chi Shi Zhi* (Hallositum), 12 g *Jing Mi* (rice) and 30 g *Da Zao* (Zizyphus Jujuba).

Author's commentary

Zhang Xi-Chun's formula *Jie Du Sheng Hua Dan* (Antitoxic Transformation Pill) contains *San Qi*, which these days is often valuable in the treatment of Crohn's disease and ulcerative colitis, especially if there is more blood than mucus in the stool (in Chinese, 'more red than white'), and is characterized by its qualities of invigorating Blood as well as stopping bleeding. *Ya Dan Zi* is also prescribed for all types of chronic dysentery and cools Heat which is evident in the rapid pulse and the bad smell of the stool. *Jin Ying Hua* cools as well; it is not only used successfully for pulmonary infections but also for bacterial dysentery. *Bai Shao* nourishes the weakened Blood and assists *San Qi* in stopping pain and cramps. Raw *Gan Cao* also cools Heat-toxins and harmonizes acute conditions.

Once this formula had taken effect and there was less blood than mucus (in Chinese, 'more white than red'), *Bai Tou Weng Tang* (Pulsatilla Decoction)

from the '*Shang Han Lun*' could be prescribed, although it can also be used if there is blood in the stool. It cools Heat-toxins in the Blood and stops dysentery. Sun Si-Miao's variation may have the same indications but is not as strong in cooling Heat, as it also contains *Gan Jiang* (dried Ginger) and *Fu Zi*.

At first glance, Blood stasis appears to be towards the background whilst Heat is the foreground. However, one should know that Zhang Xi-Chun used *San Qi* as a universal remedy for Blood stasis; for him it was like a combination of several medicinals that invigorate Blood, stop bleeding and generate new flesh ('*Yi Xue Zhong Zhong Can Xi Lu*', vol. 1, p. 86). Similarly, other authors regard *Dan Shen* as a combination of the ingredients of the Blood nourishing and Blood harmonizing formula *Si Wu Tang* (Four Ingredients Decoction).

Case Study 9.9 Pain: Blood stasis due to Liver-*Qi* stagnation (*Gan Qi Yu Jie*) (from Zhao Wen-Kui)

Patient Shi, male, 60 years old. For more than 2 years he suffered repeatedly occurring pain in the lower costal arch due to Blood stasis in the vessels, which started with Liver-*Qi* stagnation (*Gan Qi Yu Jie*). In this case Wang Qing-Ren's method of removing obstructions from the vessels and dispelling Blood stasis is regarded as most suitable.

Prescription: *Zi Su Geng* (Radix Perillae) 3 *qian*, *Jiang Xiang* (Dalbergia) 1.5 *qian*, *Yan Hu Suo* (Corydalis) 1 *qian*, *Jin Ling Zi* (Melia Toosendan) 2 *qian*, *Ou Jie* (Nelumbo) 3 *qian*, *Jiang Can* (Bombyx) 3 *qian*, fresh shavings of *Jiang Zhen Xiang* (Lignum Acronychiae) 1.5 *qian*, prepared *Bie Jia* (Amyda) 3 *qian*, prepared *Xiang Fu* (Cyperus) 3 *qian* and endroot of *Dang Gui* (Angelica Sinensis) 1.5 *qian*.

Author's commentary

This relatively short case study without pulse and tongue details is more the exception than the rule in Dr Zhao's cases. Either he did not regard more details as necessary or the case has been handed down incompletely. Maybe he regarded Ye Tian Shi's principle of chronic disease always entering the collaterals and Wang Qing-Ren's suggestions as sufficient. The latter wrote: 'There is no difference

whether accumulations and gatherings become clumps to the left or right side of the ribs or navel, or above or below the navel or whether they can freely move about. All this can be cured using this formula (*Ge Xia Zhu Yu Tang*). As long as the indication is correct, it will be effective.'

Further on, he noted: 'In all cases of abdominal pain where pain does not wander about, there is *Yu*

Author's commentary continues

Author's commentary (cont'd)

Xue (Blood stasis) and this formula *(Ge Xia Zhu Yu Tang)* can be applied successfully.'

In 1174, during the Song dynasty, Chen Wu-Ze had already written: 'Great anger causes Blood and sweat to be in excess, they accumulate without dispersing, so the area of the flanks becomes painful.'

Obviously, this information was sufficient for Dr Zhao to select the formula, which by the way is very similar to Wu Ju-Tong's in Case study 9.5. This is no coincidence: Dr Zhao was a follower of the *Wen Bing* school. Both prescribe the seldom used medicinal *Jiang Zhen Xiang* (Lignum Acronychiae). This has a warm and pungent property, goes into the Liver, causes *Qi* to descend, and expels stasis and impure Blood, but in addition stops bleeding and pain, especially in the chest and abdomen. More often one would use *Jiang Xiang* or the more expensive *Chen Xiang* for this purpose. *Jiang Xiang* was used in this case, it invigorates the Blood, moves *Qi* and stops abdominal pain. It assists *Xiang Fu* in moving *Qi*, and is particularly suited for Liver-*Qi* stagnation. The fourth medicinal to treat emotional Liver depression is *Zi Su Geng*, which removes oppression in the chest and harmonizes the Middle.

Like *Jiang Zhen Xiang*, *Yan Hu Suo* belongs to the group of Blood 'movers' in this formula. It has the same effect on stagnated *Qi* as on Blood and is one of the most potent painkillers in Chinese medicine, having 40% of the analgesic effect of opiates. The endroot of *Dang Gui* was used because, while also harmonizing Blood, it is more effective than the whole root in moving Blood. *Bie Jia*, usually chosen for nourishing *Yin*, was certainly prescribed owing to its actions in dissolving hardness and invigorating Blood. Together with the stasis breaking *Tu Bie Chong*, it is a popular combination for pain in the costal arch; the latter also, like *Ou Jie*, removes obstructions from the vessels. This action is ascribed to *Ou Jie* by virtue of its appearance. *Jiang Can* also dissolves hardness like the other ingredient with a salty property, *Bie Jia*. *Jin Ling Zi* (also known as *Chuan Lian Zi*) assists *Xiang Fu* in moving *Qi*, as it is predominantly used for pain due to Liver stagnation attacking the Stomach.

Thus, this formula invigorates the Blood, moves *Qi*, dissolves hardness, stops pain and removes obstructions from the vessels. Comparing it with Wu Ju-Tong's formula in Case study 9.5, it is interesting to note that in addition he used *Tao Ren* (Persica), *Xuan Fu Hua* (Inula), *Chen Xiang* (Aquilaria), *Huang Lian* (Rhizoma Coptidis) and *Yu Jin* (Tuber Curcuma). In this formula we can find instead the medicinals *Jiang Xiang*, *Ou Jie*, *Bie Jia*, *Jiang Can* and mainly *Xiang Fu*, which works as well as *Chen Xiang*, but is considerably cheaper. Dr Zhao used more medicinals for dissolving hardness and focused on moving *Qi*, while Dr Wu focused on Blood stasis and cooled Heat at the same time.

Case Study 9.10   Epigastric pain: combination of Blood stasis and Phlegm (*Tan Yu Hu Jie*) (from Cao Ren-Bai)

Pain in the chest that radiates to the back is called chest-*Bi* (*Bi* syndrome of the chest). The *Yang* of such a *Bi*-patient is not sufficient in the chest, so turbid Phlegm is present. In such a disease there is not only Phlegm but stagnated Blood (stasis) as well, which together with the Phlegm blocks the area around the diaphragm.

As a result there is (abdominal) hardness and pain, and pain after eating, with a dry mouth and no desire for drinks, hard, black stool and occasional vomiting of coagulated blood. The pulse is fine and choppy. As this static Blood could not follow its usual path, one must think of draining it in order to treat the disease.

Prescription: *Mu Gua* (Chaenomelis), *Xie Bai* (Allium), *Xuan Fu Hua* (Inula), *Tao Ren* (Persica), *Hong Hua* (Carthamus), *Wa Leng Zi* (Arca), *Yuan Ming Fen* (Mirabilitum). Take together with *Er Chen Tang* (Two Old Decoction).

Author's commentary

The history does not make it clear whether this is a case of gastric or heart disease, or a combination of both. However, it does not have to make a distinction as these anatomical differentiations stem from Western medicine, and were not essential for the old doctors' ways of thinking in the Qing dynasty. As Cold, *Qi* stagnation and Blood stasis are all related to coronary heart diseases as well as to many gastric diseases, the treatment was simply directed towards the syndrome, and the aim was similarly achieved.

Mang Xiao (also called *Yuan Ming Fen*) is responsible here for eliminating stagnated Blood downwards; its salty flavour can also soften hardness. *Xie Bai* warms *Yang-Qi* and assists *Xuan Fu Hua* in expelling Middle Cold and transforming Phlegm. *Xuan Fu Hua* also moves rebellious *Qi* downwards and can therefore treat vomiting. Studies have shown that it has a negative chronotropic effect on the heart. Also *Mu Gua* harmonizes the Stomach, stops abdominal pain and removes obstruction from the vessels. *Wa Leng Zi* invigorates the Blood, moves the *Qi*, transforms Phlegm and stops pain in the epigastrium. Recent findings indicate an outstanding effect on stomach and duodenal ulcers. So far, we have an eliminating, warming and hardness-softening treatment that is focused on the Stomach.

Tao Ren and *Hong Hua*, the classical pair of Blood invigorating medicinals, are used for coronary heart diseases (CHD), in other words for Blood stasis in the Heart, and pain in the chest (including angina pectoris, coronary heart disease with pain, but also epigastric pain). In addition, *Hong Hua* increases contractility of the myocardium.

Er Chen Tang (Two Old Decoction), of which there are four variations bearing the same name, always contains *Ban Xia* and mostly *Chen Pi* as well as *Fu Ling* and *Gan Cao* to harmonize the Middle, transform Phlegm and move *Qi*. It is used for oppression of the chest, nausea, palpitations and indigestion.

In total, the formula calls to mind a modified version of Zhang Zhong-Jing's *Gua Lou Xie Bai Ban Xia Tang* (Trichosanthes Allium Pinellia Decoction). The formula focuses solely on the syndromes; anatomy is irrelevant here.[5]

---

[5] If someone asks for the exact syndrome differentiation of epigastric pain, I keep to the advice given to me by the stomach specialist Gao Jin-Liang, director of the Municipal TCM Research Hospital, who gave me this simple hint during my time as a clinical trainee: 'In the case of painful stomach disorders, either *Qi* or Blood are always stagnated. In *Qi* stagnation, patients complain of a dull pressure like a clumping; in Blood stasis, they complain of a stabbing pain as if with a knife.' See also Gao Jin-Liang: 'The Research Development and Clinical Experience of Treating Chronic Atrophic Gastritis by TCM', in the special Lectures of the 2nd International Congress of TCM in Tianjin.

MODERN CASE STUDIES

Cases listed here stem from the files of well-known TCM doctors of the last 50 years or from my own records during my time as a resident junior doctor.

Case Study 9.11   Apoplexy with Blood 'Xù' syndrome (Xu Xue Zhong Feng)

From the case studies of Dr Liu Du-Zho. Patient L, male, 83 years old. First diagnosis 11th January 1993.

Present history

CHD and cardiac arrhythmias. He fell down 2 months ago; CT showed brain stem thrombosis and unilateral brain oedema. Atrophy of the brain

Case Study continues

was also recorded. After the first consultation he had great difficulties with walking and often fell. Emotionally, he was nervous and irritable, suffering from insomnia and a feeling of fullness and distension of the lower abdomen. He reported frequent urination, but only small amounts, and dry stool, with evacuation only once every few days. The tongue body was dark purple with stasis spots on the sides. The pulse was big and knotted (*Jie*) with a powerful wave, which could be felt in all levels.

Syndrome differentiation indicated Blood stasis and Blood-Heat as described in the '*Jin Kui Yao Lüe*' in the '*Tao Ren Cheng Qi Tang* syndrome' (*Qi* Rectifying Persica Decoction).

Prescription

Tao Ren (Persica) 14 g, *Gui Zhi* (Ramulus Cinnamomi) 10 g, *Gan Cao* (Glycyrrhiza) 6 g, *Mang Xiao* (Mirabillitum, add at end) 3 g and *Da Huang* (Rheum) 3 g. This should be taken on an empty stomach before meals.

Second diagnosis

In the second diagnosis three prescriptions later, the patient reported that following intake of the prescription he had diarrhoea the colour of pig's liver, but the pressure and fullness in the lower abdomen had disappeared. His appetite had improved and his sleep at night was undisturbed. The tongue still showed signs of stasis spots and the pulse remained knotted. Moreover, the patient had cold hands and feet, which suggested Blood stasis with stagnation of *Qi* which was not flowing well. Therefore, the formula was changed to *Si Ni San* (Cold Limbs Decoction) supplemented with Blood moving medicinals *Tao Ren* (Persica), *Hong Hua* (Carthamus) and *Dan Shen* (Salvia Miltiorrhiza), so in the end the principle of invigorating Blood and *Qi*, transforming stasis and relieving depression (*Yù*) was made use of.

After five prescriptions the extremities were warm, pulse and tongue were normal and the patient stopped falling.

Author's commentary

As explained in the *Xu Xue* chapters of Wang Ken-Tang (see Chapter 11) and Lin Pei-Qin (see Chapter 11), *Tao Ren Cheng Qi Tang* (*Qi* Rectifying Persica Decoction) belongs to Zhang Zhong-Jing's standard prescriptions in the case of *Xu Xue* in the *Tai Yang* stage. Zhang states: 'The lower abdomen hard and distended, the person acts as if mad.' The distinctive feature here is Heat-Blood stasis in the Lower Burner. The *Shang Han Lun* specialist Cheng Wu-Ji of the Ming dynasty explains the expression 'as if mad' as follows: 'Not as advanced as madness, but extremely agitated.' The above-mentioned patient was nervous and irritable and suffered from insomnia, which clearly matches this syndrome.

Furthermore, this case is based on a dysfunction of the vessels of the heart and brain, suggesting poor blood flow, also seen in the stasis spots on the tongue. Dry stool, distended abdomen and irritability suggest Heat, so they were treated with a purgative method whilst Blood was invigorated using *Tao Ren Cheng Qi Tang* (*Qi* Rectifying Persica Decoction). The emperor medicinal is *Da Huang*, which purges Heat in the Lower Burner and invigorates Blood. Although the formula only included five medicinals, it proved to be quite effective, which demonstrates that followers of the *Jing-Fang* school (prescriptions according to Zhang Zhong-Jing) – among whom Dr Liu is numbered – could achieve a great deal with just a few ingredients.

As well as in gynaecology, this formula is still often used in the treatment of traumas with internal injuries. Another significant point is that the medicine was taken on an empty stomach, so it could be transported directly to its target, the Lower Burner. This has already been emphasized by Zhang.

Case Study 9.12   Psoriasis (*Bai Bi*)

From the case studies of Dr Zhao Shao-Qing. Patient M, female, 32 years old.

First consultation

The patient has been suffering from psoriasis for 8 years, accompanied by skin damage and hair loss. There are yellow erosions the size of beans all over her body including the scalp. Sometimes the disease improves, sometimes it deteriorates again. She has taken both Chinese and Western drugs to no avail. In the autumn, the disease deteriorated to the extent that the patient had to scratch harder, more scales peeled off and a red surface became visible, whereupon the lesions increased.

The pulse was wiry, fine, slippery and rapid. The tongue body was red, especially the tip, and the coating was yellow, thin and dry.

Emotionally, the patient was irritable and nervous; her sleep was shallow and she had many dreams. She reported yellow urine and dry stools. After waking up her mouth and tongue were dry and there was a bitter taste.

This case also showed a longstanding Hidden Heat (*Fu Re*), for which the suitable treatment was to cool Blood and transform stasis. As regards her diet she was advised to abstain from consuming hot food and spices of any kind.

Prescription (seven bags)

Jing Jie (Schizonepeta) 6 g, *Fang Feng* (Ledebouriella) 6 g, *Di Yu* (Sanguisorba) 10 g, *Huai Hua* (Sophora Japonica) 10 g, *Dan Shen* (Salvia Miltiorrhiza) 10 g, *Qian Cao* (Rubia) 10 g, *Zi Cao* (Lithispermum) 10 g, *Zi Hua Di Ding* (Viola Yedoensitis) 10 g, *Cao He Che* (Polygonum Bistorta) 10 g, *Mao Gen* (Imperatus) 10 g, *Lu Gen* (Phragmitis) 10 g and *Da Huang* (Rheum) 1 g.

Second consultation

After taking the prescriptions no new skin damage occurred, and irritability and dream-disturbed sleep also improved. Stool and urine were normal, but Blood-Heat was still present: the pulse remained rapid, the tongue was still red. Therefore, the treatment principle above was continued.

Prescription (seven bags)

Jing Jie (Schizonepeta) 6 g, *Fang Feng* (Ledebouriella) 6 g, *Di Yu* (Sanguisorba) 10 g, *Huai Hua* (Sophora Japonica) 10 g, *Dan Shen* (Salvia Miltiorrhiza) 10 g, *Qian Cao* (Rubia) 10 g, *Chi Shao* (Paeonia Rubra) 10 g, *Bai Tou Weng* (Pulsatilla) 10 g, *Zi Cao* (Lithispermum) 10 g, *Cao He Che* (Polygonum Bistorta) 10 g, *Bai Xian Pi* (Cortex Dictamni) 10 g, *Di Fu Zi* (Kochia Scoparia) 10 g and *Da Huang* (Rheum) 1 g.

Third consultation

After the patient had taken the prescription for a month, the skin erosions were clearly reduced. On the trunk and the limbs they were flat and healing well, however, there were still several areas on the scalp with erosions about the size of beans. The pulse was still wiry, fine, slippery and rapid, The tongue was still red, but the coating had changed to white.

It is obvious that accumulated Heat cannot be eliminated in just a few days. Thus the main principle is to continue to cool Blood and transform stasis. Restrictions in diet also need to be observed to avoid a relapse.

Prescription (seven bags)

Jing Jie (Schizonepeta) 6 g, *Fang Feng* (Ledebouriella) 6 g, *Bai Zhi* (Angelica Dahurica) 6 g, *Di Yu* (Sanguisorba) 10 g, *Huai Hua* (Sophora Japonica) 10 g, *Dan Shen* (Salvia Miltiorrhiza) 10 g, *Qian Cao* (Rubia) 10 g, *Chi Shao* (Paeonia Rubra) 10 g, *Zi Cao* (Lithispermum) 10 g, *Mao Gen* (Imperatus) 10 g, *Lu Gen* (Phragmitis) 10 g, *Jiao San Xian* (The Three Immortals: *Mai Ya*, *Shen Qu* and *Shan Zha*, roasted) 10 g each and *Da Huang* (Rheum) 1 g.

This prescription was taken with slight modifications for a further 2 months. After that, all signs of the disease were gone. The patient should carry on maintaining the dietary restrictions and pay particular attention to lifestyle.

Author's commentary

Psoriasis (*Yin Xiao* or *Bai Dao*), traditionally known as *Niu Pi Xian* (ox-skin lichen), belongs to the more difficult diseases in dermatology, yet it responds well to TCM. It belongs to the *Fu Re* disorders (hidden or residual Heat) of Blood. For this reason Dr Chao used Blood cooling medicinals, such as *Lu Gen, Zi Cao, Bai Tou Weng* etc., throughout the treatment. When Blood-Heat is permitted to continue, it can cause Blood stasis, which makes the disease worse and more difficult to treat; hence Blood invigorating medicinals, such as *Dan Shen, Da Huang* and *Chi Shao* needed to be prescribed from the very beginning. The deterioration in autumn also suggests Blood stasis: as Wang Qing-Ren remarks in

the '*Yi Lin Gao Cuo*' (see Chapter 10): '*Regardless of what disease it is, if it occurs periodically at certain times of the year, the cause is Blood stasis*' (13th indication for Blood stasis).

Particularly interesting is the effect of *Huai Hua, Qian Cao, Bai Mao Gen* and *Di Yu*, which have the combined actions of invigorating Blood, stopping bleeding and cooling Blood. Medicinals such as *Di Fu Zi* and *Bai Xian Pi* are commonly used for itching skin inflammations to expel Dampness. This also counts for the slightly warm medicinals *Jing Jie* and *Fang Feng*, which can expel Wind and Dampness from the skin, too.

Case Study 9.13   Rheumatic arthritis (*Bi Zheng*)

From the case studies of Dr Li Cong-Pu. Patient S, female, 38 years old.

First consultation

At the onset of the disease the patient experienced a sensation of heat with aversion to cold together with pain developing in the joints. Later on, she had only a sensation of heat and both knee joints were markedly swollen and painful. Her body was feverish and hot for a long time, and her temperature would not decrease. One hospital diagnosed rheumatoid arthritis, while another diagnosed thrombophlebitis. The patient was treated with cortisone and thrombolytics, which improved the swelling and pain for a fairly long time.

After 3 months her temperature suddenly jumped to 40.3°C accompanied by pain in all her joints and severely swollen knee joints, so it was impossible for her to get up and move around. In the morning her face was swollen and in the afternoon both legs felt very heavy. In addition, she was short of breath, had palpitations and had no appetite. Admission to another hospital revealed the presence of lupus erythematosus (LE) cells. The patient had previously contracted extralymphatic tuberculous pyelitis.

At the time when the history was taken her pulse was soggy and weak (*Ru, Ruo Mai*) and her tongue was dark red with a sticky yellow coating. Black-brown skin pigments were visible on her face and on both lower legs; at the dorsum of the left foot, between ankle and toes, there were cyanotic-purple marks, which felt numb but were sensitive to pressure. In contrast, the right foot was very red and swollen, and it was very sensitive to pressure. This condition prevented the patient from getting a good night's sleep.

This *Bi* syndrome was caused by Damp-Heat Blood stasis with obstruction of the collaterals disturbing the free flow of *Ying* and *Wei*.

The appropriate treatment principle is: 'remove obstructions from the vessels, invigorate Blood and transform Heat, cool and disperse Damp-Heat and thus encourage the flow of *Ying* and *Wei*.' The necessary medicinals have to be handled in a flexible way: pungent and dry medicinals must not be used as they would increase Heat; on the other hand, bitter and cool medicinals are also contraindicated as they would encourage the *Bi* syndrome.

Hence the following prescription was used: *Sheng Di Huang* (Rehmannia) 13 g, *Dang Gui* (Angelica Sinensis) 10 g, *Chi Shao* (Paeonia Rubra)

Case Study continues

10 g, *Mu Dan Pi* (Moutan) 10 g, *Qin Jiao* (Gentiana Qinjiao) 10 g, *Fang Feng* (Ledebouriella) 10 g, *Yi Yi Ren* (Coix) 10 g, *Ji Xue Teng* (Jixueteng) 9 g, *Mu Tong* (Akebia) 10 g, *Han Fang Ji* (Stephania) 10 g, *Pu Huang* (Typha) 9 g, *Di Long* (Lumbricus) 6 g and *Gan Cao* (Glycyrrhiza) 3 g.

Second consultation

After the patient had taken 17 preparations the pulse was slippery and slowed-down (*Hua, Huan Mai*). The tongue was pale red and more moist; the yellow coating had disappeared. The pain in her legs had markedly decreased so she was able to sleep well again. The cyanotic-purple discolouration of her left foot turned into a more vital red and the red hot area on her right foot turned pale-red. There was frequent and scanty urination with a burning sensation afterwards. The stool was loose and sticky. Both symptoms indicate that Damp-Heat had already been dispersed through urine and stool and obstructions were being removed from the blood vessels and vessels.

Because of this, the prescription was re-applied omitting *Gan Cao* and adding 5 g of wine-roasted *Huang Bai* (Phellodendron).

Third consultation

After the patient had taken 28 preparations, the overall image of the pulse was more balanced and the tongue was pale red with a thin white coating (normal). The left foot had completely healed, and there was no more numbness or abnormal sensitivity. The pain and swelling in the right foot had also largely receded, so the patient was able to walk around the room. There was also no more feeling of awareness (palpitations) in the chest.

As a result, the same prescription was employed as after the second consultation, but with *Sheng Di Huang* (Rehmannia), *Qin Jiao* (Gentiana Qinjiao), *Pu Huang* (Typha) and *Huang Bai* (Phellodendron) taken out and 12 g *Dan Shen* (Salvia Miltiorrhiza) added. The whole root of *Dang Gui* was replaced with the middle part of the root. *Han Fang Ji* (Stephania) was increased to 12 g.

The prescription was now made up of *Dan Shen* (Salvia Miltiorrhiza) 12 g, *Dang Gui* (Angelica Sinensis) 10 g, *Chi Shao* (Paeonia Rubra) 10 g, *Mu Dan Pi* (Moutan) 10 g, *Fang Feng* (Ledebouriella) 10 g, *Yi Yi Ren* (Coix) 10 g, *Ji Xue Teng* (Jixueteng) 9 g, *Mu Tong* (Akebia) 10 g, *Han Fang Ji* (Stephania) 12 g, *Di Long* (Lumbricus) 6 g.

Author's commentary

This complex case of Damp-Heat could not be treated by conventional methods as cold medicinals would have worsened the Dampness factor of the *Bi* syndrome and hot medicinals would have exacerbated the Heat. Moreover, due to the long-standing condition of Damp-Heat, Blood stasis had developed and gradually increased to a point where it obstructed the vessels.

Therefore Dr Li used only mild medicinals to treat the Blood, such as *Sheng Di*, *Chi Shao* and *Mu Dan Pi*. To act against the Wind and pain related to the *Bi* syndrome, he added *Qin Jiao* and *Fang Feng*. *Yi Yi Ren* and *Mu Tong* can drain Damp mildly without enhancing Heat. *Han Fang Ji* also drains Damp-Heat

via the urine, but it can also reduce oedema and swellings, inflammation and pain. *Di Long* removes obstruction from the blocked vessels and *Pu Huang*, *Dang Gui* and *Ji Xue Tang* invigorate the Blood and have a harmonizing effect. *Gan Cao* is used to soothe acute conditions, so it was no longer needed at the second consultation. Instead, it was substituted with wine-roasted *Huang Bai*, because Heat in the Lower Burner had become evident. Processing it with wine focuses the effect of *Huang Bai* on the vessels. After the third consultation the action of the formula was shifted towards invigorating the Blood and the dosage of the key medicinal *Han Fang Ji* was increased.

Case Study 9.14 Chronic hepatitis (*Gan Yu Yu Xue*)

From my own case studies with Dr Su Lian, Yunnan Sheng Zhongyi Yiyuan, 13th July 1998.

Patient M, male, 24 years old, chronic hepatitis B with indigestion, no appetite, fatigue and weakness, insomnia, large tongue, slightly purple with teeth marks, wiry pulse. In a case of chronic hepatitis such as this it takes about 2–3 months of treatment to significantly improve symptoms as well as clinical findings. After 1 year patients have to return for a follow-up examination.

Syndrome differentiation indicated Liver-*Qi* stagnation attacking the Spleen and Blood stasis. The treatment principle was to strengthen Spleen-*Qi*, soothe the Liver and invigorate the Blood.

Prescription

Chai Hu (Bupleurum) 10 g, *Bai Shao* and *Chi Shao* (Paeonia Lactiflora and Rubra) 15 g each, *Fu Ling* (Poria) 9 g, *Chao Bai Zhu* (Atractylodes Macrocephala Praeparata) 12 g, *Dan Shen* (Salvia Miltiorrhiza) 15 g, *Yi Yi Ren* (Coix) 20 g, *Jian Shan Zha* (Crategus) 15 g, *Huang Qi* (Astragalus) 30 g, *Chong Lou* (also known as *Zao Xiu*) 10 g, *Suan Zao Ren* (Zizyphus Spinosa) 20 g, *Ye Jiao Teng* (Caulis Polygoni Multifloris) 30 g, *Zi Hua Di Ding* (Viola Yedoensitis) 20 g, *Sang Ji Sheng* (Sangjisheng) 30 g, *Sheng Gan Cao* (Glycyrrhiza Recens) 4 g.

Author's commentary

Spleen-*Qi* deficiency is evidenced by no appetite, fatigue and weakness and a large tongue with teeth marks. The wiry pulse suggests a Liver pattern, possibly where the Liver attacks the Spleen and is thus responsible for the Middle deficiency. The purple tongue suggests Blood stasis, which is regularly present in chronic hepatitis and many other long-lasting illnesses. Hepatitis is often associated with Damp-Heat. Dampness develops when the transporting function of the Spleen is insufficient, which in this case is influenced by an attacking Liver-*Qi*.

Amongst other factors, accumulated Heat can generate Blood stasis, which is why *Chai Hu* and *Bai Shao* are added to soothe Liver-*Qi*, *Chong Lou*, *Zi Hua Di Ding* and *Sheng Gan Cao* to cool Heat, and *Yi Yi Ren* and *Fu Ling* to dry and drain Dampness as well as strengthen the Spleen. *Bai Zhu* and *Huang Qi* strengthen Spleen-*Qi* and *Dan Shen*, *Chi Shao*

and *Shan Zha* invigorate the Blood. Another function of *Shan Zha* is to improve digestion; *Chong Lou* can also invigorate the Blood, while *Bai Shao* also calms the Liver.

Enduring Heat has damaged the *Yin*, as a result, *Sang Ji Sheng* was included in order to nourish Liver and Kidney *Yin*, as well as the two Heart-*Yin* nourishing medicinals *Suan Zao Ren* and *Ye Jiao Teng*. The last two simultaneously calm and promote sleep.

From a pharmacological point of view, virostatic medicinals such as *Zi Hua Di Ding*, immune-strengthening herbs such as *Huang Qi* and Blood invigorating herbs such as *Dan Shen* are combined with hepatoprotective medicinals such as *Chai Hu* to contain hepatitis and prevent its sequelae. At the same time digestive medicinals like *Shan Zha* and relaxing herbs like *Suan Zao Ren* are used to remove the concomitant symptoms of hepatitis.

Case Study 9.15 Thrombophlebitis (*Tuo Chang*)

From the case studies of Dr Zhu Ren-Kang. Patient N, male, 59 years old, 5th March 1958. His main complaint was cold and painful legs, which he had had for 1 year.

History
In January 1957 the patient noticed a sensation of heat in the left foot which gradually turned into a cold and numb sensation. The big toe changed colour and ached, especially when he had been walking or after standing for longer periods of time. A similar condition developed in the other leg 1 month later, so it became difficult to walk. The pain got worse, particularly in the evening. The patient had worked as a packer in a pharmacy in the north-east corner of Tianjin for 20 years, and was a heavy smoker. He had been treated previously in a hospital in Beijing, where an amputation was suggested. However, he declined this and insisted on a referral for Chinese medicine treatment.

Present history
Both legs, from the knees down, and the skin on the left big toe, are completely dark red in colour. The toes on the left foot are icy cold; the arteries on the dorsum are both palpable, but weaker on the left. The condition of the right foot is not as bad. The pulse is superficial and tight, and the tongue coating is thin white.

   TCM diagnosis: *Tuo Chuang* (gangrene).

   Western medicine diagnosis: thrombotic occluded vasculitis.

   Present symptoms are that the toes of both feet are cold, the patient is experiencing numbness and sclerotic pain, hence difficulty with walking, and the big toe on the left is blackish-purple.

   Syndrome differentiation indicates *Bi* syndrome due to Cold with clotting which has blocked the channels and collaterals.

   The treatment principle is to warm the channels, remove obstruction from the vessels – invigorate Blood and move the *Bi* blockage.

Prescription
Ma Huang (Ephedra) 4.5 g, *Dang Gui* (Angelica Sinensis) 9 g, *Chi Shao* (Paeonia Rubra) 4.5 g, *Chuan Xiong* (Ligusticum) 6 g, *Niu Xi* (Cyathula) 9 g, *Qiang Huo* (Notopterygium) 4.5 g, *Fang Ji* (Stephania) 4.5 g, *Sang Zhi* (Morus A.) 15 g, *Sang Ji Sheng* (Sangjisheng) 9 g, red *Fu Ling* (Poria) 9 g, *Rou Gui* powder (Cortex Cinnamomi) 1.5 g (to swallow with water).

Second presentation (13th March)
After the patient had taken 8 preparations, the dark discolouration of the dorsum of the foot had receded a little. The patient now complained of cough with pain in the chest and below the costal arch. Therefore *Rou Gui* (Cortex Cinnamomi) was replaced with 30 g *Gui Zhi* (Ramulus Cinnamomi); *Kuan Dong Hua* (Flos Tussilaginis Farfarae) 9 g, *Dong Gua Zi* (Benicasa Hispida) 9 g and *Xie Bai* (Allium) 4.5 g were also added. The patient was given one bag per day.

Third presentation (28th March)
After 1 month the cough had cleared and the numbness in the foot had markedly receded. The colour of the foot slowly turned reddish and the feet gradually became warmer. Further modifications of the first formula were prescribed.

   Six weeks after the treatment all symptoms had receded to a great extent, and the patient was able to walk normally. *Hu Jian Wan* (Tiger Submitting Pill) and *Hu Gu Mu Gua Wan* (Tiger Bone Papaya Pill) were prescribed thereafter. After 3 months he had largely recovered.

   Hu Jian Wan, which contains *Huang Bai*, *Gui Ban*, *Zhi Mu*, *Shou Di*, *Chen Pi*, *Bai Shao*, *Suo Yang*, *Hu Gu* and *Gan Jiang*, is a formula of Zhu Dan-Xi, which nourishes *Yin*, descends Fire and strengthens bones and sinews.

   Hu Gu Mu Gua Wan, containing *Hu Gu*, *Ru Xiang*, *Mo Yao*, *Mu Gua*, *Tian Ma*, *Rou Cong Rong* and *Niu Xi*, is indicated for Cold and Dampness in the vessels causing pain and Blood stasis.

Author's commentary

Internal Cold, which developed either from the patient's occupation of prolonged standing in the cold or simultaneously from *Yang* deficiency, causes the Blood to coagulate and thus gives rise to Blood stasis, demonstrated by the purple discolouration of the skin and the aggravation of the symptoms at night. Blockage of the vessels generates a *Bi* syndrome, which is worsened especially by cold. Bi syndromes are commonly associated with Wind-Dampness, therefore Dr Zhu prescribed *Sang Zhi* and *Han Fang Ji*, which also stop pain. *Dang Gui*, *Chi Shao*, *Chuan Xiong* and *Niu Xi* invigorate the Blood; *Dang Gui* also nourishes the weakened Blood and *Niu Xi* guides the action of the formula down towards the legs. *Sang Ji* and *Qiang Huo* expel Wind-Dampness, but *Sang Ji* also strengthens the sinews and bones. At the same time it nourishes Blood and *Yin*, which is likely to be injured by the warm properties of *Rou Gui* and *Ma Huang*. *Rou Gui* not only warms the Middle but also opens and frees the vessels. Combined with *Ma Huang* and *Qiang*

Huo it relieves the exterior, and these were used because there was an exterior pathogen evident in the pulse, which broke out in a cough a week later. *Chi Fu Ling* was added as a preventative measure against Damp-Heat, which in the case of chronic *Bi* is likely to arise from Cold-*Bi*, and because the formula has a tendency to become too warm.

For this reason, at the second presentation Dr Zhu replaced *Rou Gui* with *Gui Zhi*, which has a better effect on the exterior, and complemented it with *Xie Bai*, another exterior relieving medicinal. To treat the cough he added *Dong Gua Zi* to expel Damp and Phlegm and *Kuan Dong Hua* to stop cough and loosen Phlegm.

Once the exterior was cleared, he reverted to the original prescription at the third presentation. Following an improvement of the acute symptoms, patent pill formulas were prescribed to cool Blood, lower Heat and strengthen Kidney *Yin* and *Yang* (*Hu Jian Wan*), as well as to treat pain, *Bi* syndrome and Blood stasis.

Case Study 9.16   Coronary heart disease (*Xiong Bi*)

From the case studies of Dr Yue Mei-Zhong. Patient L, female, 32 years old.

First consultation
The patient presented on 18th December 1971 with rheumatic mitral valve stenosis and reported that on 3rd November, when she woke up in the morning, she had suffered a thrombotic apoplexy (or TIA[6]), which resulted in right-sided hemiplegia and numbness and aphasia. Due to immediate acupuncture intervention these sequelae went away after 2 hours. However, afterwards shortness of breath and oppression of the chest had developed, which had worsened and become

painful in the morning, whereupon she became very nervous and irritable. Her pulse was slippery on the left. Therefore, I treated this case with *Jia Wei Guan Xin Tang* (Modified Coronary Decoction No. 2).

Prescription
Dang Shen (Codonopsis) 12 g, *Dang Gui* (Angelica Sinensis) 12 g, *Xie Bai* (Allium) 18 g, *Hong Hua* (Carthamus) 9 g, *Yan Hu Suo* (Corydalis) 12 g, *Yu Jin* (Curcuma) 9 g, *Dan Shen* (Salvia Miltiorrhiza) 12 g, *Gua Lou* (Trichosanthis) 24 g and *Ji Xue Teng* (Jixueteng) 24 g.

After the patient had taken this prescription the shortness of breath and oppression of the chest abated, so this formula was continued on a daily basis. After she had taken 100 further preparations, a treatment break was carried out

---

[6] Transient ischemic attack: a temporal circulatory disturbance of the cerebral arteries.

Case Study continues

as the patient had already gone back to work a few months earlier, felt emotionally balanced and was eating and sleeping well.

However, on 28th September 1972 she presented again: the fingers of her right hand had become numb. It would start and travel from the tips of the small, ring and middle fingers, which made her very nervous. Her wrist became weak, she had trouble writing quickly and eventually could not bear it any longer. I prescribed *San Bi Tang*, which after several doses led to a full recovery.

San Bi Tang (Modified Three *Bi* Decoction): 3 g each of *Ren Shen* (Ginseng), *Huang Qi* (Astragalus), *Bai Zhu* (Atractylodes Macrocephala), *Dang Gui* (Angelica Sinensis), *Chuan Xiong* (Ligusticum), *Bai Shao* (Paeonia) and *Fu Ling* (Poria); 1.5 g each of *Gan Cao* (Glycyrrhiza), *Gui Zhi* (Ramulus Cinnamomi), *Fang Ji* (Stephania) and *Xi Xin* (Asarum), baked 1.5 g of *Wu Tou* (Radix Aconiti) and 2 pieces of *Hong Zao* (Zizyphus Jujuba). This formula by Zhang Lu is used for cramps in the limbs due to *Qi* stagnation, Blood stasis and a combination of Wind, Dampness and Cold.

Author's commentary

Gua Lou and *Xia Bai* have been used in the treatment of coronary diseases since Zhang Zhong-Jing's time. They transform Phlegm in the chest and free the *Qi*. *Dang Shen* tonifies *Qi* and *Dang Gui* nourishes and invigorates Blood, so the *Bi* in the chest can open up and disperse. The other Blood invigorating medicinals, such as *Yan Hu Suo*, *Hong Hua*, *Tao Ren* and *Dan Shen* have a pain relieving effect with the latter having a special influence on the heart. The pungent flavour of *Yu Jin* makes it, like *Yan Hu*, a herb that can move *Qi* whilst invigorating Blood, and thus it can assist in transforming Phlegm.

To go into more detail, this is a combination of *Gua Lou Xie Bai Ban Xia Tang* by Zhang Zhong-Jing

and *Tao Ren Hua Zhuo Tang*, which is a formula with the primary function of transforming Phlegm, and warming and moving Blood and *Qi*. When *Yang* is deficient, Cold is likely to arise in the Upper Burner. As Cold is a *Yin* pathogen which makes *Qi* and Blood flow sluggishly, inadequate flow in the Middle Burner can cause *Qi* stagnation. In the presence of stagnation the Spleen cannot perform well, so Phlegm arises. In addition, once *Qi* cannot propel Blood anymore, the latter will also stagnate and Blood stasis arises as well, which in turn combines with Phlegm. Thus both *Qi* and Blood need to be moved, Cold needs to be warmed and Phlegm transformed to remedy this situation.

Case Study 9.17   Chronic headache due to injury (*Wai Shang Yu Xue*)

From the case studies of Dr Yue Mei-Zhong. First patient: patient L, male, 61 years old.

First consultation
The patient presented on 29th July 1969. All the six pulses were hard and wiry, especially the left *Guan* pulse (Liver). The patient reported that he had suffered from headaches for years, which did not respond to any treatment. Sometimes the whole body ached as well. A degree of

arteriosclerosis was detected in his brain, for which he was permanently on Western drugs, but without any significant effect. He described his headache and body aching 'as if stabbed with nails'. This kind of pain is mostly due to Blood stasis, so I asked for the disease history. It came to light that the pain had started after an injury in a fall. Thus I was able to conclude that this was a case of headache and body aching due to Blood stasis and prescribed *Fu Yuan Huo Xue Tang*

Case Study continues

(Blood Invigorating Recovery Decoction), with the following ingredients: *Da Huang* (Rhizoma et Radix Rhei) 6 g, *Chai Hu* (Radix Bupleuri) 9 g, *Dang Gui* (Radix Angelicae Sinensis) 9 g, *Tao Ren* (Semen Persicae) 6 g, *Hong Hua* (Flos Carthami) 6 g, *Chuan Shan Jia* (Squama Manitis) 9 g, *Tian Hua Fen* (Radix Trichosanthis) 9 g. Cook with one half clear water and one half rice wine and drink when still warm.

Second consultation on 20th August 1969
The headache was fully cured, so the formula was continued. In the following consultation his body aches had disappeared as well.

Second patient: patient Z, female, 60 years old

First consultation
The patient presented on 17th April 1970. She told me that she had fallen from a great height and sustained a concussion; thereafter, she had insomnia and severe dizziness, so she has been unable to walk for 3 months.

The pulse was deep and choppy (*Chen, Se Mai*), the tongue was noticeably dark purple, all of which suggested Blood stasis. Therefore I prescribed *Fu Yuan Huo Xue Tang* (Blood Invigorating Recovery Decoction).

Second consultation on 29th April 1970
The patient was able to walk again; however, the sublingual veins were still clearly dark purple. Furthermore, she had some phlegm in her throat, so I added *Zhu Ru* (Caulis Bambusae) and *Ban Xia* (Rhizoma Pinelliae) to the formula.

After she had taken a few preparations the dizziness was gone and the patient was able to walk normally again.

Author's commentary

In the second case, the tongue and pulse of the patient, who was suffering mainly from dizziness, provided enough evidence to infer Blood stasis. In contrast, the signs and symptoms in the first case were not as obvious, but the hint of the fixed and stabbing pain from the patient's history made one think of Blood stasis, which was verified by the patient's previous head injury. Wherever there are injuries, there is *always* Blood stasis, even if the injury dates back a long time. In both cases, Dr Yue prescribed *Fu Yuan Huo Xue Tang* (Blood Invigorating Recovery Decoction). In the second case he also added Phlegm transforming medicinals, following Ye Tian-Shi's remark: 'Where there is dizziness, there is also Phlegm.'

Fu Yuan Huo Xue Tang (Blood Invigorating Recovery Decoction) is used for pain in the costal arch and traumas of every kind. It contains *Chai Hu* to move stagnated Liver-*Qi*. Wang Ang remarked on this: 'Regardless of which organ (functional entity) is affected by injury, stagnated Blood will be present under the ribs, because the Liver governs Blood.' From today's point of view we can infer this to mean that a physical trauma is always connected to emotional tension or suffering, thus external injuries will always entail Liver-*Qi* stagnation.

Tian Hua Fen acts on the chest. It guides the action of the other medicinals to the chest and cools Heat and subdues swellings at the same time. *Dang Gui* not only harmonizes the Blood, it can also prevent Blood from becoming exhausted too quickly due to the harsh actions of the Blood stasis medicinals *Tao Ren, Hong Hua* and *Da Huang*.

Chuan Shan Jia breaks Blood stasis and improves the flow of *Qi* in the *Luo* vessels. Adding alcohol has the same function, it also improves the flow of *Qi*. These two cases demonstrate that classical formulas may also be prescribed without having to make many modifications. However, this is rather the exception in present-day practice in China.

Case Study 9.18   Mediastinal tumour (*Tan Yu Hu Jie*)

From the case files of the oncology department of the Wuxi TCM Hospital, Dr Zhang Xi-Jun, on 19th April 1982. Patient J, female, 59 years old.

Main complaints
Progressive difficulties in swallowing, also partial obstructive breathing difficulties for 6 months, pleural fluid with traces of blood for 3 months.

History
Poor general condition, emaciated, weak, no energy, facial skin sagging, hard obstruction when swallowing, hence she eats only a little, breathing difficulties and a rough, asthmatic cough, easily fatigued heart and palpitations. The patient speaks with a low, weak voice. Furthermore, there is pain in the right costal arch and she is unable to lie down flat. Stools are dry and hard; often, she defecates only once every 3 days. Further signs include scanty and deep yellow urine; dark red tongue with little coating; sublingual vein varicosis is evident; pulse is deep and choppy.

Several X-rays were made, including during some taken swallowing. It was suspected that she had a growing mediastinal tumour on the right side, with fluid accumulation in the right lateral chest area, which showed traces of blood in three pleural punctures, but there were no traces of cancer cells.

Syndrome differentiation indicated a combination of Phlegm and Blood stasis, pathological water in the chest, the *Xuan-Yin* syndrome of the '*Jin Kui Yao Lüe*'.[7]

The treatment principle is to expel Phlegm and Blood stasis, disperse accumulations and drain water.

Prescription
Gua Lou (Trichosanthes) 15 g, *Ze Xie* (Alismatis) 15 g, *Zhu Ling* (Sclerotium Polypori Umbellati) 12 g,

Xie Bai (Allium) 12 g, *Sang Bai Pi* (Cortex Mori A.) 9 g, fermented *Ban Xia* (Pinellia) 9 g, *Yu Jin* (Curcuma) 9 g, *Jiu Xiang Chong* (Aspongopus Chinensis) 6 g, *Tu Bie Chong* (Eupolyphaga) 5 g, *Sha Shen* (Glehnia) 30 g, *Bai Hua She She Cao* (Herba Oldenlandia) 30 g and pulverized *Hu Po* (Succinium) 3 g (swallow with decoction).

Additionally, one daily injection of *He Kui Ye* 4 ml (a TCM patent remedy for cancer, available only in Chinese hospitals) and an intake of *Liu Shen Wan* (Six Deities Pills) and *Zhong Jie Feng Pian* (Sarcandra Tablets) was prescribed.

Second consultation (27th April)
After these remedies were taken, the stool was normal, and the pressure in the chest and the rasping cough were alleviated. The difficulties in swallowing and the lack of energy were still present.

Prescription
Ji Xing Zi (Impatiens Balsamica) 12 g, *Wei Ling Xian* (Clematis) 12 g, *Shan Dou Gen* (Sophora Subprostrata) 9 g, *Wu Mei* (Prunus Mume) 10 g, *Jiang Can* (Bombyx) 10 g, *Gua Lou* (Trichosanthes) 15 g, *Mai Men Dong* (Ophiopogonis) 15 g, *Kun Bu* (Laminaria Thallis) 20 g, *Hai Dai* (Herba Saragassi) 20 g, *Xuan Shen* (Scrophularia) 20 g, *Gan Cao* (Glycyrrhiza) 5 g.

Additionally, the patent remedy *Liu Shen Wan* (Six Deities Pills) and *Ai Tong Pian* (Cancer Pain Tablets) were prescribed.

Third consultation (25th May)
After 24 preparations of these remedies had been taken, the obstruction in the throat and the swallowing difficulties were markedly improved. The patient could eat up to three meals a day. However, she was still coughing up a large amount of white sticky phlegm, her facial skin was still sagging and she complained of lack of energy. Her tongue coating was thin yellow, and her pulse was choppy.

Prescription
Lu Gen (Phragmitis) 30 g, *Mao Gen* (Imperatus) 30 g, *Xing Ren* (Pruni Armeniaca) 30 g, *Yi Yi Ren*

---

[7] This is one of the four thin mucus syndromes of the *Jin Kui. Xuan Yin* (suspended mucus, which is a local kind of mucus hanging from the hypochondrium area) is characterized by shortness of breath and cough, pain with inability to turn around to the side and a deep or wiry pulse.

Case Study continues

(Coix) 30 g, *Dong Gua Ren* (Benincasa) 30 g, *Bai Hua She She Cao* (Herba Oldenlandia) 30 g, *Xian He Cao* (Agrimonia) 30 g, *Lü Cao* (Humulus Japonicus) 30 g, *Che Qian Cao* (Herba Plantaginis) 30 g, *Ze Xie* (Alismatis) 15 g, *Fu Ling* (Poria) 15 g, *Mai Men Dong* (Ophiopogonis) 15 g.

In addition, *Zhong Jie Feng Pian* (Sarcandra Tablets) and *Ai Tong Pian* (Cancer Pain Tablets) were prescribed.

Fourth consultation (19th August)
After the patient had taken these remedies, by 18th August, her mental capacity was restored and she was able to swallow without any further problems. She was able to consume more food and the pain in the costal arch had gone. Her facial skin and eyelids were no longer sagging. Another X-ray examination revealed that no fluid accumulations were present. No further cancer growth was detectable; however, an ultrasound examination verified some unspecified cell changes in the liver area. Still, the dysphagia (*Ye Ge*) was cured and the patient's (Upright) *Zheng-Qi* started to recover. Therefore, the treatment focused next on the abdominal masses (*Ji Ju*) due to the combined Phlegm and Blood stasis.

Prescription
Sha Shen (Glehnia) 30 g, *Yi Yi Ren* (Coix) 30 g, *Lu Gen* (Phragmitis) 30 g, *Yu Xing Cao* (Herba Houttuyniae) 30 g, *Bai Hua She She Cao* (Herba Oldenlandia) 30 g, *Gua Lou Pi* (Cortex Trichosanthis) 15 g, *Dan Shen* (Salvia Miltiorrhiza) 15 g, *E Zhu* (Curcuma Ezhu) 15 g, *Zhi Ke*

(Pericarpium Citri Aurantii) 12 g, *Sha Ren* (Fructus Amomi) 6 g, *Chuan Bei Mu* (Bulbus Fritillariae Cirrhosae) powder (swallow with decoction).

Hou Tou Jun Pian (Monkey Head Fungus Tablets), *She Dan Chuan Bei Pian* (Fritillaria Snake Gall Tablets) and *He Kui Zhen*[8] were also prescribed.

Fifth consultation (15th October)
These remedies were taken until 14th October, by which time all the symptoms had gone, the patient was mentally agile and her complexion appeared healthy. Now she eats 6–8 *liang* (approximately 180–240 g) per meal every day and can once more tend to household chores. The prescriptions mentioned above obviously had a consolidating effect: a follow-up examination 2 years later confirmed that there had not been any relapse.

---

[8] In spite of having an extensive library at my disposal, this specification still troubles me. All that could be found in all the well-known and lesser known pharmacopoeias merely suggested *Tian Kui* (Porkert, *Pharmakologie*, p 206), also known as *Tu Kui* (Semiaquilegia Adoxoides), the roots of which are used in the treatment of tumours. *Long Kui* (Solanum Nigrum) and *Zi Bei Tian Kui* (Senecio Nudicaulis), which are also used in cancer treatment, are also mentioned in the Chinese sources. However, regarding *He Kui Zhen*, this is possibly either a more recently discovered or a local herb. The only suggestion I found was in the appendix of the extremely poor English translation of Zhang Dai-Zhao's book *The Treatment Of Cancer By Integrated Chinese-Western Medicine* (Blue Poppy Press, p. 206 ff), where *He Kui Ye* is mentioned as a patent remedy that is probably derived from *He Kui Zhen*. Thus the exact botanical name will have to remain unspecified here.

Author's commentary

It is stated in the '*Jin Kui*': 'If there is an accumulation of fluids under the ribs after drinking, along with painful cough and expectoration, this is called *Xuan Yin* (suspended mucus).' This syndrome only partly matches this case, as Blood stasis is also present, (seen in the pulse, tongue, pain etc.) along with Phlegm (*Zheng* = abdominal masses), both commonly encountered in cancer. It can be assumed that *Yang-Qi*, being a constituent part of the

Zheng-Qi, was weakened due to the long disease process and reduced food intake. As a result, *Yang-Qi* was unable to warm the Spleen which then failed to transport fluids in the Upper and Middle Burner. Pathogenic Water (retention) accumulated in the chest and caused cough and inability to lie down flat.

The obstruction in the throat, which caused severe difficulties in swallowing, prevented the

Author's commentary continues

Author's commentary (cont'd)

patient from eating normally so she gradually became weaker. For this reason, Dr Zhang first prescribed medicinals to transform Phlegm and dry Dampness, such as *Gua Lou* and *Ban Xia*, and water draining herbs such as *Zhu Ling* and *Ze Xie*, as well as *Bai Hua She She Cao*, which also clears Heat (dark urine, dry stools). These were combined with the *Qi* and the Blood moving herb *Yu Jin* and stasis breaking insect medicinals *Tu Bie Chong* and *Jiu Xiang Chong*. To treat cough and Lung-Heat he prescribed the *Yin* nourishing *Sha Shen*. This and the mild *Yang* tonifying and *Qi* moving *Xie Bai* ensured a balanced formula.

Liu Shen Wan consists of *Can Su* and other cooling and Phlegm transforming substances, which work predominantly in the throat. The injections with *He Kui Ye* were probably designed to treat the root of the cancer. Sarcandra Pills are made from Herba Sarcandra Glabra and have the effect of cooling Heat, expelling Wind and removing Blood stasis (they also heal fractures).

Thus this treatment was aimed at moving *Qi*, transforming Phlegm, cooling Heat, draining water and softening masses. It focused mainly on treating the branches; however, to a lesser extent, the root cause was also addressed by the treatment.

Once the stool and the pressure in the chest were regulated and the cough was alleviated, Dr Zhang could concentrate on treating the root of the disease: the second prescription contained *Ji Xing Zi*, which softens masses and moves food stagnation, and *Wei Ling Xian*, which softens gatherings in the Middle Burner, as well as *Kun Bu* and *Hai Dai*, which can also disperse lumps and assist *Gua Lou* in transforming Phlegm.

Wei Ling Xian generates its effect in the throat, like *Shan Dou Gen* and *Xuan Shen*, which also have cooling and softening actions. *Wu Mei* assists *Xuan Shen* to recover the fluids that were dried out by the Heat and to treat cough and the fluids in the pleura. However, like *Mai Men Dong* and *Xuan Shen*, it also nourishes the *Yin*. But maybe it was too early to burden the Spleen with the sticky nature of *Mai Men Dong*. This small flaw made itself evident in the following consultation when the coughing with

phlegm and the sticky tongue coating had increased. Even *Gan Cao* could not succeed in harmonizing this kind of Phlegm-transforming and *Yin*-nourishing formula.

But when this throat-specific formula had managed to improve the swallowing, and normal consumption of food could take place, Dr Zhang decided on a specific formula for the Lung, cough and Phlegm by including *Lu Gen* and *Dong Gua Ren*, which transform Phlegm in the Lung and, together with *Bai Mao Gen*, cool Heat. The latter assisted *Xing Ren* in treating the cough, and all of them together helped to treat the fluid in the lung. As this fluid contained traces of blood, Dr Zhang added *Xian He Cao*, which focuses on the Lung and stops bleeding.

Most of these medicinals cool the Heat that was indicated by the yellow tongue coating, except *Xing Ren* which has a slightly warm property. Consequently, *Bai Hua She She Cao* was also included to ensure the overall cool character of the formula. As Heat damaged the Lung *Yin*, *Mai Men Dong* was added, and its sticky nature was moderated by *Che Qian Zi*, *Ze Xie* and *Fu Ling*. These herbs can excrete water and Heat by diuresis, whilst *Fu Ling* also strengthens the Spleen's transportation function. The uncommonly used *Lü Cao* (Herba Humulus Japonicus or Scandentis) can invigorate Blood, transform Phlegm, soften masses, cause diuresis and cool Heat, so it seems to possess all the necessary features for this formula.

As pointed out by Dr Zhang, in the absence of Heat and *Yin* deficiency and after having restored *Zheng-Qi*, the focus of the formula had to be shifted towards treating the remaining tumour, which can be accomplished with a formula that invigorates Blood, transforms Phlegm and softens masses. Amongst the Blood invigorating medicinals are found *Dan Shen* and *E Zhu*, which is often used in the treatment of cancer and has an anticarcinogenic effect like *Bai Hua She She Cao*. As cancer usually combines with Heat, another herb was added to cool toxins, *Yu Xing Cao*. *Lu Gen* cools Heat in the Lung. To strengthen the Spleen, *Yi Yi Ren* and *Sha Shen* were included – the former to

Author's commentary continues

Author's commentary (cont'd)

treat Dampness in the Middle, the latter to treat Dryness in the Lung. To combat the Phlegm and masses he added *Chuan Bei Mu* and *Gua Lou Pi*, which has a milder effect compared to the previously prescribed *Gua Lou Ren*. *Zhi Ke* also moves Middle *Qi* with a mild action, as the patient's condition did not permit use of a stronger herb such as *Zhi Shi*. The patent remedy *She Dan Chuan Bei Pian*, in my experience has a great effect against Phlegm and masses, whilst the other two patent remedies have a specific anticarcinogenic effect. This was a complicated case that involved many modifications in the prescription, but eventually the desired results were achieved.

Case Study 9.19   Alopecia areata and totalis (*Gui Ti Tou*)

From the case studies of Dr Zhao Fa-Xin, Henan province. Patient M, female, 16 years old, first consultation 11th April 1968.

History
About 5 years ago the patient's scalp started to itch and seborrhoea with white plaques developed, which eventually led to hair loss. At the start she only lost patches of hair, but over the last couple of years she has lost all her hair, including her eyebrows. Her complexion was dark and lustreless. Her menstrual cycle was prolonged, with menorrhagia.

The patient's tongue body was pale red with stasis spots at the tip and a thin white coating. Her pulse was fine and wiry (*Xi, Xuan Mai*).

Syndrome differentiation indicated that this condition belongs to a congenital Kidney weakness with Blood deficiency resulting in Blood stasis. Therefore, the principle is to nourish *Yin* and Blood, and to combine this with using Blood invigorating medicinals.

Prescription
Dang Gui (Angelica Sinensis) 15 g, *Chuan Xiong* (Ligusticum) 10 g, *Sheng Di* (Rehmannia) and *Shou Di* (Rehmannia Praeparata) 25 g each, *Sheng Shou Wu* (Radix Polygonum Recens) and *Shou Shou Wu* (Radix Polygoni Multiflori Exsiccatus) 25 g each, *Hong Hua* (Carthamus) 10 g, *Xiang Fu* (Cyperus) 12 g, *Shi Jue Ming* (Concha Haliotidis) 20 g, *Xia Ku Cao* (Prunella) 15 g, *Chi Shao* (Paeonia Rubra) and *Bai Shao* (Paeonia Lactiflora) 12 g each, *Chai Hu* (Bupleurum) 10 g, *Tao Ren* (Persica) 10 g and *Gan Cao* (Glycyrrhiza) 3 g. Method: decoction, 6 bags.

In addition, the scalp should be washed twice daily with a decoction of 60 g of ground *Sang Bai Pi* (Cortex Mori Albae), cooled down before application.

After the scalp wash and six decoctions, the scalp stopped itching and the dandruff was reduced. After 20 further decoctions a fluff of hair was starting to grow. The above-mentioned prescription was processed into pills and continued.

After 2 months black hair and eyebrows had fully regrown, the complexion was red and vital again, she was in excellent mental and physical condition, and her menstruation was regular.

Author's commentary

This young girl with a congenital Kidney weakness[9] suffered from Essence (*Jing*) and Blood deficiency, which was the root of the disease, while the branch manifested in Blood stasis. When she started to menstruate, the loss of blood worsened the situation. As the growth of hair was not nourished sufficiently by the deficient *Jing* and Blood, and as

Blood stasis easily causes dry skin and hair, a modification of *Si Wu Tang* (Four Ingredients Decoction) plus raw and prepared *Shou Wu* was given to nourish the Kidney and Blood. Due to the concurrent presence of Blood stasis and Liver-*Qi* stagnation, triggered by the emotional problems such hair loss entailed for the adolescent girl, *Tao Ren*, *Hong Hua*, *Chao Hu* and *Xiang Fu* were all included. Both *Xia Ku Cao* and *Shi Jue Ming* are cool and their effect is also directed towards the Liver. In essence, the excess is treated with cooling, Blood invigorating and *Qi* moving herbs, whilst the underlying deficiency, the root of the disease, is remedied by strengthening and nourishing.

---

[9] Deficiency of the *Zang Fu* organs is either acquired or constitutional (literally 'Pre-Heaven and Post-Heaven' in Chinese). The congenital Kidney weakness in this case means that there is a constitutional tendency for Kidney deficiency syndromes.

Case Study 9.20 Apoplexy (*Zhong Feng*)

Patient L, male, 58 years old; first consultation on 8th March 1979.

Past history
In April 1978 this patient suffered a stroke due to a thrombus, with hemiplegia on the left side, a sluggish and slow gait, and could only walk with crutches, both feet dragging when they hit the ground. The patient is overweight, shows no facial expression, has slowed responses, reduced mental capacity (dementia), tiredness during the daytime, slurred speech, and answers very slowly or misses the point of the question; he can no longer control urination and defecation.

Diagnosis
The tongue body was swollen and dark with a thick (*Ni*) white coating; the pulse was deep and wiry (*Chen, Xuan Mai*); regular heartbeat, BP 164/110 mmHg, the patient had suffered with high blood pressure for 10 years.

Syndrome differentiation indicated this syndrome belongs to Wind-stroke affecting the channels[10] (*Zhong Feng*) with underlying Kidney-*Yang* deficiency.

Prescription
Chuan Xiong (Ligusticum) 15 g, *Ge Gen* (Pueraria) 20 g, *Dan Shen* (Salvia Miltiorrhiza) 30 g, *Wei Ling Xian* (Clematis) 20 g, *Hong Hua* (Carthamus) 10 g, *Luo Shi Teng* (Trachelospermum) 15 g, *Chang Pu* (Acorus) 12 g, *Sheng Huang Qi* (Astragalus Recens) 30 g, *Yu Jin* (Curcuma) 15 g, *Chong Wei Zi* (Semen Leonuri Heterophylli) 30 g, *Tu Si Zi* (Cuscuta) 25 g, *Jin Ying Zi* (Rosa Laevigata) 15 g, *Nü Zhen Zi* (Ligustrum) 12 g to be taken as a decoction, *Wu Gong Fen* (Scolopendra Subspinipes Pulvis) 1 g,

---

[10] In TCM, Wind-stroke is differentiated into Wind-stroke affecting the channels and Wind-stroke affecting the *Zang Fu* organs. Channel-stroke is characterized predominantly by hemiplegia or physical impairment. Organ-stroke is characterized by a mental impairment, for example unconsciousness. For details, see Glossary.

Case Study continues

Quan Xie Fen (Buthus Pulvis) 1 g to be taken as powder.

2nd consultation 29th March 1979
After 16 preparations a positive change in the mental state is noticeable; overall, there is a slight improvement of all symptoms mentioned above; the patient answers questions a lot more fluently, urination is more controlled, but he still has great difficulty with walking. Severe tiredness is still present.

The tongue body is swollen with a white coating. The pulse is deep and wiry (*Chen, Xuan Mai*). Regular heartbeat, BP 170/100 mmHg.

Prescription
Chuan Xiong (Ligusticum) 15 g, *Ge Gen* (Pueraria) 20 g, *Dan Shen* (Salvia Miltiorrhiza) 30 g, *Wei Ling Xian* (Clematis) 20 g, *Hong Hua* (Carthamus) 10 g, *Luo Shi Teng* (Trachelospermum) 15 g, *Yu Jin* (Radix Curcuma) 12 g, *Tu Si Zi* (Cuscuta) 20 g, *Jin Ying Zi* (Rosa Laevigata) 15 g, *Chong Wei Zi* (Semen Leonuri Heterophylli) 30 g, *Yi Yi Ren* (Coix) 10 g, *Niu Xi* (Achyranthis Bidentata) 15 g, *Zhen Zhu Mu* (Concha Margaritaferae) 30 g, to be taken as a decoction, *Wu Gong Fen* (Scolopendra Subspinipes Pulvis) 1 g, and *Quan Xie Fen* (Buthus Pulvis) 1 g to be taken as powder.

3rd consultation 15th May 1979
After 30 preparations had been taken, a marked improvement in the mobility of the extremities was noticeable, but the patient had a feeling of weakness, sore muscles and poor fine motor skills. Now, the patient complains of a dry mouth, dry eyes and severe sleepiness. The incontinence has continued to improve. On one occasion the patient experienced a pain in the chest lasting for 1–2 minutes.

The tongue diagnosis revealed a long, dark tongue with a white coating. The pulse was fine (*Xi Mai*). BP was 160/100 mmHg.

Prescription
As above plus *Mai Dong* (Ophiopogonis) 12 g and *Yu Zhu* (Polygonatum Odoratum) 12 g to nourish *Yin*.

4th consultation 17th May 1979
The patient's facial expressions are still poor, and he only talks a little, but he listens to the radio and reads the newspaper. He is also able to go for a walk on his own outside his room. He feels his feet to be cold.

The tongue body is thick and dark, with a white coating. The pulse is deep and fine (*Chen, Xi Mai*). BP is 160/100 mmHg.

Prescription
As for the 3rd consultation, including the *Mai Dong* and *Yu Zhu*.

5th consultation 6th June 1979
The patient's general state of health has markedly improved, daytime tiredness is reduced, and his mental state is increasingly clear; he is able to give fluent answers now, without hesitating; urination and defecation are fully under his control.

Tongue diagnosis revealed a long, dark tongue with a white coating. His pulse was deep, fine and wiry (*Chen, Xi, Xuan Mai*). BP was 160/100 mmHg.

Prescription
Chuan Xiong (Ligusticum) 15 g, *Ge Gen* (Pueraria) 20 g, *Wei Ling Xian* (Clematis) 20 g, *Luo Shi Teng* (Trachelospermum) 15 g, *Tu Si Zi* (Cuscuta) 12 g, *Niu Xi* (Achyranthis Bidentata) 15 g, *Shou Wu* (Polygonum Multiflori) 12 g, *Nü Zhen Zi* (Ligustrum) 15 g , *Gou Qi Zi* (Lycium) 15 g, *Hei Zhi Ma* (Sesamum) 15 g, *Hei Sang Shen* (Fructus Mori N.) 12 g, *Ren Dong* (Lonicera) 20 g, *Ze Xie* (Alismatis) 15 g, *Dang Gui* (Angelica Sinensis) 10 g, *Che Qian Cao* (Herba Plantaginis) 10 g, to be taken as a decoction.

6th consultation 17th July 1979
Vocal articulation very clear by now, fine motor skills of the lower limbs has improved, the patient now walks around the whole hospital. Stool and urination normal. Tongue and pulse as previously. BP 170/105 mmHg.

Prescription
Dang Gui (Angelica Sinensis) 15 g, *Ge Gen* (Pueraria) 30 g, *Wei Ling Xian* (Clematis) 20 g, *Dan*

Case Study continues

Shen (Salvia Miltiorrhiza) 20 g, *Luo Shi Teng* (Trachelospermum) 15 g, *Tu Si Zi* (Cuscuta) 20 g, *Niu Xi* (Achyranthis Bidentata) 15 g, *Nü Zhen Zi* (Ligustrum) 15 g, *Gou Qi Zi* (Lycium) 20 g, *Hei Zhi Ma* (Sesamum) 12 g, *Jin Ying Zi* 20 g, *Ren Dong* (Lonicera) 20 g, *Ze Xie* (Alismatis) 15 g, to be taken as a decoction.

7th consultation 16th August 1979

The patient's mental and emotional state is vital and expressive, he is able to greet his friends when he meets them, he answers precisely and speaks fluently and he can read the paper for 30 minutes. He can consume food and drink without problems, stool and urination are normal. He can go for longer walks with the aid of a walking stick, and there is black hair growing from a previously bald patch at the crown of his head.

Tongue diagnosis showed a long, dark tongue with stasis spots. His pulse was deep, fine, wiry and slightly rapid (*Chen, Xi, Xuan, Shuo Mai*). BP was 150/100 mmHg, and he had a regular heartbeat, 90 bpm.

Prescription

Chuan Xiong (Ligusticum) 15 g, *Dan Shen* (Salvia Miltiorrhiza) 30 g, *Dang Gui* (Angelica Sinensis) 15 g, *Wei Ling Xian* (Clematis) 20 g, *Hong Hua* (Carthamus) 10 g, *Luo Shi Teng* (Trachelospermum) 15 g, *Tu Si Zi* (Cuscuta) 30 g, *Jin Ying Zi* (Rosa Laevigata) 12 g, *Shou Wu* (Polygonum Multiflori) 15 g, *Nü Zhen Zi* (Ligustrum) 15 g, *Hei Zhi Ma* (Sesamum) 10 g, *Hei Sang Shen* (Fructus Mori N.) 12 g, *Ren Dong Teng* (Ramus Lonicera) 20 g to be taken as a decoction.

Author's commentary

With strokes, normally the earlier the patient presents for treatment, the better the results. When this case came for treatment a year after the stroke, *Qi* and Blood had already been weakened and depleted by the long illness. Kidney deficiency was also evident from the weak legs and weak sphincter muscles. In TCM it is said that the Kidney rules the Sea of Marrow (the brain), which is associated with the mental fatigue, facial expression and ability to speak.

Therefore, *Huang Qi* was given initially, to strengthen *Qi*. This was an aid to the other commonly prescribed medicinals for apoplexies that remove obstruction from the *Luo* vessels, such as

Wu Gong, Quan Xie and the Blood invigorating medicinals, whose necessity became all too obvious when omitting *Chuan Xiong* resulted in stasis spots appearing on the tongue. *Niu Xi* was not only prescribed for invigorating Blood but also to guide the other herbs' effect to the legs, which were particularly weakened. To tonify the Kidneys, *Shou Wu, Hei Sang Shen, Tu Si Zi* and others were added. As the Chong-medicinals *Wu Gong* and *Quan Xie*, which were initially employed to lower the blood pressure and regenerate the mind, weakened the Blood and *Yin* somewhat, this was moderated by the later addition of *Dang Gui, Gou Qi Zi, Hei Zhi Ma* etc.

SUMMARY

A comparison of classical and modern case studies reveals that although the classical records may not have been as precise as today's, for example as regards dosages, when it comes to diagnosis, syndrome differentiation and discussion of the treatment principles, they are comparable with today's standard, at least in the Qing dynasty. Moreover, modified versions of the classical formulas as well as individual compositions are still used today. If the classical physicians had not created the foundations of modern treatment, it is questionable whether they could have been developed today in the way they were centuries ago, when one considers modern-day time constraints and the demand for immediately effective treatment.

Maybe this is the reason why studying and understanding the classics has become such a vital tool for every TCM student in China. Only in this way can the student understand and get to grips with this complex way of thinking. In this spirit, excerpts from some of the classical texts on Blood stasis are translated and published for the first time in the next chapter.

SECTION 3

Classical texts

Knowledge of the classics, literally 'old books' (*Gu Shu*), is expected of every student and doctor in China. Many old doctors can quote from the classics without effort. However, to allow space for Western medical education, students now only need to understand rather than memorize the texts. Unfortunately, there are still only a few good translations of medical classics available. Therefore, the essential classical texts on the topic of Blood stasis are translated and presented alongside each other in this section.

First, the most important book relating to Blood stasis is presented, this being the '*Yi Lin Gai Cuo*' (*Corrections of mistakes in the medical world*). It has already been quoted and mentioned above a number of times, and is translated here for the first time in history.

The author Wang Qing-Ren, also known as Wang Quan-Ren, was born in Yu Tian, Hebei province, in 1768 (Qing dynasty under the rule of Qian Long). At the age of 20 he studied medicine, but also distinguished himself through his interest in Chinese martial arts. The name of his clinic in Beijing was 'The One Knowledge Clinic', which is derived from the saying of philosopher Zhuang-Zi: 'Know the one and all is achieved' ('*Zhi Yi Wan Bi*'). Following his death, his wife and son are said to have lost all his notes, so we can assume that he was the author of other works apart from the '*Yi Lin Gai Cuo*'.

His greatest merit is his pioneering role in performing systematic anatomical studies on bodies, together with his carrying out of clinical studies and his gaining of experience in the treatment of Blood stasis and post-apoplectic hemiplegia. Although his book contains only about 120 000 characters, in it he developed almost 40 formulas, of which many are still in use today.

He died in 1831, one year after the publication of his book.

Notwithstanding the importance of his records of organs in the first part, the greatest merit of the '*Yi Lin Gai Cuo*' is his comprehensive presentation of the diagnosis and treatment of Blood stasis in the second and third parts. There is no other book in Chinese medical literature that had such influence on medicine in relation to Blood stasis syndrome.

Further classical excerpts relating to Blood stasis follow, these being: Zhang Zhong-Jings '*Jin Kui Yao Lüe*' and '*Shang Han Lun*', from the beginning of the third century; Chen Wu-Ze's '*San Yin Ji Yi Bing Zheng Fang Lun*', from the twelfth century; Wang Ken-Tang's '*Zheng Zhi Zhun Sheng*', from the beginning of the seventeenth century; Lin Pei-Qin's '*Lei Zheng Zhi Cai*', from the beginning of the nineteenth century; and Tang Zong Hai's '*Xue Zheng Lun*', from the end of the nineteenth century. The final text from the '*Yi Shu*' by Cheng Wen-Zhou was not published until the Qing dynasty, but it was originally written by Luo Chi-Cheng in the thirteenth century. These authors come from different eras of Chinese medicine, each author reflecting the essence of the contemporary views on Blood stasis of his time.

SECTION CONTENTS

Chapter 10

Wang Qing-Ren's 'Yi Lin Gai Cuo' (Corrections of mistakes in the medical world)

CHAPTER CONTENTS

WANG QING-REN'S OWN PREFACE

I have now completed this book *Corrections of mistakes in the medical world*. Although it contains both methods for the treatment of illnesses, and notes on the anatomy of organs, it is in some places neither complete nor set out in exhaustive detail. Thus everyone who has the opportunity to examine the anatomy of the organs at first hand, should add his own suggestions to any incomplete descriptions in order to achieve further improvement.

Apart from the descriptions of organs, some notes on disease syndromes are given. These include guidelines to show the reader which internal diseases and external infections can cause damage to man, and in what ways. So, for example, excess and deficiency are described; but how do they manifest themselves?

The meanings of many terms in this book are often explained superficially, and even amongst practising physicians knowledge may be either deep or shallow. When frequently used words and phrases are encountered again and again, there is the danger that a superficial reader will fail to bring these into context.

For example, there are about 40 different syndromes for hemiplegia due to *Qi* collapse and 20 different syndromes for *Qi* collapse in infantile Wind convulsion (*Feng Jing*). If one comes across mixed syndromes of these two types, then at least 60 different references must be looked up to avoid a faulty diagnosis. Therefore I hope that the reader of this book will exercise the necessary care.

Wang Qing-Ren
Yu-Tian (Jade Field), Hebei province, 1830

PART 1.[1] WANG'S ANATOMICAL STUDIES

CORRECTION OF THE MEDICAL WORLD WITH REGARD TO INTERNAL ORGANS (*ZANG FU*[2])

In ancient times, it was said: 'One who fails to become a good state official might as well strive to become a good physician.' Arguably, this is supposed to mean that being a good physician is simple whilst being a good state official is difficult. Yet in my opinion, this is by no means the case. For generations, there have been excellent ministers ruling the country. However, there has not been a single perfect book-writing physician.

The reason why physicians could not be flawless is that their predecessors had written medical books containing errors with regard to internal organs, and their successors accepted these already established theories without question, so proper understanding of the causes of diseases was lost.

Once this knowledge is lost, it will not matter how advanced in his thinking a writer might be or what great skills he might possess;[3] he will still fail to grasp the disease mechanisms with regard to the internal organs. For that reason medicine was not able to produce a flawless physician.

In order to diagnose diseases, one must be familiar with the organs. I often read classical theories about the organs with their corresponding illustrations and find that they are inconsistent.

For example, with regard to the Spleen and Stomach the classical texts say: 'Spleen belongs to the element Earth (within the Five Phases), Earth governs stillness and so does not belong to motion. If the Spleen moves, it will be restless.' If

---

[1] The chapter headings did not exist in the original edition; they were added later to achieve an improved overview.

[2] The unintentional ambiguity of the term '*Zang Fu*' (storage organs, labour organs) should be noted here. As long as the anatomical organs of Western medicine and the functional entities that are the TCM organs are differentiated, this ambiguity does not come into play. In his theory, Wang of course refers to Chinese medicine; however, he also describes his knowledge of the anatomical characteristics of the internal organs, which he has gained over the course of time from studying dead bodies. Before the time of Wang there were hardly any studies that highlighted the (seeming) contradictions between TCM concepts and anatomical findings. Today the two concepts are no longer confused with each other and the contradictions are no longer a cause for debate. As Wang was primarily concerned with the anatomical organs that he was investigating, the term '*Zang Fu*' is translated as 'internal organs', unless the *Zang Fu* TCM organs are specifically being referred to.

[3] Literally: 'To stitch dragons and engrave tigers', and 'To cut out of the clouds in order to stuff the (not round) mouth'. Two Chinese idioms.

'Spleen in motion is restless', why does it say later on in the text that if the Spleen perceives noises, it will move and rub against the Stomach to aid digestion, and if the Spleen fails to move, then ingested food will not be digested? There is a contradiction here as far as motion and stillness are concerned.[4]

With regard to the Lung, it is said to be hollow, similar to a beehive full of combs. It is described as having no aperture towards the abdominal cavity, and is said to be full on inspiration and empty on expiration. However, if it is said to have no lower aperture, why is it mentioned elsewhere that the Lung is supposed to have twenty-four holes, which criss-cross in every direction to disperse the organs' Qi. There is a contradiction here concerning the holes and apertures of the Lung.

As far as the Kidney is concerned, there are said to be two which together are called 'Kidneys'. The Qi moving between them is supposed to be the Ming Men ('Gate of Life'). If the Qi moving between the two Kidneys is called Ming Men, why is it said elsewhere that the left Kidney is called Kidney, but the right Kidney Ming Men? If the Kidneys are one organ, why were they given two different names? What is the basis for this? If the moving Qi in the middle is called Ming Men, and if on the other hand the moving Qi is stored in the Ming Men, what exactly case is the Ming Men? This is the contradiction regarding the Kidney.

The Liver is said to have a channel both to the left and to the right, thus vessels, which are supposed to begin laterally at the ribs (i.e. Liver channel), extend up to the eyes and run downwards from the lower abdomen, winding around the genital organs, finally reaching the big toe. So, if the Liver is said to have two channels with a symmetrical course, why does it say elsewhere that the Liver resides on the left and the left ribs belong to the Liver? Here is a contradiction, as far as left and right are concerned, with regard to the Liver.

The Heart is said to be the monarch amongst the organs and the Mind (Shen) arises from it. Intention (Yi) is said to be stored there, and is a function of the Heart. Intention is said to transform into Will Power (Zhi), the movement and change of this Will Power is said to be Reflection (Si), long-term Reflection is described as Planning (Lü), and the utilization of this Planning to arrange one's affairs is said to be Wisdom (Zhi).[5]

All these five arise from the Heart. If all of them are stored in the Heart, why is it said elsewhere that the Spleen governs intentional wisdom, the Kidney governs skill, the Liver governs planning and the Gallbladder governs decisiveness? At all times and in all places the Mind (Ling Ji) is stated to be the only source. According to these theories the Mind (Ling Ji) is present everywhere, but it is never explained what Mind (Ling Ji) really is, where it comes from and what it looks like. All theories about the Heart are thus as nebulous as those quoted here.

The Stomach is said to govern the processing of food and drink. Furthermore, it is stated that the movement of the Spleen generates digestion in the Stomach, that the Stomach opening is called the 'injection gate' (Pen Men) and food arrives in the Stomach via this gate; the subtle, rarefied Qi (extracted from food) passes through the Pen Men to the Spleen and Lung from where it is distributed to all the vessels. This part of the theory is neither clear nor logical.

The exit of the Stomach is called the 'deep gate' (You Men, pylorus). It is the upper beginning of the Small Intestine. The Small Intestine is said to be responsible for receiving and transformation; this means food enters the Small Intestine, where it is transformed into excrement, finally arriving at the frame gate (Lan Men, ileocecal valve), which forms the lower exit of the Small Intestine. When the pure and impure are separated, feces are supposed to enter the Large Intestine and become excreted by the anus (Gang Men), while the fluids are passed to the Bladder in the form of urine.

According to this theory urine is filtered from excrement, so its smell should be bad. I use baby urine (in treatment), and I have also made enquiries of patients who used their own urine for treating themselves: its taste is supposed to be merely salty, but by no means is there a bad smell.

---

[4] In this and the following paragraph he uses the word 'Wu', i.e. mistake, misconception.

[5] Wisdom 'Zhi', although it is a homophone with Will 'Zhi', is a different character.

Moreover, if food and drink are mixed with excrement, would not the stool be thin and runny like diarrhoea? This may be true of chicken and ducks, which do not pass urine, but for horses and cattle this is certainly not the case, let alone for humans. To read the words 'The Small Intestine transforms food, water passes through the 'frame gate' (*Lan Men*, ileocecal valve)' is to accept the most ridiculous story of all time.

The Pericardium (*Xin Bao*) is said to have fine sinews like silk and to be connected to the Heart and Lung. Elsewhere it is said that the Pericardium is the yellowish fat located at the outside of the Heart, or that the yellowish fat between the horizontal membrane below the Heart and the hard membrane [diaphragm; translator's note] is the Pericardium, and finally that the middle of the chest (*Tan Zhong*) only bears a name but has no substance. Now, if on the one hand the Pericardium is said to merely have a name but no substance, why on the other hand is the channel on the middle finger claimed to be the Pericardium channel? Having heard so much (contradictory information) about the Pericardium, what is the Pericardium after all, and where does all this knowledge come from?

Discussing the Triple Burner is even more ridiculous. In the *'Ling Shu'* (The Yellow Emperor's Classic, Spiritual Pivot), it is stated: 'The Triple Burner of the hand governs all that is above, the Triple Burner of the feet governs all that is below.' This suggests there are two Triple Burners.

In the *'Nan Jing'* (The Classic of Difficulties), it is stated in the thirty first question: 'The Upper Burner is above the Stomach and governs the interior and does not excrete. The Middle Burner is in the middle of the abdomen and governs the digestion of food. The Lower Burner is below the navel and governs the distribution of pure and impure essences.'

It also says: 'The Triple Burner is the digestive tract.' This suggests that the Triple Burner is a concrete object. Further on, it says: 'The *Qi* moving between the Kidneys is the source of the Triple Burner.' So here the Triple Burner is insubstantial *Qi*.

Thus, according to the *'Nan Jing'*, sometimes the Triple Burner has a shape, sometimes it has not and sometimes there are two of them!

Wang Shu-He[6] is most likely the author of the passage in which it is stated that the Triple Burner bears a name but has no solid form; likewise, it is Chen Wu-Ze who claims that the Triple Burner is the membrane below the navel, and Yuan Chun-Pu who considers the Triple Burner to be a layer inside the body that is the reddest of all in shape and colour, Wu Tian-Min who states it is the body cavity and Jin Yi-Long who theorizes that there are both an anterior and a posterior Triple Burner. There are more theories of the Triple Burner, including theories on shape or no shape, than there are fingers on the hand. If these revered masters cannot agree on one standard, why is it said that the channel on the small finger is the Triple Burner channel?

There are many contradictions which various people have exposed and criticized, but these critics were not right either. All things considered: once the original source is in error, every subsequent explanation is also doomed to fail.

I would have liked to correct these errors, but I had no opportunity to observe organs. Writing a book without having seen the internal organs would be like a psychopath describing his dreams. Treating diseases without knowing the organs, is like a blind man feeling his way through the dark streets at night. No matter how exact one's thoughts and how good one's perception, how will it be of any use?

I had spent 10 years on this subject when I came to Luanzhou (today's Tang Shan near Tianjin), as a 30-year-old man in the year 1798. An infectious colitis epidemic with a mortality rate of 80–90% had affected many children. In poor families it was customary to bury the children in grass matting instead of coffins. Furthermore, it was also the custom not to bury them too deep, so that wild dogs could get to the bodies. According to this superstition, the next child would not die.

Therefore, the bodies of hundreds of eviscerated children were lying in the cemetery. I passed

---

[6] The following paragraphs mention the theories and explanations of several historic physicians. Wang Shu-He, also known as Wang Xi, is the famous author of the Pulse Classic (*Mai Jing*) and editor of the modern version of Zhang Zhong-Jing's *'Shang Han Lun'* and *'Jin Kui Yao Lüe'*.

them every day on horseback. At first I held my nose, but later on I thought of all the classical authors' erroneous ideas about the internal organs, which I had never seen myself. So I stopped avoiding the filth and ugliness, and every morning I went to the cemetery to study the bodies of these eviscerated children. Amongst the bodies the dogs had partially devoured, most still had stomach and intestines, but only a few had hearts and livers. Only three in ten were sufficiently complete for comparisons to be drawn.

In 30 days I was able to study just over 30 bodies, and I started to realize that the pictures of internal organs in medical books did not correspond with the internal organs of the human being at all. Even the stated number of organs was wrong.

To my disappointment, the membrane in the chest [diaphragm] that I was the most keen to see, was as thin as paper and thus was destroyed in every case, so I could not gain any clear knowledge about its location, whether it was above or below the heart, or whether it was oblique or straight. This was most regrettable.

Two years later, in the year 1799, a 26-year-old woman from Liaoyang province had lost her mind and murdered her husband and father-in-law. She was brought to Fengtian [today's Shengyang] to be executed by dismemberment. I went to the execution ground, where I suddenly became aware of the fact that this was not about a man, but a woman. So I did not dare to approach any further. Shortly after wards, when the executioner showed me the heart, liver and lung, I noticed on closer inspection that these organs matched those I had seen before.

Later, in the year 1813 in Beijing, a man who had killed his mother was condemned to death by dismemberment. The execution took place outside the Zhai Wen gate, south of the suspension bridge. I could not get any closer and see the organs, and the diaphragm was already destroyed, so I was unable to see it.

In the year 1829, when the condemned criminal Zhang Ge-Er was brought there, I could not attend. So I wasn't having any success, but I could not give up.

However, on the night of the 13th in the twelfth month of the year 1829, when I was called for a diagnosis to the house of the Heng family in the Ban Chang alley off An Ding Gate Street, to my surprise I met the imperial army officer Heng of the city government of Jiang Ning. He told me that he had led the army from his headquarters in Hami (in Xinjiang) to Geshegeer, where scores of dead bodies were to be found on the battlefield, so he knew what he was talking about when it came to diaphragms.

When I heard this I was extremely pleased and implored him to enlighten me. He had mercy on me and described every detail to me.

Finally, after 42 years, I had certainty about the internal organs and was able to carry out a complete study. Originally, I wanted to publish it much earlier, but at first I feared that ensuing generations, if they had not seen any organs for themselves, might criticize me for finding faults in the classic texts. On the other hand, it seemed to me that it could cause great damage to medicine if passing on the information was to be delayed for hundreds or thousands of years.

When I thought about this more closely I couldn't help thinking of the Yellow Emperor, who when he wanted to ease the suffering of his people did not hesitate to put trivial questions (considering his position) to his advisors Qi Bo and Gui Yu Ou; indeed this led to the name 'Su Wen', which means 'common questions'.

If the two officials had the correct information, then their answer to the emperor would indeed be right. But if they did not know, further enquiry was necessary. How can one just answer carelessly, without having the proper knowledge? This causes great damage to ensuing generations.

I also thought of Qin Yue-Ren's 'Nan Jing' (Classic of Difficulties) and Zhang Shi-Xian's 'He Tu Luo Shu' (Diagrams and Notes) with commentaries, where it is claimed that the heart, liver and lung were weighed and measured precisely; every organ was weighed, the large and small intestines had their length measured in Cun (Chinese inch); the length and size of every organ, for example the liver and the stomach were all measured, including their volume in cups and litres, all of which sounds very authentic and credible. In reality, these organs were never looked at; it was just empty talk amounting to deceit, because it served the writer's own reputation; but it caused damage to humanity. If we call someone who steals money a thief, then equally we must call someone who acquires fame in such a way a criminal! Never mind, even if it takes hundreds or thousands of years, can the truth be concealed forever?

I am preparing these prints today not to further my own reputation nor to criticize the classical authors' inadequacy; I am not hoping to make a name for myself for posterity, nor do I want to be condemned as a heretic later on. All this is solely to improve the understanding of the medical reader, so that when he sees these pictures, hopefully everything will become clearer and his knowledge will be increased. Then, when he is treating patients, he will have at hand a precise methodology, rather than relying an guesswork and a lack of clear answers, and can thereby reduce losses due to disease.

The esteemed reader should think about this and understand that this is my greatest hope!

ILLUSTRATIONS OF THE ORGANS FROM THE CLASSICS

Illustrations of the organs from classical works are shown below in Figures 10.1–10.12.

Lung

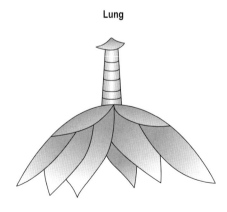

The lung has six leaves and two upper lobes, so it is often depicted with eight leaves

Figure 10.1   Lung.

Large intestine

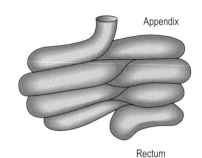

Appendix

Rectum

Figure 10.2   Large Intestine.

Stomach

Stomach opening

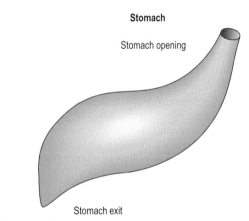

Stomach exit

Figure 10.3   Stomach.

Spleen or pancreas *(Pi)*

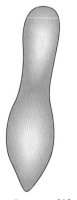

Figure 10.4   Spleen or Pancreas *(Pi)*.

Heart

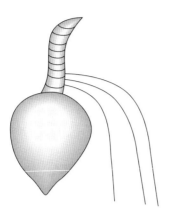

Figure 10.5 Heart.

Pericardium

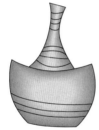

Figure 10.6 Pericardium.

Small intestine

Stomach exit

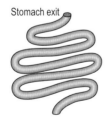

Figure 10.7 Small Intestine.

Urinary bladder

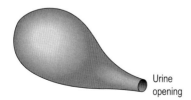

Urine opening

Figure 10.8 Urinary Bladder.

Kidneys

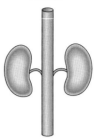

Figure 10.9 Kidneys.

Triple warmer

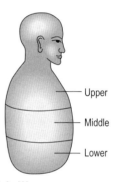

Upper

Middle

Lower

Figure 10.10 Triple Warmer.

Liver

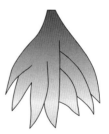

The liver has three lobes on the left and four on the right

Figure 10.11 Liver.

Gall bladder

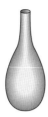

The gall bladder is mostly depicted
as a short outgrowth from the liver

Figure 10.12   Gall-Bladder.

Heart

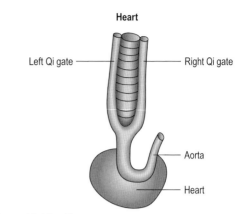

Left Qi gate — — Right Qi gate

— Aorta

— Heart

Figure 10.13   Heart.

Lung

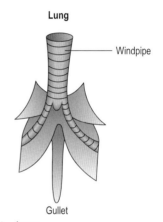

— Windpipe

Gullet

Figure 10.14   Lung.

Figures 10.13–10.24 show the corrected illustrations of the organs that I was able to study personally.

The right and left Qi gates[7] (see Fig. 10.13) are two vessels that converge in the middle of the heart, and running transverse at the heart meet in the *Wei* main vessel (main vessel of Protective *Qi*) towards the left at the back[8] of the heart. The heart is located below the windpipe, not below the bronchi. At the top, the heart and lung lobe press against each other.

The windpipe forks out to the left and right along the Lung (Fig. 10.14), and each branch enters one of the two lung lobes; the branches extend, in the shape of hollow vessels, to the end of the lobes. Throughout the lung are clasps of cartilage. Inside there are whitish bubbles[9] everywhere, similar to soya milk bubbles. These are shaped but have no substance. Towards the back, the leaves of the lung have a larger surface whilst towards the chest they have a smaller surface. Both the upper and lower tips point toward the chest. The outer skin of the lung is firm and has neither openings towards the body cavity nor 24 holes[10] for *Qi* to flow through.

[7] Wang mentions the 'left and right *Qi* gate' but not in the meaning of openings as they are usually called in TCM. Judging from his drawings, he describes two tube-like vessels at both sides of the trachea merging at the level of the heart; probably he is referring to the two carotid arteries.
[8] Supposedly, the aorta.
[9] Supposedly, the appearance of the alveoli resembling bubbles.
[10] Depending on where the terminal segments of the bronchioles are detached, there are in fact 10–30 'holes', which in historic sources are arguably represented by the '24 holes' in the form of air passages.

The stomach (Fig. 10.15) has an opening (injection gate) at the top, which lies exactly in the middle; at the bottom it has an exit (deep gate); above to the right, about one inch to the left of the deep gate, lies the *Jin* gate (fluid gate, papilla of the major pancreatic duct). To the left of the *Jin* gate, inside the stomach,[11] are small bulbs similar to berries, called *Zhe Shi* (food cap, probably the bulbus duodeni, the superior part of the duodenum). Outside the stomach, to the left of the *Jin* gate, at the so-called *Zong Ti* (main link, i.e. pancreas), the stomach borders the liver. The stomach lies within the abdomen, stretched horizontally lengthwise; its opening points to the backbone, its exit points to the right, its base lies towards the abdomen and it opens into the fluid tract.

[11] Wang regards the superior and ascending division of the duodenum as an extended part of the stomach.

Stomach

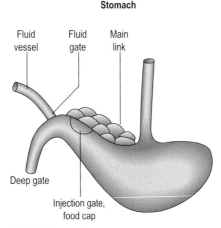

Figure 10.15 Stomach.

Liver with liver lobes

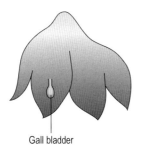

Figure 10.16 Liver with liver lobes.

The liver (Fig. 10.16) consists of four segments. The gallbladder is situated behind the second liver lobe.[12] Overall, the liver lies superior to the stomach. From its base it points upwards; towards the back it is connected to the part that lies against the backbone. The liver is solid and full, not hollow like intestine, stomach and bladder, therefore it can definitely not store Blood.[13]

Above **the diaphragm** (Fig. 10.17) the lung and heart are the only organs, with both *Qi* gates to the left and right. All the other organs are situated below the diaphragm, which makes the diaphragm a border separating the upper and lower halves of the body.

The spleen (Fig. 10.18) has a passage inside like a tube. Its substance is very delicate and

Diaphragm

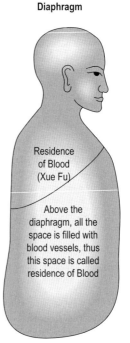

Figure 10.17 Residence of Blood (*Xue Fu*).

it emits fluids slightly; its name is 'delicate passage'.

The length of the spleen is almost equal to that of the stomach. In the middle, there is a passage like a tube, the delicate passage. This and the *fluid vessels* are shown in the next illustration.

The delicate passage runs along the middle. From there, the fluid runs in both directions and seeps into the fluid canal, which leads to the bladder where it is collected as urine. One part leads back from the fluid canal to the blood vessels; this part also belongs to the fluid canal.

The *Qi* organ (Fig. 10.19) (residence of *Qi*), also commonly known as cockscomb fat, is situated below the small intestine.[14] *Yuan Qi* is stored within the *Qi* hollow organ, but outside the small intestine. *Yuan Qi* is the source of human life, and also aids digestion. The *Qi* hollow organ belongs to the small intestine, which the *Qi* hollow organ adheres to.

Two *Qi* vessels meet at the inner sides of both **kidneys** (Fig. 10.20). These vessels are connected to the *Wei* main vessel. Both kidneys are solid and full, and do not have chambers inside, so they can not store essence (as stated in the '*Nei Jing*').

---

[12] According to the drawing, this describes the anterior segment of the right liver lobe.

[13] According to the *Yellow Emperor's Classic*, the Liver stores Blood in the same sense as the Urinary Bladder stores urine.

[14] This should be the mesentery.

Spleen

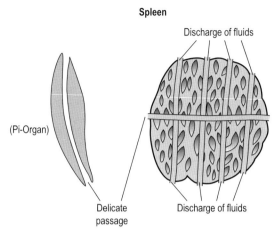

(Pi-Organ)

Discharge of fluids

Delicate passage

Discharge of fluids

Figure 10.18   Spleen.

The Qi organ
(residence of Qi)

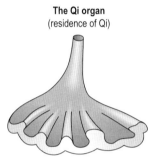

Figure 10.19   The *Qi* organ.

Kidneys

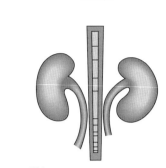

Figure 10.20   Kidneys.

Leading to the Wei main vessel

Leading to the backbone

Bladder

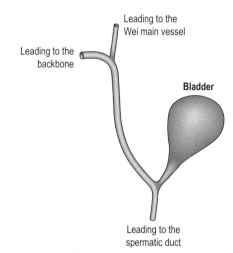

Leading to the spermatic duct

Figure 10.21   Bladder.

The bladder (Fig. 10.21) has a lower but no upper passage. The lower passage opens into the penis (jade stem). The tube of the spermatic duct (*Jing Dao*) also leads to the penis. In women, the spermatic duct is called the uterine tube.

The large intestine (Fig. 10.22) starts at the end of the small intestine.

It is also called the appendix. The large intestine ends at the rectum.

The white cap at the back end of **the tongue** (Fig. 10.23) is called the epiglottis. It is situated above the left and right *Qi* gates, and is part of the throat.

Formerly, the channels and *Luo* vessels (*Jing Luo*) (Fig. 10.24) were said to be identical with the blood vessels and every organ was said to have two blood vessels leading outwards; only the bladder was found to have four. I myself have seen hundreds of organs and none of those had any blood vessels leading outwards; that is why I have prepared this written text and illustrations.

Towards the small intestine

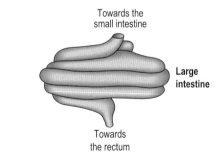

Large intestine

Towards the rectum

Figure 10.22   Large intestine.

Epiglottis   **Tongue**

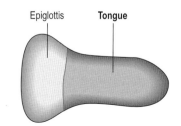

Figure 10.23   Tongue.

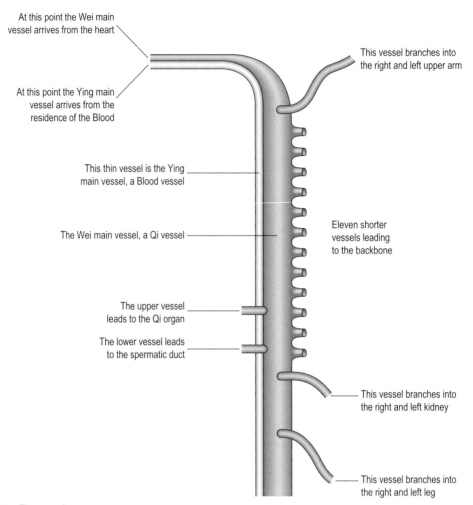

At this point the Wei main vessel arrives from the heart

At this point the Ying main vessel arrives from the residence of the Blood

This vessel branches into the right and left upper arm

This thin vessel is the Ying main vessel, a Blood vessel

Eleven shorter vessels leading to the backbone

The Wei main vessel, a Qi vessel

The upper vessel leads to the Qi organ

The lower vessel leads to the spermatic duct

This vessel branches into the right and left kidney

This vessel branches into the right and left leg

Figure 10.24 The vessels.

NOTES ON THE EPIGLOTTIS, LEFT AND RIGHT *QI* GATES, *WEI* MAIN VESSEL, MAIN CONSTRUCTION VESSEL, RESIDENCE OF *QI* AND RESIDENCE OF BLOOD

In order to appreciate the nature of the organs, one should first have a clear picture of the entry and exit of air[15] and the digestive tract that receives food and drink. In ancient times, the space behind the root of the tongue was called the windpipe-throat (*Hou*). The throat is located at the back, where the air streams in and out, at the start of the windpipe. Even further back in the throat lies the gullet-throat (*Yan*). Swallowing takes place here. Ingested food and drink pass into the stomach, via the stomach opening.

The gullet-throat (*Yan*) is therefore said to receive food and the windpipe-throat (*Hou*) to receive air. This is seen as an unalterable fact. For 4000 years, from the *Yellow Emperor's Classic* ('*Huang Di Nei Jing*') to this day, nobody has recognized and corrected the mistake.

Everybody knew that ingested food and drink got into the stomach, but there was still ambigu-

---

[15] Literally, '*Qi*', which as usual can have many meanings, amongst them 'air'. In this and the following chapter I will therefore translate *Qi* as air, which is the commonly used meaning today.

ity about the precise entry and exit gate of air within the throat.

The fact that both greater parts of the lung present towards the back and the small part towards the chest, was unknown. The windpipe branches first into both lung leaves, where it divides again into nine small branches, each forking out into numerous other smaller branches. At the end of these small branches there are absolutely no holes. The entire structure is similar to the Qilin vegetable (Eucheuma muricatum). The outer skin of the lung has no holes or cavities either. All that it does contain is a light, whitish foam, but no connection ducts (to the abdominal space). The 24 holes in which *Qi* is supposed to move are also not there.

The revered masters from ancient times explained that the lung is full after inspiration and empty after expiration. But this and all similar statements are incorrect, and there is no need to explain this in any more detail.

During inhalation, a man's abdomen expands so it becomes full and larger, but not the lung. Once he exhales, his abdomen becomes empty and smaller again, but not the lung itself. Exhaled and inhaled air, spitting out phlegm or secretions, and salivation are in no way influenced by the lung.

Behind the windpipe, in front of the gullet, within two cavities on the left and right side lie the two *Qi* vessels (aorta carotis communis), which have about the same diameter as chopsticks. Their upper end is situated below the epiglottis; the left one is called left *Qi* gate, the right one right *Qi* gate. Phlegm, secretions, spit and saliva exit via the *Qi* tubes.[16]

In ancient times it was falsely assumed that cough, shortness of breath, asthma and so on were lung diseases, because they were all observed to affect the chest.

The reason that this was believed was that exterior infections were successfully treated with diaphoretic and releasing medicinals; dry Phlegm was successfully treated with refreshing and cooling medicinals; accumulated Heat was successfully treated with purgative medicinals; the collapse of *Yin* was treated with *Yin* nourishing medicinals, which was effective; and Blood stasis was treated with stasis dispelling medicinals, which also worked, affording the doctors great satisfaction. In this way their own theories became established and books were written saying that without any doubt, these must be diseases of the lung.

But in reality nobody knew that the left and right *Qi* vessels on both sides of the windpipe proceed downwards and converge in front of where the windpipe forks out, just like the way the branches of a tree meet at the trunk. The width of the *Qi* vessels matches that of chopsticks. After having merged, the *Qi* vessel continues into the heart. It then rotates and emerges at the left side of the heart, having about the size of a writing brush. From here it runs along to the rear left, passes the windpipe on the left and leads to the backbone, and from there, down to the tailbone. This section is called the *Wei* main vessel, and is also commonly known as the hip vessel. Below the hip it divides into two vessels, the thickness of chopsticks. The upper vessel leads to the *Qi* organ, also commonly known as cockscomb fat because it looks like a cockscomb turned upside down.

The *Qi* organ wraps around the small intestine which runs across in front of the *Qi* organ.

Outside the small intestine, but within the *Qi* organ, is the place where *Yuan Qi* is stored. *Yuan Qi* is the physiological Fire, the body's Fire: this is the true *Yuan Qi*,[17] the Fire which is the (energy) source of human life.

Ingested food gets from the stomach into the small intestine. There, it is heated up and transformed, aided by the action of *Yuan Qi*. If there is sufficient *Yuan Qi*, food will be digested easily. If there is a lack of *Yuan Qi*, digestion will become difficult. Thus we have considered the vessel that branches off upwards to the abdomen.

The vessel branching off downwards probably leads to the spermatic duct in men and to the uterus in women. It is a single cord which so far I have not been able to examine closely. For this reason there are still uncertainties about it, which physicians who come after me should correct and

---

[16] What Wang defines as *Qi* gates are probably the tubal tonsils or arytenoid cartilages of the larynx, interpreted as the exit of the carotid arteries, which are visible from outside, so they are regarded as one structure.

[17] Literally: 'Yuan-Qi is Fire – Fire is Yuan-Qi'.

verify provided they get an opportunity for close observation of the vessel.

Also behind the heart, the *Wei* main vessel branches into two pencil-sized vessels that lead to the shoulders. There is a further branching at the height of the hip, from which two vessels lead to the kidneys, and another branching below the hip, from which two vessels lead to the thighs.

Above the hip, centred right in front of the backbone, there are 11 short vessels that are connected to the backbone. All of these serve for the transportation of *Qi* and body fluids.

If there is sufficient *Qi* and blazing Fire, the Body Fluids will become very concentrated, and this resulting fluid is then called Phlegm (*Tan*). If *Qi* is deficient and Fire is weak, then it will not be able to heat up the Body Fluids (*Jin Ye*), and a thinner fluid will develop, which is called thin mucus (*Yin*).[18]

If there is Phlegm or thin mucus within the *Qi* vessel, then the *Qi* inside the vessel will propel it upwards, i.e. past the heart to be expelled eventually through both *Qi* gates, from within the *Qi* vessel running in front of the windpipe. Phlegm and thin mucus are both present within the *Qi* vessels. Formerly, it was falsely claimed that these are substances present in the lung, because nothing was known about the two *Qi* vessels running in front of the windpipe. It was only known that Phlegm, thin mucus, secretions and saliva arise from the middle of the chest. The reason for describing them as substances coming from the lung was purely because the internal organs had not been inspected before.

The fact that the hands can grasp, the feet can walk, the head can turn and the body can twist, indeed all movement, all the body's yielding and giving, is based solely on this *Qi*.

If *Qi* is inhaled, the *Qi* organ will be filled up and the abdomen will expand. If *Qi* is exhaled, the *Qi* vessel will empty, and due to its emptiness the abdomen will become smaller as well.

The *Wei* main vessel is an organ that moves *Qi*, thus it does not contain any Blood. If Blood

gets into the *Qi* organ, then it will be expelled together with the *Qi*: it goes upwards in the form of vomiting Blood or nose bleeding, or downwards in the form of blood in the urine or bloody stool.

Running parallel in front of the *Wei* main vessel there is a vessel, about as thick as a chopstick, that is called *Ying* main vessel and this is a Blood vessel. It is filled with Blood and has the same length as the *Wei* main vessel. The Blood inside comes from the residence of Blood, which is a membrane in the lower chest area, as thin as paper, but very stable.

Towards the front it nestles in to the curvature of the tip of the heart, extending to the sides from both arches of the ribs like a cliff to the hip, so at the front it is further up and at the back it is further down. The lower part towards the back is concave like a pond, so Blood which is derived from the essence of fluids, can be stored in it. Therefore, this space is known as the residence of Blood.

For more about essence and fluids, the reader is directed to the next section, where the 'gate of fluid' is discussed. The epiglottis mentioned earlier is a light-coloured plate behind the root the tongue and serves to close both *Qi* gates to the left and right as well as the lower throat area.

ON THE GATE OF FLUIDS, THE FLUID PASSAGES, THE 'FOOD CAP', THE PANCREAS, THE DELICATE VESSELS AND THE WATER VESSEL

Below the throat is the gastric area, which is called the crop in birds, the maw in quadrupeds and simply the stomach in humans. In classical illustrations the stomach opening, called the 'injection gate' (*Pen Men*), is on top, and the stomach exit, called 'deep gate' (*You Men*), is below. Only these two gates were described, in ignorance of the fact that the stomach has a third opening. The stomach was depicted as a lengthy tube running downwards, in ignorance of the fact that it runs horizontally. However, not only does it lie in a horizontal position, it also runs along the broad side of the body. The upper opening, the injection gate, is tilted toward the backbone and the fundus of the stomach is located downwards, facing the

---

[18] *Yin* in the 3rd tone is not identical with the *Yin* (1st tone) in *Yin* and *Yang*. It is also defined as Rheum (Wiseman), fluid retention (various Chinese authors) and thin mucus (Clavey). See also Chapter 9, footnote 7.

abdomen. The deep gate of the stomach exit points upwards and to the back right, along the flanks towards the backbone.

Within the deep gate, a few inches further back, there is a third opening, which I call the 'gate of fluids'. A passage ends at this gate, which I call the 'fluid passage' (major pancreatic duct). This is the route that the concentrated essence of fluids takes to leave the stomach. Anatomically, the fluid passage is very difficult to find, because the 'food cap' of the 'main link' is located above it. The common name of the main link is the pancreas. It is located running lengthwise to the right of the injection gate and to the left of the deep gate, exactly above the fluid gate.

Below the main link is the *Qi* organ (residence of *Qi*, mesentery), connected to the small intestine at the front and to the large intestine at the back. Above the stomach, the *Qi* organ is connected to the liver, which itself is connected to the backbone, but below the diaphragm.

Thus, the tube of the pancreas is connected to the stomach, the liver, the large intestine and the small intestine. Whenever food and drink enter the stomach, the solid food remains at first inside the stomach. The essence of the watery fluids runs through the fluid gate into the fluid passages. A few inches further on from the fluid passages, there is a threefold junction (probably cystic duct, and left and right hepatic duct).

From here, the refined clear fluids pass into the residence of the Marrow and are transformed into Marrow, whilst the refined turbid fluids pass into the residence of Blood and are transformed into Blood. The watery fluids flow through the lower branch, which is situated behind the midline of the liver, into the spleen.

There is a passage in the middle of the spleen, which runs across in a very fine and regular fashion and is therefore called the delicate vessel. From this passage, the watery fluids flow in two directions and go into and out of the water vessel (larger lymph glands). Behind the water vessel, the tissue appears like a mesh and is therefore called mesh fat tissue. The watery fluids are filtered inside the water vessel and from here flow into the bladder, where they are transformed into urine. This tissue behind the water vessel is the most difficult of all the structures to recognize.

In 1798 I was able to see the organs for myself. The water vessel contains many small bubbles filled with clear liquid (lymph follicles), but there are also some without liquid. Their function was not entirely clear to me.

When I was diagnosing diseases at a later stage, I was able to inspect the bodies of patients who had died after a long illness; of these, some had drunk quite a lot not long before death, some had drunk only a little and some had drunk nothing at all. However, there was still water to be found in their abdomens. I compared this with the descriptions from the section about the water vessel but still could not determine anything with certainty. After this, I made a comparative study using animal experiments; I performed an autopsy directly after feeding and found the mesh fat tissue to be full of liquid, whilst that of those animals not fed for 3–4 days contained no liquid. From this I was able to conclude without doubt that the water vessels have the function of distributing water (i.e. lymph) in the body.

As I mentioned before, when food and drink arrive in the stomach, the food remains there whilst the clear fluids exit through the fluid gate. The width of the fluid gate is about the diameter of a chopstick, so how is it possible that, if the clear fluid can pass through, thin chyme (food pulp) cannot enter at the same time?

Although the fluid gate is the same width as the diameter of a chopstick, the stomach tissue at this point is very thick; its walls lie closely pressed together, so that only fluid and no food can pass through. Furthermore, a few millimetres to the left of the fluid gate is a berry-like bulb called the food cap (*Zhe Shi*). This holds the solid food back and only allows thin-fluid substances to pass through, so the solid food is kept in the stomach, where it can be digested slowly and then gradually passed on to the small intestine, where it is transformed into excrement.

But how is food transformed into excrement in the small intestine? The *Qi* organ (mesentery) lies outside the small intestine. Its *Qi* encloses the entire small intestine. Outside the small intestine, but inside the *Qi* organ, *Yuan Qi* is stored, which is capable of transforming food. One should compare this with the earlier account of the *Qi* organ.

After transformation, excrement reaches the large intestine, from where it is excreted through the anus.

This section has mainly focused on how the fluid essence passes from the stomach through the fluid gate, and how it contributes to the production of essence (*Jing*) and Blood; how watery fluid flows from the delicate vessels into the water vessel and from there into the bladder, where it becomes urine; and how food arrives in the small intestine from the stomach and is then transformed into excrement by the action of *Yuan Qi*.

CONCERNING THE BRAIN AND SPINAL MARROW

Consciousness and memory are anchored not in the heart, but in the brain, which goes without saying. Yet although it seems obvious, it is still difficult to prove. But if this were not mentioned, the cause of many diseases might remain unknown. In consideration of this, one cannot remain silent about this.

It's all the same whether it's medical books stating that consciousness belongs to the heart, or Confucians debating morals: they all ascribe personality and behaviour to the heart. The reason for this is that in the past people did not know about the position of the heart in the chest, and its functions. They did not know about the two *Qi* vessels that are rooted in the neck on the left and right (carotid arteries), which run along in front of the windpipe, converging and passing into the heart. The vessel that emerges from the heart towards the left and runs past the lung, which is connected to the backbone, is called the *Wei* main vessel (aorta). To the front, it is connected to the residence of *Qi* (mesentery) and the spermatic ducts; to the rear, it is connected to the backbone; above, it is connected to the arms, in the middle to the kidney and below to the legs. This vessel contains the *Yuan Qi* and Body Fluids (*Jin Ye*). The entry and exit of *Qi* goes through the heart, and as the heart functions as a gate for *Qi*; where then is consciousness supposed to arise from, and where is memory supposed to be stored?

Consciousness and memory are located in the brain. Food and drink generate Blood and *Qi*, which allow the muscles and flesh to grow; and

the essence of the clear fluids is transformed into marrow, which reaches from the backbone up to the brain, where it is called brain marrow (medulla oblongata).

The area that houses the brain and brain marrow is called 'Sea of Marrow'. The bone on top is called 'roof of the soul'. Both ears are also connected to the brain. All sounds that are heard also go to the brain.

If the *Qi* of the brain is deficient, then the brain will shrink. If the connection between the *Qi* of the brain and the *Qi* of the ears is impeded, then hardness of hearing will develop.

The eyes also develop from brain matter and are connected to the brain by (nerve) cords. This means that everything one sees goes into the brain. If the brain fluid flows downwards into the eyeballs, the pupils change to a whitish colour, which is called 'brain fluid flowing into the eyes'. The nose is also connected to the brain, which is why all good and bad smells enter the brain. If the brain is attacked by pathogenic Wind-Heat factors, it will excrete a turbid, unpleasantly smelling liquid through the nose, which is called 'brain leak' (*Bi Yuan*). Looking at newborns we see that their brains are not yet fully grown, the fontanelles still feel soft, the eyes do not move voluntarily, the ears cannot hear clearly yet, the nose cannot smell accurately and the tongue cannot articulate. After 1 year the brain has steadily grown; gradually, the fontanelles become closed, the ears understand how to hear and the eyes can move skilfully; the nose knows a little more about how to tell bad from good smells, and the tongue can already utter one or two words.

When the child is aged 3 or 4 years old, brain and marrow are nearly complete, the fontanelles have fully closed, the ears can hear, the eyes can see deliberately, the nose can differentiate bad from good smells, and the child can form whole sentences and speak.

The reason for lack of memory in infants, then, is that the brain is not yet fully developed, whereas memory disturbances in old age are due to brain and marrow decreasing in size. Li Shi-Zhen remarks on this: 'The brain is the residence of the original soul (*Yuan Shen*).' And Jin Zheng-Xi explains: 'Man's capacity for remembering lies entirely in the brain.' Finally, Wang Ren-An comments: 'When someone wants to remember a past situation, he has to close his eyes or stare upwards in order to think. If the supply of *Qi* to the brain and marrow stops for just a short time, and also if the brain has no consciousness, it will die, regardless of whether the period is short or long.'

One only has to look at epilepsy, generally known as 'squealing-like-a-goat' Wind: this is exactly what happens when *Yuan-Qi* cannot reach the brain for a short period. During the fit it appears almost as if the person were alive, but his brain is about to die. The person is alive, because he has air[19] in his chest and can breathe, and his limbs twitch in convulsions; his brain seems to be dying because it is without air, the ears are deaf and the eyes have turned upwards like a dead person's.

First, a cry is released; only then does the convulsion set in, because at first the brain no longer has any air, and so the air in the chest is inhaled and exhaled in an uncontrolled manner, finally being released explosively. Then, during the convulsion, a bubbling noise due to the fluid in the *Qi* vessels develops inside the chest, originating from the absence of air in the consciousness of the brain. The fluid is vomited and swallowed and flows into the *Qi* vessels, which brings about the noise.

After the fit, headache and a faint-like sleep exist, because there is not sufficient *Qi* available yet, although it is flowing into the brain again.

Convulsions in children following a long illness, along with sudden faints in adults, are caused by *Qi* deficiency (here, lack of air) in the brain. Patients have no memory of the time immediately preceding an attack.

If all this is considered together, how can there be any doubt that consciousness is seated in the brain?

ON QI VESSELS AND BLOOD VESSELS

I will give an honest account here of the shape of the vessels. May heaven punish me if I should make any deliberately wrong statements in order to be considered a 'superman', and my conscience shall never rest.

The residence of *Qi* stores *Qi* and the residence of Blood stores Blood. The *Wei* main vessel sends

Qi from the residence of *Qi* to the entire body. That is why it is called *Wei* main vessel. The *Ying* main vessel sends Blood from the residence of Blood to the entire body. That is why it is called *Ying* main vessel.

The *Wei* main vessel is thick and large and runs along in front of the backbone, to which it is also connected. Furthermore, it branches out to the head and the limbs and reaches to the muscles and bones, thus to every *Qi* vessel in the body.

The *Ying*[20] main vessel is thin and fine. It runs along in front of the *Wei* main vessel and is also connected to it. It branches out into the head and the four limbs and also into the flesh and skin, so it connects all Blood vessels in the body.

Qi dwells in the residence of *Qi*, where it can enter and exit, which it does through breathing. Vision, hearing, turning one's head and moving one's body, grasping with the hands and walking are all only possible by virtue of the movement of *Qi*. Blood dwells in the residence of Blood, from where it flows into the *Ying* main vessel and from there into all other body tissues. It can also enter the muscles and flesh outside the Blood vessels.

The *Qi* vessels also pass into sinews and bones as well as into the internal organs, but this is not easy to recognize. As *Qi* moves inside the *Qi* vessels, the *Qi* vessels move too; however, the Blood vessels are filled with Blood, so they cannot move.[21]

All the 'pulsating' vessels on the head, face and limbs are *Qi* vessels, not Blood vessels. For example, at the end of the eyebrow there is a concave area, commonly known as *Tai Yang*,[22] where the flesh is thin and the skin is close to the bone. When this area is palpated, a pulse is felt, which comes from a *Qi* vessel leading up to the head and face. When the space between the big

---

[19] Literally, 'Qi'. See footnote 15.

[20] Wang uses the character *Rong* instead of *Ying*, which is interchangeable in this context. I have translated it as *Ying*, because the pair *Wei-Qi* (Protective *Qi*, defensive energy) and *Ying-Qi* (Nutritive *Qi*, constructive energy) should be well known. As everyone who is familiar with the basics of Chinese medicine should know, *Wei-Qi* has more affinity to *Qi* whilst *Ying-Qi* has more affinity to Blood, which is what Wang wants to express here.

[21] Now it becomes obvious that Wang clearly differentiated arteries and veins and defined them as *Qi* vessels and blood vessels.

[22] The extra point *Tai Yang*, M-HN 9 according to Deadman's nomenclature, is named after this location.

and second toes at the dorsum of the foot, where the skin is thin and lies directly on the bone, is palpated, one can feel a pulse. This is due to the *Qi* vessels penetrating both feet. A pulse can be felt at the transverse crease of the wrist, on the radial styloid process, where little flesh is found and the skin is close to the bone. This originates from the *Qi* vessels passing into both hands.[23]

These vessels are sometimes thick, sometimes thin, sometimes straight or winding; the constitution is different in every person. At the part of the forearm, where the flesh is thick, the protruding *Qi* vessels are short, whereas at the part between elbow and wrist, where the flesh is thin, the protruding *Qi* vessels are long. If an exterior infection permits Wind to invade the *Qi* vessels, they will swell. If palpated, the tension will be felt. If Cold invades the *Qi* vessels, the fluids inside will contract, which obstructs the flow of *Qi*. If this pulse is felt, it must therefore appear slow. If Fire invades the *Qi* vessels, this will heat up the *Qi*. The pulse will appear to be very accelerated if it is felt.

If the person is strong and his *Qi* is in excess, then there will be plenty of *Qi* inside the *Qi* vessels. Thus there will be an ample and powerful pulse. However, if he is weak and his *Zheng Qi* is deficient, there will be little *Qi* inside his vessels. Thus the pulse will feel weak and without energy.

In a patient suffering from chronic disease with no prospect of recovery the *Yuan Qi* is diminished, *Qi* does not reach the head and hands, and it does not descend, so it cannot be felt at the foot. If the *Qi* vessels at the hand can be felt, then it will appear as if sometimes there is a pulse and sometimes not, or else the pulse is narrow and thin like silk, or a very weak movement is felt under one's fingers. All these signs indicate a collapse of *Qi*.

In this section I have talked about the *Qi* vessels, which can be different in every individual, i.e. thicker, thinner, straight or winding. Their length also depends on whether there is much or little flesh at the wrist. By feeling the vessels' size one can determine excess and deficiency. Cold and

Heat (Fire) syndromes are determined by feeling a rapid or slow pulse.

What I described carefully earlier are of course the Blood vessel pulses (the German version uses the term 'Ader' here; translator's note) of pulse diagnosis. But I did not call them vessel pulses, because in the past nobody knew about the right and left *Qi* gate, the residence of Blood, the residence of *Qi*, the *Wei* main channel, the *Ying* main vessel, the fluid gate, the fluid vessels, the *Zhe Shi* (food cap), the *Zong Ti* (pancreas), the *delicate passage* and the water vessel. This means that they did not know about the structures in the body cavity, and their purposes. In any case, when theories were produced regarding the organs and vessels, no clear definitions were given. With regard to the channels and the Triple Burner, what they actually constitute was not clearly defined. They could not explain at all that in fact the channels and *Luo* vessels are *Qi* and Blood vessels.

Thus, when theorizing about pulse diagnosis, one must first talk about the Blood vessels ('Adern'; translator's note), which permeate the entire structure of the body, as the residence of Blood. Formerly, the '*Mai*' (pulses) were believed to be blood vessels, in which *Qi* and Blood were circulating all the time. However, if a circulation of Blood is assumed, then it will have to flow from one place to another, so it will first have to flow into an empty space, where there is no Blood, which would lead to (pathogenic) Blood deficiency. On the other hand, if there is no space, where is Blood supposed to flow to?

In earlier times, nobody knew that the Blood vessels of the pulse are *Qi* vessels, but many different pulses were described, and although a lot was written, the pulse locations were unique for every human and could not be compared.

A theory with 27 different pulses was proposed. I do not want to question this in every detail, nor do I want to claim that the classics are wrong in this matter. My only fear is that those who come after us will not understand the relationship between syndromes and pulses, because while it is easy to make a favourable or unfavourable prognosis on the basis of the pulse, diagnosing a disease is difficult. In order to correctly recognize a disease, one must first be clear about *Qi* and Blood. It doesn't matter whether there are exterior

---

[23] Wang describes three of the traditional pulse locations that were conventional before the '*Nan Jing*' (*Classic of Difficulties*): the temporal pulse (*Shang Guan*, Gb 3), the Kidney pulse of the foot (*Tai Xi*, Ki 3) and the Lung pulse or wrist pulse (at the styloid process).

pathogens or internal damage, it is always the case that at the beginning of every disease, before the organs have been affected, when sinews and bones remain uninjured, and before the skin and flesh have been damaged, *Qi* and Blood are the first to be harmed.

Qi can be in excess or deficient. If in excess, there will be excessive pathogenic *Qi* in addition to one's own *Qi*. If deficient, there is a deficiency in one's own *Qi*. When it comes to *Qi* deficiency syndromes, there are about 40 different types for hemiplegia and 20 further types in relation to convulsions in children, which should be compared with each other.

Blood can be empty or stagnated. In the case of Blood deficiency there must be a reason for the deficiency: sometimes it is due to vomiting blood, sometimes it's due to nose bleeding, sometimes it's due to blood in the urine or stool or it may be due to injuries, not forgetting metrorrhagia and excessive lochia. The Blood stasis syndrome can be identified diagnostically. Further on in this book 50 different Blood stasis syndromes are given for reference.[24] Blood stasis of the blood in the chest area (residence of Blood) is the only one that is very hard to differentiate. Fever in the second half of the day which continues to rise in the first half of the night, falling again in the second part and disappearing in the first part of the day, indicates Blood stasis in the residence of Blood. If the Blood stasis is only mild, these four different phases will not be present; the fever will only last for about 4 hours before and after sunset. In even milder cases it will only last for 2 hours. This kind of fever is perceived as a sensation of heat by the patient.

In contrast, a sensation of chilliness after midday and fever of short duration points to a *Qi* deficiency syndrome, for which Ginseng and Astragalus can be given. If the body does not feel hot at sunrise and the fever has disappeared for a while, then this *Yang* exhaustion syndrome indicates the prescription of Ginseng and Aconite Decoction (*Shen Fu Tang*).

These syndromes must not be confused with each other.

---

[24] See Part 2 Wang's famous formulas and their indications.

ON HEART BLOOD DEFICIENCY

I have a friend with the name Yu You-Xue, called Lang Zhai, from Tong Zhou, who is quite proficient in medicine. In the tenth month of the year 1830 he came to my house to say goodbye because he had to go to Shan Dong on business. We chatted about the classical theories regarding the origin of Blood: about the fact that sometimes Blood is said to be created in the Heart, while the Spleen is said to hold it inside the blood vessels; and sometimes it is said to be created in the Spleen and the Heart is said to be responsible for its position in the blood vessels. But which should we believe? I told him the following: none of these theories. Blood is an essence created in the chest (residence of Blood), whilst the Heart is an organ which *Qi* passes in and out of. It does not contain any Blood.

Lang Zhai replied: 'What my old friend is saying cannot be quite right; since all animals have Blood in the Heart, how could it be that only humans have no Blood in the Heart?'

In reply I said: 'How do you know that all animals have Blood in the Heart?'

He said: 'Amongst the classical formulas is *Sui Xin Dan* (Euphorbia Heart Pill), which can cure manic-depressive psychosis. It contains Euphorbia Kansui Powder, which is processed into a pill using the blood from a pig's heart. Is this not proof that the Heart contains Blood?'

Then I replied: 'This is a mistake in the classics. Blood does not come from the Heart, but flows in after the heart has been cut with a knife. When you look at an undamaged heart, it does not contain any Blood. I have seen plenty of those hearts. When you witness a sheep being killed, you will see that when its throat is slit open without injuring the heart, no blood will be found in its heart afterwards.'

He continued to ask: 'If it is not stabbed in the heart, why does it still die so quickly?'

My answer was: 'All the Blood in the chest flows quickly out through the wound, then the remaining Blood returns to the chest from the peripheries; this means that later, the Blood will flow slower. But as Blood is depleted and *Qi* dispersed, death sets in quickly. If somebody is injured in battle and loses a lot of Blood, *Qi* will also be dispersed and Blood will be depleted, so gradually cramps develop. In ancient times this was called *Po Shang Feng* (literally wound wind, i.e. tetanus). Wind dispersing medicinals were used to treat the dying. The killer planned to escape his punishment with the doctor's help. But anyone treated in this way was dying already and so both killer and victim had to die. If the principle of *Qi* dispersed due to Blood deficiency had been known, 320 g Astragalus and 160 g Codonopsis would have been prescribed and thus *Qi* would have been strengthened. Thus if the victim had been rescued, two lives could have been rescued, could they not?

Hereupon Lang Zhai nodded and said goodbye.

DISCUSSION ON THE EFFICACY OF FORMULAS AND THE ORIGINS OF MISTAKES IN THE CLASSICS[25]

(This includes a treatise on the misconception of 'Blood transforms into sweat'.)

My nephew Zuo Li came to Beijing, where he caught sight of the *Zang Fu Tu Ji* (organ illustrations). He asked me this question:

In my revered uncle's illustrations, all the channels are Qi *vessels, arising from the* Zong Wei Guan (Wei *main vessel). From there, they are distributed throughout the whole body, forming a complete network of channels, rather than rising as two channels from one* Zang Fu *organ pair. Therefore, your nephew wonders how, if the classical texts did not have exact knowledge about the channels, was Zhang Zhong-Jing in his 'Shang Han Lun' able to develop the diagnosis of the six channels, draw up 113 formulas, differentiate 397*

---

[25] In this section, Wang anticipates us in a misconception that happens frequently today, by comparing the similar names of the *Zang Fu* organs and their respective channels with the anatomical organs or with the channel-related diagnostic methods employed in the *'Shang Han Lun'*. Today we realize that we shouldn't make this mistake, because the [anatomical] bladder is not the same as the (TCM organ) Bladder, nor can it be equated with the Bladder channel, or the *Zu Tai Yang* Bladder channel syndrome described in the *'Shang Han Lun'*. Wang explains that the examples he mentions are typical for 'the theory is incomplete, however the formulas are still effective'. But from a contemporary point of view, the same applies to Wang's formulas, which is why we can learn from him in spite of all his anatomical shortcomings.

therapeutic methods and still compose such excellent formulas? Your nephew does not understand how this can be.

I told him:

Just have a thorough look at the first section of Zhang Zhong-Jing's book, and it will become clear to you why the formulas are effective but the explanations wrong. For example, in the first section he talks about the Zu Tai Yang *Bladder channel. If this channel is affected by* Shang Han *(Cold pathogen), the patient will have a headache, sore limbs, a stiff neck, a raised temperature, chilliness; dry retching, but no sweating as signs of Cold damage. Then,* Ma Huang Tang *(Ephedra Decoction) is employed for treatment. If similar symptoms appear with sweating at the same time, then Wind damage is the cause and* Gui Zhi Tang *(Cinnamon Decoction) is employed for treatment.*

So, only the Zu Tai Yang *Bladder channel is mentioned, which flows in both legs, but not in the hands. When he discusses the transmission of the pathogen into a different channel, he discusses the six leg channels, but not the arm channels. Have a look at the initial symptoms of* Shang Han: *headache, body pain, stiff neck, fever, chilliness; nothing is said about the arms, the arms have neither pain nor fever nor chilliness. If* Ma Huang Tang *(Ephedra Decoction) is employed now, the whole body is treated and not just the arms or hands. Doesn't this show that the formula may work, even though that the theory is wrong?*

If the organs had already been known before the time of Zhang, people would have known that the channels go throughout the body. Then, Zhang would have written in the 'Shang Han Lun' that pathogenic Cold invades all the channels of the body, and that by using Ma Huang Tang *(Ephedra Decoction) the pathogenic Cold is expelled from the whole body by diaphoresis. That would have been clear and comprehensible.*

When it comes to the concept of 'in the case of sweating pathogenic Wind is the cause' and the resulting treatment with Gui Zhi Tang *(Cinnamon Decoction), which contains Cortex Cinnamomi, Radix Paeoniae Lactifloriae and Radix Glycyrrhizae, then there has not been a single case yet where a recovery was achieved, because* Gui Zhi Tang *(Cinnamon Decoction) does not work* here. The reason is that headache, sore limbs and fever with sweating are not a disease due to Wind, which is why Wu You-Ke had to come up with the concept of febrile infectious diseases.

Then, he asked:

If the Cold pathogen is at the superficial level (extima, Biao, exterior), of course symptoms such as headache, sore limbs, fever and chilliness without sweating will occur, because all of them are exterior symptoms. If in this initial stage of Shang Han the disease has not yet invaded the interior (intima, Li), where does the interior symptom of retching come from? Neither Zhang Zhong-Jing nor Wang Shu-He nor many others explained the cause of retching. Your nephew cannot explain this and therefore asks his uncle for advice.

I used to think that you might have gained a good deal of textbook knowledge but no practical medical understanding. The questions you ask today show that you can both think logically and act with the necessary caution, so that you will not put anyone's life at risk. Well, you ask how a typical interior symptom like retching can develop in the presence of an exterior Cold pathogen. I will explain it to you in detail. At the beginning the Cold pathogen invades through the pores; from the pores it reaches the skin and from the skin it reaches the finest branches of the Luo vessel channel network (Sun Luo). From the finest Luo vessels it invades the Yang Luo vessels and from the Yang Luo vessels it invades the main channels. From the channels it invades the Zong Wei Guan (Wei main vessel) and from there it runs horizontally towards the Heart. From the Heart it ascends into the left and right Qi vessel and there it strikes upwards against the left and right Qi gate in the throat, which eventually causes the retching and thus is the cause for retching in connection with this exterior syndrome.

If Ma Huang Tang (Ephedra Decoction) is administered now, this will reach the stomach and from there the liquid substance of the medicine will pass through the fluid gate into the vessels, flowing into the liver and spleen and into their delicate passages, where the water is filtered and then reaches the bladder in the form of urine.

When it comes to the Qi of the decoction, namely its active ingredients, these go from the vessels into the Zong Wei Guan (Wei main vessel) and from there into the channels; from the channels they go into the Luo vessels and from the Luo vessels into the finest Luo network vessels. From here, the medicine-Qi continues into the skin and from the skin into the pores, from where it expels the Cold pathogenic factor. This generates sweating. As the pathogenic factor leaves, together with the sweat, it is dispersed by the sweating and the retching ceases, too.

This is the sequence of vessels for the entire body, connecting the interior and exterior, through which Ma Huang Tang (Ephedra Decoction) disperses the pathogenic factor in the exterior by causing sweating.

He further asked:

Zhang Zhong-Jing explains that eye pain, dry nose and insomnia are symptoms of the Zu Yang Ming stomach channel and are therefore treated using Ge Gen Tang (Pueraria Decoction). The formula contains Ge Gen (Pueraria) but also Ma Huang (Ephedra). I do not understand the exact reason for this.

I answered:

Cold pathogen invades the channels from the exterior. Due to the pathogen's conflict with the body's own Zheng Qi (physiological or Upright Qi), Heat is generated, which is then called pathogenic Heat. If this pathogenic Heat surges upwards to the roof of the skull, it will irritate the brain, which causes the insomnia. The eyes are connected directly to the brain, so the Heat hits the eyes from the brain and causes pain. As the nose is also connected to the brain, the Heat will also pass into the nasal cavities, which will thus become dry. All this creates a typical picture of Heat blazing upwards, which causes a Fire syndrome, not an exterior Cold pathogen of the Zu Yang Ming Stomach channel. If Ge Gen Tang (Pueraria Decoction) is used, the patient will be cured. However, this should not lead one to believe that Ge Gen (Pueraria) is a warming and dispersing medicinal. Ge Gen is still a cooling and dispersing medicinal. The formula employs Ma Huang (Ephedra) to disperse the pathogenic Cold at the exterior, which so far has not invaded and transformed into Heat. This is another example of a false theory of the channels along with a formula that is still effective.

Next he asked:

Zhang Zhong-Jing explains that pain in the costal arch, hardness of hearing, a bitter taste in the mouth and alternating heat and chills with retching is a half-exterior half-interior syndrome, thus a syndrome of the Zu Shao Yang Gall-Bladder channel and he uses Xiao Chai Hu Tang (Small Bupleurum Decoction) with great success. Your nephew now thinks the following: if the disease is not in the Gall-Bladder channel, why does the formula work so well? On the other hand, if the disease is in the Gall-Bladder channel, and the Gall-Bladder is situated below the diaphragm, why does the chest area ache? This section is not comprehensible to me.

I explained to him:

On the 'Illustrations of the organs', take a look at the chest area above the diaphragm, then it will dawn on you: the Heat pathogen invades this 'residence of Blood' (Xue Fu) and attacks the Blood contained in it, which causes the pain in the chest. The pathogenic factor attacks the interior from the exterior and Zheng Qi defends the outside from the inside. This is attack and defence, which generates the alternating sensations of hot and cold. Heat irritates the left and right Qi gate in the throat and the upper and lower Qi cannot flow freely. What results is the retching and a bitter taste in the mouth. If the pathogenic Heat surges upwards it will cause hardness of hearing and dizziness. Xiao Chai Hu Tang (Small Bupleurum Decoction) can release the Heat in the 'residence of Blood', which leads to sweating. Heat disappears together with the released sweat and there will be a speedy recovery. This is also an example of a false channel theory but a formula that is still effective.

Despite all the variations, basically all this points to is interior, exterior, excess and deficiency. If you want to understand the 'Shang Han Lun,' you will have to take a look at Wu You-Ke's book 'Wen Yi' (Febrile Diseases); you will only be able to recognize more than Cold or Heat if you read widely.

Yesterday evening, when a guest was present, you mentioned the classical theory that the sweat inside the skin is actually Blood and only becomes sweat once it has left the skin, or in other words, sweat is a form of Blood. You could not explain the reason for this. But to avoid too much talk I did not give you an explanation, because our guest had only little knowledge of medicine, without a deeper understanding. I avoided an explanation for that reason.

The theory that sweat is a transformation from Blood comes from Zhu Dan-Xi, also named Zhu Zhen-Hou. Although Zhang Jing-Yue regards it as false, he cannot think of a better explanation for the origin of sweat. The mistakes of the classics are derived from the fact that they did not know about Qi and Blood having two different kinds of vessels. The Qi vessels (channels) lead into the opening of the pores to release the sweat. The Blood vessels, however, do not reach into the pores, therefore they cannot form sweat.

How do I know that blood vessels do not reach into the pores? Just take a look at the yellow fluid that flows out from seeping boils; their toxins come from the Qi vessels. Every day, when the yellow fluid seeps out, the skin remains unreddened. If the disease toxin came from the blood vessels, the skin would be reddened from the start, and if the boils broke open, blood and pus would have to seep out. When you have a look at Wen Du (febrile toxins), exanthemas, illnesses such as measles and childhood diseases like smallpox, then there may be a reddening of the skin, but no discharge of blood. Is this not proof of the fact that blood vessels do not reach into the skin?

When my nephew came to Beijing and chatted to me about these issues, this book was already in the printing press. Therefore this section had to be added at the end of the book.[26]

PART 2. WANG'S FAMOUS FORMULAS AND THEIR INDICATIONS

RELIEF THROUGH PRESCRIPTIONS

I am not going to write about the Triple Burner here, because anatomically it does not exist. I

---

[26] As the Chinese copy of the 'Yi Lin Gai Cuo' originally did indeed include this paragraph at the end, I took the liberty of following his intention and inserting it before the section on anatomy, rather than at the end of the book.

divide the body externally into the head, face and limbs, which are all permeated internally by blood vessels, and into the two internal regions above and below the diaphragm. Above the diaphragm are the heart, lungs and throat organs, as well as the *Qi* gates to the left and right (carotid arteries).[27] All the other organs lie below the diaphragm.

To treat Blood stasis in the vessels of the head, face and limbs, the Orifices Opening, Blood Invigorating Decoction (*Tong Qiao Huo Xue Tang*)[28] is suitable. For treating Blood stasis in the upper chest area the Anti-Stasis Chest Decoction (*Xue Fu Zhu Yu Tang*, literally 'Dispelling Blood Stasis of the Residence of Blood Decoction') is suitable. To treat Blood stasis below the diaphragm the Anti-Stasis Abdomen Decoction (*Ge Xia Zhu Yu Tang*, literally 'Above the Diaphragm Blood Stasis Dispelling Decoction) is suitable.

Diseases can be subdivided into thousands of nuances and manifestations, which cannot all be listed here. For further reference regarding syndromes see Wang Ken-Tang's *Manual of Diagnosis and Treatment* ('*Zheng Zhi Zhun Sheng*'), regarding formulas see Zhu Su's *General Prescriptions* ('*Pu Ji Fang*') and regarding medicinals see Li Shi-Zhen's *Systematic Materia Medica* ('*Ben Cao Gang Mu*'). I regard these three books as profound sources of medicine to be read and studied. Many effective formulas are to be found amongst the works of our medical ancestors: they are a real treasury of medicine. For example, when talking about febrile diseases, one may think of Wu Ju Tong ('*Wen Bing Tiao Bian*'). Although at that time the anatomy of the internal organs was not yet known, sedatives and laxatives, tonifying and draining formulas, had been developed and many of these were very effective.

But this is not my topic. Having corrected some of the errors in the medical world with regard to anatomical drawings, I would now like to describe some simple guidelines for the treatment of *Qi* deficiency and Blood – *Yu Xue* (Blood stasis) syndromes.

However, this account is by no means exhaustive and only the superficial reader would demand completeness from my book. This would not be my fault; it would arise from a false interpretation of my motives.

LIST OF INDICATIONS FOR *TONG QIAO HUO XUE TANG*[29] (ORIFICES OPENING, BLOOD INVIGORATING DECOCTION)

1. Hair loss

Hair loss setting in after febrile disease. All medical books describe this as a consequence of

---

27 See footnote 7.

28 The consecutive formula names are translated according to my concept of clarity and brevity. This was done consistently, for example *Zhu Yu*, literally 'stalking the stasis', was always translated as anti-stasis. *Xue Fu*, literally 'residence of blood', was translated as chest according to its meaning. Thus, Wang's famous formulas ending with '. . . *Zhu Yu Tang*' bear the following names:

Xue Fu Zhu Yu Tang = Anti-Stasis Chest Decoction
Ge Xia Zhu Yu Tang = Anti-Stasis Abdomen Decoction
Shao Fu Zhu Yu Tang = Anti-Stasis Lower Abdomen Decoction
Shen Tong Zhu Yu Tang = Anti-Stasis Pain Decoction
Hui Yan Zhu Yu Tang = Anti-Stasis Epiglottis Decoction
Tong Jing Zhu Yu Tang = Anti-Stasis Exanthema Decoction
Gu Xia Yu Xue Tang = Anti-Stasis Ascites Decoction

29 The quantities mentioned in the original are related to the *qian* unit (in the Qing dynasty this was 3.125 g). In China, 3 *qian* are usually rounded to 9 grams; however, as this appears too little to me when lower herb quality due to today's mass production, and the comparatively stronger physique, especially of Caucasians due to today's improved nutrition are taken into consideration, I define a quian as 4 g instead of 3.125 g.

Therefore the values mentioned in this book are subject to a little flexibility. In China, many modern physicians increase classical dosages for the same reasons mentioned above, as is clear in Dr Shang Xianmin's *Practical Experience in Treatment with Chinese Medicinals*. In his work, *Chi Shao* (Radix Paeoniae Rubrae) in *Ge Xia Zhu Yu Tang* is increased from 2 *qian* (given as 6 g in modern Chinese textbooks) to 15 g, emphasizing the anti-stasis effect, which is legitimate *as long as it is indicated for the patient*. Of course, this can only be decided for each case individually by thorough syndrome differentiation (*Bian Zheng Lun Zhi*). On the other hand, it is an established fact that many (Western) patients initially react more strongly to Chinese medicinals than Chinese patients do, who have been used to these medicinals since childhood. Therefore, one should start with small dosages in the beginning.

The final but nevertheless crucial factor is the quality of the medicinal, which is often lower in Chinese clinics than in exported goods. In essence, the place of origin of the medicinals is very important.

damage to the Blood. They clearly do not know that there is Blood stasis in the skin covering the flesh. In cases like these, the vessels are blocked, so Blood cannot nourish the hair sufficiently and the hair falls out.

After three prescriptions (of this formula) it will stop falling out. After 10 prescriptions new hair will have grown.

2. Reddened, painful eyes

Reddened, painful eyes, also commonly known as 'sudden eye fire' (inflammation of the eye). Blood is irritated by pathogenic Fire and coagulates in the eyes, which redden as a result. Regardless of whether the patient has blurred vision or not, one preparation of this formula should be prescribed to start with, and later on *Jia Wei Zhi Tong Mo Yao San* (Supplemented Pain Relieving Myrrh Powder) should be given twice daily. After 2–3 days everything should be fine.

Jia Wei Zhi Tong Mo Yao San *(supplemented pain relieving Myrrh Powder)*
1. Myrrha (*Mo Yao*)   9 g
2. Sanguis Draconis (*Xue Jie*)   9 g
3. Rhizoma Rheum (*Da Huang*)   9 g
4. Mirabilitum (*Pu Xiao*)   6 g
5. Concha Haliotidis (*Shi Jue Ming*)   9 g

3. Rosacea of the nose

The red veining points towards Blood stasis. Even if this illness has been in existence for decades, just three prescriptions of this formula will have an effect. There should be a full recovery after a few more prescriptions. Apart from this formula, there are no other effective prescriptions.

4. Chronic hardness of hearing

The small ear passages reach into the brain. When there are external signs of *Yu Xue* (Blood stasis), the vessels are narrow and clogged, leading to hardness of hearing. This formula should be taken in the evening. In the morning, *Qi* Passage Powder (*Tong Qi San*) should be taken, one dose twice daily. This is effective even if the hardness of hearing has lasted for decades.

5. Vitiligo (white spot disease)

This is Blood stasis under the skin, so a handful of prescriptions will not suffice to remove it. Approximately another 30 prescriptions should be taken to achieve recovery.

6. Chloasma (blue spot disease)

In this case, *Yu Xue* (Blood stasis) lies in deeper skin layers. The same therapy as for vitiligo. Very effective.

7. Bluish facial marks

The face shows bluish marks as if caused by blows. The marks are bluish-purple or the whole face may show a bluish-purple discolouration. This syndrome is due entirely to Blood stasis. If the problem is of a few years standing, 10 prescriptions will suffice. With a history of more than 10 years, there should be a correspondingly greater number of doses.

8. Dark blue birth marks on the face

This Blood stasis syndrome often occurs in members of the imperial court. About 30 prescriptions should suffice.

9. Ulcerative–necrotic inflammation of the gum

The teeth are closely connected to the bones. Blood nourishes the teeth.

Infections like *Shang Han*, febrile diseases, pox and abdominal neoplasms all contribute to 'heating' the Blood (today we would say that they contribute to releasing inflammatory factors and increasing viscosity). Blood stasis of this kind gives the gum a blue-purple shading. When the Blood is dead (necrosis) the gum turns black and the teeth fall out. How can anyone continue to live in this state? Even if the patient takes cooling medicinals, the Blood will clot and death will set in even more quickly.

In such cases, *Tong Qiao Huo Xue Tang* (Orifices Opening, Blood Invigorating Decoction) should be taken in the evening, and *Xue Fu Zhu Yu Tang* (Anti-Stasis Chest Decoction) in the morning. Furthermore, 8 *qian* (approximately 30 g) of Astragalus *Huang Qi* Decoction should be taken in small sips throughout the day, about three prescriptions daily. After 3 days the patient should feel some effect; after about 10 days there is a clear improvement and after 1 month recovery is complete. Some teeth will be lost occasionally, but all patients will survive, except those cases where the ulcer ruptures.

10. Offensive smell from the mouth (foetor ex ore)

This is *Yu Xue* (Blood stasis) in the chest. Blood must be stagnated in the local vessels. The windpipe[30] and the blood vessels are connected to the expulsion of air, so why should the air not smell unpleasant? It is similar to the way that the wind can carry the scent of flowers.

This formula (Tong Qiao Huo Xue Tang) should be taken in the evening, but in the morning *Xue Fu Zhu Yu Tang* (Anti-Stasis Chest Decoction) should be taken. The effect should be visible within a few days. Regardless of the original illness, the formula should be used as long as there is bad breath.

11. Amenorrhoea

No menstruation for 3–4 months or even 5–6 months. Cough, shortness of breath, poor appetite, little thirst, no strength in the limbs, often a raised temperature at midday, which continues to rise until the evening.

Three to six prescriptions of this formula should be used, nine in severe cases. I have yet to experience a lack of success with this treatment.

12. Exhaustion in men (also consumption, tuberculosis)

In the initial stage, there are symptoms of heavy and aching limbs, and gradual muscle atrophy. Decreasing appetite and thirst, yellowish-white facial colour, frothy cough, increased nervousness

---

[30] TCM also states 'Qi Xue Tong Yuan' (Qi and Blood arise from the same source). Here the wording is literally 'Qi Guan' (Qi vessel), but in this instance too Wang is talking about anatomical realities, thus 'windpipe' is used.

and irritability, afternoon fever and night sweating (are also symptoms).

Physicians were consulted to correct the situation. At first they prescribed *Yin* nourishing, and later *Yang* strengthening medicinals, but without any success. Eventually, they said: 'This is deficiency that is unable to accept tonification (*Xu Bu Shou Bu*). How does this come about?'

This is just ridiculous. It fails to differentiate between weakness due to disease and disease due to weakness. For example, *Shang Han* (Cold infections), febrile diseases and other severe diseases can all weaken the *Qi* and Blood and cause deficiency. Patients whose constitution originally showed syndromes of *Qi* and Blood weakness, are prescribed tonifying medicinals to replenish the deficiency, and they recover. However, in patients with no deficiency, the weakness is caused by the longstanding disease itself. Thus, if the disease is fought, *Yuan-Qi* will return by itself. But if one looks for the disease, neither exterior nor interior syndromes can be identified. All that can be identified are Blood stasis syndromes. I often treat such cases: for simple cases I prescribe nine preparations to restore health, in more severe cases I prescibe 18.

If there is still considerable *Qi* deficiency (weakness) after three prescriptions, approximately 30 g (8 *qian*) of Astragalus is prescribed, taken in sips over the day. If there is no *Qi* deficiency one can forego the Astragalus. Once the disease is defeated, *Yuan-Qi* (the original vitality) will return by itself.

13. Diseases with cyclical episodes

Whatever disease it is, as long as it occurs periodically at certain times of the year (*Jie Qi*), it is due to Blood stasis. How is Blood stasis recognized? Every time I get to see cases of vomiting blood and clotted blood, these symptoms occur at certain times; that is how I know. After three prescriptions it will not reoccur.

14. Infantile malnutrition (Gan–syndrome)

The initial stage of infantile malnutrition: turbid and milky urine, raised temperature which peaks in the afternoon, markedly protruding blood vessels, hard and distended abdomen, yellowish-cyanotic complexion and muscle atrophy. Skin and hair are lustreless and dry, the eyes are expressionless.

This kind of syndrome used to be called exhaustion (*Lao*) in adults, but malnutrition in children (*Gan*). So-called *Gan* deficiency syndromes are termed according to the type of deficiency, literally 'This-and-that-deficiency'. For example, there are Spleen *Gan* deficiency syndrome, *Gan* diarrhoea and oedema, *Gan* dysentery deficiency syndrome, Liver *Gan* deficiency syndrome, Heart *Gan* deficiency syndrome, diabetic *Gan* deficiency syndrome, Lung and Kidney *Gan* deficiency syndrome, *Gan* Heat syndrome, brain *Gan* deficiency syndrome, backbone *Gan* deficiency syndrome, roundworms *Gan* deficiency syndrome, *Wu Gu* (induced by vomiting milk) *Gan* deficiency syndrome, *Ding Xi* (extreme emaciation) *Gan* deficiency syndrome and *Pu Lu* (febrile colitis induced) *Gan* deficiency syndrome: there are 19 types in total, for which there are 50 formulas.

Most formulas contain *Zhi Zi, Huang Lian, Ling Yang Jiao* (Siberian Antelope Horn), *Shi Gao* and Jujube, because in most cases the cause of the disease is overfeeding with milk. If too much fatty and sweet food cannot be absorbed any more, it will stagnate in the stomach, the transport of food will be impeded and the gastrointestinal tract is gradually damaged. In this way, stagnating Heat is generated. If this Heat becomes greater, the *Gan* deficiency syndrome develops, *Qi* and Blood are reduced and Body Fluids (*Jin Ye*) run dry.

Due to the presence of Heat syndromes, I initially used very cooling medicinals, which were supposed to clear away the stagnated Heat, but I had no success. After that, I reconsidered the aetiology and the progression of this disease. In the case of excessive intake of food with subsequent blockage in the abdomen, cold medicinals are unsuitable. When I saw this syndrome on another occasion, it analysed more precisely/as follows. Afternoon fever which peaks in the evening points towards *Yu Xue* (Blood stasis). But protruding blood vessels are not sinews (literally *Qing Jin Bao Lu*, greenish sinews [*Jin*] protrude), rather these are veins lying under the skin which protrude more obviously, which also suggests *Yu Xue*

(Blood stasis). An abdomen that gradually becomes larger and harder with palpable masses allows us to conclude that this is clumping stasis in the abdomen.

Therefore I used *Tong Qiao* (Orifices Opening, Blood Invigorating Decoction, *Tong Qiao Huo Xue Tang*) to remove obstructions from the vessels, *Xue Fu* (Anti-Stasis Chest Decoction, *Xue Fu Zhu Yu Tang*) to lower the afternoon fever and *Ge Xia* (Anti-Stasis Abdomen Decoction, *Ge Xia Zhu Yu Tang*) to dissolve the lumps in the abdomen. Since then I have not seen any cases where the combination of these three formulas did not show any effect.

TONG QIAO HUO XUE TANG[31] (ORIFICES OPENING, BLOOD INVIGORATING DECOCTION)

Tao Ren 10 g Se. Persicae	*Hong Hua* 10 g Fl. Carthami Tinct.
Sheng Jiang 10 g Rh. Zingiberis Officinalis. Recens	*Cong Bai* 10 g Bu. Alli Fistulosi
Chi Shao 4 g Rx. Paeoniae Rubrae	*Chuan Xiong* 4 g Rx. Ligustici Wallichii
Hong Zao 7 pc. Fr. Zizyphi Jujubae	*She Xiang* 0.5 g Moschus[32] 0.15 g dissolved in 300 ml yellow wine

Briefly cook the first seven medicinals in wine, sieve, and add Moschus to the slightly warm mixture. Bring back to the boil twice more and

---

[31] See footnote 29.

[32] Moschus secretions are no longer obtained by killing the musk deer, but rather by scraping out the musk gland that is newly formed every year. Nevertheless, Moschus is still one of the most expensive substances within the Chinese materia medica, which is why it is often faked. One cannot praise its value too highly, because it is rich in hormonal, cardiotonic, antibiotic and other properties.

If it is unavailable, Maciocia recommends approximately 9 g of Acorus Graminei (*Shi Chang Pu*) per prescription. Yet Wang emphasizes that to achieve an excellent result an excellent Moschus is necessary. As shown by clinical experiments in China, its use can even cure long-term tinnitus and loss of hearing.

take before going to sleep. The *Liang*[33] measurement for the yellow wine is different in each location. Therefore, the patient had better take the larger measurement, rather than take too little. After the first boiling the wine loses its taste, so even people who do not like wine can drink it.

You can often buy fake Moschus on the market, and one *liang* (approximately 32 g) of this is the same price as one *qian* (approximately 3.2 g) of the real Moschus, but it is no alternative to the real thing. The Moschus contained in this formula is of greatest importance, so no expense must be spared to purchase the highest quality product and achieve success.

FORMULA RHYME[34]

Orifices-opener dispels stasis	= Orifices opening Blood invigorating decoction
Headache, eyes, ears, nose:	= for headache, red eyes, deafness, sinusitis
Saffron flower, shallots,	= *Hong Hua, Cong Bai*
Peach kernels and ginger, too	= *Tao Ren, Sheng Jiang*
12 grams each; but Peony	= all 12 g each. But *Chi Shao*
like Chuanxiong four, Jujubae seven	= and *Chuan Xiong* 4 g, seven pieces of *Hong Zao*
and wine-dissolved zero-three Moschus	= add 0.3 *She Xiang* dissolved in wine
brings Blood in the head into flow!	= Removes Blood stasis in the head (alopecia, dizziness, etc.)

The literal translation of the rhyme is:

[The effect of] Orifices opening is based predominantly on the excellent Moschus,[35] peach, saffron, jujube, old [i.e. stored] scallion, ginger, Chuanxiong, wine and red peony;
[whether] outside [or] inside, [it makes all] vessels penetrable, the first formula [amongst them all].

ANALGESIC MYRRH POWDER, SUPPLEMENTED

Indicated in eye pain in the initial stage and reddened inflamed eyes covered with mucus.

Myrrha (*Mo Yao*) 9 g

Sanguis Draconis (*Xue Jie*) 9 g

Rh. Rhei (*Da Huang*) 6 g

Mirabilitum (*Mang Xiao*) 6 g

Concha Haliotidis (*Shi Jue Ming*) 9 g

Make into a powder and divide into four portions, dissolve in warm water and apply in the morning and evening. This is one of the best formulas in ophthalmology for exterior conditions of the eye.

QI PASSAGE POWDER

Indicated in pronounced hardness of hearing. A proven formula for 30 years.

Chai Hu 38 g

Xiang Fu 38 g

Chuan Xiong 38 g

---

[33] A Chinese *liang* used to be about 32 g in the Qing dynasty, 16 *liang* amounted to one *jin*. Wang states that one half *jin* of yellow wine should be used. It may be replaced with white wine, which is the closest match to Yellow wine.

[34] In China, from antiquity to modern times, so-called *Tang-Tou-Ge* (formula rhymes or songs) have always been the best way to memorize formulas. There is not a single TCM doctor in China who cannot recite the principal formula rhymes by heart. I myself also learnt a few by heart, but with much less success. The Chinese find them a lot easier to learn as they naturally have a better feel for their native language. Certainly, no foreigner is expected to learn these rhymes by heart in Chinese in order to become proficient in TCM; the ambiguous nature of the characters alone and the presence of differing characters which share the same sounds would require tremendous effort. With this in mind, I have tried to show how these formulas combine indications, dosages and ingredients as well as the name of the formula, in a succinct, 'concentrated' rhyming composition with a metre that is easy to retain. In short, a venture like this would be nearly impossible in our language. I ask for the reader's tolerance if this part of the translation lacks precision.

[35] Compare with Wang's note on the importance of genuine and pure (not fake) Moschus in the preceding paragraph.

Make into a powder, then rinse with 10 g both in the morning and evening.

LIST OF INDICATIONS FOR *XUE FU ZHU YU TANG* (ANTI-STASIS CHEST DECOCTION)

1. Headache

Headache due to a cold is characterized by exterior symptoms such as raised temperature and chills at the same time. Diaphoretic medicinals are indicated. The syndrome of accumulated Heat manifests in connection with a dry mouth (dry tongue) and thirst. In this case, *Cheng Qi* decoctions (purgative and other similar formulas) are effective. *Qi* deficiency syndrome manifests in feeling ill without a (real) locatable pain. Ginseng (*Ren Shen*) and Astragalus (*Huang Qi*) are the medicinals of choice.

If the patient is still suffering from headache, with no internal or exterior syndromes, if neither *Qi* deficiency nor Phlegm accumulation can be diagnosed, no method proves helpful and all the formulas mentioned above have no effect, then a prescription of *Xue Fu Zhu Yu Tang* (Anti-Stasis Chest Decoction) will be effective.

2. Retrosternal pain

Pain in the right side of the chest is treated with *Mu Jin San* (Wood Metal Powder).[36] Pain that radiates through to the back indicates the use of *Gua Lou Xie Bai Bai Jiu Tang* (Trichosanthes Allium Rice Wine Decoction). For chest pain that is due to infection with Cold pathogens, *Gua Lou* [*Tang*] (Trichosanthes decoctions), *Xie Xin* [*Tang*] (Heart Relieving decoctions, e.g. with Pinellia) or *Chai Hu* [*Tang*] (Bupleurum decoctions)[37] and so on are useful. However, if there is sudden chest pain, and none of the formulas mentioned above are indicated, then one should use *Xue Fu Zhu Yu Tang* (Anti-Stasis Chest Decoction). The pain will stop immediately.

---

[36] No formula of this name could be found in modern or classical sources. Possibly a spelling mistake.
[37] Wang is referring to some of the well-known formulas from Zhang Zhong-Jing's '*Shang Han Lun*'.

3. Dislike of pressure on the chest

A 74-year-old civil servant from Jiang Xi, called A-Lin Gung, could only sleep if his chest was left uncovered at night. As soon as he was covered, even with a thin blanket, he experienced a sensation of pressure on the chest and could not sleep. This condition had been present for 7 years, so he asked me for a diagnosis. Five prescriptions of this formula sufficed to achieve a complete recovery.

4. A liking for pressure on the chest

A 22-year-old woman could only sleep once she had ordered the house servant to sit on her chest. She had had this condition for 2 years. Three prescriptions of this formula were successful.

If these two patients were to ask me for the cause of the disease, what answer could I give them?

5. Sweating in the morning

Sweating after waking up is called spontaneous sweating; when it occurrs before waking up it is called thievish sweating (night sweating), because in the long run it will reduce the body's *Qi* and Blood. This is a traditional theory. If the (in this case commonly used) formulas for tonifying *Qi*, sealing the exterior, nourishing *Yin* and reducing Fire do not show any effect, or if they exacerbate the condition, then this is due to ignorance of the fact that *Yu Xue* (Blood stasis) can also lead to spontaneous or thievish sweating. The sweating will stop as soon as *Xue Fu Zhu Yu Tang* (Anti-Stasis Chest Decoction) is given rather than the formulas mentioned above.

6. Difficulties in swallowing (when swallowing, food slips into the right abdomen, feeling of pressure in the gullet)

Food normally slips straight down through the gullet, which is the middle of the throat. However, there are cases where swallowed food noticeably slips down to the right. As the gullet lies behind the windpipe, it must arch to the front at the side of the lung. Below the lung, it passes the liver and penetrates the diaphragm, to reach the abdomen.

The windpipe lies exactly in the middle. If there is Blood stasis in the chest, the gullet will be pushed to the right side. Simple cases that do not involve great difficulty in swallowing are easier to treat than those where the gullet has already become crooked and thin-walled. These patients have great difficulty, and it is not easy to cure them with this formula.

7. Sensation of Heat in the chest ('lantern disease')

The name 'lantern disease' comes from the fact that on the outside, the body is cool, while inside the chest there is a sensation of Heat. There is Blood stasis internally. If it is now wrongly assumed to be an empty Heat (*Xu Re*) syndrome, tonification will make the stasis worse. If it is wrongly assumed to be a syndrome of excess Fire, more and more Blood will stagnate due to the prescription of cold medicinals. A few prescriptions of this formula will bring the Blood back into flow and repel the Heat.

8. Depressive gloominess

The slightest thing causes the patient to become withdrawn: this is also Blood stasis. Three prescriptions of this formula rectify the condition.

9. Nervous irritability

When the patient is healthy, everything is all right, but as soon as he is ill, he becomes nervous and irritable. This consequence of Blood stasis should improve after a few prescriptions.

10. Many dreams

A light sleep at night with many dreams. This is due to Blood stasis. A few prescriptions of this formula will rectify the condition. There is no better formula for this.

11. Hiccups

If there is *Yu Xue* (Blood stasis) in the chest, both the left and right carotid arteries, which converge at the heart (aorta), and the windpipe will be compressed and the inhaled air cannot flow freely. The

air is pressed back upwards, resulting in hiccups.[38] If the *Yu Xue* (Blood stasis) is pronounced, the windpipe may even become constricted, so no air at all can pass through it, and the patient dies from suffocation. In ancient times nothing was known about the causes of this disease. Thus, prescriptions such as *Chen Pi Zhu Ru Tang* (Aurantium Bambusa Decoction), *Cheng Qi Tang* (*Qi* Ordering Decoction), *Du Qi Tang* (Pathogenic *Qi* Decoction), *Ding Xiang Shi Di Tang* (Caryophyllus Kaki Decoction), *Fu Zi Li Zhong Tang* (Aconite Centre Regulating Decoction), *Sheng Jiang Xie Xin Tang* (Zingiber Heart Relief Decoction), *Xuan Fu Dai Zhe Tang* (Inula Haematite Decoction), *Da Xian Xiong Tang* (Great Chest Relieving Decoction) or *Xiao Xian Xiong Tang* (Small Chest Relieving Decoction) and so on were given, but without any success. People say that those who get hiccups due to *Shang Han* (Cold induced) or *Wen Bing* (febrile infection) diseases will die. As there was no effective medicine in former times, doctors refrained from treating this disease. Regardless of whether *Shang Han* or *Wen Bing* or any other disease is present, as soon as hiccups are encountered as a concomitant symptom, this formula (i.e. *Xue Fu Zhu Yu Tang*) should be prescribed. Regardless of whether the hiccups are slight or severe, one prescription is sufficient, according to my personal experience.

12. Choking on drinking liquids

Choking on drinking liquids is caused by pressure on the cap of the glottis, induced by Blood stasis. This formula provides excellent help. The theory from ancient times about this is absolutely mistaken; details can be found in the section on pox-

---

[38] Even if Wang's theory on the development of hiccups and several other of his anatomical descriptions do not correspond to our present-day standard of knowledge, it is still remarkable that someone tried to propose explanatory models at the beginning of the nineteenth century. Today we know that hiccuping is a diaphragmatic reflex due to irritation of the phrenic nerve, often occurring in pericarditis, bronchial asthma and hiatus hernia – diseases for which Wang recommends *Xue Fu Zhu Yu Tang*. However, we have only been aware of these diseases for a few decades, since the advent of specific diagnostic methods such as contrast X-rays and ECG.

like diseases (see 'Discussion about choking on drinking liquids in smallpox', p. 218).

13. Insomnia

Sleeplessness at night in patients where calming and Blood nourishing medicinals have been unsuccessful; this medicine works wonders.

14. Infantile crying at night

If children only cry at night, but not during the day, they have Blood stasis. One or two prescriptions of this formula will bring them back to health.

15. Palpitations, panic palpitations

In patients with palpitations and panic palpitations where *Gui Pi Tang* (Spleen Recovering Decoction) and *An Shen* (calming) medicinals were used to no avail, this formula is a hundred per cent effective.

16. Restlessness at night

Patients suffering from restlessness at night get up as soon as they go to bed, and feel tired again as soon as they are awake and sit down. In this way, they hardly ever get a quiet 15 minutes in bed. In severe cases, the bed is wrecked. This is due to *Yu Xue* (Blood stasis). Using a little more than 10 prescriptions of this formula, the disease can be completely eradicated.

17. So-called short temper

When a patient suffers from angry outbursts for no apparent reason, this is due to *Yu Xue* (Blood stasis) in the chest. One should definitely not tonify *Qi*, but use this method instead.

18. Nausea

If there are no other symptoms except nausea without vomiting, then this is due to *Yu Xue* (Blood stasis). When we use this formula, Blood will move again and nausea will stop.

19. Sensation of Heat in the evening

Every evening the patient feels too hot internally and at the same time the skin feels temporarily hot. In such cases one prescription of this formula suffices, but use two in severe cases.

XUE FU ZHU YU TANG (ANTI-STASIS CHEST DECOCTION)

Dang Gui 12 g Rx. Angelica Sinensis	*Sheng Di* 12 g Rx. Rehmannia
Tao Ren 16 g Se. Persica	*Hong Hua* 12 g Fl. Carthami
Zhi Ke 8 g Pc. Citri Aurantii	*Chi Shao* 8 g Rx. Paeoniae Rubrae
Chai Hu 6 g Rx. Bupleurum	*Gan Cao* 6 g Rx. Glycyrrhizae
Jie Geng 6 g Rx. Platycodi	*Chuan Xiong* 6 g Rx. Ligustici Wallichii
Niu Xi 12 g Rx. Achyranthis	

FORMULA RHYME

Chest Decoction for pressure of the heart	= Anti-stasis chest decoction for a sensation of pressure in the thorax
No sleep, head and stomach pain,	= insomnia, headache, heart/stomach pain
Twelve Saffron and Rehmannia,	= 12 g *Hong Hua*, *Sheng Di*
Also Achyranthes, Angelica,	= *Niu Xi* and *Dang Gui*
But Chuanxiong, Liquorice, Bupleurum	= *Chuan Xiong*, *Gan Cao*, *Chai Hu*
Six grams as Platycodum	= and *Jie Geng* 6 g each.
Of peaches sixteen; red peony	= *Tao Ren* 16 g, *Chi Shao*
Only eight as well as bitter lemon.	= and *Zhi Ke* 8 g each.

The literal translation of the rhyme is:

Chest [decoction contains] Angelica, Rehmannia, Peach kernels, Saffron, Liquorice, Bitter Orange, Red Peony, Bupleurum, Chuanxiong, Platycodum and so on Invigorated Blood flows (again) downwards (and) does not exhaust (the body any more).

LIST OF INDICATIONS FOR ANTI-STASIS ABDOMEN DECOCTION (*GE XIA ZHU YU TANG*)

1. Accumulations and gatherings

To avoid getting into endless debates, we will not discuss classical terms such as 'the five accumulations', 'the six gatherings', 'the seven concretions' and 'the eight conglomerations' here, nor will we discuss mistakes to these terms. We will simply ask what these accumulations in the abdomen actually are. If something gathers in the stomach, it must be food; if it gathers in the intestine, it must be waste products. If such accumulations have been there for a longer period of time, but food and drink are still consumed as usual, then (the clumps) cannot be in the stomach and intestine, but must exist somewhere outside them. Everywhere outside the stomach and intestine, regardless of which part of the body, are *Qi* and *Xue* (Blood). *Qi* flows in the *Qi* vessels (channels), and Blood in the blood vessels. *Qi* is insubstantial, therefore it cannot gather and form lumps. The gatherings must therefore be formed from *Xue* (Blood).

If the pathogenic factor Cold clashes with Blood, then Blood will coagulate into clumps. This will also happen if the pathogenic factor Heat clashes with Blood.

If vessels that run up and down the body become clogged, vertical swellings will develop, but if vessels that run across the body become clogged, horizontal swellings will develop. If Blood coagulates in both vessel types, those that run vertically *and* horizontally, then discoid (two-dimensional) swellings will develop. If the formation of layers of discs continues over a prolonged period of time, they will become thicker and eventually form (three-dimensional) clumps. Once these lumps have developed, there will be fever.

To check whether there is *Yu Xue* (Blood stasis) in the chest area, check whether there is any fever (raised temperature). The chest area is the origin of *Xue* (Blood); once there is stasis in here, life will be endangered.

If there is *Yu Xue* (Blood stasis) in the abdomen, no fever develops. The abdomen is where Blood ends (i.e. it is consumed here), so Blood stasis in here will not endanger life.

It makes no difference whether accumulations and gatherings become clumps on the left or right side of the ribs or navel, above or below the navel, or whether they can freely move about. All of these can be cured using this formula. As long as the indications are correct, it will be effective.

Mild cases are given fewer prescriptions, more severe ones are given more accordingly. If the patient's *Qi* is too weak to tolerate dispersing formulas, then instead of sticking rigidly to the dogma one may add 10–15 g of *Dang Shen* (Radix Codonopsis) to tonify *Qi*.

2. Abdominal masses in children

Abdominal masses in children who have a swollen body and protruding greenish veins are entirely due to *Yu Xue* (Blood stasis), from the beginning to the end. If this formula is used in alternation with the two described earlier, *Tong Qiao Huo Xue Tang* and *Xue Fu Zhu Yu Tang* (Senses Opening Blood Invigorating Decoction and Anti-Stasis Chest Decoction), then success will be apparent after about one month.

3. Pain that is always in the same location

All cases of abdominal pain where pain does not move about indicate *Yu Xue* (Blood stasis) and this formula can be applied successfully in these cases.

4. Feeling of heaviness in the abdomen during sleep

On going to sleep, the patient feels as if there is something heavy in his belly. When he is lying on the left side, it pulls downwards to the left (i.e. towards the floor) and if he is lying on the right side, it pulls downwards to the right. This is due to internal Blood stasis. This formula should principally be used (supplemented by appropriate formulas) when there are other symptoms.

5. 'Kidney-induced' diarrhoea

The syndrome of 'several times diarrhoea at dawn' was defined classically as 'cockcrow diarrhoea'. This describes a deficiency of Kidney-*Yang*. *Er Shen Wan* (Two Deities Pill), *Si Shen Wan* (Four Deities Pill) and so on are prescribed. If there is no success, this syndrome may be present for many years without becoming better. Ignorance about the condition is based on lack of awareness of *Yu Xue* (Blood stasis), which has been mentioned above; during sleep, the *Jin Men* (*gate of fluids*) is clogged up by stasis, and the watery liquids cannot exit through the gate. Instead, they flow through the deep gate (pylorus) into the small intestine, where they join the remaining chyme and thus make the stool more fluid. Repeated morning diarrhoea is the result.

If this formula is used to dissolve the above-mentioned *Yu Xue* (Blood stasis), Blood will be invigorated, the gate of fluids will no longer be blocked and the watery fluid will no longer be discharged together with the diarrhoea. A few prescriptions should bring about a total recovery.

6. Chronic diarrhoea

Prolonged chronic diarrhoea that has been unsuccessfully treated with all kinds of formulas is due to the occurrence of Blood stasis and can also be treated with this formula.

ANTI-STASIS ABDOMEN DECOCTION (*GE XIA ZHU YU TANG*)

Dang Gui 10 g Rx. Angelicae Sinensis	*Tao Ren* 10 g Se. Persica
Hong Hua 10 g Fl. Carthami	*Gan Cao* 10 g Rx. Glycyrrhizae
Mou Dan Pi 7 g Cx. Moutan	*Wu Ling Zhi* 7 g Faec. Trogopteri
Chuan Xiong 7 g Rx. Ligustici Wallichii	*Chi Shao* 7 g Rx. Paeoniae Rubrae
Wu Yao 7 g Rx. Lindera	*Zhi Ke* 5 g Pc. Citri Aurantii
Xiang Fu 5 g Rh. Cyperi	*Yuan Hu* 3 g Rh. Corydalis

FORMULA RHYME

Abdomen decoction for abdominal pressure	= Anti-stasis abdomen decoction for a sensation of pressure in the abdomen
Pain, clumping, diarrhoea too,	= pain, abdominal masses and diarrhoea
Saffron, Liquorice, Persica,	= Of *Hong Hua*, *Gan Cao*, *Tao Ren*
Ten each as well as Angelica,	= and *Dang Gui* 10 g each
Chuanxiong, Moutan, Lindera,	= *Chuan Xiong*, *Mu Dan Pi*, *Wu Yao*,
Trogopterus, red peony	= *Wu Ling Zhi* and *Chi Shao*
Seven each; three Corydalus,	= 7 g each plus *Yan Hu Suo* 3 g
Five bitter lemon, Cyperus.	= finally, *Zhi Ke* and *Xiang Fu* 5 g each

The literal translation of the rhyme is:

Abdomen [decoction contains] Angelica, Liquorice, Persica, Bitter Orange, Red Peony, Saffron, Ligusticum, Trogopterus, Corydalis etc.
Masses dissolve and invigorated Blood flows on.

PART 3. WANG'S CLINICAL STUDIES AND METHODOLOGY

FOREWORD TO THE THEORY OF ONE-SIDED PARALYSIS (HEMIPLEGIA)

Physicians write books basically and attempt to help people. Such an attitude is very commendable. To do this the physician must himself treat the patient, and develop methods and expertise, so that failures can be avoided. Only then can one's formulas be left for posterity. If a type of syndrome is not identified correctly, then one must leave it up to the next generation to complete it.

Against this background, it is totally wrong to establish a theory only on the basis of one's reputation, or to compose a formula for a disease which one has never seen before. Given that the fundamentals of the disease are unknown, then the formula will be unsuitable. Human lives are surely put at risk by this, rather than being saved. Isn't this utterly terrifying?

In ancient times, there were, for example, specialists in *Shang Han* (Cold induced diseases), *Wen Bing* (febrile infectious diseases), various syndromes and gynaecology. Adequate formulas were applied, most of which were successful. Although there was the occasional inaccuracy, in most cases the flaws were minor.

But when it comes to one-sided paralysis, which was also described in former times, there have been only a few amongst more than 400 medical schools who put forward theories on it, and amongst those not even one who described its origin. However, if the origin of the diseases is unknown, how can one compose the correct formula?

I got to see this syndrome early in my career and followed the theories of the '*Ling Shu*' and '*Su Wen*' (*The Yellow Emperor's Internal Classic*) as well as Zhang Zhong-Jing's theory ('*Shang Han Lun*' and '*Jin Kui Yao Lüe*'), but without any success. After that I applied the theories of the He Jian school, which are the theories of Li Dong-Yuan and Zhu Dan-Xi, but again the medicinals failed to show any effect. Thus I was going around in circles without getting any further.

However, Zhang Zhong-Jing's *Shang Han* theory and Wu You-Ke's *Wen Bing* theory were totally self-contained, in other words they were conceived independently of the classical works. I just had the will to help people, but not the means.

So for 40 years, whenever I came across this disease, I researched deficiency or excess of *Qi* and Blood and differentiated as to whether the channels were obstructed or unobstructed. I wanted to publish the results of these studies to benefit posterity, but at first I did not dare to criticize the classical methods by suggesting a new method.

However, my friends said: 'If you can sincerely suggest a beneficial and approved method that will complement the classical methods, then you will help to solve problems in the future. Not only that, at the same time, you will be contributing towards improving the classical methods. How could that be wrong?'

Thus I came to write in great detail about hemiplegia in men, women and children, paralysis of the legs and atrophy of the muscles, cramps and convulsions, about causes and characteristics, approved formulas, favourable or unfavourable prognoses as well as about all the earlier, incorrect descriptions of the vessels, organs and channels. I explained every single detail, and now I hope that all necessary amendments will be made by the good physicians of the future, who will unquestionably come after me.

THEORIES ON ONE-SIDED PARALYSIS (HEMIPLEGIA)

Although it is only one disease, theories about hemiplegia vary according to the author. We start with the '*Ling Shu*' (*The Yellow Emperor's Internal Classic*, Spiritual Pivot, Chapter 75), which explains:

When the pathogenic factor Deficiency has penetrated into one side of the body and damages the well-nourished Wei-Qi (Defensive Qi) in the deeper levels, this infiltration naturally diminishes Wei-Qi and the body's own Qi will vanish from there. This means that the pathogenic Qi stays there on its own and one-sided withering presents.

The withering disease is hemiplegia.

In the '*Su Wen*' (*The Yellow Emperor's Internal Classic*, Plain Questions, Chapter 42) it is said:

When pathogenic Wind penetrates through the acupuncture points of the five storage organs and six labour organs (five Zang and six Fu) deep into the interior – it is then called Zang Fu Wind – it leads to one-sided Wind, according to the weakest point at which it invades.

Zhang Zhong-Jing[39] said: 'In apoplectic Wind stroke (*Zhong Feng*) one side of the body cannot move voluntarily.'

---

[39] Author of the classical and foundational works '*Shang Han Lun*' and '*Jin Kui Yao Lüe*'. The quotation is taken from the latter work, Chapter 5, first line (modern classification).

All three theories relate the disease to pathogenic Wind. Thus, the classical formulas had no effect, until Liu He-Jian[40] finally appeared and, after he had witnessed the lack of effect of the classical formulas, proposed a new theory:

> Apoplectic Wind stroke (Zhong Feng) is not due to unrestrained Liver-Wind, i.e. internal Wind, neither is it due to exterior pathogenic Wind. The cause is that physiological Fire inside the body is stirred by an excessively active lifestyle. Its counterpart, physiological Water, is slowly consumed and unable to restrain Fire, so eventually the mind becomes impotent and the patient dies, without regaining consciousness.

Li Dong-Yuan noticed the contradiction in Liu's theory and formula and thus proposed his own theory:

> Wind stroke (Zhong Feng) commonly affects patients with Qi deficiency, who are attacked by exterior pathogenic Wind. The disease occurs mostly after the age of 40 years, and more frequently in fat than in thin people, including obese patients with a whitish skin and debility due to Qi deficiency.

He differentiated Wind stroke of the storage organs (Zang) and the labour organs (Fu), of the Blood vessels and channels, and hypothesized that the cause of pathogenic Wind affecting the patient in the first place was to be found in the underlying deficiency of Qi.

Zhu Dan-Xi, however, perceived Li's formulas and syndromes to be inadequate, and supplemented them with another theory. He explained that in the cold climate in the North, Wind stroke (Zhong Feng) would exist, but that in the damp and warm climate in the South the disease would not be a genuine Wind stroke (Zhong Feng). The disease is said to develop mainly from underlying internal Qi or Blood deficiency, as well as from (pathogenic) Phlegm that is derived from pathogenic climatic Dampness. In turn, such Phlegm would cause Heat, and Heat would cause internal

Wind.[41] Thus his theory discusses Phlegm and explains Dampness and Phlegm to be the cause.

Wang An-Dao, having read Zhu's theory that the disease occurring in the damp South was no genuine Wind stroke, added that the disease mentioned in The Yellow Emperor's Internal Classic and Zhang Zhong-Jing's work was the genuine Wind stroke, whereas the disease mentioned by Liu He-Jian, Li Dong-Yuan and Zhu Dan-Xi was a disease similar to Wind stroke (Lei Zhong Feng).

Yu Tian-Ming commented on this:

> Wang An-Dao differentiates genuine Wind stroke and the disease similar to it. But to put it this way is not correct. Looking at these diseases, they can all be put down entirely to Qi deficiency, Dampness and Phlegm in connection with Wind. Has anyone ever heard about the differentiation of genuine and similar Wind stroke?

Only Zhang Jing-Yue has the vision of a great physician. He recognizes that in most cases one-sided paralysis is related to Qi deficiency, and that it may be called Wind stroke but cannot be put down to Wind. Instead, he quotes the 'Nei Jing' (The Internal Classic) and associates Wind stroke with the syndrome of syncope (Jue Ni) mentioned there, which is linked with Heat, Cold, Blood deficiency and the twelve channels; but of course these do not match with the symptoms of Wind stroke, and consequently the corresponding for-

---

[40] Also Liu Wan-Su, one of the great physicians of the Jin and Yuan dynasty. The other are also mentioned in the text: Zhang Zi-He, Zhu Dan-Xi, Li Dong-Yuan.

[41] Whilst this logic may appear incomprehensible to the beginner, any practitioner familiar with the foundations of TCM will surely recognize the aetiology of diseases here. However, I would like to emphasize again that although damp weather is a concrete and substantial phenomenon, the pathogenic factors generated from it (Dampness, Phlegm, Heat and Wind) suggest specific models in TCM, i.e. they are descriptions of clearly defined physical situations. For example, pathogenic Phlegm may also manifest as concrete 'phlegm' in the throat, nasal cavities or bronchi, but at the same time it is a term for a general syndrome that can be related to symptoms such as lassitude and heaviness, mental disorders, swollen lymph nodes and lipomas, and even arthritic deformations of the bones. A more detailed analysis of Phlegm can be gained from Maciocia's Foundations of Chinese Medicine, Chapter 19, Porkert's Klinische Chinesische Pharmakologie and especially from Clavey's excellent analysis in Fluid Physiology and Pathology in Traditional Chinese Medicine, Chapters 7 and 8.

mulas do not work. It is a shame that the master only saw a few of these cases.

All these famous physicians suggest only Wind, Fire, *Qi* or Phlegm as the cause of this disease. As a result, all formulas either expel Wind, cool Fire, invigorate *Qi* or transform Phlegm.

Thus it is always suggested that for Wind stroke due to Blood and *Qi* deficiency one should use Wind expelling and Fire cooling formulas and add *Qi* strengthening and Blood nourishing medicinals; while for Wind stroke due to *Yin* deficiency collapse one should use *Yin* nourishing medicinals and add *Qi* tonifying and Phlegm transforming ones. Sometimes health is considerably strengthened and the disease is attacked a little, sometimes health is only a little strengthened and the disease is strongly attacked. This is then proudly called a strategy of simultaneously strengthening and attacking.

But when these methods are used, they simply fail to show any effect. Yet the possibility of errors in the classics is still not discussed; instead, it is claimed that the classical formulas do not suit present-day diseases, because it is convenient to say that a typical present-day constitution is not equivalent to one in ancient times. But if we assume that the formulas do not suit the diseases because constitutions differ, why is it then that *Ma Huang* decoctions (containing Ephedra), *Zheng Qi* (*Qi* ordering) decoctions, *Xie Xiong* (chest relieving) decoctions and *Chai Hu* (containing Bupleurum) prescriptions[42] work excellently for *Shang Han* (diseases due to Cold), but as soon as we talk about Wind stroke, formulas such as *Dao Tan*, *Qin Jiao* and *San Hua* decoctions (i.e. expelling Wind and Phlegm decoctions) suddenly have no effect?

Clearly nobody thought of these two possibilities concerning the composition of classical formulas: namely that some are effective and some are ineffective. Effective formulas were composed with the aid of accumulated personal experience of successfully treating patients. Ineffective formulas were devised mostly through guesswork on the subject of theoretically existing diseases.

If the theory is merely guesswork, and if the formulas are based only on such theories instead of on experience, then how can the cause of the disease be known at all? How can we explain hemiplegia and one-sided facial paralysis, and the post-apoplectic muffled speech and the uncontrollable drooling at the corner of the mouth? What is the explanation for the dry stools and urinary incontinence at the same time? From that day to this, nobody had the slightest idea, everything was mere guesswork! If more attacking medicinals are prescribed for a disease which incapacitates half of the body, and these have an additional reducing action, how could this be anything but wrong?

When we look for the cause, we will find the actual mistake not in the physicians themselves but in the people who published such theories. Confound it! How can one attempt to unravel such a life-threatening matter by guessing?

DISCUSSION OF ONE-SIDED PARALYSIS (HEMIPLEGIA)

Looking at all the teachings that discuss Wind, Fire, Dampness and Phlegm as the cause of hemiplegia, what concrete evidence can we find? I see it the following way. In the section *Zhong Feng* of the 'Shang Han Lun', Zhang Zhong-Jing wrote that Wind stroke (*Zhong Feng*) causes headache and body pain, as well as fever with aversion to cold and dry retching with spontaneous sweating. He wrote in the 'Jin Kui Yao Lüe' that Wind damage causes sneezing and blocked nose as well as loud coughing and a runny nose with thin secretions. In the chapter on Wind stroke he writes: 'This disease caused by Wind makes people paralysed on one side.'

Shouldn't we be asking ourselves these questions: what Wind (*Feng*) and stroke (*Zhong*) are these that cause headache and body pain, as well as fever with aversion to cold and dry retching with spontaneous sweating; what Wind (*Feng*) and stroke (*Zhong*) are these that cause sneezing and a blocked nose as well as loud coughing and a runny nose with thin secretions; and, what Wind

---

[42] These quotations refer to Zhang Zhong-Jing's 'Shang Han Lun', in which specific modifications such as those mentioned (*Ma Huang Tang* (Ephedra Decoction), *Xiao Chai Hu Tang* (Small Bupleurum Decoction) and *Zheng Qi* (*Qi* ordering decoctions), *Xie Xiong* (chest relieving decoctions)) very often occur and were used in Wang's time as frequently as nowadays.

(*Feng*) and stroke (*Zhong*) are these that cause one-sided paralysis?

If one-sided paralysis is really due to pathogenic Wind, which attacks people in the form of a stroke, then it must[43] travel through the skin into the channels and cause traceable syndromes on its way from the exterior into the interior. Now, when confronted with hemiplegia, one will not find any exterior syndromes such as headache and body pain, fever with aversion to cold, eye pain accompanied by a dry nose or alternating sensations of heat and cold,[44] in its initial stage. If no such exterior symptoms (*Biao Zheng*) can be found, then the conclusion is that hemiplegia cannot be caused by a pathogenic factor invading from the exterior, such as Wind.

Moreover, there is even more confusion among those who theorize about Wind, Fire, Dampness and Phlegm. This is because regardless of whether Wind, Fire, Dampness or Phlegm are involved, or whether internal or external factors are involved, they all need to be transported through the vessels. In turn, the vessels contain either *Qi* (in the channels and *Luo*-vessels) or Blood (in the blood vessels). Now, when Wind, Fire, Dampness or Phlegm give rise to *Qi* stagnation or Blood stasis, the symptom that develops is pain. Pain suggests *Bi* syndrome,[45] but not hemiplegia. In hemiplegia, there is no pain as a concomitant symptom. Among all the cases of hemiplegia that I have treated in my entire life, I have never seen anyone in whom hemiplegia developed as a result of painful *Bi* syndromes. This consideration leads us to conclude that Wind, Fire, Dampness or Phlegm do not cause hemiplegia.

THE CAUSE OF ONE-SIDED PARALYSIS (HEMIPLEGIA)

Some people ask me this: 'You claim that the cause of hemiplegia lies in the collapse of *Yuan-Qi*. If that is the case, why does this disease occur when only half of *Yuan-Qi* has collapsed? That is a very interesting question.'

To this, I can say the following: *Yuan-Qi* flows in the channels through out the whole body and half of it is distributed to the left and half to the right. *Yuan-Qi* is always needed, whether a person is walking, standing or moving. If there is sufficient *Yuan-Qi* a person will have enough energy for all this; however, if *Yuan-Qi* is weak, he will be powerless. When there is no *Yuan-Qi*, death will set in.

If we assume that if two out of ten parts are lost from the entire energy of *Yuan-Qi*, then there will still be eight left, this means four out of eight parts (of *Yuan-Qi*) for each half of the body. One-sided paralysis will not develop from this. However, if five out of ten parts of *Yuan-Qi* are lacking, then two and a half parts will remain for each side. Although there is still no one-sided paralysis at this point, there *is* a deficiency of *Qi*, even if the patient cannot feel it because there is neither pain nor itching.

When the *Yuan-Qi* system collapses, the channels are not sufficiently supplied with *Qi*. So, under these circumstances, there is an opportunity for the *Yuan-Qi* of one side to combine with the *Yuan-Qi* of the stronger side and to fully supply that one, at least. If the two and a half parts from the right flow to the left, then of course there is no *Qi* on the right; and vice versa, if the two and a half parts from the left flow to the right, then of course there is no *Qi* on the left side of the body. When there is no longer any *Qi* energy left, then movement will not be possible. When the ability to move is lacking, this is called paralysis, and this means that the person can no longer use one side of the body at will.

If the merging of the remaining *Qi* takes place during sleep, the patient will be unaware of this. Once awoken, however, he will be unable to turn over one side of the body. If *Qi* moves while the patient is awake, then he will feel as if the ill half of his body were moving towards the other half; the noise of this is louder than the noise of waves in flowing water.[46]

On the other hand, if this takes place when the person is sitting, then the body will tilt towards

---

[43] According to Chinese Medicine theory.

[44] Sensations of alternating heat and chills are the typical symptoms of a disease invading the interior from the exterior, as would be the case for a pathogenic factor coming from the outside.

[45] According to Western definition, *Bi* syndrome belongs to diseases of the rheumatic sphere. For a precise definition, see Glossary.

---

[46] It is not clear from this comparison whether Wang is referring to the sound of the disturbed, flaccid side of the body or the typical rushing noise that appears after strokes affecting the vertebrobasilar circulation.

one side; if one half of the body is depleted of *Qi* during walking, then the person will collapse. People usually say that the paralysis is due to the fall, because they are unaware that this is not true. In fact, the one-sided paralysis is due to the collapse of *Qi*, and this is why the patient fell down.

DISCUSSION ON DEVIATION OF THE MOUTH AND EYE (FACIAL PARALYSIS)

People often ask, if hemiplegia is not caused by Wind, how about deviation of the mouth and eye (facial paralysis)? I can say the following: the reason for calling it 'deviation' in former times lies solely in the fact that this symptom was not observed well enough. In deviation of the mouth and eye there is by no means an actual deviation, but rather, after the Wind stroke half of the face no longer has any *Qi*, so one side appears smaller: an eye that has no *Qi* can no longer fully open, thus one corner of the eye is pulled downwards. If one side of the mouth has no *Qi*, it can no longer open, thus one side of the mouth is pulled upwards, so that when the mouth is closed it may first appear as if it was deviated, although in fact there is no genuine deviation between the left and the right side.

Mostly, this disease behaves like this: if the left side of the body is hemiplegic, the right side of the face deviates. Conversely, if the right side of the body is hemiplegic, the left side of the body deviates. This makes us look in vain for explanations. There are no hints in the books either, so what is to be done about it?

Some channels come from the left side of the torso and cross over in the face or on the head towards the right, or they come from the right and go to the left side of the face or head, so left and right cross over. Still, I do not venture to postulate this as an explanation; obviously, we will have to wait until this explanation can be complemented by more precise and better examination.

DISCUSSION ON 'WHY DROOLING FROM THE CORNER OF THE MOUTH IS NOT A SIGN FOR PHLEGM SYNDROME'

When I am asked why drooling from the corner of the mouth is not a sign for Phlegm syndrome, I

reply that if such cases are looked at in detail, we find that the saliva running from the corner of the mouth is in fact a clear secretion, and not thick liquid phlegm. To understand this we must study the theory 'Qi deficiency causes loss of control of Body Fluids' most precisely. If this should still fail to make it clear, then we should observe infants with *Qi* deficiency syndrome: nine out of ten have drooling. If these symptoms are accurately compared yet again, it will become clear that this type of drooling belongs to the category of deficient *Qi* failing to consolidate.

DISCUSSION ON 'WHY DRY STOOL IS NOT A SIGN FOR WIND AND FIRE SYNDROME'

It is often said that if the patient suffers from paralysis and at the same time the stool is dry and hard, then in former times this was called Wind-Dryness; this means the disease is due to Wind and Fire. Is this explanation correct?

I can say the following: provided that it is due to Wind and Fire, then one can just prescribe Wind dispersing, Fire cooling and Dryness moisturizing purgative medicinals. Once the stool is regulated, Wind will be dispersed and Fire cooled and the symptoms typical of Dryness will also cease to occur. However, if this disease is encountered and purgative medicinals are incorrectly prescribed, the stool will only become harder after purgation.

Apparently, nobody has ever considered the fact that normally the stool does not flow out of the digestive tract, but rather it is pushed out with force. Now, if the body is paralysed on one side, and, due to the absence of *Qi*, neither arms nor legs can be moved and the tongue has no power to speak, how can *Qi* be provided to push out the stool? Thus we can infer that neither Wind nor Fire are involved, but rather that the *Qi* required to push out the stool is lacking. The longer stool stays in the large intestine without moving, the harder it will become.

DISCUSSION ON URINARY INCONTINENCE AND FREQUENT URINATION

It is often said that if urine flows in large quantities, frequently and involuntarily, then this is a

Fire or deficiency syndrome. How can they be differentiated?

To this, I can say the following: if the urethra hurts during urination and urine is passed merely in drips and is red at the same time, then this is a sign of a Fire syndrome; if an elderly person or someone of a weaker constitution passes a lot of clear urine without any pain, then this belongs to a deficiency syndrome; if urine leaks from the end of the urethra without the person being aware of it, then this is called involuntary urination; if urine flows even though the person tries to hold it, and they are unable to, then this is called incontinence. So much for diseases in relation to urine.

Hemiplegia accompanied by frequent and involuntary passing of large amounts of urine, or incontinence, but with no concomitant pain in the urethra, can be ascribed to a lack of control due to *Qi* deficiency.

DISCUSSION ON 'WHY MUFFLED SPEECH IS NOT A SIGN OF PHLEGM AND FIRE SYNDROME'

It is said: 'In former times, dysphasia, classically also known as 'muffled speech', was related to Phlegm or Fire inhibiting the root of the tongue. Is this explanation wrong?' I am convinced that no Phlegm or Fire syndrome comes into play here. There are two tubes in the middle of the tongue, which are connected to the *Qi* of the brain. These are *Qi* vessels through which *Qi* moves to and fro.[47] In this way the tongue can move and speech becomes possible.

If one half of the body is without *Qi* and cannot move, then one side of the tongue also lacks *Qi*, and the tongue cannot move fully, hence the affliction dysphasia, which develops in this way.

---

[47] It is of course very tempting to describe the *Qi* vessels as nerve fibres and the *Qi* flowing through them as chemo-electric energy for transmitting information. However, then *Qi* would have to be redefined for every new context. Therefore, in the more recent publications, *Qi* is usually not translated.

DISCUSSION ON TRISMUS AND TEETH GRINDING

It is said: 'How can lockjaw and teeth grinding exist if there is no Wind and Fire syndrome?' To this, I say the following: trismus on its own is the symptom 'lockjaw', teeth grinding on its own is the symptom 'teeth grinding'. Thus in the classics, two different symptoms were just thrown together. How can anyone be so negligent when they are two such different symptoms? Lockjaw presents in deficiency syndromes, teeth grinding in excess syndromes. Lockjaw is when the teeth are clenched and do not open; teeth grinding is the sound of teeth rubbing against each other.

Within the scope of *Shang Han* (Cold induced diseases), *Wen Bing* (febrile infectious diseases), various other syndromes and gynaecology, we see patients with lockjaw due to a deficiency syndrome and teeth grinding due to an excess syndrome. However, in hemiplegia we only see lockjaw, but definitely not teeth grinding. If the teeth are clenched together very tightly a sound similar to teeth grinding may be produced, but in fact this is not genuine teeth grinding, but rather points to a deficiency syndrome.

If there is no hemiplegia and no syndrome associated with it, but lockjaw suddenly presents, then this is related to pathogenic Wind, which blocks the channels so *Qi* cannot flow there. If medicinals that remove obstructions are given in such cases, the problem will be removed.

THE CONDITION BEFORE THE DISEASE (APOPLECTIC PRODROMAL SYMPTOMS)

Is it possible to diagnose a deficiency syndrome after *Yuan-Qi* has collapsed, but before hemiplegia occurs?

Of all the diseases, this is the one I have treated most often and know best. Every time I treat [stroke], I ask the patient what his condition was like before the disease. In most cases the patient says that he had a feeling of dizziness; some also say that all of a sudden their head felt very heavy; others suddenly experienced a rushing noise in the ears or a high-pitched buzzing noise like the sound of cicadas.

Some people describe how their lower eyelid twitched frequently, others tell how one of their eyes gradually became smaller,[48] or how their eyes suddenly started staring, or how something like a whirlwind twisted in front of their eyes.

Some say it felt as if a cold draught passed into their nose, others felt their upper lip twitching, or had the sensation of their lips being pulled together. Several say that during sleep they were drooling from the mouth; some patients with a usually good memory said that they had suddenly forgotten something or that when they were talking they suddenly did not know where the beginning and end of the sentence were, or they suddenly found themselves talking nonsense.

Some report that they felt short of breath for no reason, or a hand twitched or both hands trembled; or their ring finger arched by itself once a day, without the patient being able to straighten it, or their thumb moved by itself or their arm suddenly went numb.

Others say that their leg suddenly went numb, or their muscles suddenly twitched, and some say that time and again they had a sensation of cold in the tips of their fingers or below their toenails. Yet others say that it felt as if a cold draught was coming out from their knees, or their thigh suddenly became weak so they twisted outwards, whilst others gave an account of occasional cramps in the legs or in the toes, or said that during walking it felt as if their legs were hollow and empty like bent onion stalks.

Several say that they had a sensation in the middle of the chest as if air had got stuck, or as if their chest was suddenly hollow and their breath would get stuck, whilst others told of a sudden feeling of fear in the middle of the chest.

Some report that their neck suddenly got stiff or that when they were sleeping their body suddenly felt very heavy.

All these are signs for the collapse of *Yuan-Qi*; however, as there is no pain or itching, and no sweating or chills, and their daily life is not affected, these signs are usually ignored.

DISCUSSION ON HEMIPLEGIA IN CHILDREN

Can children also become affected with one-sided paralysis? I can report the following. There are a considerable number of children ranging from the age of 1 year to later childhood who will suddenly become affected with this disease. In most cases this is the consequence of *Shang Han*, *Wen Bing*, pox-like infectious diseases, dysentery-like diseases and so on. After the disease the *Yuan-Qi* is damaged, the complexion is cyanotic-pale, the hands and feet are gradually less able to move, and in severe cases there are cramps in the limbs. The limbs themselves are as stiff as clay. All this is the consequence of *Qi* not reaching the limbs. Formerly, it was treated as Wind syndrome because there was insufficient experience of this disease.

THEORY OF PARALYSIS AND ATROPHY

When it is said that *Yuan-Qi* flowing together to one side from the left and right causes one-sided paralysis, could it not also arise from *Qi* flowing together from above and below?

I can explain it as follows: if one half of *Yuan-Qi* collapses and 50% of *Qi* is lacking in the lower body half, then after *Qi* has gone a collapse must take place somewhere. If *Qi* suddenly converges in the upper half of the body, then it will not be able to supply the lower part and both legs will become paralysed and suffer atrophy.

The classics relate this atrophy syndrome solely to Damp-Heat in the Stomach channel, which steams upwards and causes Heat in the Lung, and they explain that if the lung leaves are damaged due to Heat, then the skin and pores wither and atrophy will take its course. According to this theory one should prescribe cooling and purgative formulas. However, whenever *I* talk about cooling and purgative formulas, I am thinking about the treatment of painful *Bi* syndrome[49] due to Damp and Heat, rather than about the treatment of paralysis and atrophy of the legs, as such formulas are totally unsuitable here.

---

[48] This probably means that the eyelid gradually closed.

[49] See Glossary.

Does nobody realize that although painful *Bi* syndromes may eventually lead to paralysis of the legs after a long period of time, they nevertheless continue to be painful after the paralysis? The atrophy syndrome which we are discussing here causes the legs to become paralysed suddenly, but from start to finish there is no pain involved at all. If the cause of the disease and its consequences are not clearly distinguished, and if deficiency and excess syndromes are confused, surely this will lead to problems for ensuing ages?

BU YANG HUAN WU TANG (FIVE TENTH DECOCTION OR YANG TONIFYING FULL RECOVERY DECOCTION)[50]

This formula is used for hemiplegia, facial paralysis, dysphagia, uncontrollable drooling, dry and hard stool, polyuria and urinary incontinence.

Huang Qi 160 g	*Dang Gui* 9 g
Rx. Astragali	Rx. Angelicae Sin.
Chi Shao 6 g	*Di Long* 4 g
Rx. Paeoniae Rubrae	Lumbricus
Tao Ren 4 g	*Hong Hua* 4 g
Se. Persicae	Fl. Carthami
Chuan Xiong 4 g	
Rx. Ligustici Wallichii	

At the onset of hemiplegia, 4 g of *Fang Feng* (Ledebouriella) need to be added to these ingredients, which can be discontinued after 4–5 prescriptions. If the patient is alarmed on the basis of reports that the dosage of Astragalus could be too high, then one should let him have his way and prescribe only 40–80 g at first. Later on, the dosage can be gradually increased to 160 g and if the effect still fails to be satisfactory, it can even be increased to 160 g twice daily, but only for 5–6 days; after that return to one dose once a day.

If the condition has been present for several months and previous physicians using classical methods prescribed too many cooling medicinals, then 16 g of *Fu Zi* (Aconite) can be prescribed. If too many Wind dispersing medicinals were previously prescribed, then one may add 16–20 g of *Dang Shen*. If no other medicinals were taken, then one should not add any of this.

This formula may be an excellent method of treatment, but if the disease has been present for a long time, so that *Qi* has collapsed and there are symptoms such as a very loose-hanging arm and shoulder with spasms and inability to straighten the limbs, an ankle that is twisted outwards, or aphasia with inability to speak but a single word, then this signifies that the disease cannot be cured completely. Although a full recovery may not be possible, a prescription of this formula can prevent exacerbation.

Even if the patient has fully recovered, the intake should not be discontinued, and it should not be interrupted for a few days or taken irregularly. This is because once the intake has been interrupted, it is to be feared that syndromes of *Qi* collapse will appear again. With regard to Astragalus (*Huang Qi*), its place of origin does not play a role; as the effect is the same, all varieties of Astragalus may be used.

FORMULA RHYME

After Wind-stroke, this restores,	= For post-apoplectic loss of one body half
Skilfully supplementing *Yang*,	= the *Yang* supplementing decoction recovers
One-six-zero Astragalus,	= it contains 160 g *Huang Qi*, and
6 grams red peony plus	= 6 g *Chi Shao* and
Dang Gui 9, but Lumbricus,	= 9 g *Dang Gui*, but only 4 g of: *Di Long*,
Chuanxiong-peach, Carthamus,	= *Chuan Xiong*, *Tao Ren* and *Hong Hua*
4 grams each and there, it works:	= 4 g each only
Hemiplegia be gone!	= which can treat hemiplegia.

The literal translation of the rhyme is:

Bu Yang Huan Wu Tang, Chi Shao, Xiong,
Dang Gui, open the channels with *Di Long,*
4 *liang* of *Huang Qi* main medicinal,
Blood stagnation, standstill take *Tao Hong.*

---

[50] Literally *Yang* supplementing, the (lacking) five returning decoction. Wang explains hemiplegia as being due to five of the ten parts of *Qi* being missing, which explains the name.

ON THE FEBRILE INFECTIOUS DISEASES WITH DIARRHOEA AND VOMITING CAUSING CONVULSIONS

Diarrhoea and vomiting with convulsions was known as cholera in former times. The imperial health authority of the Song dynasty established so-called official formulas, including *Huo Xiang Zheng Qi San* (Patchouli *Qi* Rectifying Powder), in order to combat this disease. In a disease where the pathogenic *Qi* damages the Vital *Qi* (*Zheng Qi*), if one incorrectly uses medicinals that diminish Vital *Qi*, does this not mean that one shames the good name of the imperial health authority?[51]

In the year 1821 of our current dynasty, an epidemic of febrile infectious diseases (*Wen Du*) broke out, and in many provinces there were sick people with diarrhoea, vomiting and convulsions. It was particularly serious in the capital. So many people were affected that the government provided money for the poor, who had no means to afford a funeral, to buy coffins; within the space of one month this had cost 100 000 gold bars.

The physicians of this period say they observed that Ginseng (*Ren Shen*), Rhizoma Atractylodes Macrocephalae (*Bai Zhu*), Ginger (*Jiang*) and Tuber Aconiti Sinensis (*Fu Zi*) were effective, so they conveniently concluded that *Yin*-Cold was the cause. Other physicians had success using the 'Three Yellows'[52] (*Huang Qin, Huang Lian, Huang Bai*) and Fructus Gardeniae (*Zhi Zi*), so they said the disease was a Fire syndrome.

I said that it was neither Heat nor Cold, as women and men, old and young were all affected, and great numbers of people became ill at the same time, so it must have been an infectious epidemic. I was asked the question why, if it was an infectious epidemic, did the hot medicinals Ginger and Aconite have the same good effect as the cold medicinals Radix Scutellaria and Rhizoma Coptidis (*Huang Qin* and *Huang Lian*)? I explained that Scutellaria and Coptidis show an effect at the beginning, when the person still has a strong defence against the epidemic, whereas the hot medicinals Ginger and Aconite are effective when the sick person's *Qi* is already weakened.

Some people asked me about a few cases where neither Scutellaria and Coptidis, nor Ginger and Aconite were effective; on the contrary, the illness became worse. What could be done in those cases? My advice was to try needling pricking,[53] which will be helpful because the blood is completely dark-purple, so how could it be anything other than excessive Heat in the Blood due to an infectious epidemic?

The infection enters the breathing vessels via the mouth or nose; from there it reaches the Blood vessels, where it stagnates and coagulates *Qi* and Blood, and thus it blocks the *fluid gate* (*Jin Men*); thus fluid cannot be separated any more and will exit upwards in the form of vomiting or downwards as diarrhoea.

First the blood vessel in the elbow crease is punctured and the dark-purple blood is allowed to come out. In this way the disease toxin is expelled together with the blood and the disease is cured.

Question: which acupuncture point is needled? Please explain in detail.

Answer: I am also proficient in acupuncture, so there is no doubt that this is the point *Chi Ze* (LU 5). The human body is permeated everywhere by *Qi* vessels (channels) and blood vessels. The acupuncture point *Chi Ze* (LU 5) is surrounded by numerous vessels, which all bleed when punctured, achieving the desired effect. Needle pricking above and below *Chi Ze* will also lead to success.

All in all, needle pricking in this way will achieve a recovery in every case, provided that the disease is caused by Wind, Fire and excess syn-

---

[51] Wang criticizes the prescription of medicinals for severe infections similar to cholera that exhaust the patient, i.e. reduce his Vital *Qi*, (though otherwise, in case of e.g. summer diarrhoea, these are excellent). The formula relieves the exterior (*Biao*), a method which may also be described as attacking (*Gong Fa*). However, the main effect of this formula is drying pathogenic Dampness with warm, drying, but also *Qi* regulating medicinals. According to TCM theory, this will also have a reducing effect on *Qi*, which should be avoided in patients already weakened by a severe infection.

[52] *Huang* means yellow. As these three medicinals are often used together they are often called the 'Three Yellows'.

[53] This is not to be understood as bloodletting in the Western medical sense, but rather as *Fang Xue*, a method applied in acupuncture where only a few drops of blood are drawn from specific acupuncture points.

dromes. However, if there is a deficiency syndrome, it will worsen every time needle pricking is employed. This is a secret of the acupuncturists, which on the whole they are unwilling to discuss.

This acupuncture method is very practical in very urgent cases. By needling and prescribing *Jie Du Huo Xue Tang* (Detoxifying, Blood Invigorating Decoction) simultaneously, Blood is invigorated and at the same time the toxin is expelled. There are hardly any patients for whom this method would not achieve a recovery.

This disease develops very quickly and thus damages *Yuan-Qi* extremely rapidly; after one and a half days the patient's life is already in danger. After one or two hours of diarrhoea and vomiting, or after half a day when leg spasms or arm spasms can be observed, *Qi* in the legs and, *Qi* in the arms are reduced respectively. If the eyes (being dehydrated) have sunk and the patient is streaming sweat, then in most cases the limbs are freezing cold. Here, cooling medicinals would be harmful, so I have developed the effective formula *Jie Du Huo Xue Tang* (Detoxifying, Blood Invigorating Decoction).

In this disease, if the mouth is dry with a dry tongue and there is a great thirst for cool drinks, with several bowls of water being drunk every hour, then without further hesitation *Ji Qiu Hui Yang Tang* (Emergency Yang Recovery Decoction) can be used, which has a life-saving effect. This method is virtually unknown amongst mediocre physicians.

FORMULA RHYME

Detox decoction invigorates Blood	= Detoxifying, Blood Invigorating Decoction
for vomiting and diarrhoea it does well	= for acute febrile vomiting and diarrhoea
three two peach, citrus four	= contains 32 g *Tao Ren*, 4 g *Zhi Ke*,
Rehmannia, Saffron, twenty here,	= 20 g each of *Sheng Di* and *Hong Hua*
Red peony, Bupleurum	= 12 g each of *Chi Shao* and *Chai Hu*
Twelve; but Forsythia	= but *Lian Qiao* and
Angelica, Liquorice, Pueraria	= *Dan Gui*, *Gan Cao*, *Ge Gen*
These four eight each that's for sure.	= of these four medicinals 8 g each.

The literal translation of the rhyme is:

Jie Du Huo Xue: Forsythia, Persica
Carthamus, Dang Gui, Citrus, Pueraria, Paenoia
Bupleurum, Glycyrrhiza as well as Rehmannia
In diarrhoea and vomiting, decocted is a good formula.

This formula is used at the onset of diarrhoea and vomiting. If heavy sweating, cold limbs and sunken eyes are already apparent, then it must *not* be used; instead, use the following formula.

JIE DU HUO XUE TANG (DETOXIFYING, BLOOD INVIGORATING DECOCTION)

Lian Qiao 8 g Fr. Forsythia	*Ge Gen* 8 g Rx. Puerariae
Chai Hu 12 g Rx. Bupleuri	*Dang Gui* 8 g Rx. Angelicae Sin.
Sheng Di Huang 20 g Rx. Rehmanniae	*Chi Shao* 12 g Rx. Paeoniae Rubrae
Tao Ren 32 g Se. Persicae	*Hong Hua* 20 g Fl. Carthami
Zhi Ke 4 g Pc. Citri Aurantii	*Gan Cao* 8 g Rx. Glycyrrhizae

JI QIU HUI YANG TANG (EMERGENCY YANG RECOVERY DECOCTION)

This formula must be used in cases of diarrhoea and vomiting with convulsions, cold body and pronounced sweating, even if the patient has a great thirst and wants to consume lots of cold drinks.[54]

---

[54] Wang means that when the patient desires cold most physicians will conclude that there is Heat in the body and therefore they will not risk prescribing the hottest of all drugs, *Fu Zi* (Radix Aconiti carmichaeli). In respect to modern pharmacology however, this method is justifiable.

Fu Zi 32 g
Rx. Aconiti

Gan Jiang 16 g
Rh. Zingiberis

Bai Zhu 16 g
Rh. Atractylodes M.

Gan Cao 12 g
Rx. Glycyrrhizae

Tao Ren 8 g
Se. Persicae

Ren Shen or Dang Shen 8 g
Rx. Ginseng or
    Codonopsis[55]

Hong Hua 8 g
Fl. Carthami

FORMULA RHYME

Emergency decoction for vomiting and diarrhoea	= Emergency Yang Recovery Decoction
Dehydration and convulsions,	= for vomiting and diarrhoea with dehydration and convulsions,
Of Aconite take three two grams,	= Take 32 g of Fu Zi
Peach, Ginseng and Saffron,	= of Tao Ren, Ren Shen and Hong Hua
Eight each; but twice as much	= take 8 g each; but take 2 × 8, thus 16 g of
Of ginger and Atractylodes,	= Gan Jiang and Bai Zhu
Finally, take 12 grams of Liquorice	= finally take 12 g of Gan Cao
This warms the limbs, strengthens Blood.	= this warms cold limbs due to shock and invigorates Blood

The indications for Ji Qiu Hui Yang Tang (Emergency Yang Recovery Decoction) and Jie Du Huo Xue Tang (Detoxifying, Blood Invigorating Decoction) must be distinguished *precisely*, then they cannot fail in their effect. Therefore, caution is advised.

---

[55] In the original version, Radix Codonopsis is mentioned; however, this herb was commonly used to replace the more expensive Ginseng, even in the nineteenth century. If available, in an emergency it is recommended to use Ginseng instead, as earlier formulas used to combine Ginseng and Aconite, especially for shock and cold limbs. Such as Shen Fu Tang, Si Ni Jia Ren Shen Tang and Hui Yang Qiu Ji Tang.

DISCUSSION ON 'WHY WIND-CONVULSION[56] IN INFANTS IS NOT WIND SYNDROME'

Nowadays, so-called Wind-convulsion is treated with relatively little success. However, this is not the fault of our contemporaries, but due to the fact that the classical formulas concerning this syndrome lead to false conclusions. There are countless examples of such diseases where the classical formulas were merely deduced from previous theories about the diseases, and in this way have led to confusion. This also accounts for the name 'Wind-convulsion', where the word 'Wind' is particularly misleading.

Furthermore, there is the term 'slow Wind shock', which is derived from the fact that most of these syndromes are caused by Shang Han, Wen Bing, pox-like diseases, diarrhoea and vomiting and so on and can lead to convulsions in the case of prolonged duration of the disease. When these three words in a row 'slow Wind shock' are read as a term, they become all the more ridiculous. Apart from being contradictory, on closer inspection they also demonstrate that the cause of the disease was completely unknown.

If this was a genuine Wind syndrome with a person being attacked by pathogenic Wind, it would have to pass into the channels via the skin. In addition, there should be visible symptoms where the disease moves from the exterior (Biao, surface) to the interior (Li).

Why did people in former times have to ascribe each and every superficial symptom to Wind, even if no exterior pathogenic factors were detectable, eventually writing about them and composing formulas? The reason for ascribing this disease to Wind is that in an attack there are symptoms such as stiff neck and arched back, eyes turned upwards, lockjaw with drooling, a 'phlegmy' rattling sound in the throat and fainting. To ascribe

---

[56] The term Chou Feng (translated here as Wind-convulsion, also called Chi Zong) stands for clonic convulsions of the limbs, also occurring in epilepsy and tetanus as a result of febrile infectious diseases. The following paragraph mainly refers to tetanus, especially in children.

this to Wind stroke is certainly down to a lack of attention.

Was it completely unheard of that stiff neck and back and cramps of the limbs with clenched fists are related to *Qi* deficiency with loss of control over the limbs? Eyes turned upwards and lockjaw also belong to *Qi* deficiency, where the *Qi* does not reach the head. Drooling with bubbles in the front of the mouth is due to deficiency of *Qi* which is thus unable to consolidate the fluids, and the rattling sound in the throat is not due to Phlegm but also to *Qi* deficiency, *Qi* being unable to complete its circulation and failing to return to its origin.

Anyone who does not understand this explanation should have a look at elderly patients with protracted disease in the final stage. They also have a stiff neck and heaviness of the body, protruding eyes or mouth cramps with drooling, phlegmy rattling breathing or cold streaming sweat, all of which are signs for *Qi* becoming depleted – clearly and plainly signs of *Qi* deficiency.

When *Yuan-Qi* is so empty and unable to supply the blood vessels sufficiently, Blood will lack the driving force of *Qi*; it becomes stagnant and Blood stasis develops. That is why it is wrong to apply Wind dispersing and Fire cooling formulas in this Blood stasis syndrome due to *Qi* deficiency. If Wind dispersing medicinals were used where no Wind syndrome is present, one would instead disperse *Qi*; if Fire cooling medicinals were used where no Fire syndrome is present, the cold nature of the medicinals would cause the Blood to stagnate further. In general, when attacking and reducing formulas are used, *Qi* is diminished and Blood is damaged. How can there be any hope for life under these circumstances?

But let us return to the beginning: the deadly outcome of this disease is not the physicians' fault, but rather the patients die because of those irresponsible authors. Specialists in paediatric diseases who often get to see this disease do not even attempt to cause further damage. Because they know about the classical formulas' inefficacy, they would rather not treat these cases. There are also some excellent physicians who when diagnosing the children already know in advance that a Wind-convulsion syndrome will develop. Even if they cannot do anything about it, at least they inform the relatives about the true state of the disease, i.e. that the development of a Wind-convulsion must be feared.

But how can such an attack be anticipated? In general, before the Wind-convulsion attack occurs, there will be evidence for the existence of a Wind-convulsion syndrome, such as sunken fontanelles, unconscious state of sleep with half-opened eyes, tongue movements, absence of crying or crying with no tears, flaring of the nose, phlegmy rattling in the throat, drooping head which cannot be lifted, closed mouth, muteness, cold arms and legs, outpouring of frothy saliva, barrel chest, panting with shortness of breath, pale, cyanotic complexion, streaming sweat, no desire to be nursed, greenish stool, abdominal noises, cough and diarrhoea, muscle twitching. All these are prodromal symptoms of Wind-convulsion. These twenty symptoms do not all have to present together, but if a few of them occur, one knows that Wind-convulsion will follow.

The children who can be cured and those who cannot are listed next, followed by the formula to be used. Children who have protruding eyes where the white of the eye is visible, who have no appetite and do not cry, and who have a phlegmy rattling noise in the throat and panting, can be healed, although the disease is serious. In those cases where the forehead is grey, the testes are pulled upwards, and some have a weak and fine pulse,[57] while others do not have a pulse, no treatment is possible, although the disease appears uncomplicated.

KE BAO LI SU TANG (GUARANTEED RESUSCITATION DECOCTION)

This formula is effective in all children who have *Qi* deficiency syndromes after a protracted disease duration of Cold induced diseases (*Shang Han*), febrile infectious diseases (*Wen Yi*), pox- or measles-like diseases, diarrhoea and vomiting and so on. Symptoms include, for example, cramps in the limbs, stiff neck or opisthotonus, eyes turned

---

57 Literally *Mai Wei Xi*, in Porkert: pulsus evanescens et minutus.

upward, outpouring of frothy saliva and dead faint.

Huang Qi 60 g[58] Rx. Astragali	*Dang Shen/Ren Shen* 12 g Rx. Codonopsis/Ginseng
Bai Zhu 8 g Rh. Atractylodes M.	*Dang Gui* 8 g Rx. Angelicae
Bai Shao 8 g Rx. Paeoniae Lactiflorae	*Suan Zao Ren* 12 g Se. Zizyphi Spinosae
Gou Qi Zi 8 g Fr. Lycii	*Gan Cao* 8 g Rx. Glycyrrhizae
Bu Gu Zhi 4 g Fr. Psoralea	*Shan Zhu Yu* 4 g Fr. Corni

Add one walnut, ground together with the shell (*He Tao*).

For 4-year-olds this dose is divided into two parts (one in the morning and one in the evening); for 2-year-olds one half of the dose is divided into two parts and administered daily; for 1-year-olds a third of the dose is divided into two parts and administered daily; for children who are only a few months old a fourth of the dose is divided in two parts and administered daily.

These dosages are merely suggestions. When I prescribe this formula, it often happens that cramps cease to occur after a few preparations, but then it is imperative to tell the parents to carry on with the formula. On must not stop under any circumstances once the cramps have ceased, but continue to give several more preparations until there is enough *Qi*; then the formula may be discontinued.

FORMULA RHYME

Febrile convulsions in children: take	= For clonic convulsions in children after febrile infections
Guaranteed resuscitation elixir!	= we recommend *Ke Bao* *Li Su Tang*

---

58 In a Shanghai publication of this book 2.5 instead of 1.5 *liang* (25 instead of 15 *qian*) are mentioned. One *qian* (see Glossary) is the equivalent of 3.125 g, which I (the author) would round up to 4 g, which would mean 100 g instead of 60 g of Astragalus.

60 grams Astragalus,
Ginseng,
    sour-Zizyphus
	= take 60 g *Huang Qi*
	= of *Ren Shen* and *Suan*
	    Zao Ren

Twelve of these, but
    four Fructus
Psoralea and Cornus,
	= 12 g each, then 4 g of
	
	= *Bu Gu Zhi* and
	    Shan Zhu Yu

Eight Liquorice,
    Angelica, Lycii
Atractylodes, Peony,
Both white; a final
    addition
Ground finely,
    walnut.
	= 8 g each of *Gan Cao*,
	    Dang Gui, *Gou Qi Zi*,
	= *Bai Zhu* and *Bai Shao*
	= (not to confuse with
	    Cang Zhu and *Chi Shao*)
	= finally add a whole
	    walnut with the shell,
	    ground.

The Literal translation of the rhyme is:

Guaranteed quickly resuscitating Psoralea,
Atractylodes, Angelica, Paeonia, Ginseng, Astragalus, Liquorice,
Cornus, Lycium cooked in water,
One walnut with shell, pounded.

DISCUSSION ON 'WHY POX-DISEASES ARE NOT FOETAL TOXINS'

There have been countless books and formulas from the Han dynasty until the present day about infectious children's diseases with exanthema (*Dou Zhen*, pox and measles). Most of these merely differentiated between favourable, dangerous and unfavourable cases, so they categorized them into minor and major disease with moribund and recovering patients. But nobody explained the causes of these diseases. Therefore, physicians who came afterwards kept to *Bao Yuan Tang* (Origin Protecting Decoction) with Astragalus and Ginseng, or *Gui Zong Tang* with radish root and calcium sulphate, or *Jie Du Tang* with Rhinoceros horn and Coptis,[59] but the medicinals used for this single disease had different characteristics.

In favourable and less serious cases, the pox was examined to see if the child was strong or weak, in order to assess whether draining or

---

59 The meaning of these formulas: *Bao Yuan Tang* is Origin Protecting Decoction, *Gui Zong Tang* is Return to Origin Decoction, *Jie Du Tang* is Detoxifying Decoction.

strengthening, cooling or cold methods would be suitable. In this way, a recovery could be expected.

Only for the severely ill was there no adequate formula. Then it was said, 'Well, that's just fate', just because the origin of the pox was unknown. But one may counter: if the origin of the pox was unknown in those times, why were they still able to accurately predict an unfavourable prognosis?

My answer goes as follows: it was not because they knew the cause of the disease, but rather because they had sufficient experience gained from frequently treating pox to predict when exanthemas would appear, what shape they would have and what colour, which concomitant symptoms would present, when treatment would not help, and, finally, when an unfavourable outcome was imminent. Thus they also knew after how many days of the extreme stages of the disease death would occur. How could it be that they knew the cause of the disease, but were unable to apply any formula for it?

So I was asked: going by what you say, does this mean that you can even treat the most severe cases of pox? I answered as follows. With regard to the less serious cases, they are easy to treat, so I will not mention them any further. With regard to the severe cases, the question is rather: if the cause of the disease is known, and one is able to make a clear diagnosis (syndrome differentiation), why should one not be able to treat it?

These are some of the symptoms: restlessness; exanthemas that barely surface and are distributed over the whole body, that are fine and dense like silkworm cocoons, smooth like snakeskin, and appear before the fever; and small dark-purple dots, coalescing densely without demarcation, with grey-whitish gaps. Other symptoms are light-headedness, stiff mouth and neck, swollen lymph nodes of the neck, but with the skin not swollen, fluid-filled vesicles all over the body, blisters that do not swell yet contain a thick fluid, no formation of pustules, but scarring. There may also be persistent cramps, light blood flow from all body orifices, cough and loss of voice, choking on every drink, 6–7 days itching of the skin with bleeding when scratched, 7–8 days of diarrhoea, and no appetite. Finally, in the most dangerous stage, the head droops, the legs cannot be held straight, the eyes turn upwards, are opisthotonos

and other unfavourable signs are present. But it is possible to cure these cases.

At the beginning of the diagnosis one must clearly differentiate deficiency and excess for there to be hope of saving the person's life. When the principles are clear, we can compensate for the inadequacies of our predecessors, and the problems of present-day people can be solved. However, when the principles are not clear, one may assess these problems incorrectly and state that I am talking nonsense. But it is not me who is talking nonsense, as I am familiar with the causes of pox.

Those who do not understand the causes always theorize that pox belongs with the foetal toxins.[60] Furthermore, they say that there was no pox before the Han dynasty (206 BC–220 AD). If the cause of pox is foetal toxin, then it follows that people before the Han dynasty did not originate from mothers and fathers.

This is the most ridiculous theory. Assuming it refers to the classical theory according to which the so-called foetal toxin is stored in the organs, why do the organs not become ill before the pox appears? Somewhere else it is mentioned that foetal toxin is stored in the skin and muscles. So why does the skin not have purulent pustules before the pox appears?

Yet others say that foetal toxin is stored in the bone and marrow, and it would then, sometimes as a result of fright occasioned by a fall, or after a cold due to undernourishment, become stimulated and appear in the form of pox. If this is to be believed, then it is their own fault that people become ill, because they are negligent, and are responsible for own their fright, fall, cold or poor diet.

When we think this over clearly, it becomes apparent that when pox emerges it's not just one person who becomes ill, but at the very least an area is affected or, in the worst case, several provinces. So, is it possible that the people of

---

[60] Foetal toxin can have two meanings: (1) congenital syphilis and (2) a pathogenic factor that is linked to the foetus. In most cases this is a toxin caused by Heat during pregnancy, which after delivery leads to the development of exanthematous skin diseases in the child.

several provinces were all negligent at the same time? Such a theory does not make sense.

According to the physicians who vaccinate against pox,[61] there is not one single case following vaccination, regardless of whether a large or small number of people were vaccinated, that does not run smoothly. If foetal toxin was the cause of pox, and since there are both severe and mild cases, then those cases with a lot of toxin should turn out to be correspondingly dangerous; so how could it be possible then that there is not a single case that does not run smoothly?

When we look at it this way, it is incomprehensible that we cannot separate ourselves from these two words, 'foetal toxin'. Didn't anybody know that pox diseases are not foetal toxins, but rather that they are present in the foetus within the blood in the form of 'impure *Qi*' (virus)?

Developing from a drop of sperm, a child grows inside the womb, and all his organs and limbs arise from the mother's blood. Thus, the blood of the foetus contains impure *Qi*, which can also be found in the blood after birth. This gets into contact with the naturally present impure *Qi* of a febrile disease (*Wen Yi*). This latter reaches the airways via the mouth and nose; from the airways it is passed into the blood vessels, where it meets the local impure *Qi*, and together they reach back into the skin.

Since the colour (of the toxin) is red as in flowers, these pox diseases are also called 'flower heaven disease'; because of their bean-like shape they are called 'bean pox'.

In summary, if there is a mild infection with a febrile infectious disease (*Wen Yi*), this will then come out in the skin eruptions (exanthema). After the exanthema the prognosis is good. If the infec-

tion with the febrile infectious disease is severe, it will remain in the interior and is not expelled with the pox exanthema. This indicates danger. If the infection with the febrile infectious disease is extremely severe, it will generate internal Heat pathogens in the Blood and make the blood coagulate. Coagulated blood is purple, and necrotic blood is black. How the pathology is identified depends on whether there is purple or black blood with the pox.

Necrotic blood clogs the vessels, so the toxins of the febrile infection cannot be expelled outwards via the skin, and therefore they attack the organs in the interior. When the organs are irritated by the Heat-toxin, a corresponding and unfavourable pathology will develop in each organ.

As the textbooks on the subject describe it, it is precisely this idea of an unfavourable pathology of pox in a particular channel that disregards the fact that if a *particular channel* shows signs of pox, then it must be influenced by febrile infectious disease (*Wen Bing*) in the stage of blood (Xue) – which is present in the *whole* body. The good or bad prognosis of pox is therefore related to the severity of the febrile infectious disease (*Wen Bing*).

Thus the most important issue in treating pox is the treatment of the febrile infectious disease. If this is not treated, the disease will be fatal even with little exanthema; whereas if the febrile infection is removed, life will be in no danger, in spite of widespread exanthema.

The textbooks on pox only mention treatment of foetal toxin. Treatment of the infection is unknown. In cases where there *is* such knowledge, then it is not known that the source of the infectious toxin is in the Blood. Now, if mild and severe infection are clearly differentiated, likewise stasis or flow of Blood, excess or deficiency of *Qi*, then in no time at all the treatment becomes quite simple. If this crucial point is known, then the problem is solved.

---

[61] Immunization with the pox virus has been known in China since 600 BC. At that time, the infectious agent was inoculated through the mucous membranes of the nose. For centuries, other diseases were also successfully vaccinated against. In his book *'Zhou Hou Lüe Ji Fang'* (*Practical Formulas for Emergencies*, Chapter 7, clause 54), Ge Hong (281–341 AD) recommends this for a rabies infection due to a dog bite: 'The dog is brought back and killed, its brain taken out and put on the wound. After this, the disease will not break out again.' Because the theoretical basis for immunization was still lacking, this was just regarded as another, not always successful method.

DISCUSSION ON 'WHY PUS INSIDE PUSTULES IS NOT BLOOD'

Initially, the pox pustules are red; after 5–6 days a clear fluid forms, which later on turns milky, then transforms into yellowish pus and eventually scars. In ancient times, pus secretions were said to be transformed Blood. But if this is transformed Blood, then red must be able to turn itself white. So, if we take a bowl of blood and test this by adding vitriol or by cooking it, does it first become like clear water, then white, milky and turbid fluid or purulent yellow?

The impure *Qi* of pox inside the blood vessels now meets the impure *Qi* of the febrile infectious disease from the outside, which reaches the airways via the mouth and nose, and from there enters the blood vessels. Now, if the impure *Qi* and the Blood inside the blood vessels together with fluids inside the *Qi* vessels[62] are pushed through the pores towards the outside, reddish round skin lesions form. About 5 or 6 days later, Blood returns from the pox blisters to the blood vessels. What remains in the blisters is the impure *Qi* fluid, which is clear and is known as clear secretion. When this clear secretion is heated by the febrile infectious toxin (*Wen Du*), it will become thick and whitish. Then it is called white secretion. When this white secretion is heated further, it will thicken even more and become turbid. This is then called turbid secretion. When heated further the turbid secretion becomes tenacious like the pus inside ulcers, then it's called yellow pus. If it continues to be heated, this yellow pus will become dry and form scars.

If the secretion inside the pustules fails to regress, then this is due to the fact that Blood is not flowing back into the vessels; and the Blood isn't flowing back into the vessels because the infectious toxin continues to generate febrile Heat in the vessels, so the Blood coagulates and the passages are clogged up. Once the Blood stasis in the vessels is removed, one need not fear a delayed regression of the secretions in the pustules.

DISCUSSION ON CHOKING WHEN DRINKING LIQUIDS IN POX DISEASE

If the disease had been present for a few days and the patient had always choked when drinking, it was said in ancient times that this was related to Heat-toxin blocking the throat and pharynx, but this was not treated. However, the left and right *Qi* gates (common carotid arteries) were unknown.

Behind the tongue is the pharynx, where the windpipe begins, and behind the pharynx is the gorge, where the gullet begins. In between, in front of the gorge and behind the pharynx, in two spaces arched inwards, lie two tubes, the left *Qi* gate and the right *Qi* gate. Behind the root of the tongue is a light flap, about the size of a coin: it is called the epiglottis and covers the entire opening of the windpipe. To the left and right lie the upper openings of the *Qi* gates.[63]

When someone swallows food or drink, these need to be pushed down by the tongue, so that the epiglottis closes the windpipe and the *Qi* gates. Then food can pass the windpipe and *Qi* gates, and so reach the gullet.

It can be observed how, during a meal, if someone who has food or drink already in his throat, which has not yet reached the pharynx, gives a sudden short laugh with his mouth closed, air will shoot forth, the epiglottis opens and either a few rice grains or a few drops of water slip into the *Qi* gates and are propelled out of the nose. This is the pathology described above.

When the infectious toxin produces febrile Heat, Blood in the epiglottis will coagulate, so it cannot cover the *Qi* gates. As soon as water gets into these, one chokes. Food cannot be swallowed as the tiny gaps only allow water to pass, but will not let chunky bits of food penetrate, so swallowing does not take place. Once Blood stasis in the epiglottis is removed, the choking will quickly cease.

DISCUSSION ON THE ITCHING OF PUSTULES AFTER SEVERAL DAYS

In patients with pox whose pustules are very itchy, one must first differentiate skin and flesh.

---

[62] These fluids inside the *Qi* vessels could be lymph inside the lymph vessels, as channels are probably not implied here.

[63] As the carotid arteries do not open into the middle of the throat, and as Wang talks about the upper openings (*Shang Kou*), it can be concluded that he studied this part of anatomy on the torso of decapitated people, to which he had had access, as described earlier in the text.

Pi-skin is the upper skin, *Fu*-skin is the deeper skin tissue. If the two are not clearly differentiated, how can the cause of itching in pox pustules be recognized?

When someone has burns or scalds, a blister may form, but it is as thin as paper. This comes from the *Pi*-skin (epidermis). Below the *Pi*-skin there is a thick layer above the flesh, which is the *Fu*-skin (dermis).

After about 6 or 7 days of pox, the infectious toxins, the impure *Qi* and the fluids, all lying above the *Fu*-skin, reach into the *Pi*-skin. *Zheng Qi* is deficient in the pox pustules; it has no power to move the secretion of the pustules, transform them into pus and dry them out. The infectious toxin can neither get outside through the *Pi*-skin nor can it return inwards into the *Fu*-skin. Thus, it lies between the *Pi* and *Fu* and as a result produces itching.

The medical establishment holds in high regard the comments of the '*Su Wen*' (*The Yellow Emperor's Classic*, Simple Questions), where it is said: 'Pain and itching in inflammations is always related to Fire pathogen.' Accordingly they use Heat cooling and cold medicinals, which weaken the person's own *Qi*. With this treatment, whether the itching stops or not, the Stomach *Qi* is always weakened. However, when *Qi* tonifying medicinals are used, *Qi* will be strengthened, but Blood will stagnate as a result. When there is Blood stasis, *Qi* will be even less able to reach the skin. In such cases, both *Qi* tonifying and Blood stasis breaking formulas need to be used to remove obstructions from the vessels. Once *Qi* can get directly to the skin, no further medicinal is necessary and the itching stops.

TONG JING ZHU YU TANG (ANTI-STASIS EXANTHEMA DECOCTION)

This formula can be used for densely distributed pox exanthema, covered or surfacing, but also for fine and pointed pustules on the whole body, which become flat platelets, or with interjacent measles-like or spotted exanthema or for blisters filled with secretions. The colour can be purple, dark or blackish. Concomitant symptoms can be an urge to vomit, irritability, insomnia at night and by day as well as unfavourable signs and symptoms of every kind.

These symptoms are a result of the impeded Blood in the blood vessels due to Blood stasis, and thus they all indicate this syndrome. The medicinals in this formula are neither too cold nor too hot; their action is neither too attacking nor too purging. It is truly a good formula.

Tao Ren 32 g Se. Persicae	*Hong Hua* 16 g Fl. Carthami
Chi Shao 12 g Rx. Paeoniae Rubrae	*Chuan Shan Jia* 16 g Squama Manitis
Zao Jiao Ci 24 g Spina Gleditsiae Sin.	*Lian Qiao* 12 g Fr. Forsythia
Di Long Lumbricus	*Chai Hu* 4 g Rx. Bupleuri
She Xiang 0.3 g Moschus	*Tong Jing Hiu Yu Tong* *Di Long* 9 g

If the stool is also very dry, 8 g of Rhizoma Rhei (*Da Huang*) needs to be added in the last 2–5 minutes of decocting, but not if the stool is normal. After several days, when blisters with clear or white secretions can be seen, Moschus (*She Xiang*) must be omitted and replaced with 20 g of Astragalus (*Huang Qi*), and the amount of Squama Manitis (*Chuan Shan Jia*) and Spina Gleditsiae (*Zao Jiao Ci*) should be reduced by half. Eventually, after 7–8 days, the amount of Semen Persica (*Tao Ren*) and Flos Carthami (*Hong Hua*) should also be reduced by half, and 32 g of Astragalus (*Huang Qi*) may be used.

In 4- to 5-year-olds this formula is valid as it stands. For children who are only 1–2 years old, it can be halved. But if the children are 8 or 9 years old, another half of the amount specified above may be added.

The literal translation of the rhyme is:

Vessels [made] penetrable by Manitis, Gleditsia, Moschus, Lumbricus,
Anti-stasis [effect have] Paeonia, Persica and Carthamus,
Forsythia, Bupleurum dislodge the toxin,
[in case of] dry stools take a little Rheum to purge.

HUI YAN ZHU YU TANG (ANTI-STASIS EPIGLOTTIS DECOCTION)

This formula is for the treatment of frequent choking when drinking liquids after about 5–6 days of pox.

Tao Ren 15 g Se. Persicae	*Hong Hua* 15 g Fl. Carthami
Gan Cao 9 g Rx. Glycyrrhizae	*Jie Geng* 12 g Rx. Platycodi
Sheng Di 12 g Rh. Rehmanniae	*Dang Gui* 6 g Rx. Angelicae
Xuan Shen 3 g Rx. Scrophulariae	*Chai Hu* 3 g Rx. Bupleuri
Zhi Qiao 6 g Pc. Citri Aurantii	*Chi Shao* 6 g Rx. Paeoniae Rubrae

Where convulsions developing after pox lead to choking, then *Qi* deficiency leading to the epiglottis not closing fully is the cause. In cases like this, the reader is referred to the section on the treatment of convulsions (p. 211).

The literal translation of the rhyme is:

[In] Anti-Stasis Epiglottis Decoction Blood stasis [is] the cause,
Persica, Carthamus, Glycyrrhiza, Platycodi, Rehmannia, Angelica, Scrophularia,
Bupleurum, Pericarpium Aurantium, Paeonia Rubra,
Choking on water [due to] Blood stasis will become better at once.

ZHI XIE TIAO ZHONG TANG (ANTI-DIARRHOEA CENTRE REGULATING DECOCTION)

This formula treats persistent diarrhoea that presents after approximately 6–7 days of pox; it is equally effective in treating diarrhoea that has lasted more than 10 days.

Huang Qi 32 g Rx. Astragali	*Dang Shen* 12 g Rx. Codonopsis
Gan Cao 8 g Rx. Glycyrrhizae	*Dang Gui* 8 g Rx. Angelicae

Bai Zhu 8 g Rh. Atractylodes M.	*Bai Shao* 8 g Rh. Paeoniae Lactiflorae
Chuan Xiong 4 g Rx. Ligustici Wallichii	*Hong Hua* 12 g Fl. Carthami
Fu Zi 4 g Rx. Aconiti	*Gao Liang Jiang* 2 g Rh. Alpinia Offz.
Rou Gui 2 g Cx. Cinnamomi	

This formula treats the kind of diarrhoea that presents after about a week of pox. It can also be used when convulsions that develop after pox present together with diarrhoea. It is not suitable for diarrhoea at the onset of pox.

The literal translation of the rhyme is:

Stops diarrhoea, regulates the centre [decoction, take] Codonopsis, Glycyrrhiza, Astragalus,
Atractylodes, Angelica, Paeonia Lactiflora, Ligusticum and Carthamus,
China Aconite, high quality ginger and a little cinnamon,
[in cases of] *Qi* deficiency with diarrhoea [it is] always suitable.

BAO YUAN HUA CHI TANG (ORIGIN PROTECTING ANTI-DYSENTERY DECOCTION)

Huang Qi (Astragalus) 80 g and *Hua Shi* (Talc) 40 g with 20 g of sugar
Take in the evening.

This is one of my most tested and approved formulas. Not only is it effective for pox diseases in children, but also for infectious colitis (dysentery), and for acute or chronic dysentery in adults. At the onset of dysentery in adults, 60 g of Talc should be used with 40 g of sugar; Astragalus can be omitted. For sufferers of chronic dysentery, Astragalus must be employed and 60 g of Talc again.

The literal translation of the rhyme is:

Origin protecting, stagnation transforming, [both] tonifying [and] attacking formula,
one *liang* of Astragalus is decocted for this preparation,
one *liang* of pulverized Talc is needed,

all this is swallowed together and colitis will be stopped without damaging the *Qi*.

(Translator's note: today's prescriptions use different dosages.)

ZHU YANG ZHI YANG TANG (ANTI-ITCHING YANG TONIFYING DECOCTION)

This is for the treatment of incessant itching that presents for about 6–7 days after pox, with no bleeding after scratching the skin. At the same time, the formula is also effective for loss of voice.

Huang Qi 40 g Rx. Astragali	*Tao Ren* 8 g Se. Persica
Hong Hua 8 g Fl. Carthami	*Zao Jiao Ci* 4 g Spina Gleditsiae Sin.
Chi Shao 4 g Rx. Paeoniae Rubrae	*Chuan Shan Jia* 4 g Squama Manitis

The literal translation of the rhyme is:

Yang tonifying, stopping itching [decoction contains] Astragalus, Persica, Carthamus, Gleditsia, Paeonia Rubra, Manis together,
it can also be used [in cases of] hoarse voice, loss of voice,
[in cases of] external deficiency syndrome (*Biao Xu*) [and] stagnation of *Qi* [causing Blood stasis in the skin] due to interior *Qi* [deficiency of Wei *Qi*].

ZHU WEI HE RONG TANG (*WEI* AND *YING* STRENGTHENING DECOCTION)

This is used for the treatment of convulsions after pox disease, which presents with eyes that are turned upwards, lockjaw, uncontrollable frothy salivation, deep unconsciousness and purulent ulcerating abscesses all over the body.

Huang Qi 80 g Rx. Glycyrrhizae	*Gan Cao* 8 g Rx. Astragali
Bai Zhu 8 g Rh. Atractylodes M.	*Ren Shen* 12 g Rx. Ginseng
Bai Shao 8 g Rx. Paeoniae Lactiflorae	*Dang Gui* 4 g Rx. Angelicae

Suan Zao Ren 8 g Se. Zizyphi Spinosae	*Tao Ren* 6 g Se. Persicae
Hong Hua 6 g Fl. Carthami	

This formula is particularly suitable for the treatment of convulsions after pox and for purulent ulcerating abscesses all over the body. However, when the convulsions are due to Cold-induced diseases (*Shang Han*), febrile infectious diseases or chronic diseases with other syndromes such as *Qi* deficiency, then special formulas can be found for these types in the section on 'convulsions' p. 211.

The literal translation of the rhyme is:

Wei and Ying harmonizing [decoction contains] Astragalus, Glycyrrhiza, Atractylodes, Ginseng, Paeonia Lactifloria, Angelica, Zizyphus Spinosa, Persica, Carthamus, [has an effect] for [those diseases] falsely described as Wind-convulsion by the ancestors, when this [formula] is used, *Yang* will return [and] life becomes normal again.

DISCUSSION ON *SHAO FU ZHU YU TANG* (ANTI-STASIS LOWER ABDOMEN DECOCTION)

This formula treats gatherings and accumulations in the lower abdomen, both with and without pain. It is also effective for pain in the lower abdomen without abdominal masses, and for distension and fullness in the lower abdomen, as well as for dysmenorrhoea starting with back pain and distended lower abdomen.

The formula can also be used for oligomenorrhoea (scanty bleeding) with multiple consecutive bleedings per month: a bleeding has scarcely stopped before the next one begins. The blood may be dark or purple, with clots. The formula is also effective for uterine bleeding with pain in the lower abdomen or for light blood with leucorrhoea. These are all indications for *Shao Fu Zhu Yu Tang* (Anti-Stasis Lower Abdomen Decoction), which works excellently in these cases.

The astonishing effect this formula has on fertility is also remarkable; when it is started on the first day of menstruation, and five further prescriptions are taken without interruption, pregnancy will be achieved after about 4 months.

During the treatment the wife and husband must choose the appropriate month for impregnation according to their age and whether the month is an 'even' or 'uneven' one. If one of them is of an even-numbered age and the other one is of an uneven-numbered age, an even-numbered month[64] must be chosen for intercourse. However, if both are of an even-numbered or uneven-numbered age, then an uneven-numbered month is suitable. In doing this, the time of impregnation should not be chosen according to the usual beginning of the month, but according to half-month (i.e. 15 days) cycles. When more than 20 days have passed after impregnation, the date should be noted. If the suitable month was calculated incorrectly, and a daughter (instead of a larged-for son) is born, then I cannot be blamed for this. So far, I have used this formula with unfailing success.

In the year 1823 the 60-year-old honourable master Su Na of the government in Zhi Li (Tianjin) came to me for a consultation, because he had no children and was very sad about this. I comforted him by saying: 'This situation is not too difficult.' Starting from the sixth month, he prepared five prescriptions of the formula every month for his wife according to my instructions; in the ninth month pregnancy was achieved and in the following year on the twenty-second day of the sixth month he had a small son. The child is 7 years old now.

Furthermore, this formula has another amazing effect, in that it appears to be dangerous, but in fact it removes danger.[65] Pregnant women with a strong constitution, who indeed have enough *Qi* and who do not suffer from a poor appetite or have any injuries, may suddenly have a miscarriage round about the third or fourth month. Despite the fact that a good deal is written in medical books about these cases suffering from habitual abortion, they are usually advised to nourish and tonify *Yin* and Blood, to strengthen and nourish the Spleen and Stomach, to calm the foetus and to employ protective methods; but hardly any of the formulas work.

What they fail to realize is that while the embryo is growing in the uterus, Blood stasis has already taken up some space there. In the third month, as the unborn child continues to grow, there is no more room in the uterus, and space becomes constricted. Blood cannot flow into the placenta, and flows past it downwards, which causes gestational bleeding. As blood cannot flow into the placenta, the foetus lacks nourishment and miscarriage follows.

Thus, whenever there is another pregnancy after a miscarriage around the third month or after a number of consecutive abortions, several preparations (between three and eight) of this formula should be prescribed in the second month to invigorate the stagnated Blood in the uterus. As the foetus continues to grow, it will have enough space and miscarriage will not occur.

---

[64] Nowadays, the months in Chinese are named according to their number: first month (January), second month (February) and so on. In Wang's time, however, the moon calendar was prevalent. For more details see Granet, *La Pensée Chinoise*; Needham, *Science and Civilization in China* vols 2 and 4; Porkert, *Theoretische Grundlagen der Chinesischen Medizin*; and to a lesser extent also Schipper, *Le Corps Taoïste* and Maspero, *Le Taoïsme et les Religions Chinoises* (see Appendix 7). Wang emphasizes a preference for the even more ancient farmer's almanac of the 24 half-moons. Also see Glossary, 24 seasonal periods.

[65] According to the principles of Chinese medicine and pharmacology, to avoid an undesired abortion Blood invigorating formulas should not be prescribed during pregnancy. Therefore, the use of *Shao Fu Zhu Yu Tang* (Anti-Stasis Lower Abdomen Decoction) appears contraindicated at first. However, as the paragraph goes on it becomes obvious that if used properly it can actually prevent a threatened abortion. This makes *Shao Fu Zhu Yu Tang* (Anti-Stasis Lower Abdomen Decoction) one of the common gynaecology formulas that are still in use nowadays. See Nanjing College of Traditional Chinese Medicine *Concise Traditional Chinese Gynecology*, p. 172ff. and Shao *The Treatment of Knotty Diseases*, p. 357ff (see Appendix 7).

Wang's explanation may not be convincing according to present-day anatomy and pathology, nevertheless his formula has an excellent effect, which has been confirmed to me by many gynaecologists. This is just one example of the 'Paracelsus principle' (whoever cures is right) in Chinese medicine, which after all is successfully treating a quarter of humanity at present.

Several preparations can also be given following a miscarriage to secure later foetuses and ease successive pregnancies.

This formula treats diseases, achieves fertility and protects the foetus; absolutely effective and useful, it is truly an excellent formula.

SHAO FU ZHU YU TANG (ANTI-STASIS LOWER ABDOMEN DECOCTION)

Xiao Hui Xiang 2 g Se. Foeniculi	*Pao Jiang* 1 g Rh. Zingiberis Officinalis
Yuan Hu Suo 4 g Rh. Corydalis	*Mo Yao* 8 g Myrrha
Dang Gui 12 g Rx. Angelicae	*Chuan Xiong* 4 g Rx. Ligustici Wallichii
Rou Gui 4 g Cx. Cinnamomi	*Chi Shao* 8 g Rx. Paeoniae Rubrae
Pu Huang 12 g Pollen Typhae	*Wu Ling Zhi* 8 g Ex. Trogopterori

FORMULA RHYME

Gynae-potion, for the menses also,	= A gynaecological formula for menstrual disorders,
Lower abdominal pain be gone,	= commonly used for lower abdominal pain
Also from the hypogastrium take:	= it is Anti-Stasis Lower Abdomen Decoction
Ginger, Fennel, Chuanxiong, Cinnamon,	= containing *Pao Jiang*, *Xiao Hui Xiang, Chuan Xiong, Rou Gui*
Corydalis, Peony	= *Yan Hu Suo, Chi Shao*
Myrrh, Trogopterus,	= *Mo Yao* and *Wu Ling Zhi*; of these take
1, 2, '3 times 4 and 8',	= 1 g, 2 g, 4 g, 4 g, 4 g and 8 g, 8 g, 8 g
Pollen, Angelica 12 – completed!	= plus *Pu Huang* and *Dang Gui* 12 g each.

The literal translation of the rhyme is:

Lower abdomen: Fennel and roasted Ginger,
Corydalis, Trogopterori, Myrrha, Chuanxiong, Danggui,
Typhae, Cinnamomum, Paeonia Rubra,
the number one formula for offspring and to calm the foetus [in cases of impending miscarriage].

ON PREGNANCY (AND ON PROBLEMS WITH DELIVERY AND THE PLACENTA)

In ancient times it was said that the foetus was in the uterus and was nourished by the channels in turns: in the first month it is nourished by the Liver channel, in the second month by the Gall-Bladder channel, in the third month by the Heart channel, in the fourth month by the Triple Burner channel, in the fifth month by the Spleen channel, in the sixth month by the Stomach channel, in the seventh month by the Lung channel, in the eighth month by the Large Intestine channel, and in the ninth month by the Kidney channel.

So the foetus is nourished by the Liver channel up until the beginning of the second month, and then the Gall-Bladder channel takes over. Realistically, such a theory is neither clear nor sensible. The child inside the womb is nourished entirely by the mother's blood. It doesn't require much explanation to grasp this. So why promote such a theory except to deceive people?

In the *Zi Ti Men* (*On Crying in Children*) it is reported: 'The child is in the womb, and in its mouth it has the umbilical cord, through which it is nourished with Blood.'

How on earth is the foetus supposed to be nourished in the beginning, when the mouth has not yet developed? I simply do not understand why these authors do not ask a woman at home, or a midwife first, and then only start writing when they are sure of the facts. At least in that way they would not be a laughing stock among those who come after them.

One should be aware of the fact that the foetus does not have a placenta in the first month. The placenta is formed not until after the first month and into the second month. By the time the placenta has developed, the body of the foetus is already established. The placenta itself has two components: a double-walled, thick layer containing plenty of blood vessels, and a thinner, single-layered chamber, in which the foetus grows. A cord arises from between the thick and thin layers. This is called the umbilical cord and it leads to the foetus's navel. The mother's blood flows into the placenta and from there into the umbilical cord.

The body, limbs and organs all grow at the same time, not this organ first and then that one next. When abortion happens in the first month there is no placenta, but abortion in the second month presents with a placenta in the shape of a *Cheng-Chui*-balance,[66] narrow at the top and broad at the bottom. Usually, its length is no greater than the width of three fingers. An aborted foetus in the third month already has ears, eyes, mouth and nose; only the fingers and toes have not yet separated.

In the last month, when the birth is imminent, the child ruptures the placenta and is born head first. In most cases, the placenta comes away at the same time as the birth, and the blood above the placenta also flows out. So this is how the child develops in the womb and is born.

However, in a difficult delivery, it is extremely important to realize that *Kai Gu San* (Bone Expanding Powder), which was described in ancient times, is sometimes effective and sometimes not. In general, its bone expanding (obstetric) effect is based on its Blood invigorating action, so no further effort is needed by the mother in labour. When I use this formula I always add a large amount of Astragalus, so the child emerges within a short space of time.

In cases when the placenta does not come away, *Mo Jie San* (Myrrha Draconis Powder) was always employed in ancient times. When it was first used it was sometimes successful and sometimes unsuccessful. When it had no effect, it was recommended to try again with double the amount; then the afterbirth would instantly come away. The components of a formula are very important, but the dosage is even more important.

GU KAI GU SAN (BONE EXPANDING POWDER)

This formula is for the treatment of difficult deliveries.

Dang Gui 40 g	*Chuan Xiong* 20 g
Rx. Angelicae Sinensis	Rx. Ligustici Wallichii
Gui Ban 64 g	*Xue Yu Tan* 8 g
Plastrum Testudinis	Crinis Carbonisat.

Also add 160 g Radix Astragali (*Huang Qi*).

GU MO JIE SAN (CLASSIC MYRRHA DRACONIS POWDER)

Mo Yao 12 g	*Xue Jie* 12 g
Myrrha	Sanguis Draconis

Add the powder to boiled water and administer.

HUANG QI TAO HONG TANG (ASTRAGALUS PERSICA CARTHAMUS DECOCTION)

For postpartum convulsions (including puerperal fever) as well as for symptoms such as eyes that roll upwards, uncontrollable salivation, opisthotonos, deep unconsciousness).

Huang Qi 320 g[67]	*Tao Ren* 12 g
Rx. Astragali	Se. Persicae
Hong Hua 8 g	
Fl. Carthami	

For these problems, the '*Ji Yin Wang Mu*' (*Catalogue of Gynaecology*) is the most sound text; its formulas and theories were collected in the '*Yi Zong Jin Jian*' (*Golden Mirror of Medicine*) and rewritten into formula rhymes, so they are easy to read and memorize. However, the formulas are not very effective when it comes to convulsions, so I have supplemented the ones in that area.

---

[66] The *Cheng Chui* is a set of hand scales with a scale stick for units and a weight that can be moved to and fro. Physicians used to weigh medicinals with them, hence it could be folded up into a box and carried along. This wooden box had the shape of a pear, a comparison that Wang refers to in this sentence.

[67] In present-day China, any larger amount than 120 g of Astragalus is only prescribed in individual cases, therefore this appears to be a very high dose. On the other hand, Astragalus is a very safe medicinal with an LD 50 in laboratory rats reported as 40 g/kg (intraperitoneal). As it stimulates the immune system (increases lymphoblastogenesis as well as leukocytes and polymorphic nuclear granulocytes), this dose seems to be adequate for a severe sepsis such as in puerperal fever.

GU XIA YU XUE TANG (ANTI-STASIS ASCITES DECOCTION)[68]

This formula treats ascites due to Blood stasis. But how do we identify it? An abdomen that is distended like a drum with the skin showing protruding greenish blood vessels indicates ascites syndrome due to Blood stasis.

Tao Ren (Persica) 32 g	*Da Huang* (Rheum) 2 g
Tu Bie Chong (Eupolyphaga) 6 g	*Gan Sui* (Gansui) pulverized 2 g or whole 4 g

If taken alternately with *Ge Xia Zhu Yu Tang* (Anti-Stasis Abdomen Decoction) (previously described), the effect is increased.

CHOU HU LU JIU (GOURD EXTRACT)

This treats ascites and generalized oedema. A dried gourd (Lagenaria Siceraria, *Ku Hu Lu*) is roasted until it can be pulverized. After that, the powder is mixed with 12 ml of yellow wine. If the gourd is very large, the yellow wine can be poured into it and heated for 1 hour; then, the wine should be drunk. This method is supposed to draw water out of the body.

MI CONG ZHU DAN TANG (ONION, HONEY AND PIG'S GALLBLADDER DECOCTION)

This formula is for oedema without ascites.

Zhu Dan 1 pc.	*Bai Mi* 120 g–132 g
Cong Tou 4 pc.	*Huang Jiu* approx. 300 ml

(A pig's gall-bladder, mixed with pale honey, four shallots including approximately 2 cm of the stalks and yellow wine)

CI WEI PI SAN (CORIUM ERINACEI POWDER)

For the treatment of all sorts of spermatorrhoea, wet dreams and loss of semen, regardless of whether caused by excess or deficiency.

The skin of Erinaceum Europaeus or Dauricus is roasted in a clay pot until dry, made into a powder, mixed with yellow wine and administered in the morning. This formula is absolutely affective, but it tastes truly vile.

XIAO HUI XIANG JIU (FENNEL TINCTURE)

This formula treats milky urine (including gonorrhoea), also known as *Xia Lin*, in cases of Wind and Cold affecting the spermatic duct, when other formulas prove ineffective.

40 g of *Xiao Hui Xiang* (fennel seed) are made into a coarse powder, about 300 ml of quickly-boiled yellow wine are poured on top, and left to brew. Sieve and administer.

TREATISE ON BI SYNDROME[69] AND BLOOD STASIS

Normally, symptoms such as shoulder pain, hip pain, arm and leg pain or even pain throughout the body are described universally as *Bi* syndrome. One should know that for Wind-Cold syndrome, medicinals of a warming or hot and dispersing nature are mostly ineffective, and that for Damp-Heat syndrome, Dampness draining and Fire descending medicinals also achieve little success. When the muscles atrophy after long-term disease, this is attributed to collapse of *Yin* and so *Yin* nourishing medicinals are prescribed, also to no avail.

People say about this stage that if the disease is in the skin and vessels, success is easy to achieve; but once the sinews and bones are diseased, success will be difficult to attain. But this is only because the location of the pain has not been thoroughly considered. Wind, Cold, Dampness and Heat invade via the skin; when these pathogenic factors invade the channels, a 'wandering' pain

---

[68] Not to be confused with *Xia Yu Xue Tang* (Purging Blood Stasis Decoction).

[69] The term '*Bi* syndrome' is hardly translated these days. Although its significance overlaps to a large extent with diseases of the rheumatic sphere, its meaning is much broader, including other diseases which in Western medicine are classified as heart diseases or arthritic conditions. For a extensive discussion of all *Bi* syndromes see Vangermeersch & Sun, *Bi-Syndromes*.

(are which changes location) develops. On the other hand, when they invade the Blood vessels, the pain is fixed. When it comes to excess and deficiency, deficiency is a result of the disease, it does not cause the disease. So, if only *Yin* is nourished, what should be done about the pathogenic factor?

If only Wind and Cold are expelled, and Heat and Dampness attacked, then the already thickened Blood is considerably less able to move. When water is exposed to Wind and Cold, it freezes: after the ice has formed, Wind and Cold are long gone.

Why should the treatment of *Bi* syndromes still be difficult, once the principles have become clear to us? There are quite a large number of classical formulas; if these fail to show any effect, then the formulas below should be used.

SHEN TONG ZHU YU TANG (ANTI-STASIS PAIN DECOCTION)

Qin Jiao 4 g Rx. Gentianae Qinjiao	*Chuan Xiong* 8 g Rx. Ligustici Wallichii
Tao Ren 12 g Se. Persicae	*Hong Hua* 12 g Fl. Carthami
Qiang Huo 4 g Rx. Notopterygii	*Mo Yao* 8 g Myrrha
Dang Gui 12 g Rx. Angelicae Sinensis	*Wu Ling Zhi* 8 g Ex. Trogopterori
Xiang Fu 4 g Rh. Cyperi Rotundi	*Niu Xi* 12 g Rx. Achyrantes
Di Long 8 g Lumbricus	*Gan Cao* 8 g Rx. Glycyrrhizae

If there is evidence of a slight Heat syndrome, add *Cang Zhu* (Rhizoma Atractylodes Lanceae) and *Huang Bai* (Cortex Phellodendri). With deficiency and weakness, a large amount of *Haung Qi* (Astragalus) must be added, approximately 40–80 g.

FORMULA RHYME

Anti-Stasis pain, acute	= Anti-Stasis Pain Decoction for acute pain

12 grams work well for arthritis:	= is effective for arthritis, taking 12 grams each of:
Peach, Saffron, Achyranthes,	= *Tao Ren*, *Hong Hua*, *Niu Xi*,
Angelica, all well-known,	= *Dang Gui*, which are well-known medicinals;
8 grams Myrrh, Ligusticum, Lumbricus,	= 8 g *Mo Yao*, *Chuan Xiong*, *Di Long*,
Liquorice and Trogopterus,	= *Gan Cao* and *Wu Ling Zhi* as well as
4 grams Notopterygi – plus	= 4 g each of *Qiang Huo*,
Qinjiao – Gentian, Cyperus.	= *Qinjiao* and *Xiang Fu*.

The literal translation of the formula rhyme is:

Pain, stasis dispersing Achyrantes, Lumbricus, Notopterygium, Qinjiao, Cyperus, Glycyrrhiza, *Dang Gui*, Chaunxiong,
Astragalus, Atractylodes Lancea, Phellodendri in addition,
If acute Trogopterus, Persica, Myrrha, Carthamus.

NAO SHA WAN (SAL AMMONIAC PILL)

This formula treats scrofula, lymphadenitis, neck ulcers and ulcers on the chest, which ulcerate and contain liquid pus. This formula works excellently.

Nao Sha 8 g
Sal ammoniac, pulverized

Zai Jiao approx. 100 seeds
Fr. Gleditsiae

Gan Cu approx. 600 ml
Vinegar

The first two ingredients are added to the vinegar and allowed to steep for 3 days. Subsequently, the mixture is boiled in an earthenware pot until dry. The ammonium chloride crystals on the bottom of the pot are turned over with a spatula and are scooped on top of the Gleditsia seeds until everything is dried (over a low flame). It can also be dried slowly close to the hob.

Five to eight pills are taken every evening with water, or every morning and evening, or at other times twice daily. The dried Gleditsia seeds are quite tough due to the drying process, so they may also be pulverized.

In nature, there are red and white variants of Sal ammoniac. I use the red variety, so I do not know how effective the other one is. Red Sal ammoniac comes from the pit on the North Mountain; in the summer fire burns from this cave, so it cannot be approached. In winter, Muslim people enter the cave unclothed and mine the Sal ammoniac.

In the 'Ben Cao Gang Mu' (Systematic Materia Medica) it is stated that the medicinal is derived from drying turbid salt water in Xinjiang, but this is not correct.

DIAN KUANG MENG XING TANG (PSYCHOSIS DECOCTION)

In cases of manic-depressive psychoses, with continuous crying, laughing, yelling, singing and swearing, regardless of who is present, and with many deranged states of mind, the fundamental pathology is still Blood stasis and Qi stagnation, where the Qi of the brain is not harmonized with the Qi of the organs, so there is a state of confusion as if the patient is in a dream.

Tao Ren 32 g Se. Persicae	Chai Hu 12 g Rx. Bupleuri
Xiang Fu 8 g Rh. Cyperi	Mu Tong 12 g Cs. Akebiae Mutong
Ban Xia 8 g Rh. Pinelliae	Da Fu Pi 8 g Pc. Arecae
Qing Pi 8 g Pc. Citri Reticulatae Vir.	Chen Pi 12 g Pc. Citri Reticulatae
Sang Bai Pi 12 g Cx. Mori A.	Chi Shao 12 g Rx. Paeoniae Rubrae
Su Zi 16 g Fr. Perillae	Gan Cao 20 g Rx. Glycyrrhizae Ural.

FORMULA RHYME

Psychosis Decoction helps when ill
Thanks to Liquorice, Peach kernel,
Cortex Morus, two Citrus,
Bupleurum and Betel Nut,
Red Peony, Mutong plus,
Pinellia and Cyperus,
Perilla, too, that will do:
There will be no mania nor depression!

The literal translation of the formula rhyme is:

[From] the psychosis nightmare one awakes by
   virtue of Peach kernels,
Cyperus, Citrus Reticulata Viride, Bupleurum,
   Pinellia, Mutong,
Citrus Reticulata, Pericarpium Catechu, Paeonia
   rubra, Morus Alba, Perilla,
In the company of Liquorice which calms the
   Centre.

LONG MA ZI LAI DAN (DRAGON HORSE PILLS)

Ma Qian Zi 320 g Se. Strychni	Di Long 8 pc. Lumbricus

Xiang You approx. 600 ml
Sesame oil

Pour the sesame oil into the pan and heat until it boils. Now fry the nux-vomica seeds until they make loud cracking noises.[70] If you take a seed, open the gap on its side with a knife and split it into two halves, the inner part should look reddish-purple when done. After that it should be ground into a fine powder and mixed with the pulverized Lumbricus. Then, with a little liquid it is formed into pills the size of green soy beans (mung beans).

---

[70] Nowadays, nux-vomica seeds are heated together with sand in a pan in order to eliminate their toxicity. This process is explained on page 13 of Philippe Sionneau's 'Pao Zhi'. Whilst at university, I also prepared nux-vomica seeds in this way, but noticed that only top quality seeds produce the cracking noise described by Wang. If they are moist or even mouldy, they will char slowly without a sound.

However, these days the preparation of raw medicinals does not fall to doctors but to pharmacologists and drug experts. This is to maintain standards of potency and to prevent poisoning which might happen if non-professionals were involved. Therefore, I strongly discourage any layperson from carrying out the preparation method described above.

Each dose of about 1 g should be taken with a little salty water before going to bed. Children aged 5–6 years should take half the dose and a small amount of sugary water. Vegetarians may leave out Lumbricus.

This formula treats epilepsy, traditionally also called 'squealing-like-a-goat' Wind. *Huang Qi Chi Feng Tang* should be given every evening, and one pill of this formula before going to bed. The decoction may be stopped after 1 month; the pills should be continued. The recovery will be evident after a while, but the pills should be taken for 1–2 years to treat the root of the disease and maintain the effect.

The aetiology of this disease was discussed in the section 'On the brain and spinal marrow'.

HUANG CHI QI FENG TANG (ASTRAGALUS RED WIND[71] DECOCTION)

Huang Qi 80 g
Rx. Astragali

Chi Shao 4 g
Rx. Paeoniae Rubrae

Fang Feng 4 g
Rx. Ledebouriellae

This is taken as a decoction, but use half the amount for children. To treat paralysis of the limbs another dose is taken until the legs can move by themselves; after that no more should be prescribed.

This formula can be used for the treatment of all sorts of ulcers and diseases, or *Qi* deficiency or weakness caused by illness.

If no disease is present when the formula is prescribed, there will not be any negative effects. This formula cannot be praised too highly, as it is effective for so many diseases. It makes the whole body's *Qi* come into flow and avoids stagnation. In addition, it invigorates the Blood and prevents the formation of stasis. Thus, if *Qi* and Blood are vigorous and vibrant, how could any disease continue to exist?

---

[71] 'Red Wind' consists of red peony (*Chi Shao*) and windscreen (*Fang Feng*). For easy memorization, I shortened the herb names, as was also the case with Dragon Horse Decoction (Earth-dragon (*Di Long*), Horse nux vomica (*Ma Qian Zi*)) and Psychosis Decoction, which should actually be called 'from the (bad) dream of psychosis awakening decoction'.

HUANG QI FANG FENG TANG (ASTRAGALUS LEDEBOURIELLA DECOCTION)

This formula treats prolapsed rectum; even if it has been present for 8–10 years, the effect is surprisingly complete.

Huang Qi 120 g
Rx. Astragali

Fang Feng 4 g
Rx. Ledebouriellae

Children take half the dose.

HUANG QI GAN CAO TANG (ASTRAGALUS LIQUORICE DECOCTION)

This treats urinary incontinence in elderly people as well as knife-like stabbing pain in the urethra. It has an immediate effect, even if the disease has been present for months or years.

Huang Qi 120 g
Rx. Astragali

Gan Cao 32 g
Rx. Glycyrrhizae

Two preparations per day may be prescribed for more severe cases.

MU ER SAN (WOOD FUNGUS POWDER)

This treats suppurating ulcers and various abscesses with incomparable success. This formula should not be underrated.

Mu Er 40 g
Auricularia auricula

Granulated sugar 20 g

First, the pulverized black *Mu Er* Wood fungus is soaked in warm water for a while until a kind of paste has formed. This is applied to the affected area which is then bandaged. This formula like *Ci Wei Pi San* (Corium Erinacei Powder), treats loss of semen, and, like *Chou Hu Lu Jiu* (Gourd Extract), treats ascites, because it employs the same principle. Only those who understand this principle can study and apply Chinese medicine successfully.[72]

YU LONG GAO (JADE DRAGON PASTE, ALSO CALLED SHEN YU GAO)

Applied externally, this treats sprains and traumatic injuries.

---

[72] I will not spoil the fun of solving this little puzzle in Wang's book. Whoever is interested in giving it a try may send me a letter or an e-mail, and I will return a letter with the solution. GN.

Bai Lian 16 g
Rx. Ampelopsis jap.

Dang Gui 16 g
Rx. Angelicae Sin.

Jin Yin Hua 16 g
Fl. Lonicerae

Chuan Wu 16 g
Rx. Aconiti Carm.

Ru Xiang 6 g
Gummi Olibanum

Qing Fen 12 g
Calomelas

She Xiang 1 g
Moschus

Xiang You 800 ml
Sesame oil

Sheng Ma 16 g
Rh. Cimicifugae

Lian Qiao 16 g
Fr. Forsythiae

Shan Jia 16 g
Squama Manitis

Xiang Pi 16 g
Corium eleph.

Mo Yao 6 g
Myrrha

Bing Pian 1 g
Borneol

Bai Zhan 80 g
White vinegar

The first eight medicinals are fried in oil until they are dry. Impurities are removed and the oil is mixed with three boxes of Minium [lead oxide, Translator's note], taken from the fire and cooled down. Then, Olibanum, Myrrha, Calomelas, Borneol and Moschus are stirred in and finally white vinegar. The paste is then distributed evenly and dispersed.

If Minium is omitted, the formula is called 'Medical Paste' and is very effective for open abscesses and ulcerations.

Mu Er San (Wood Fungus Powder) and *Yu Long Gao* (Jade Dragon Paste) are both very reliable formulas for the treatment of suppurating ulcers and abscesses of every kind. They should by no means be underestimated.

Table 10.1 Formulas that invigorate Blood used in the '*Yi Lin Gai Cuo*'

Effect	Chinese name	English name
Anti-Stasis decoctions (6)	*Xue Fu Zhu Yu Tang*	Anti-Stasis Chest Decoction
	Ge Xia Zhu Yu Tang	Anti-Stasis Abdomen Decoction
	Shao Fu Zhu Yu Tang	Anti-Stasis Lower Abdomen Decoction
	Shen Tong Zhu Yu Tang	Anti-Stasis Pain Decoction
	Tong Jing Zhu Yu Tang	Anti-Stasis Exanthema Decoction
	Hui Yan Zhu Yu Tang	Anti-Stasis Epiglottis Decoction
Blood invigorating decoctions (2)	*Tong Qiao Huo Xue Tang*	Orifices Opening Blood Invigorating Decoction
	Jie Du Huo Xue Tang	Detoxifying, Blood Invigorating Decoction
Qi moving and Blood invigorating decoctions (3)	*Dian Kuang Meng Xing Tang*	Psychosis Decoction
	Tong Qi San	*Qi* Passage Powder
	Shi Xiao San	Sudden Smile Powder
Qi tonifying or *Yang* tonifying and Blood invigorating decoctions (7)	*Bu Yang Huan Wu Tang*	*Yang* Tonifying Five-Tenth Decoction
	Tong Qi San	*Qi* Passage Powder
	Huang Qi Tao Hong Tang	Astragalus Persica Carthamus Decoction
	Zhu Wei He Rong Tang	*Wei* and *Ying* Tonifying Decoction
	Huang Qi Chi Feng Tang	Astragalus Red Wind Decoction
	Zhu Yang Zhi Yang Tang	Anti-Itching *Yang* Tonifying Decoction
	Ke Bao Li Su Tang	Guaranteed Resuscitation Decoction

Box 10.1   Medicinals employed in the 'Yi Lin Gai Cuo'

- Blood invigorating medicinals
  - Blood harmonizing medicinals
    Dang Gui (Angelica Sin.), *Chi Shao* (Paeonia Rubra), *Mu Dan Pi* (Moutan), *Niu Xi* (Achytanthis Bidentata)
  - Blood moving and Blood stasis dispelling medicinals
    Chuan Xiong (Ligusticum), *Hong Hua* (Carthamus), *Wu Ling Zhi* (Trogopterus), *Pu Huang* (Typha), *Mo Yao* (Myrrha), *Ru Xiang* (Olibanum), *Yuan Hu* (Corydalis)
  - Stasis breaking and attacking medicinals
    Da Huang (Rheum), *Tu Bie Chong* (Eupolyphaga), *Gan Sui* (Gansui)
  - Blood stasis breaking medicinals
    Tao Ren (Persica), *Xue Jie* (Sanguis Draconis), *Chuan Shan Jia* (Manitis), *Gan Qi* (Lacca), *Wu Ling Zhi* (Trogopterus)
- *Qi* tonifying medicinals
  - *Qi* tonifying medicinals
    Huang Qi (Astragalus), *Dang Shen* (Codonopsis), *Bai Zhu* (Atractylodes Macrocephala), *Gan Cao* (Glycyrrhiza)
  - *Qi* moving medicinals
    Zhi Qiao (Citrus), *Xiang Fu* (Cyperus), *Qing Pi* (Citrus Retic. Vir.), *Chen Pi* (Citrus Retic.), *Da Fu Pi* (Areca), *Xiao Hui Xiang* (Foeniculum), *Wu Yao* (Lindera)
- Other medicinals
  - Orifices opening medicinals
    She Xiang (Moschus), *Cong Tou* (Allium)
  - Exterior relieving medicinals
    Lian Qiao (Forsythia), *Qiang Huo* (Notopterygium), *Fang Feng* (Ledebouriella), *Chai Hu* (Bupleurum)
  - Pain stopping medicinals
    Qin Jiao (Gentiana), *Ru Xiang* (Olibanum),[a] *Mo Yao* (Myrrha)[a]
  - Centre warming medicinals
    Gui Zhi (Cinnamomum), *Gan Jiang* (Zingiberis), *Gao Liang Jiang* (Alpinia)
  - *Yang* recovering medicinals
    Fu Zi (Aconitum), *Rou Gui* (Cinnamomum Cassia)
  - *Yang* tonifying medicinals
    Shan Zhu Yu (Diocurides), *Hu Tao Ren* (= *He Tao Ren*) (Persica)
  - Blood tonifying medicinals
    Gou Qi Zi (Lycium), *Niu Xi* (Achyranthis Bidentata),[a] *Bai Shao* (Paeonia Lactiflora)
  - *Yin* tonifying medicinals
    Gui Ban (Testudinus)
  - Liver calming medicinals
    Di Long (Lumbricus), *Shi Jue Ming* (Halotidus)
  - Phlegm transforming medicinals
    Ban Xia (Pinellia), *Jie Geng* (Platycodon), *Sang Bai Pi* (Cort. Mori), *Zao Jiao Ci* (Gleditsia), *Su Zi* (Perilla)

[a] according to the latest pharmacological research, these medicinals also have blood invigorating qualities (see Part 2).

Table 10.2   Treatment principles employed in the 'Yi Lin Gai Cuo'

Classification of diagnostic methods	Syndromes	Treatment principle of the formula
Arranged according to cause of disease	Pronounced Blood stasis Qi deficiency and Blood stasis Qi stagnation and Blood stasis Internal Cold and Blood stasis Yang deficiency and Blood stasis Fever toxin and Blood stasis	Invigorate Blood, remove stasis Tonify Qi, invigorate Blood Move Qi und invigorate Blood Warm the Centre and invigorate Blood Recover Yang and invigorate Blood Detoxify and invigorate Blood
Arranged according to cause and location of disease	Liver-Qi depression and Blood stasis Kidney deficiency and Blood stasis Blood stasis in the vessels Abdominal masses (Ji Ju or Zheng Jia)	Soothe the Liver and invigorate Blood Strengthen the Kidneys and invigorate Blood Remove obstructions from the vessels and remove Blood stasis Soften masses and remove stasis
Arranged according to deficiency and excess	Excess syndrome and Blood stasis Deficiency syndrome due to Excess	Purge and invigorate Blood Tonify and attack simultaneously (e.g. tonify Qi and invigorate Blood, strengthen the Kidneys and invigorate Blood, invigorate Yang and Blood, warm the Centre and invigorate Blood etc.)
Arranged according to Wang's own anatomical division of the body	Blood stasis in the pharynx Blood stasis in the head, face and the limbs Blood stasis in the chest Blood stasis in the abdomen Blood stasis in the lower abdomen	Anti-Stasis Epiglottis Decoction Orifices Opening Blood invigorating Decoction Anti-Stasis Chest Decoction Anti-Stasis Abdomen Decoction Anti-Stasis Lower Abdomen Decoction

APPENDIX: 'YI LIN GAI CUO'

What follows in Box 10.1 and Tables 10.1 and 10.2 is a summary and analysis of the medicinals used by Wang Qing-Ren, their combinations, the formulas and finally the principles of differential diagnosis. Through this my aim is to give the reader an overall impression of Wang's own conception of Blood stasis.

Twenty-three out of Wang's 33 formulas were predominantly designed for invigorating Blood. These formulas can be arranged as in Table 10.1.

Chapter 11

Excerpts relating to Blood stasis from six other classical texts (in chronological order)

1. EXCERPTS FROM ZHANG ZHONG-JING'S 'JIN KUI YAO LÜE'[1] AND 'SHANG HAN LUN' (BEGINNING OF THE THIRD CENTURY AD)

Zhang Zhong-Jing (150–219 AD) was the first to use the name 'Yu Xue' for Blood stasis, which is also used today, and to describe a few of the typical syndromes caused by Blood stasis. His frequently used formulas that are still in use today are *Di Dang Tang* (Resistance Decoction) and *Tao Hong Cheng Qi Tang* (Qi Rectifying Persica Carthamus Decoction), both purgative formulas. Aetiologically, he regards Heat excess syndrome as the predominant cause of Blood stasis, therefore it can be removed by purgation.

The original work 'Shang Han Za Bing Lun' was lost and only Wang Shu-He's edited version is now available, which he had rendered into the 'Shang Han Lun' and the 'Jin Kui Yao Lüe'. Thus the excerpts listed below are outlined according to Wang Shu-He.

Wang Shu-He is also the author of the 'Mai Jing' (Pulse Classic), in which he attempts to classify Zhang's pulse qualities as well, failing at times in this as Zhang's pulse specifications were often also synonymous with the corresponding syndromes.

The now standard classification into 28 pulse qualities originated much later, namely in Li Shi-Zhen's (1518–1593 AD) 'Ping Hu Mai Xue' (The

---

[1] Also called 'Jin Gui Yao Lüe' in South China

Pulse Studies of Ping Hu), which means that the inexperienced should exercise great care when adopting Zhang's pulse specifications literally. But keeping this premise in mind, Zhang's '*Shang Han*' and '*Jin Kui*' prove to be indispensible classics for all practitioners of Chinese medicine.

'JIN KUI YAO LÜE'

Chapter 16 Xue Xu

The patient has a sensation of fullness in the chest, has a bluish tongue and dry mouth, is thirsty, but keeps fluids in his mouth with no desire to swallow. There is no sensation of heat or cold. There is no abdominal distension, but the patient feels as if there were. The pulse is minute (*Wei*), but also slow (*Chi*) and comes in big waves (*Da*).

If the patient feels feverish, full and irritable, has a dry mouth and feels thirsty, while the pulse indicates no Heat (this means it is not rapid, so it points towards a *Yin* syndrome), then this signifies residual Heat (of a past disease that has remained in the Blood) with Blood stasis at the same time. In this case, a purging method should be commenced.

'SHANG HAN LUN'

Clause 124

After approximately 7–8 days of *Tai Yang* syndrome:[2] the exterior syndrome is still present, the pulse is weak, yet it is deep (instead of superficial, as is characteristic for an exterior syndrome). There is no feeling of oppression in the chest (i.e. the Upper Burner) but the patient acts as if mad due to stagnation of Heat in the Lower Burner. The

---

[2] Tai means 'the greatest, the utmost', *Yang* is one pole of the bipolar entity *Yin/Yang*. Thus, *Tai Yang* may be translated as 'the greatest *Yang*' in symbolic contrast to *Tai Yin* 'the greatest *Yin*'. The meaning of these terms stems from the *Yi-Jing* school of the eastern Zhou dynasty (770–256 BC). In modern Chinese the combination '*Tai Yang*' has another meaning, i.e. 'sun'. It is very strange that some authors in English-speaking countries, who can obviously read dictionaries but otherwise lack any understanding of the Chinese language, chose to translate *Tai Yang* channel with 'Sunlight' channel. In my translation the original term is preserved to avoid causing even more confusion.

lower abdomen feels hard and tense; however, urine is passed without difficulty (this means there is no abdominal water retention but rather Blood stasis). Once the stagnated Blood is dispelled by purgation, the patient will recover.

The pathological mechanism is as follows: pathogenic Heat reaches the interior via the *Tai Yang*, where it generates Blood stasis. Therefore, *Di Dang Tang* (Resistance Decoction) is appropriate.

Clause 237

Yang Ming syndrome: If the patient is forgetful, then Blood stasis is evident. This is due to the fact that chronic Blood stasis can lead to forgetfulness as well as to hard and dark stools, which are, unexpectedly, passed without effort. Purging with *Di Dang Tang* (Resistance Decoction) is suitable.

Clause 257

The patient has no exterior-interior syndromes (i.e. no *Shao Yang* 'half-interior half-exterior syndromes). There is fever for about 7–8 days and despite the presence of a superficial and rapid pulse, the purging method can be employed.

If the pulse is still rapid after purgation, this indicates that Heat has accumulated in the interior (i.e. also in the Blood and Stomach), leading to accelerated digestion and to the patient feeling hungry (which is a typical sign for Stomach-Heat).

However, if there is still no stool after 6–7 days, Blood stasis has formed (due to Heat in the Blood) and the prescription of *Di Dang Tang* (Resistance Decoction) is appropriate.

2. EXCERPT FROM CHEN WU-ZE'S 'SAN YIN JIN YI BING FANG LUN' (TREATISE ON THREE CATEGORIES OF DISEASE CAUSES, 1174 AD)

Fractures and traumata with (acute) Blood stasis and their treatment

When the patient has suffered traumata, the bad (extravasated) Blood flows inside. Or great anger causes excess of Blood and sweat, they accumulate without dispersing, and so the area of the flanks becomes painful. There are leg cramps, sometimes the joints become swollen, *Qi* ascends but fails to descend; all this is due to Blood stasis in the interior. There are formulas available for each symptom.

Ji Ming San (Cock Crow Powder) treats falls and pressure injuries caused by stone and wood. In every case where damage was caused by traumata, or by accumulations due to coagulated Blood, where *Qi* does not flow any more and life is in danger; or in cases where Blood stasis has accumulated for a long time, with agitation and pain accompanied by crying out loud, this formula can remove all these symptoms by dispelling Blood stasis. It dispels the old and encourages the formation of the new (tissue). It is also very effective for fractures.

Ji Ming San (Cock Crow Powder): 2 *liang* (approximately 60 g) *Da Huang* (Rheum) steamed in wine, 37 kernels of *Xing Ren* (Prunus Armeniaca)[3] with the tips removed. Grind them and cook in wine until the liquid is reduced to 60%, bottle it and remove the residue. Take in the morning at the first cock crow. Blood stasis will be eliminated the same day the formula is taken, and the patient will be cured.

In acute cases, when life is in danger and the casualty is unable to speak, and there is no time to prepare the formula, it is possible to open his mouth and pour in heated urine.[4]

Blood stasis as the consequence of (long standing) disease and its treatment

Due to absence of sweating or haemorrhaging the patient suffers from stasis and internal Blood accumulation, so a waxen complexion and pale lips develop. There are further symptoms such as black stool, weak legs and shortness of breath. In

severe cases there may be mania or depression. All this is due to Blood stasis and can be treated with a specific formula: *Niu Jiao Di Huang Tang* (Rhino Rehmannia Decoction).

For the treatment of both *Shang Han* (Cold induced diseases) and *Wen Bing* (febrile infectious diseases), the patient should start to sweat, if not, the (hot) internal accumulation of Blood turns into Blood stasis. In the case of nose bleeding and vomiting Blood when not all (coagulated) Blood has been discharged and remains in the interior, the complexion becomes yellowish-waxen and the stool becomes black like tar.

Niu Jiao Di Huang Tang (Rhino Rehmannia Decoction): pulverize 2 *liang* Rhinoceros horn powder,[5] 8 *liang Sheng Di* (Rehmannia), 3 *liang Chi Shao Yao* (Paeonia Rubra), 2 *liang Mu Dan Pi* (Moutan); for a dose of 4 *Qian* take 1.5 litres of water, bring to the boil and reduce to 70%, and sieve. In the case of mental disorders add 2 *liang Da Huang* (Rheum) and 3 *liang Huang Qin* (Scutellaria).

If the patient's pulse is big and slowed down, and if the abdomen is not swollen but the patient feels pressure inside the abdomen, then no Heat is present, so the formula mentioned above may be used without these additions.

3. FROM THE ENCYCLOPAEDIC COLLECTION OF THE QING DYNASTY '*YI SHU*', COMPILED BY CHENG WEN-YOU (ORIGINAL TEXT BY LUO CHI-CHENG, YUAN DYNASTY, 1206–1308 AD)

Sometimes people ask what experience has been gained regarding the combination of Phlegm and Blood stasis. My opinion is as follows.

There are many who know how Blood stasis develops from Phlegm, but they do not know how Phlegm develops from Blood stasis:

---

[3] The number 37 is very uncommon. I suspect a numerological significance which describes a relationship to the medicinal *San Qi* (meaning '37') and injuries due to Blood stasis.

[4] This may appear very unappetizing, nevertheless the urine of infants and children to the age of about 6 was already in use in Li Shi-Zhen's '*Ben Cao Gang Mu*' (*Systematic Materia Medica*) and even before that time. Today we know that normally sterile urine – especially that of infants – contains urokinase and hormones such as 17-ketosteroids, oestrogen, 17-oxycorticosterone and gonadotrophins, but also vitamins (B[1], B[2], B[6] and C) and essential minerals.

[5] There were still sufficient rhinoceroses in the year 1174, well before the invention of the rifle and its sale to African and Asian nations by Western countries. Safari hunting was also unknown, so rhinoceros horn powder was destined for one single use: to save lives. Today, Water Buffalo horn, of which 100 times the amount is needed, may be used.

1. If injury causes Blood to flow into the other direction, Blood will stagnate. The *Qi* that is stagnated due to the trauma generates Phlegm and as Blood is stagnated here too, it is then called Blood stasis generating Phlegm. The diseased body part is painful on pressure; other symptoms are vomiting Blood, nose bleeding or tarry stools. The pulse is slippery (*Hua*) in the superficial layer and choppy (*Se*) in the deep layer.[6] To treat such a syndrome, one must eliminate Phlegm and break stasis. First, one needs to use *Dao Tan Tang* (Guide Out Phlegm Decoction) plus *Cang Zhu* (Atractylodes), *Xiang Fu* (Cyperus), *Zhi Qiao* (Citrus) and *Bai Jie Zi* (Sinapis) to dispel stagnation and eliminate Phlegm. After that, *Chuan Xiong* (Ligusticum), *Dang Gui* (Angelica Sinensis), *Tao Ren* (Persica), *Hong Hua* (Carthamus), *Su Mu* (Sappan), *Mu Dan Pi* (Moutan) and *E Zhu* (Curcuma Ezhu) are employed to break stasis.

2. If Phlegm has accumulated first, which is often the case, resulting[7] in Blood stasis that combines with the Phlegm, it is then called Phlegm with Blood stasis. In this case, the diseased body part may ache but not always at the same point, and there are symptoms such as fullness and oppression in the chest, sometimes signs of Heat or Cold, the pulse is like an onion stalk (*Kou*) above and slippery (*Hua*)[8] below. In such cases one must first break stasis and transform Phlegm consecutively or treat both at the same time.

Sometimes, this is treated wrongly by tonifying or using cold medicinals; this only results in the disease being held back, and the chronic stagnation will lead to lung cavities (*Cao Nang*). Such a lung cavity is painful and one is unable to turn to the side; sometimes the pleura is swollen and has Heat, cough and shortness of breath are present, and the sputum is malodorous. Zhu Dan-Xi remarks on this: 'Phlegm containing stagnated Blood leads to lung cavities, which are untreatable.'[9]

4. EXCERPT FROM WANG KEN-TANG'S 'ZHENG ZHI ZHUN SHENG' (*MANUAL OF DIAGNOSIS AND TREATMENT*, 1602 AD)

Chapter *Xu Xue* (Blood accumulation)

Regardless of whether food, drink or habitation are involved, if daily lifestyle is inappropriate, it can result in lack of movement of Blood and Blood stasis. For this reason bad Blood is responsible for numerous diseases.

In medical books all information is classified appropriately; the seven affections[10] are mentioned amongst the syndromes, but stagnated Blood is not mentioned. And for that reason I will add this to it.

Blood that is discharged from the nose and mouth suggests Blood accumulation in the Upper Burner. If pressure in the space below the Heart cannot be tolerated, Blood accumulation in the Middle Burner is evident. However, if the abdomen is slightly distended and painful, Blood accumulation is in the Lower Burner.

Blood accumulation in the Triple Burner can always be diagnosed on the pulse of the left hand.[11] In the case of Blood accumulation in the Upper Burner *Hou Ren Xi Jiao Di Huang Tang* (Hemp Rhino Rehmannia Decoction) should be taken. In the case of Blood accumulation in the Middle Burner *Tao Ren Cheng Qi Tang* (Qi Rectifying Persica Decoction) should be taken. In the case of Blood accumulation in the Lower Burner *Di Dang Tang* (Resistance Decoction), *Di Huang Tang*

---

[6] The fact that the pulses called 'slippery' and 'choppy', which may contradict each other in their definition, can exist in the same location at different levels, is proven by experience, although only if one differentiates as precisely as Luo did 77 years ago.

[7] Phlegm hinders the flow of *Qi*, and when *Qi* stagnates, it fails to propel Blood.

[8] This pulse is even more complex: the pulse is straight and firm in the superficial layer, is absent in the middle, and is slippery in the deep layer.

[9] This is substantial Phlegm that is coughed up, containing extravasated and thus stagnated Blood. The whole pathology of '*Cao Nang*' (literally: slimy nests in the lung) points to lung tuberculosis and emphysema.

[10] In the '*Huang Di Nei Jing*' the seven affections are: Cold, Heat, Joy, Anger, Fear, Pensiveness and Worrying, i.e. the five emotions of the *Zang Fu* organs plus Cold and Heat.

[11] As the left hand reflects Blood and the right hand reflects *Qi* (Author's note).

(Han's Rehmannia Decoction) or *Sheng Qi Tang* (Raw Euphorbia Decoction) should be taken.

Thus it is stated in the 'Hai Zang': Zhang Zhong-Jing's *Di Dang Tang* or *Wan* can be used for Blood accumulation. However, it is feared that a less able practitioner may not know precisely the temperature properties of the medicinals and may prescribe too much, which if taken continuously can eventually damage the Blood, especially in the old, weak or those with a deficiency syndrome. For this reason *Sheng Di Huang Tang* (Shen's Rehmannia Decoction) was developed, which apart from the ingredients of *Di Dang Tang* (Resistance Decoction), namely *Meng Chong* (Tabanus), *Shui Zhi* (Hirudo), *Da Huang* (Rheum), *Tao Ren* (Persica) also contains *Sheng Di Huang*, *Gan Qi, Sheng Mu Li, Da Qing Ye* (Rehmannia, Lacca Sinica Exsiccate, Isatidis Folium Daqingye).

With regard to *Sheng Qi Tang* (Raw Euphorbia Decoction), it must also be feared that its effect will be too strong, as with *Di Dang Tang/Wan* (Resistance Decoction/Pill). *Sheng Qi Tang* is a formula to break Blood stasis, but with a milder effect than *Di Dang Tang* (Resistance Decoction). If it proves successful, larger dosages may be prescribed. Nevertheless, its effect in dispelling abdominal masses may be too strong, as it contains *Gan Qi* and *Nao Sha* (Lacca Sinica Exsiccate, Sal ammoniac), so one must first confirm the presence of a *Qi* excess syndrome, otherwise it is contraindicated.

In the case of symptoms like rotting teeth and suchlike that have been existent for years, which points at Blood accumulation in the *Yang Ming* channels,[12] *Tao Ren Cheng Qi Tang* (*Qi* Rectifying Persica Decoction) should be commenced. The ingredients of this formula should first be ground into a fine powder and processed into honey pills, about the size of dates. This method always works excellently for alcoholics presenting with this syndrome.

In the case of internal injuries resulting from falls from a great height, blows and stab wounds, where non-dissolving Blood accumulations can be found in the chest and abdominal area, Upper,

Middle and Lower Burner must be differentiated respectively. Then, it is easy to drain Blood using approved formulas like *Xi Jiao Di Huang Tang* (Rhino Rehmannia Decoction), *Tao Ren Cheng Qi Tang* (*Qi* Rectifying Persica Decoction) or *Di Dang Tang/Wan* (Resistance Decoction/Pill). Adding a mixture of the patient's cooked urine and alcohol can also serve the same purpose. Alternatively it is effective to add *Sheng Di Huang* (Rehmannia) and *Dang Gui* (Angelica Sinensis) or *Da Huang* (Rheum) to the formulas mentioned above.

Another method: in patients with a deficiency syndrome who cannot tolerate purging formulas, *Si Wu Tang* (Four Ingredients Decoction) plus *Chuan Shan Jia* (Squama Manitis) are prescribed, with excellent results. *Hua Rui Shi San* (Ophicalcitum Powder) dissolved in the urine of children[13] or in alcohol can also be used in such cases. However, the cold property of this formula must be observed, *Yin* and *Yang* must be differentiated, and an exact syndrome differentiation (*Bian Zheng*) is essential.

5. EXCERPT FROM LIN PEI-QIN'S 'LEI ZHENG ZHI CAI' (COLLECTION OF DIFFERENTIAL DIAGNOSIS AND TREATMENT, 1839 AD)

Chapter *Xu Xue* (Blood accumulation)

Traumata and injuries of every kind, exhaustion and overstrain, fits of anger with rebellious *Qi*, all these causes force the Blood to cease its flow and stagnate. Hints for diagnosis are, for example, sensations of heat and cold, yellowish complexion, pressure-sensitive and painful areas or tension in the chest, below the ribs or in the abdomen.

It is recommended that the treatment is divided according to upper, middle and lower section. For example, vomiting Blood or nose bleeding with Blood stasis belongs to the upper section. The typical syndrome of 'thirst with desire to rinse one's mouth but aversion to swallowing' will also be present = *Xi Jiao Di Huang Tang* (Rhino Rehmannia Decoction). If Blood accumulates in the area of

---

[12] See also 'Shang Han Lun' clause 237 Blood stasis in the *Yang Ming* channels and usage of *Di Dang Tang*.

[13] See footnote 4.

the diaphragm, this belongs to the middle section. The syndrome 'thirst and irritability accompanied by talking nonsense' will be present = *Tao Ren Cheng Qi Tang* (*Qi* Rectifying Persica Decoction). If the abdomen feels hard and distended and there are tarry stools, this belongs to the lower section. The syndrome: 'forgetfulness and mental confusion' will be present = *Di Dang Tang* (Resistance Decoction), *Dai Di Dang Tang* (Substitute Resistance Decoction).

In the case of Blood accumulation in the Triple Burner there are certainly mania and mental disorders accompanied by constipation = *Sheng Di Huang Tang* (Shen's Rehmannia Decoction).

In cases of Blood accumulation in the initial stage with pain in the chest or abdomen *Xiang Ke San* (Cyperus Citrus Powder) is prescribed.

In cases of trauma resulting from a fall from a great height with stagnated, coagulated Blood (*E Xue*), which is not dissolved and causes unbearable pain in the chest and flanks, *Fu Yuan Huo Xue Tang* (Blood Invigorating Recovery Decoction) is prescribed.

In cases of stagnated Blood due to exhaustion/fits of anger[14] *Chen Xiang Jiang Qi San* (Aquilaria Directing *Qi* Downwards Decoction) and cases of Blood stasis in the chest area shallot juice (or spring onion juice) mixed with baby urine is prescribed.

In bleeding conditions where the Mind is also affected, *Dang Gui Huo Xue Tang* (Blood Invigorating Angelica Decoction) is prescribed. In cases of sensations of heat and cold as well as a yellowish complexion and a wiry fine pulse, according to the '*Qian Jin Fang*' (*A Thousand Ducats Prescriptions* by Sun Si-Miao) medicinals such as *Da Huang* (Rheum), *Mang Xiao* (Mirabilitum), *Dang Gui Wei* (tail of Angelica Sinensis), *Tao Ren* (Persica), *Ren Shen* (Ginseng) and *Gui Xin* (Cortex Cinnamomi)

---

[14] While Liu initially refers to both exhaustion (*Nu*) and anger (*Nu*) causing Blood accumulation, here he only uses the first character '*Nu*' for exhaustion, whereas in the formula section below he uses the second character '*Nu*' for anger. The spelling of both words is almost identical. As the name of the formula indicates, lower *Qi* and the medicinals have the action of moving Liver-*Qi* stagnation, I assume that in fact Blood accumulation due to anger is meant, so this is probably a spelling or printing mistake.

are prescribed as a powder and administered with a little wine.

However, there is grave danger when Blood accumulation presents as tarry black stool. But if the mental condition and pulse remain normal, treatment with formulas may certainly be commenced. In the case of clumping due to Dryness *Yu Zhu San* (Polygonatum Odoratum Powder) is prescribed.

In cases with a yellow discolouration of the face, head or body, the skin is rubbed using a silken cloth soaked in raw ginger juice. This is my own recommendation.

Formulas

- Upper section: *Xi Jiao Di Huang Tang* (Rhino Rehmannia Decoction)
- Middle section: *Tao Ren Cheng Qi Tang* (*Qi* Rectifying Persica Decoction)
- Lower section: *Di Dang Tang* (Resistance Decoction)
- Lower section: *Dai Di Dang Tang* (Substitute Resistance Decoction)
- Triple Burner: *Sheng Di Huang Tang* (Shen's Rehmannia Decoction)
- Pain in the chest: *Xiang Ke San* (Cyperus Citrus Powder)
- Pain in the flanks and abdomen: *Fu Yuan Huo Xue Tang* (Blood Invigorating Recovery Decoction)
- Damage due to fits of anger: *Chen Xiang Jiang Qi San* (Aquilaria Directing *Qi* Downwards Decoction)
- Mental confusion as if due to seeing ghosts: *Dang Gui Huo Xue Tang* is prescribed (Blood Invigorating Angelica Decoction)
- Clumping due to Dryness: *Yu Zhu San* (Polygonatum Odoratum Powder)

6. EXCERPTS FROM TANG ZONG-HAI'S '*XUE ZHENG LUN*' (*TREATISE ON BLOOD SYNDROMES*, 1884 AD)

1. Blood stasis syndromes and formulas from the chapter 'Blood stasis'

Regardless of whether vomiting Blood, nose bleeding, bloody stools or lochias are involved, in these symptoms Blood always moves out of its course. And in all cases of Blood outside the Blood vessels, this destroyed Blood can no longer combine with the nourishing (*Ying-*) Blood, which flows everywhere throughout the body. If it reaches the Stomach, it must be removed by emesis or purgation. That (clotted Blood) which is still in the Blood vessels but not in the stomach, should be dispelled with medicinals immediately or eliminated via the urine or stool, so it cannot become static and pathogenic.

If this Blood is still present inside the body, it cannot combine with the good Blood; it actually impedes the normal activity of Blood. Therefore, one should be always aware of transforming stasis as well.

In general, static Blood is described as a Blood clot and fresh Blood as not static. In the same way, blackish blood is described as static but bright coloured blood as not static, but this way of thinking is not adequate: as soon as blood moves out of the blood vessels, including fresh and bright coloured blood, then this is called blood outside the blood vessels, and even if it is fresh or bright, it has now become static (i.e. no longer circulating). Evidently, a while after it has left the blood vessels, this blood also turns dark.

For example, in the case of skin lacerations, blood shed from the wound is initially light in colour and turgid. It is obvious that blood is flowing out of the blood vessels, yet it is fresh blood. After a few days the wound turns blackish-purple, which makes it clear that blood becomes dark once it has been out of the blood vessels for a longer period of time.

If Blood is still in the blood vessels but has already become blackish-purple, it still constitutes fresh blood and has not yet turned into clotted blood, because it can still be moved by *Qi* and reach the stomach or intestines. From there, it can be discharged by emesis or purgation. If it was clotted inside the blood vessels, how could it travel into the stomach and intestines? As for blood clots, as soon as this blood reaches the stomach or intestines, it will coagulate there within a short time. One only needs to observe when sheep or pigs are slaughtered how blood coagulates within a short time when it drips into the bowl. You can easily see this for yourself.

In all cases of bleeding, regardless of whether the blood is clear or clotted, fresh or blackish-purple, Blood stasis was always present beforehand. Moreover, when Blood stasis is present, there should also be clear signs of a Blood stasis syndrome, so the physician may always start the treatment based on this syndrome without any further hesitation.

When Blood stasis attacks the Heart, symptoms such as heart pain, dizziness, fainting and deep unconsciousness are present. It doesn't matter whether child-bearing mothers or patients vomiting Blood are involved: whenever such a syndrome is present, danger is nearby. One should be quick to calm the Blood and protect the Heart by prescribing *Gui Xiong Shi Xiao San* (Sudden Smile Powder with Angelica and Ligusticum) and adding *Hu Po, Zhu Sha* and *She Xiang*.[15] Alternatively, *Gui Xiong Tang* is prescribed with the addition of *Xue Jie* (Sanguis Draconis) and *Ru Xiang* (Olibanum), which also works very well.

When Blood stasis is located in the Lung, there is a retching irritable cough and shortness of breath with sooty blackish nostrils; mouth and eyes are also of a dark colouring. In this case, *Shen Su Yin* (Codonopsis and Perilla Drink) is prescribed to protect the Lung and remove Blood stasis, as this a very dangerous syndrome.

Generally, coughing up Blood is a life-threatening sign, because in many cases it can be related to Blood stasis in the Lung, and because Blood clots can clog up the windpipe. This formula is balanced mostly towards Lung deficiency with otherwise sufficient amount of *Qi*. If there is Lung excess and *Qi* stagnation, the Lung should not be tonified any further, but instead Blood stasis should be removed so *Qi* can move freely again. To save someone's life, prescribe *Ting Li Da Zao Tang* (Lepidium and Jujube Decoction) plus *Su Mu* (Sappan), *Pu Huang* (Pollen Typhae), *Wu Ling Zhi* (Trogopterus) and *Tong Bian* (Infantis Urina).[16]

When Blood stasis is located between the *Zang Fu* organs and the channels, there is pain in the whole body. Stasis blocks *Qi*, which should move, and this depression of *Qi* generates pain, known

---

[15] Succinum, Cinnabaris and Moschus.
[16] See footnote 4.

as the so-called 'pain due to obstruction' syndrome. *Fo Shou San* (Buddha Hands Powder) plus *Tao Ren* (Persica), *Hong Hua* (Carthamus), *Xue Jie* (Sanguis Draconis), *Xu Duan* (Dipsacus), *Qin Jiao* (Gentiana), *Chai Hu* (Bupleurum), *Zhu Ru* (Bambusa) and *Gan Cao* (Glycyrrhiza) with alcohol should be prescribed.

Alternatively, prescribe *Xiao Chai Hu Tang* (Small Bupleurum Decoction) plus *Dang Gui* (Angelica Sinensis), *Chi Shao* (Paeonia Rubra), *Mu Dan Pi* (Moutan), *Tao Ren* (Persica), *Jing Jie* (Schizonepeta), for internal and external use. This formula is more balanced.

When Blood stasis is in the Upper Burner, there is hair loss with a bald patch, and sometimes a stubborn, stabbing pain in the arms and the chest, and blurred vision. Then, prescribe *Tong Qiao Huo Xue Tang* (Orifices Opening Blood Invigorating Decoction). In addition, *Xiao Chai Hu Tang* (Small Bupleurum Decoction) plus *Dan Gui* (Angelica Sinensis), *Chi Shao* (Paeonia Rubra), *Tao Ren* (Persica), *Hong Hua* (Carthamus) and *Da Ji* (Cirsium) can be prescribed.

When Blood stasis is in the Middle Burner, there is pain in the sides and abdomen and a fixed stabbing pain between navel and hip. The prescription is *Xue Fu Zhu Yu Tang* (Anti-Stasis Chest Decoction) or *Xiao Chai Hu Tang* (Small Bupleurum Decoction) plus *Xiang Fu* (Cyperus), *Jiang Huang* (Curcuma Longa), *Tao Ren* (Persica) and *Da Huang* (Rheum).

When Blood stasis is in the Lower Burner, there is pain in the costal arch, the abdomen is distended, with stabbing pain, and the stools are blackish, so the prescription is *Shi Xiao San* (Sudden Smile Powder) plus vinegar-processed[17] *Da Huang* (Rheum) and *Tao Ren* (Persica), or *Ge Xia Zhu Yu Tang* (Anti-Stasis Abdomen Decoction).

When Blood stasis is in the interior, there is thirst. *Qi* and Blood are interdependent: with Blood stasis in the interior, *Qi* is blocked; it cannot propel fluids upwards and so thirst develops; this is known as also Blood-induced thirst. The patient should take *Si Wu Tang* (Four Ingredients Decoction) plus *Suan Zao Ren* (Zizyphus Spinosa), *Mu*

Dan Pi (Moutan), *Pu Huang* (Pollen Typhae), *San Qi* (Notoginseng), *Hua Fen* (Trichosanthes), *Yun Ling* (Poria), *Zhi Qiao* (Citrus) and *Gan Cao* (Glycyrrhiza). *Xiao Chai Hu Tang* (Small Bupleurum Decoction) plus *Tao Ren* (Persica), *Mu Dan Pi* (Moutan) and *Niu Xi* (Achyranthis Bidentata) may also be taken. On the other hand, *Wen Jing Tang* (Menses Warming Decoction) contains warming medicinals for removing Blood stasis, so it is also suitable for long-term abdominal masses. All formulas mentioned above should be used according to their indications.

When Blood stasis is located in the pores, *Ying-Qi* and *Wei-Qi* are not balanced; there are sensations of heat with aversion to cold. The pores are situated between the exterior and interior, where *Qi* and Blood pass constantly. If there is Blood stasis in this region, *Ying-Qi* will be damaged, which generates aversion to cold, whereas if *Wei-Qi* is damaged, there will be aversion to heat, so eventually there is alternating heat and cold as in *Nüe Ji* (a syndrome similar to malaria). The prescription is *Xiao Chai Hu Tang* (Small Bupleurum Decoction) plus *Tao Ren* (Persica), *Hong Hua* (Carthamus), *Dang Gui* (Angelica Sinensis) and *Jing Jie* (Schizonepeta).

When Blood stasis is in the muscles and flesh, there is persistent high fever, with spontaneous or night sweating. The muscles and flesh are dominated by the *Yang Ming* channels (Stomach and Large Intestine). If Dryness in the *Yang Ming* channels concentrates the fluids thus leading to Blood stasis, *Bai Hu Tang* (White Tiger Decoction) and *Xi Jiao Di Huang Tang* (Rhino Rehmannia Decoction) are appropriate. *Tao Ren* (Persica) and *Hong Hua* (Carthamus) must be added to cure this disease. Also effective is *Xue Fu Zhu Yu Tang* (Anti-Stasis Chest Decoction) plus vinegar-processed[18] *Da Huang* (Rheum).

When Blood stasis is between the *Zang Fu* organs and channels, there are also concretions (*Zheng*) and conglomerations (*Jia*).

Conglomerations (*Jia*) sometimes gather and sometimes dissipate. These gatherings form because *Qi* is stagnated due to Blood being stagnated. Conversely, Blood stasis will be dispelled once *Qi* moves, so no more masses will be present or visible. In such cases of clumping the *Qi* dis-

---

[17] *Da Huang* processed with vinegar. When the laxatives are removed by the cooking procedure, *Da Huang*'s effect is focused on invigorating Blood in the liver area.

[18] See footnote 17.

persing method is suitable to move Blood, so *Jiu Qi Wan* (Nine *Qi* Pill) can be prescribed.

If this syndrome is present in the chest area above the diaphragm, one must add *Ge Gen* (Pueraria), *Zhi Ke* (Citrus), *Mu Gua* (Chaenomelis), *Sheng Jiang* (Zingiberis) and *Gan Cao* (Glycyrrhiza). If it is located on the right, add *Su Zi* (Perilla), *Sang Bai Pi* (Cortex Mori Albae) and *Chen Pi* (Citrus Reticulata), but if it is located on the left, add *Qing Pi* (Citrus Immaturus), *Mu Li* (Concha Ostrae) and *Dang Gui* (Angelica Sinensis).

If it is present in the abdominal area of the Middle Burner, one prescribes *Hou Po* (Magnolia), *Zhi Ke* (Citrus), *Fang Ji* (Stephania), *Bai Shao* (Paeonia Lactifloria) and *Gan Cao* (Glycyrrhiza). If it is present in the lower abdomen, add *Ju He* (Citrus seed), *Xiao Hui Xiang* (Foeniculum), *Li Zhi He* (Litchii), *Bing Lang* (Areca), *Chuan Lian Zi* (Melia) and *Wu Ling Zhi* (Trogopterus).

If *Qi* is dispersed again after this, stagnated Blood will also be dispelled and will not form any more gatherings. However, if it is feared that after dispersion of *Qi*, gatherings may form anew, then the most appropriate method is to regulate Blood in order to harmonize *Qi*. In this case the *Qi* of the conglomerations is dispersed in the Blood, so if Blood is regulated the dispersed *Qi* will be harmonized again and no new gatherings will form. The prescription is *Xiao Yao San* (Easygoing Walk Powder) plus *Mu Dan Pi* (Moutan), *Xiang Fu* (Cyperus) or *Gui Pi Tang* (Spleen Recovering Decoction) with *Chai Hu* (Bupleurum) and *Yu Jin Zi* (Semen Curcuma).

On the other hand, concretions (*Zheng*) are gatherings of a permanent nature that do not disperse easily. They consist of more Blood than *Qi*. As *Qi* is weaker here, it is unable to disperse the Blood. Sometimes there is only stagnated Blood or a mass of stagnated Blood may enclose Water. Blood may accumulate for some time and then transform into Phlegm and Water, of which the latter may also stand for *Qi*.[19]

Concretions (*Zheng*) arise from a concentration of Blood and *Qi*. One must break Blood stasis to bring *Qi* back into motion and remove clumping. The origin of the disease is of paramount importance: it must not be neglected.

However, in weakened patients with chronic abdominal masses, one should not only attack the actual syndrome, one must also tonify at the same time to cure the ill successfully. Prescriptions for attacking Blood stasis are *Di Dang Tang* (Resistance Decoction), *Xie Yu Xue Tang* (Blood Stasis Purging Decoction) or *Dai Di Dang Wan* (Substitute Resistance Pill). The prescription for attacking Phlegm and Water is *Shi Zao Tang* (Ten Jujube Decoction). If both Blood and Water are to be attacked at the same time, suitable prescriptions are *Da Huang Gan Sui Tang* (Rheum Kansui Decoction) or *Mi Fang Hua Qi Wan* (Secret Prescription for Transforming *Qi* Pill).[20] For external application, *Guan Yin Qiu Ku Cao* (*Kuanyin Overcomes Suffering Ointment*)[21] is suitable.

When Blood stasis is in the *Zang Fu* organs and the channels, Blood stasis may engage in combat with *Qi*, to the effect that the clotted mass starts to rot and pus may form. Further details can be found under purulent sputum, purulent stool and purulent abscesses.

Where there is Blood stasis in the *Zang Fu* organs and channels, the heated *Qi* concentrates Blood stasis into dry Blood. This *Qi* is the fiery *Yang* between the Kidneys (*Ming Men*). If *Yin* is weak the fiery *Yang* will blaze upwards, so that its hot *Qi* will combine with the Fire of the Heart. As a result, the excess of *Qi* will generate an excess of Fire. Thus, fiery *Qi* coagulates the stagnated Blood, which is therefore too dry. For this reason, this syndrome presents with a condition of exhaustion and fever, dry, brittle skin or scaly lichenifications of the skin. This is then termed 'exhaustion due to Blood Dryness' (*Gan Xue Lao*). A third of the patients presenting with this syndrome can be cured using Zhang Zhong-Jing's *Da*

---

[19] Tang's definition of Fire and Water differ from the common meaning. He emphasises the *Yang* aspect and the *Yin* aspect of the body. In this sense, he explains: 'Yin and Yang are Water and Fire; Water and Fire are *Qi* and Blood. Water transforms into *Qi* and Fire into Blood.' His interpretation of Water corresponds to Kidney Water, which is transformed into *Yuan-Qi* and *Wei-Qi* by the Fire of the Heart.

[20] Even within the 10 volumes of *Zhong Guo Yao Fang Da Zi Dian* (Great Encyclopaedia of Chinese Formulas) there is no formula of this name. Therefore, it is assumed that a mistake has been made and that the Blood invigorating and abdominal masses dissipating formula *Mi Fang Hua Chi Wan* is implied.

[21] Seldom used nowadays. Contains *Lue Dou Fen*, *Huang Lian* and *Huang Bai*.

Huang Bie Chong Wan (Rheum Eupolyphaga Pill). Such symptoms belong to the syndrome of Blood Dryness. The usual Blood moving formula does not suffice here because Vital *Qi* is already depleted. This is why animal drugs[22] are chosen in order to break up dry Blood in Blood stasis.

Due to the fact that Blood stasis already impedes the flow of fresh Blood in the tissues, the presence of a Blood Dryness syndrome makes any flow of Blood impossible. Therefore the treatment of Blood Dryness syndrome is the top priority, even if a deficiency syndrome presents at the same time.

Because of the deficiency, some people risk using these medicinals exclusively.[23] They can still use nourishing and strengthening medicinals and add to them *Da Huang Bie Chong Wan* (Rheum Eupolyphaga Pill), which is an effective trick too.

2. Blood stasis syndromes and formulas from the chapter 'Upper Blood syndrome and its treatment'

On how Blood stasis is removed

Having come to a standstill, one part of the Blood has already left the vessels and cannot return. If this Blood is extravasated in the upper area, it will stagnate between the diaphragm and backbone, or if further down, at the border of the ribs and the hip. It is almost certain that pain will develop in those places.

Sometimes, this condition manifests in the limbs, so they will also present as painful and swollen. Sometimes, it stagnates under the skin or in the muscles and as a consequence sensations of heat or cold will arise.

In every case, Blood stasis blocks the flow of *Qi*. In the long run, such an obstruction of vital mechanisms generates conditions like 'bone-steaming'

fever,[24] dry Blood (*Gan Xue*) and fatigue syndrome (*Lao Zai*). Treatment must start immediately. Moreover, stasis that is stuck in the vessels obstructs the passage of fresh Blood; as a result, this has no other choice but to move out of the vessels and to erupt in the form of haematemesis or other haemorrhaging. Thus, removing Blood stasis is the most immediate method employed to treat Blood in its entirety. *Hua Rui Shi San* (Ophicalcitum Powder) is prescribed to transform stasis into fluid and drain it. It also does not damage the *Qi* of the five *Zang* organs, making it an excellent prescription for Blood stasis.

If *Hua Rui Shi San* (Ophicalcitum Powder) cannot be used, the following medicinals are rcommended: *San Qi* (Notoginseng), *Yu Jin* (Curcuma), *Tao Ren* (Persica), *Niu Xi* (Achyranthis Bidentata) and *Cu Da Huang* (vinegar-processed Rheum), which also has a fine and quick eliminating action.

If the old clotted Blood fails to leave, new Blood will be unable to develop; but if there is not enough new Blood, the old Blood cannot be washed away. In a manner of speaking, if the good fails to grow, the bad will not retreat. One must therefore know that new Blood must be generated daily once Blood stasis is removed. When stasis is being removed, it must be eliminated via the urine or the large intestine, so that it does not collect in any other place. *Hua Rui Shi* discharges stasis via the urine, *Cu Huang San* (Vinegar-processed Rheum Powder) discharges it via the feces.

However, if Blood stasis is merely removed without engendering new Blood, then this is like trying to win a battle without knowledge of the General. Upright *Qi* (*Zheng Qi*) is responsible for expelling pathogenic influences, but how can stasis be fully removed without new Blood propelling it outwards?

---

[22] Most of the animal drugs in the treatment of Blood stasis belong to category III (breaking Blood stasis), like the above-mentioned *Tu Bie Chong* (Eupolyphaga). For further details on research about Blood stasis see Chapter 7 'Blood stasis related medicinals, their application and combination'.

[23] Literally: 'Someone who does not have the mouth and the knowledge for this . . .' This means that Blood stasis breaking medicinals, on account of their potency, may theoretically further drain a weak patient with *Qi* deficiency.

---

[24] Bone-steaming syndrome (*Gu Zheng*) is a *Yin* deficiency syndrome with hyperactivity of internal Heat (as if the bones themselves are cooked), characterized by fever, night sweating, lethargy, irritability, insomnia, sensation of heat in the palms and soles and so on. This could be related to a dysregulation of the internal second clock spoken of in chronobiology. Further information can be obtained from my essay on 'Lily Disorder' (*Bai He Bing*), which was originally described in the '*Jin Kui Yao Lüe*' (see Bibliography).

The recommended method is to use *Sheng Yu Tang* (Wise Healing Decoction) to strengthen the Blood, plus *Tao Ren* (Persica), *Hong Hua* (Carthamus), *Mu Dan Pi* (Moutan), *Zhi Ke* (Citrus), *Xiang Fu* (Cyperus), *Fu Ling* (Poria) and *Gan Cao* (Glycyrrhiza) to achieve an eliminating and a strengthening effect at the same time. Using this method removes Blood stasis whilst Upright *Qi* remains unharmed.

The general treatment of Blood stasis should proceed in this way. In some cases, however, warming medicinals may be prescribed as well, for it is stated in the '*Nei Jing*' (*The Yellow Emperor's Internal Classic*): 'Blood needs *Yin* but it fears Cold. Cold stagnates its flow. Warmth loosens it and facilitates its flow.'

Moreover, there are cases where cooling medicinals have no effect, because there is still some pathogenic residual Heat (*Fu Re*) hidden in the *Yin*. In this case, one must combat like with like by expelling *Yang* (using warmth) from the *Yin*, using Zhang Zhong-Jing's *Bai Ye Tang* (Biota Decoction). The principle is to expel Blood stasis caused by Cold, or Blood stasis which has remained in the *Yin*. The three medicinals in the decoction are all warm in nature.

However, this formula is by no means suitable for Blood stasis due to pathogenic Fire, unless one plans to balance the formula with further medicinals, in which case *Si Wu Tang* (Four Ingredients Decoction) or *Xie Xin Tang* (Heart Relieving Decoction) can be added. The medicinals of these formulas have a counteracting (i.e. cooling) effect.

The methods described above are generally considered as the treatment for Blood stasis. Blood stasis can linger anywhere in the body, above, below, deep inside or more superficially. But it does not matter where it lies, as long as the treatment is aimed at the location, it will always be effective.

If the diagnosis identifies Blood stasis in the Upper Burner, with symptoms of pain in the shoulders, breast or back, deafness, fullness or nausea, this can be treated with *Xue Fu Zhu Yu Tang* (Anti-Stasis Chest Decoction) or *Ren Shen Xie Fei Tang* (Ginseng Lung Relieving Decoction) plus *San Qi* (Notoginseng), *Yu Jin* (Curcuma) and *Jing Jie* (Schizonepeta). This can free the Upper Burner from Blood stasis.

With Blood stasis in the Middle Burner there is distension and fullness of the abdomen and pain in the hip below the costal arch. The *Dai Mai* (Girdle Vessel) runs around the hip and is connected to the internal organs below, in women to the Uterus and the ovaries, and in men to their source of vitality, so it is responsible for the blood vessels in this area. This means that whenever the Blood is diseased, the *Dai Mai* is also affected. If there is Blood stasis in this area, the treatment will also have a good effect on the *Dai Mai*. As the Spleen functional entity is located in the area of the *Dai Mai*, the recommended treatment is to treat the Spleen. An example of this is Zhang Zhong-Jing's *Shen Zhuo Tang* (Blocked Kidney Decoction), which treats the Spleen and thus the *Dai Mai*.

So, if Blood stasis occurs in the area of the *Dai Mai*, *Jia Ji Hua Tu Tang* (Paeonia Glycyrrhiza Decoction) is recommended, plus *Tao Ren* (Persica), *Dang Gui* (Angelica Sinensis) and *Jiang Huang* (Curcuma Longa). For severe hip pain, *Lu Jiao Jiao* (Gelatinum Cornu) should be added, and for pain below the costal arch *Pu Huang* (Pollen Typhae) and *Wu Ling Zhi* (Trogopterus).

Blood stasis in the Lower Burner, with symptoms such as pain below the hip, tension and distension in the lower abdomen, indicates Blood stasis either of the Liver or the uterus. Thus, the lower abdomen (*Xue Hai*, Sea of Blood) is painful. The recommended prescription is *Gui Xiong Shi Xiao San* (Sudden Smile Powder with Angelica and Ligusticum).

If there is constipation at the same time, *Da Huang* (Rheum) is added. Amongst Zhang Zhong-Jing's especially effective formulas for Blood stasis are *Di Dang Tang* (Resistance Decoction), *Tao Ren Cheng Qi Tang* (Rectifying *Qi* Persica Decoction) and others. All of them contain bitter and cold medicinals that have a purgative and dispersing effect to expel this kind of Blood stasis.

However, if warm medicinals need to be used, *Sheng Hua Tang* (Generate Change Decoction) and *Niu Xi San* (Achyranthis Powder) are more appropriate. These formulas were dispensed originally in gynaecology in the treatment of postpartum residual Blood in the uterus and retained afterbirth. But in my opinion they can be used for both genders in spite of the differences, as Blood is stagnated in the Lower Burner affecting both genders in the same way. This is why in this case these two formulas usually achieve very good results.

Apart from that, the Lower Burner belongs to the *Yin* part of the body and Heat in the Upper Burner belongs to the *Yang* Heat syndromes, so no warming medicinals should be employed in this case. Blood stasis in the Lower Burner belongs primarily to *Yin* syndromes, which explains why a woman in childbed perceives warmth as pleasant and cold as unpleasant. When this is considered, it should be clear why predominantly warming medicinals are prescribed for the treatment of Blood stasis in the Lower Burner.

Still, one must always first diagnose a syndrome of Blood stasis due to Cold before using warming medicinals. If there is Heat in the Lower Burner instead, one must keep to *Tao Ren Cheng Qi Tang* (*Qi* Rectifying Persica Decoction).

When Blood stasis is accompanied by painful swollen limbs, stasis and swelling must be removed by prescribing *Xiao Tiao Jing Tang* (Small Menses Regulating Decoction) plus *Zhi Mu* (Anemarrhena), *Yun Ling* (Poria), *Sang Bai Pi* (Cortex Mori Albae) and *Niu Xi* (Achyranthis Bidentata).

In cases of Blood stasis in the skin and muscles, where the flow of *Ying-Qi* and *Wei-Qi* is disturbed, sensations of heat and cold arise, and there are fits of vomiting and diarrhoea, 'bone-steaming' fever, night sweating and an alternating urge to cough and retch, *Xiao Chai Hu Tang* (Small Bupleurum Decoction) plus *Dang Gui* (Angelica Sinensis), *Tao Ren* (Persica), *Mu Dan Pi* (Moutan) and *Bai Shao* (Paeonia Lactiflora) can be used.

If the Cold syndrome is very pronounced, one should add *Ai Sui* (pulverized Artemisia) and *Xi Xin* (Asarum); if the Heat syndrome is very pronounced, one should add *Hua Fen* (pulverized Trichosanthes), *Ge Gen* (Pueraria), *Zhi Mu* (Anemarrhena) and *Qing Hao* (Artemisia Qinghao).

In cases of cough with Phlegm and Heat one should prescribe *Gua Lou Shuang* (pulverized condensed Trichosanthes), *Xing Ren* (Pruni Armeniaca), *Mai Men Dong* (Ophiopogonis), *Wu Wei Zi* (Schisandra), *Yun Ling* (Poria) and *Zhi Mu* (Anemarrhena).

In cases of thin-fluid mucus ascending, *Ting Li Zi* (Lepidium) may be added.

Xiao Chai Hu Tang (Small Bupleurum Decoction) has the action of soothing Liver-*Qi* transversely from the centre, to relieve it of stagnation, so *Ying-Qi* and *Wei-Qi* can flow unobstructed through skin and muscles. If Blood invigorating medicinals are added to this formula, its effect will focus on removing Blood stasis. Now, if stasis blocks *Ying-Qi* and *Wei-Qi* in the skin and muscles, as described above, such a formula will achieve impressive and immediate results.

In summary, when Blood stasis is located in the *Zang Fu* organs and channels, it easily turns into dry Blood (*Gan Xue*) and consumption worms.[25] When Blood stasis is located more in the exterior parts of the body, hemiplegia and abscesses develop. In the case of Blood stasis in the skin and bones, bone-steaming fever accompanied by dry skin and dry hair develop. All these symptoms are caused by the damaging effects of Blood stasis. Therefore, in the treatment of Blood diseases it is the top priority to focus on treating Blood stasis.

3. Blood stasis syndromes and formulas from the chapter 'On the transformation of stasis and formation of new Blood'

Blood inside the uterus is renewed every month; the old is shed, the new is formed. Old Blood is static Blood; if it is not discharged, it will block the formation of new Blood.

All physicians know the method of breaking stasis in order to regulate the menses. But if men or women vomit Blood or bleed from the nose, nobody thinks of applying the method of transforming Blood stasis so that new Blood is formed. When the circulation of Blood is disturbed by stasis, it impedes the entire process of Blood formation. The comparison with menstruation should make this clear.

In abscess treatment in traumatology, first the putrid flesh is removed so new flesh can form. If it is not removed, it will impede the formation of

---

[25] Due to the fact that smaller microorganisms were still unknown in Tang's era, he proposed the theory that tuberculosis and similar diseases were caused by contagious 'worms' (*Chong*). After the study of microscopic biological and pathological agents had been introduced to China, they were still translated as 'worms' due to the traditional familiarity with the term. In addition, the term comprises all tiny organisms such as insects, worms, protozoa and even smaller organisms.

new flesh and Blood as well. In the treatment of purulent fistulae, the decayed tissue must be opened to let the pus drain, otherwise the new tissue cannot be generated.

Treating loss of Blood without removing stasis is like encouraging new tissue growth without removing the putrid flesh! For this reason, one cannot separate the treatment of stasis from the treatment of Blood deficiency. Blood cannot be renewed until stasis is removed, so treating Blood stasis and tonifying Blood must be undertaken together, in the same way that menstruation expels old Blood and at the same time causes the regeneration of Blood. When Blood is expelled, another pregnancy can take place in the Sea of Blood soon afterwards; one does not have to wait for the end of menstruation. So we can recognize that if stasis is removed, Blood can regenerate, but also that if Blood is regenerated, stasis can be removed.[26]

As described above, regeneration of Blood takes place, while the source of it is the Spleen and Stomach. The classics say: 'Qi and fluids are collected in the Middle Burner. These two form a red fluid that is Blood.' This statement can also be backed up by observation: in women, the milk in the mammary glands arises from food and drink; in other words, it is a liquid that is also derived from the collected Qi and fluids in the Middle Burner. Once milk is formed in the breast, menstruation ceases, because the fluid is discharged from the breast in the form of milk rather than from the uterus in the form of Blood.

It is a well known fact that in order to stimulate the flow of milk, one has to tonify Spleen and Stomach; however, nobody realizes that in order to nourish Blood one has to tonify Spleen and Stomach as well. As Blood and milk are from the same source and as the method of stimulating the flow of milk is well known, one may use this method for nourishing Blood, too.

However, when Spleen and Stomach are tonified, one must differentiate *Yin* and *Yang*. In Spleen-*Yang* deficiency, there is a failure to transform food and drink. In Spleen-*Yin* deficiency, proper transformation of food and drink similarly fails to arise. This can be compared to cooking rice in a pot. If there is no fire, the rice will not be cooked. If there is no water, it will not be cooked either. I have often found it to be the case that lack of appetite due to Spleen deficiency became worse when warm medicinals were used, but better when cool medicinals were prescribed.[27] I also found that lactation increased when *Huang Qi* (Astragalus), *Bai Zhu* (Atractylodes Macrocephala) and *Lu Rong* (Cornu Cervi) were used to stimulate it, but I also saw that lactation decreased following the prescription of these medicinals. One time the prescription was correct, another time it was not!

Suitable medicinals for tonifying Spleen-*Yang* are *Gan Jiang* (Zingiberis) or *Fu Zi* (Aconitum), which stimulate the fluids. Suitable medicinals for nourishing Spleen-*Yin* are *Zhi Mu* (Anemarrhena) or *Shi Gao* (Gypsum).

Authors in earlier times used to discuss the method of strengthening Spleen-*Yang*, but the method of nourishing Spleen-*Yin* was not explained. Therefore, I would like to emphasize at this point that the Spleen has both *Yin* and *Yang*; (in treatment) one should not consider only one of them in isolation.

---

[26] Although his examples are logical, sometimes they are rather strangely arranged in the light of modern physiology. His explanations may not always match those of present day physiology; nevertheless they are good memory hooks for TCM treatment principles, as is also shown in the following paragraph.

---

[27] Usually it is the other way round, because Spleen deficiency always refers to either Spleen-Qi deficiency or Spleen-*Yang* deficiency.

1. COMPARISON OF SURFACE AND BOTTOM OF THE TONGUE

Figures 1a–1c show the surface and bottom of the tongue of 3 patients.

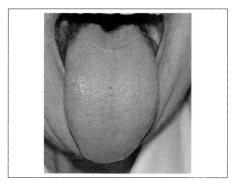
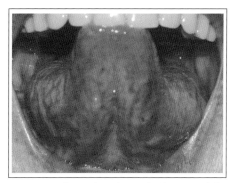

1a left and 1a right: In a purple tongue (shown on the left) you can also expect to see signs of stasis on the bottom of the tongue (right: with stasis spots)

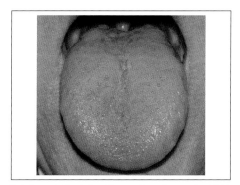
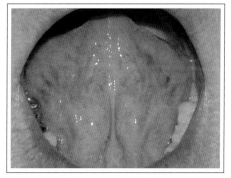

1b left and 1b right: Signs of stasis can be hidden under a red or red-purple tongue as well, as shown in this example.

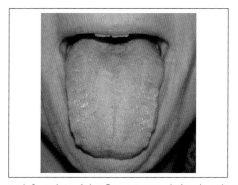
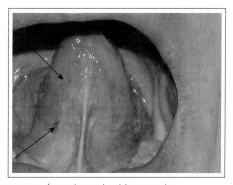

1c left and 1c right: But even an obviously pale tongue can indicate stasis (see arrows), as shown in this example.

2. COMPARISON OF VARIOUS PURPLE TONGUES

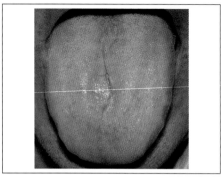 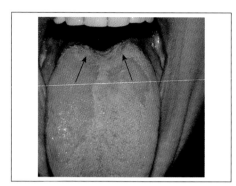

2a left and 2a right: On the left, a red-purple tongue showing a scarred crack in the centre; on the right, parts of the tongue without coating can be seen, and convex cup-shaped papillae behind the sulcus terminalis, often seen in fungal infections of the nasal cavity.

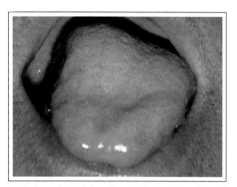 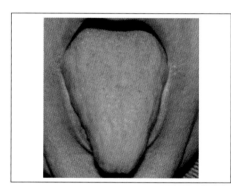

2b left and 2b right: On the left, a flaccid, pale purple tongue with a slippery coating found in cases of *Qi* deficiency with Dampness and Blood stasis; on the right a stiff, dry, purple tongue as in *Yin* deficiency Blood stasis.

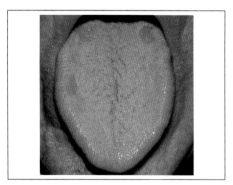 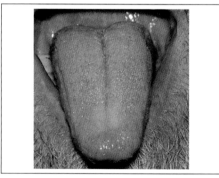

2c left and 2c right: To the left, a tongue that is pale red at the front and purple at the back – below the parts without coating; to the right a dark red-purple tongue with red tip, which is almost completely covered with a thick coating.

3. VARIOUS SUBLINGUAL VEINS

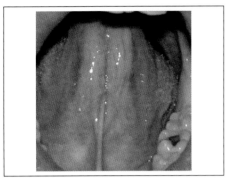 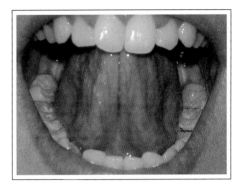

3a left: Pale sublingual vein with thickened mucosa ('cellophane' or 'shower curtain' vein) is often a sign for Dampness or Phlegm.

3a right: If the sublingual veins are reddish or show reddish branches, Heat is more likely.

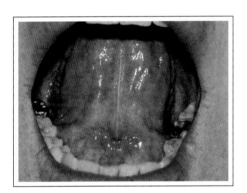 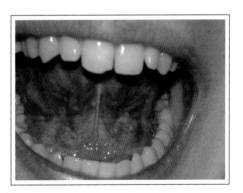

3b left: Every dilation of the venules/capillaries suggests Heat or febrile infections.

3b right: In such cases, the floor of the tongue should also be inspected.

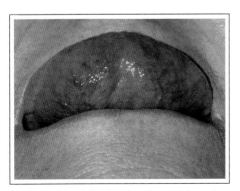 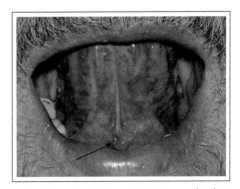

3c left and 3c right: Surging Heat with stasis can also be identified in the vessels all over the bottom of the tongue (left). If stasis is stronger than Heat, then the red colouration of the bottom of the tongue turns blue. Stasis spots on a thickened tongue knot on the frenulum (right, below) can point towards tumour formation.

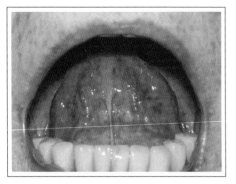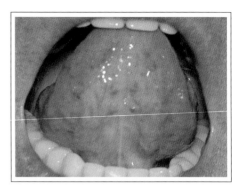

3d left: In the case of Cold with stasis, there is usually a dark blue or blackish shading.
3d right: If the sublingual veins are hardly visible and the spots red, Heat-Dryness prevails over Blood stasis.

4. INDICATIONS OF SUBLINGUAL DIAGNOSIS

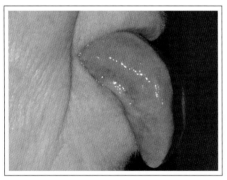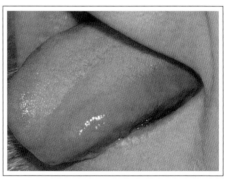

4a left and 4a right: If the sides are clearly spotted (left), then you should look for Liver signs; thus sublingual diagnosis gives particular importance to comparison, as stasis spots on the sides are often hard to recognise (right, a different patient).

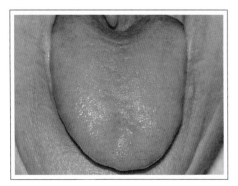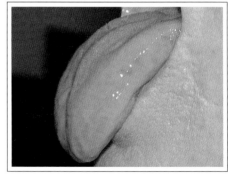

4b left and 4b right: In this picture (left) stasis spots are hardly visible, but inspected from the side they can be seen more clearly (right: same patient).

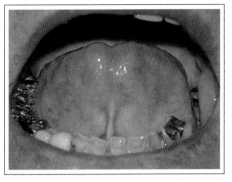
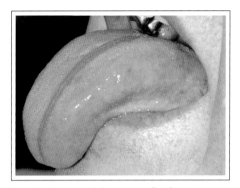

4c left and 4c right: Important exceptions: stasis that is difficult to recognize from the bottom of the tongue (left) can become more obvious once the sides are inspected (right, same patient). Thus the sides should always be included in inspection.

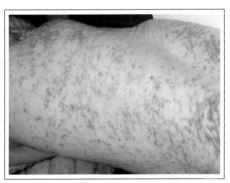
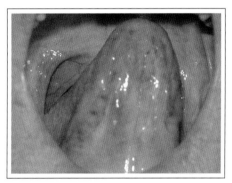

4d left and 4d right: When stasis signs appear on the skin (often behind the ears as well), in this case due to a drug reaction, they will always appear on the tongue (same patient) as well.

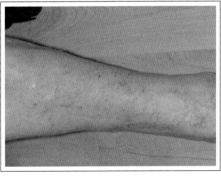
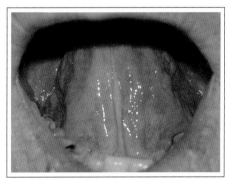

4e left: In cases of poor circulation, varicose veins or arteriosclerosis (as shown in illustration), the bottom of the tongue should also be assessed.

4e right: The same patient, tongue. Enlarged but flaccid sublingual veins are often found in patients with arteriosclerosis and elderly people.

5. COMPARISON OF THE TONGUE BEFORE AND AFTER TREATMENT

The same tongue is illustrated, before and after treatment.

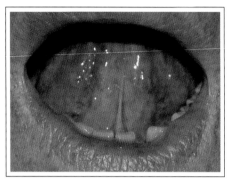 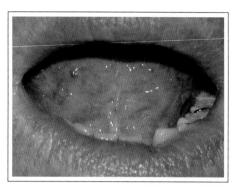

5a left and 5a right: After just a short treatment period (approximately 2 weeks) Blood stasis spots begin to dissolve. Left: before; right: after 2 weeks of Blood invigorating prescriptions.

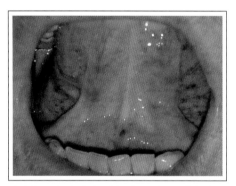 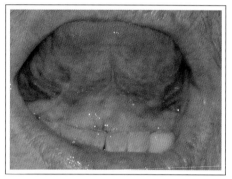

5b left and 5b right: Blood stasis medicinals can dissolve tongue spots within a few weeks. Left: before; right: after about 3 weeks.

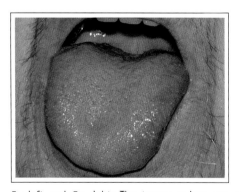 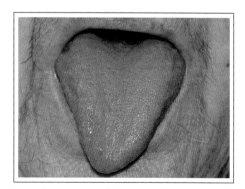

5c left and 5c right: The tongue colour can also revert from pale purple back to pale red (same patient as above). Left: before; and right: after.

6. COMPARISON OF VARIOUS DEGREES OF STASIS ON THE BOTTOM OF THE TONGUE

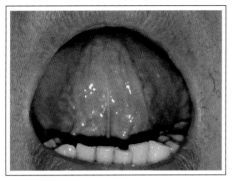 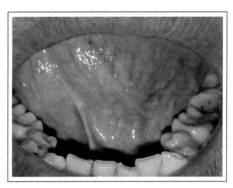

6a left: 1st degree: almost normal tongue with three sublingual vein branches reaching into the second zone (see left of illustration).

6a right: Minor elongation of the veins on the left side with up to three stasis spots, approaching 1st degree.

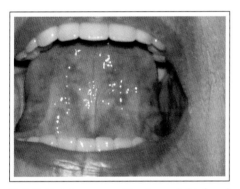 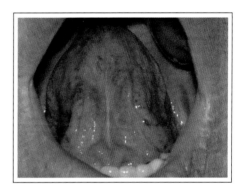

6b left: 2nd degree: reaching beyond the frenulum into the third zone.

6b right: Although there are no elongated veins this is still 2nd degree, with between 3 and 10 stasis spots.

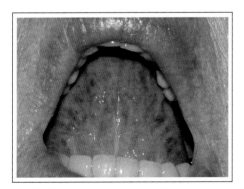 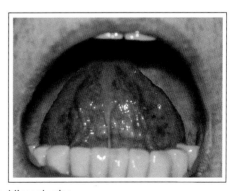

6c left: 3rd degree: more than 10 stasis spots in the presence of elongated sublingual veins.

6c right: 3rd degree due to the dark colour and the crooked and enlarged veins, despite only a few Blood stasis spots.

7. COMPARISON OF VARIOUS SUBLINGUAL VEINS (I)

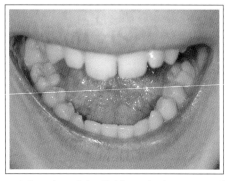 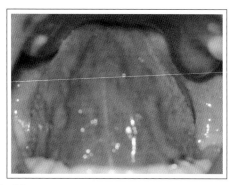

7a left and 7a right: Sublingual veins are not always indicative of Blood stasis. Dilated capillaries with a red shading can also hint at fever or Heat (left). However, if there is also a dark shading of the sublingual veins (right), Blood stasis with Heat is present.

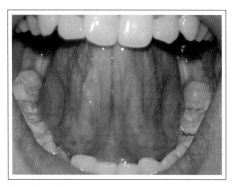 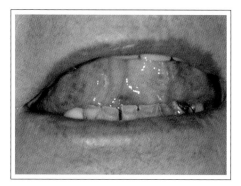

7b left: If Phlegm or pronounced Dampness obscure the sublingual veins, stasis spots still remain as a clear sign of Blood stasis.
7b right: Left: chronic asthma; right: chronic hepatitis

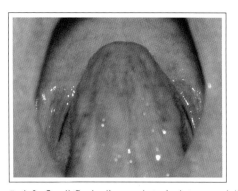 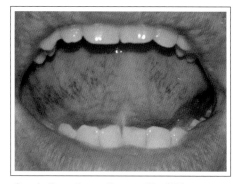

7c left: Small finely dispersed stasis dots, especially at the tip of the tongue, often indicate heart diseases like CHD.
7c right: Left: initial stage; right: different patient, advanced stage.

Comparing stasis dots, stasis spots and stasis areas (enlargement)

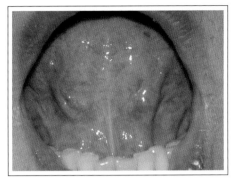 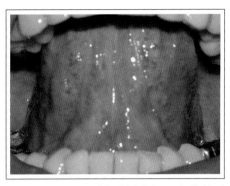

8a left and 8a right: Stasis dots that are flat and therefore do not fade when pressed, often found in *Qi* deficiency. Individual spots (left) and covering an entire area (right).

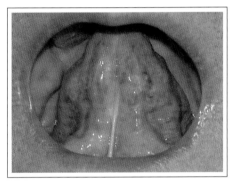 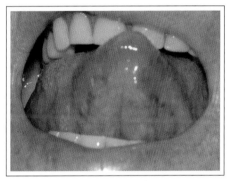

8b left and 8b right: Transition between stasis dots that fade when pressed and protruding stasis spots (left). If they cover an entire area, they can point towards pronounced stasis as seen in high blood pressure, CHD or liver cirrhosis (right).

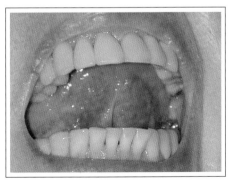 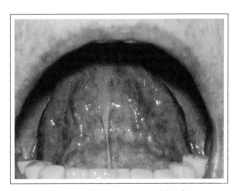

8c left and 8c right: Stasis areas can merge and become dark streaks, which can be isolated (left) or extensive (right). In these cases, there is often Cold or loss of *Zheng-Qi* with Blood stasis.

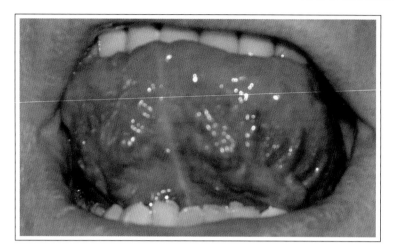

9a (top): Case of CHD, high blood pressure and arteriosclerosis: typical engorged veins obscure stasis spots.

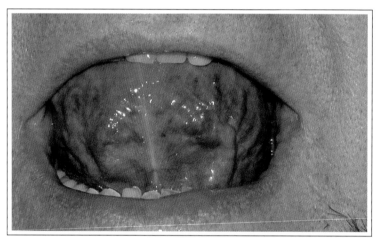

9b (middle) and 9c (bottom): After treatment the now decongested veins allow inspection of the stasis spots (middle), which in the course of the treatment will gradually fade away (below).

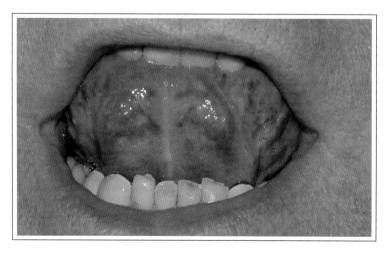

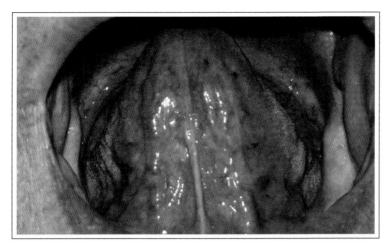

10a (top): Typical sublingual varices as is often the case in arteriosclerosis, with crooked dark blue sublingual veins and 1st degree stasis spots.

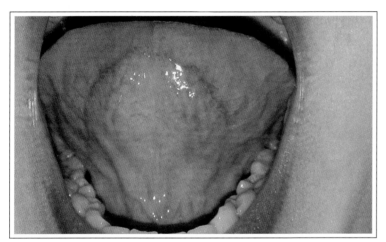

10b (middle): In this patient with myomas full extension of the tongue clearly demonstrates the formation of red Heat spots at the crown of the skin fold above the dark sublingual veins, which have reached beyond the frenulum: this is minor Blood stasis with Heat.

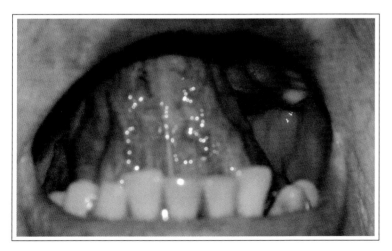

10c (bottom): In this elderly patient with pain and circulatory problems one can observe an advanced stage of Blood stasis with enlarged sublingual veins and a dark stasis area.

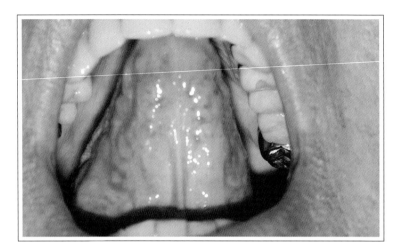

11a (top): In this patient with hepatitis, while the upper area is nearly clear, there are stasis spots accumulating almost exclusively on the sides.

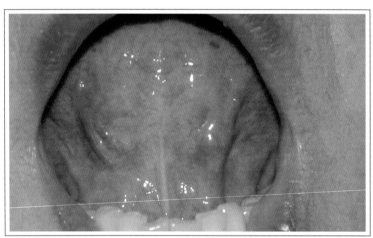

11b (middle): This patient first contracted Lyme disease and then developed rheumatic pain. Apart from a generalized enlargement of the capillaries, only one stasis spot and sublingual veins reaching beyond the frenulum can be recognized. Nevertheless, she responded well to the Heat and Blood stasis decoction.

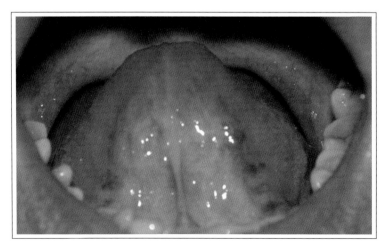

11c (bottom): In this Chinese patient with CHD (*Qi* deficiency and Blood stasis) the sublingual veins are hardly visible. Still, one can clearly see the three-dimensional enlargement of the veins, which becomes evident when the stasis spots are pressed with a spatula, and thus temporarily caused to fade.

Appendices

Appendix 1

Glossary of essential TCM terms

This glossary marks only the beginning of a bigger project of mine, in which I am trying to standardize TCM terms in German, as they are relatively uniform in the Chinese language. This was done in a similar way in the works of Andrew Ellis and Nigel Wiseman in the first published version of *Fundamentals of Chinese Medicine* in 1986.

As a result of my experiences in the translation of specialized TCM texts whilst residing in Taiwan, I occasionally like to seek advice from professional translators. I orientate myself predominantly but not solely by the functional translation theory, as suggested by Reiss and Vermeer (1984) with their application of the so-called Skopos theory. In my view, this approach, resulting from a reorientation within translation theory,[1] seems to be the most suitable for purposeful translation in the professional practice of Chinese medicine.[2]

Nevertheless, such an undertaking is extremely difficult (see my remarks about styles of translation and terminology in the Preface) and is still in its infancy. **Therefore all suggestions are welcome and, if sound and convincing, will be incorporated into later editions.**

As explained in the Preface, since this book is concerned mainly with Chinese medicine, designations such as Liver, Heart, Spleen, etc. usually denote the TCM organ function including the anatomical organ. If, in an exceptional case, the anatomical organ as defined by Western medicine is meant, this will be pointed out.

A

Anuria: *Long Bi*

Long Bi is defined as difficult urination or slowly dripping urine as well as reduced urine or pain. *'Long'* means difficult urination and dripping of a reduced amount of urine, which indicates a slow or chronic illness. *'Bi'* means total anuria with a few drops of urine at best and indicates an acute condition. Nowadays, all kinds of organic or functional changes in the bladder or the urinary system, leading to dripping or no urine, as well as every kidney related disorder with the same symptoms, are included under this heading.

According to TCM, this disease is located primarily in the Urinary Bladder, but Lung, Spleen, Kidney or Triple Burner are also involved. The transformation (*Qi Hua* in this case) of urine takes place in the Triple Burner and is supported by the Lung, Spleen and Kidney. The Lung is responsible for dispersing and descending *Qi* as well as for

---

[1] Compare Snell-Hornby 1986 (see footnote 2).
[2] Literature: Koller W (1992) *Einführung in die Übersetzungswissenschaft*. Stuttgart, Universitätstaschenbücher für Wissenschaft; Nord C (1993). *Einführung in das funktionale Übersetzen*. Stuttgart, Universitätstaschenbücher für Wissenschaft; and Snell-Hornby M (ed) (1986) *Übersetzungswissenschaft: eine Neuorientierung*. Stuttgart, Universitätstaschenbücher, Francke

regulating the water passages. If its function of dispersing and descending is disturbed, the regulation of the water passages will also become confused. The Spleen regulates transportation and transformation, including that of fluids and food. If this function is disturbed, the clear and the turbid parts of food will not be separated, the clear will not ascend and the turbid will not descend. The Kidney regulates all the water in the body and is responsible for opening and closing. If the transformation (*Qi Hua* in this case) of urine by the Kidney is disturbed, the transportation and discharge of water will be disturbed and the function of opening and closing will be impaired. *Long Bi* may arise from any dysfunction in any of the named organs. In addition, Liver-*Qi* depression (*Yü*) due to emotional upset, blockage of the arteries and vessels, external injuries, cancer and urinary stones may also affect the transformation (*Qi Hua* in this case) of urine in the Triple Burner and thus lead to *Long Bi*.

Anuria may occur suddenly or develop gradually. Defined as *Long Bi* it comprises impaired urination with dripping or total anuria that is characterized by absence of pain. When there is pain involved, the syndrome belongs to '*Lin Zheng*', painful urination.

Compare with **painful urination** and **haematuria**.

Ascites: *Fu Shui*
This is accumulation of pathogenic water in the abdomen. Wang Qing-Ren, however, calls this '*Gu*', i.e. drum, which is easily confused with meteorism, where the abdomen is swollen due to accumulation of air rather than water. The characteristic distended veins (caput medusae) described by Wang in the section *Gu Xia Zhu Yu Tang* (the 'classic' Anti-Ascites Decoction) also suggest ascites. Also see **tympanites** and **Phlegm-rheum**.

Attack, to: *Gong*
A treatment method in TCM, characterised by decimating pathogenic *Qi*, for example by using purgative medicinals that attack the pathogenic factor and expel it downwards.

B

Bi syndrome: *Bi Zheng*
A condition where pathogenic factors, such as Wind, Cold, Dampness or Heat, cause a blockage of *Qi* in the channels or organs.

1. *Bi* syndrome of the channels manifests anatomically in the limbs or joints as strong pain and partly as swelling, feeling of heaviness or signs of inflammation. Diseases belonging to the rheumatic sphere, for example soft tissue rheumatism, rheumatic arthritis and so on, may not fully correspond to the *Bi* syndrome, however many similarities and overlaps exist.

   Other painful blockages are defined according to topographical position, for example chest-Bi (heart diseases), bone-Bi or skin-Bi.

2. Furthermore, there is the rather uncommon classification, *Bi* syndromes of the *Zang* organs. They are defined as Liver-*Bi*, Heart-*Bi*, Spleen-*Bi*, Lung-*Bi* or Kidney-*Bi*.

   Also see **blockages**.

Bind, to: *Jie*
This term relates to the localized accumulation of pathogens that adopt a concrete form. Belonging to these bindings are **masses and gatherings, concretions and conglomerations**.

Binding: *Jie*
Localized accumulation of pathogens (e.g. Phlegm). Pathologically, binding overlaps with tissue hardening and swelling of the lymph nodes.

Block pattern: *Bi-Zheng*
A term used in conjunction with Wind stroke, which belongs to the **Blockage** syndromes. Generally included are disorders such as menstrual block (amenorrhoea) and intestinal block (constipation). More specifically, it denotes the block pattern after a Wind stroke, characterized by unconsciousness, convulsions, and a rapid and wiry pulse. Also see **Wind stroke** and **blockages**.

Blockage(s): *Bu Tong*

Blockages generally comprise all the stagnated products of body structures that are usually in a state of constant flow, such as *Qi*, Blood and Body Fluids (*Jin* and *Ye*). The latter when concentrated may generate Phlegm and **Phlegm-rheum**. A previously flowing substance that becomes blocked may in the long term also bring other substances to a halt, as for example *Qi* stagnation and Blood stasis may be both cause and effect of each other.

Stagnation is a blockage of *Qi*, stasis is a blockage of Blood. Liver-*Qi* depression or Liver depression is a particular form of stagnation caused by emotions or occasionally by internal Heat. See **Liver-*Qi* depression**, **Blood accumulation** and **emotional stagnation**.

Blood amassment: *Xù Xue*

This term was first used in Zhang Zhong-Jing's '*Shang Han Za Bing Lun*' (today's '*Shang Han Lun*') to describe a type of Blood stasis due to pathogenic Heat in the Lower Burner presenting with pain in the lower abdomen and sometimes also with psychological disorders (see translation of *Jin Kui Yao Lüe*, Chapter 16 and *Shang Han Lun* clause 124 in Section 3 Chapter 11.

After Zhang the term was generalized and used as a generic term for all types of **Blood stasis** as well as for **Blood depression**. It was only after Wang Qing-Ren and Tang Hong-Zai that the term was used in its more original meaning again.

Blood depression: *Xue Yù*

Blood accumulation is a kind of **blockage** belonging to the **six depressions**. In most cases it is the result of excessive anger, internal injuries or exhaustion. In his book '*Yi Xue Zhong Zhong Can Xi Lu*' (*Essential Notes on Chinese and Western Medicine*), in the section 'Concerning *San Qi*', Zhang Xi-Chun describes the case of a young shepherd from a neighbouring village, to whom befell all three causes of Blood depression at the same time when his fellow shepherd friends played a dirty trick on him.

After he had been held down and his hands tied behind his back, he was bent far over and his head stuck in his codpiece, which was then laced up.

For hours he had to remain in this position, which is traditionally called 'watching one's gherkin', in the summer heat on the meadow. When he was found, he had already fainted, but he was helped to regain consciousness. Afterwards, he suffered from a constant sensation of pressure in the chest and could not take deep breaths any more. Occasionally, he fainted again.

During the treatment, Zhang concluded that the young man's helpless struggling to free his head from the trousers, together with anger and Heat in the Blood due to the heat of the sun, had caused Blood to ascend to the chest and stop there, because it could no longer circulate; thus Blood depression was generated.

After two preparations of *San Qi* powder (Radix Notoginseng) Blood could move again and no more symptoms occurred.

This case study shows that pathogenic Heat in the Blood, exhaustion, Liver-*Qi* depression due to anger, and maybe internal injuries (Zhang did not tell us whether the boy was beaten up as well, but it appears as if he quite certainly was) were present in this case, so one could equally conclude Blood stasis to be the syndrome. It is not always possible to distinguish whether the author is referring to Blood stasis or Blood depression, since the latter was not precisely defined until after the time of Wang Qing-Ren. However, as long as the history is taken and a syndrome differentiation is made, there is no problem regarding the treatment itself. Also see **blockage**, **six depressions**, **Blood amassment** and **Blood stasis**.

Bloodletting; needle pricking: *Fang Xue*, *Ci Luo Fa*

Ci Luo Fa (small vessel pricking method) or *Fang Xue* (bloodletting), as it is called in Taiwan, may be older than acupuncture itself. Professor Unschuld holds the opinion that acupuncture points were mainly manipulated in this way at the time of the '*Nei Jing*' in ancient China, because the usage of fine needles was disseminated at a later stage. The method of bloodletting that was widely practised in the Middle Ages in the West but later became proscribed as an 'unscientific miraculous cure' has only little in common with the Chinese method.

The method described in detail in the 'Huang Di Nei Jing' ('Ling Shu': Xiao Zhen Jie etc.) remains one of the quickest and most effective varieties of manual technique. Thus, Zhang Zi-He, one of the four masters of the Jin/Yuan dynasty (twelfth century), explained that out of all methods, needle pricking achieves the speediest recovery for symptoms of dizziness, eye diseases and head-Wind (trigeminal neuralgia, facial paralysis etc.).

This method is still very popular in Taiwan and South China. For fear of infection with HIV or hepatitis viruses it could not be spread very far in the West. However, if due care is not taken, infection could equally be caused when blood samples are taken or acupuncture carried out.

Blood *Lin* syndrome: *Xue Lin*

Painful urination with cloudy and bloody urine. See *Lin* **syndrome**.

Blood stasis

Blood flow that slows down or is brought to a standstill. This can arise from exogenous factors such as traumata, pathogenic Cold and Heat as well as internal deficiency syndromes such as Blood deficiency due to loss of blood but also *Qi* deficiency, *Yang* deficiency, fatigue due to long illness, weakness after exhaustion, and internal excess syndromes such as *Qi* stagnation, emotional fits and physical overexertion.

Blood may accumulate in the blood vessels and thus it has numerous pathogenic influences on the body and its organs. It may also leave the blood vessels and present as haemorrhagic diathesis (tendency to bruise and bleed easily) with bleeding under the skin, or as haemorrhaging, which includes bloody stools, heavy menstruation, nose bleeding etc.

Also see **hyperviscosity** in the Glossary on haemorheology (Appendix 2).

Body Fluids: *Jin Ye*

General definition for all fluid substances of the body such as saliva, sputum, tears, sweat, urine, nasal secretions, but in the modern sense it may also include hormones, blood constituents, cerebrospinal fluid etc., in effect all secretions, excretions and fluid substances that are bound in an aqueous solution.

These can be further differentiated as the finer and thin fluids *Jin* (e.g. sweat, urine) ascribed to *Yang* and the coarser thick fluids (*Ye*) (e.g. sputum, nasal secretions) ascribed to *Yin*.

Therapeutically, this differentiation makes no difference as one may be able to differentiate between Blood tonifying and Body Fluids generating medicinals, but not between *Jin* and *Ye* generating medicinals. The Chinese may literally say *Sheng Jin* (i.e. generating *Jin*), however this abbreviated form is always defined as *Sheng Yang Jin Ye* (i.e. generating and nourishing *Jin and Ye*).

According to the Five Phases doctrine, the five secretions relate to the following Phases (Elements): tears relate to the Liver (Wood), sweat relates to Heart (Fire), thin-fluid saliva relates to the Spleen (Earth), nasal secretion relates to the Lung (Metal) and thick-fluid sputum relates to the Kidney (Water). For a differentiation of sputum and saliva see **sputum** and **saliva**.

As Blood and Body Fluids nourish each other, deficiency affecting Blood may cause Body Fluids to become deficient as well and vice versa. For example, excessive chronic sweating damages the Blood (= Blood deficiency); on the other hand loss of blood due to prolonged and heavy menses and other conditions may lead to internal Dryness or Body Fluids deficiency, which mostly coincides with *Yin* deficiency, as both Blood and Body Fluids belong to the *Yin* part of the body. Also see **generate fluids** and *Yin-Yang* **of the Body Fluids**.

Bone steaming fever, bone Heat syndrome: *Gu Zheng Chao Re*

Yin deficiency fever with afternoon peak, where there is a sensation of heat and noticeably hot limbs that feel as if they were heated up from the inside. The skin is cold, but if touched it warms up 'from the inside' as if it were isolated from the deeper, warmer layers. At the same time there are other *Yin* deficiency symptoms such as night sweating, hot palms and soles, pale face with red cheeks etc.

Boost, to: *Yi*
Strengthening or tonifying treatment method. Boosting (*Yi*) is commonly used in connection with tonifying *Qi*. See **tonification**.

Break, to: *Po*
See **disperse**.

C

Calm Liver–Wind: *Pin Gan Xi Feng*
A therapeutic method to treat hyperactivity of Liver-*Yang*. Most medicinals that calm Liver-Wind also lower blood pressure. Although ascending (also blazing) Liver-*Yang* (*Gan Yang Shang Kang*) is not absolutely identical with high blood pressure, there are still many matching symptoms (headache or sensation of pressure in the head, dizziness, red eyes etc.). Liver-Wind resulting from ascending Liver-*Yang* or extreme Heat (*Re Ji Sheng Feng*) may also, apart from the previous symptoms mentioned, present with tremor or convulsions of the limbs.

Calm the Mind: *An Shen*
A therapeutic method where calming or tonifying medicinals are prescribed to treat nervousness, irritability, insomnia etc. Most medicinals in this group do not have the same effect as sedative or hypnotic drugs in Western pharmacology, thus fewer side effects (e.g. daytime drowsiness) can be expected.

Chest–Bi: *Xiong Bi*
The *Chest-Bi-disease*, described as *Xiong-Bi* in the '*Jin Kui Yao Lüe*', is characterized predominantly by a sensation of pressure or tension in the chest, and to a lesser extent by intensive pain. This corresponds to mild prodromal symptoms of CHD or to untypical conditions, such as bouts of pain-free angina pectoris or silent myocardial ischemia and infarction. More severe conditions and such like, characterized by increased pain, coincide more with the syndromes of 'heart pain' – '*Xin Tong*', as described in the '*Nei Jing Su Wen*' (central chest pain reaching under the ribs, pain radiating to the shoulders and back, etc.), or with 'crushing pain' – '*Jue Xin Tong*', which is mentioned in the '*Ling*

Shu' (pain as if stabbed into the heart, accompanied by cold hands and feet, cold sweating and weakness . . .). Both these types coincide more with unstable angina pectoris or acute myocardial infarction.

Even worse is the 'absolute (literally "true") heart pain' – '*Zhen Xin Tong*', which in its pathology coincides entirely with acute infarction. It was also described in the '*Ling Shu*': 'Cyanosis of the hands and feet as far as the joints, extreme pain, starting in the morning it will lead to death at night, and starting in the evening it will lead to death in the morning . . .'. The diseases' names mentioned in the classics are thus classified according to their degree: chest-*Bi*, heart pain, crushing pain and absolute heart pain.

Chong medicinals (drugs), insect drugs: *Chong Lei*
Medicinals derived from reptiles, arthropods and crustaceans. Most are regarded as highly effective for invigorating Blood or breaking Blood stasis.

Clear: *Qing*
Pure or immaterial (e.g. clear food essences from the Spleen), in contrast to turbid which refers to impure and substantial properties.

Clumping: *Pi*
Sensation of a gathering in the upper abdomen (not palpable in most cases) or of a 'clumping in one's stomach'. The cause is Spleen-*Qi* deficiency or stagnation or, if palpable, Blood stasis or hardening. Also see **masses and gatherings** and **concretions and conglomerations**.

Cold: *Han*
1. (adj.) Property of certain medicinals that are used for cooling Heat.
2. (noun) One of the six pathogenic excesses. Also see **six excesses**, **Heat** and **Fire**.

Cold syndrome: *Zheng Han*
Pathogenic Cold causes signs like aversion to Cold, a preference for warmth and warm drinks, cold limbs, lying in a curled up position etc.

Concretions and conglomerations: Zheng Jia Ji Ju
See **masses and gatherings**.

Congealing, thickening: Ning
Heat and Cold (and sometimes Dampness) can congeal and slow down the flow of Blood, thus causing Blood stasis.

Cool, to; clear, to: Qing
A therapeutic method to remove pathogenic Heat.

Course, to: Shu
Therapeutic method with two meanings:

1. To open a blocked canal, for example a *Luo* vessel, through which no *Qi* is flowing after a Wind stroke, the vessel thus becoming numb and immobile.
2. Promoting the flow of depressed Liver-*Qi* (*Gan Qi Yu Jie*) which due to emotional upset (repressed anger) manifests as a syndrome. Also see **emotional stagnation**.

Cun, finger inch: Cun
A proportional measurement used for finding the approximate position of acupuncture points. One *Cun* corresponds to about the length of the medial phalanx of the middle finger.

Cun, Guan, Chi or 'Cun Kou' (Cun opening)
Three pulse positions superior to the radial artery: *Cun* is the distal, *Guan* is the middle and *Chi* is the proximal position. *Guan* is located directly over the styloid process of the radius above the artery, *Cun* lies distal and *Chi* proximal.

Cupping: Ba Guan
Complementary method of acupuncture. While in ancient times animal horns were applied, nowadays glass or plastic cups are applied on specific areas of the skin and acupuncture points. The resulting suction generates local stimulation, increased circulation and a partly artificial haematoma. The effect is based on a kind of 'auto-haemotherapy' which stimulates the immune system by means of macrophage activity, increased metabolism and lymph drainage, and by a reflex zone therapy on the dermatomes. The speed by which the haematoma forms reveals diagnostic clues to the permeability of the vessels. Cupping, as shown in the laboratory, increases local monocyte activity 2–5-fold as compared to areas not treated with cupping.

D

Damage: Sun
Loss and impairment, for example of Blood and fluids due to dryness, overexertion, pathogenic factors and so on.

Dampness: Shi (Shi Xie)
One of the six pathogenic factors. It may also arise from Kidney- and/or Spleen-*Yang* deficiency, when water is not sufficiently metabolized and thus leads to fluid retention. Typical symptoms are digestive disorders such as bloatedness, borborygmi, nausea, loss of appetite, heavy limbs and lethargy, a slippery or thick tongue coating and a slippery pulse.

While Heat, Cold and Dryness are easier to understand with regard to physiology and pathology, the meaning of Dampness in modern medicine is not easily interpreted. In recent years, however, more research has been carried out, with the result that Dampness is now more comprehensible to patients and TCM laymen.

In 1992, Dr Li Lian-Cheng from the town of Shijiazhuang in Hebei province examined a total of 1005 patients of whom 10.55% were ascertained to be suffering from Dampness syndrome. As the capital of Hebei province has a dry climate that is typical for North China and as the patients did not show any significant differences regarding sex, age and occupation, it can be concluded that not so much the climate but rather temperament (stagnated Liver *Qi* impairs the Spleen function) and diet (excessive, irregular and excessively fast eating habits as well as a high proportion of fat and sugar) caused Dampness.

In the humid South of China, climate plays a bigger role in the development of Dampness. The symptoms of patients in a trial there developed very slowly and primarily affected the Spleen and secondarily the Lung; the tongue had a thick sticky coating, and other key symptoms of

Dampness such as tiredness and weakness, a feeling of having a turban wrapped around the head, a sensation of clumping in the stomach and a distended abdomen occurred in 70% of the affected patients.

Dampness in this trial belongs to 'internal Dampness', which did not arise from climatic factors. But 'external Dampness' is also mentioned in TCM, outlined in the reports described below. In 1995, in a TCM hospital in Hubei province, a humid climate was artificially generated in a large-scale experiment, and live laboratory animals were observed within this high humidity climate, over a long period of time. Typical symptoms of Dampness as in humans also occurred here; for example a reduced urge to move and weakened motor ability, poor appetite, swollen joints, leg oedema, thin and unformed stool and even (as far as could be observed) a white moist tongue coating. This demonstrated that internal as well as external circumstances can lead to Dampness syndrome, as indicated in TCM theory.

As a result of these studies, in the following years (1994–1996) the mechanisms of what was happening in an organism affected by Dampness were closely examined. It was concluded that Dampness can be examined in four different areas of the body, namely the intestinal flora (digestion), the immune system (defence), energy metabolism (mental and physical activity) and pathomorphology of the lung, intestines, liver and joints.

In my personal experience, indicators of Dampness are often mycoses of the skin, mucous membranes and the intestines, which therefore respond well to medicinals that treat Dampness.

Dampness-induced generation of Cold:
Shi Cong Han Hua
Kidney- and Spleen-*Yang-Qi* are responsible for the transformation and transportation of water. In the event of Kidney- or Spleen-*Yang* deficiency or exogenous Cold invasion, the excess of unprocessed water and the Cold cause a Cold-Dampness syndrome in the lower Burner, because both are *Yin* pathogenic factors and tend to affect the lower region of the body. Typical symptoms are, for example, leg oedema or leg pain, difficult urination etc.

Dampness-induced generation of Heat:
Shi Cong Re Hua
Dampness can lead to the generation of Heat and Fire as well. In such a case, pathogenic Dampness can be both exogenous and endogenous. The latter occurs more often due to the consumption of a lot of sweet and greasy food resulting in **Phlegm** or **Dampness**. While Dampness predominantly affects the Middle Burner (Spleen and Stomach), causing indigestion, Damp-Heat tends to accumulate in the Lower Burner and creates symptoms typical for Dampness, such as heaviness and a thick 'curd-like' tongue coating, as well as symptoms typical for Heat, such as a yellow tongue coating and fever (as Dampness has a *Yin* nature, fever peaks in the late afternoon, when *Yang* declines).

Similar consequences arise from exogenous Dampness due to damp living conditions, as in basement flats or at the seaside. Thus the proportion of patients with Dampness in Taiwan (average humidity 85–95%) is very high, whilst in Tianjin (average humidity 25–55%), Dampness occurs fairly seldom as an exogenous factor.

Dampness-induced generation of Phlegm:
Shi Tan
Due to a poor transporting action caused by Spleen deficiency, Body Fluids accumulate and generate pathogenic Dampness at first. If the Dampness continues to accumulate, Phlegm may arise. Typical symptoms are thin white phlegm and oppression of the chest or abdomen, nausea and sometimes cough and shortness of breath, but in every case there is an enlarged tongue body with teeth marks, the tongue itself being shiny or slippery (*Hua Tai*).

Decoction: *Tang*
A therapeutic preparation where the medicinals are cooked in water to draw out their active ingredients.

Dehydration: *Ku*
A condition caused by the loss of Body Fluids (bleeding, sweating, diarrhoea etc.), which in TCM can also describe a chronic latent condition.

This is then called *Yin* deficiency or – more specifically – *Jin-Ye* deficiency.

Diaphoresis: *Fa*
Effluence of pathogenic factors with the sweat, either due to the body's reaction to pathogenic factors or due to treatment with diaphoretic (sweat inducing) medicinals.

Disease process: *Bing Ji*
This is the process where a disease develops and progresses. This is always mentioned in internal Chinese medicine. (For example, in the school of febrile diseases some formulas are prescribed to act on the subsequent disease level. This means, if the disease is still on the *Wei-Qi* level, the formula prescribed is designed to prevent the pathogenic factor from advancing to the *Ying* level).

Disharmony: *Bu He*
Functional imbalance between organs or regions (*Ying*, *Wei*, *Qi* and Blood).

Dispel, to: *Jie*
General term for the elimination of pathogenic factors or pathogenic energetic influences, such as toxins (detoxify = *Jie Du*).

Disperse: *San*
Therapeutically dissipating stagnated *Qi* or pathogenic factors. (The German word for *San* is 'dispergieren' for which the closest match in English is 'disperse'; the reader is reminded that the term '*San*' is also translated as 'dissipate' by Wiseman and Maciocia – Translator's note.)

Disperse, to; dispel, to: *Xiao Fa*
General therapeutic method in which pathogenic factors are eliminated, mostly Blood stasis or Phlegm. A stronger method of dispelling is breaking Blood stasis, for which Blood stasis breaking medicinals (group 3) are employed. Also see **eight methods**.

Drain, to: *Xie*
Either a pathological state in which there is a loss of body fluids, for example diarrhoea; or, more often used in the sense of the therapeutic draining of a pathogenic factor by inducing a downwards-draining action, either diuretic or purgative. If used as a therapeutic measure, translated as draining. See also **purge**.

Drink: *Yin* (third tone, contrary to '*Yin*' from '*Yin* and *Yang*', which is first tone)
A medicinal extract which is consumed cold, as often cooling medicinals were used in its production, e.g. *Xian Fang Huo Ming Yin* (Invigorating Drink of the Immortals), which is used for furuncles, skin infections etc.

E

Eight methods: *Ba Fa*
The eight methods of treatment in Traditional Chinese Medicine: Sweating (*Han Fa*), Vomiting (*Tu Fa*), Purging (*Xia Fa*), Harmonizing (*He Fa*), Warming (*Wen Fa*), Heat Clearing (*Qing Fa*), **Dispersing** (*Xiao Fa*), **Tonifying** (*Bu Fa*).

Eight principles: *Ba Gang*
The eight major principles of syndrome differentiation used in the classification of symptoms. These are the two main principles *Yang* and *Yin* and the subordinated principles of Exterior and Interior, Heat and Cold, Excess and Deficiency.

Elixir: *Dan*
Originally a definition of alchemistic formulas for prolonging life, which were used by the so-called *Wai-Dan* (Exterior Elixir) school and were mainly comprised of partly poisonous metals. Later on the definition '*Dan*' represented the processing of medicinals into pills or powder, manufactured from especially high-grade or expensive components. This designation is still valid today, so patent formulas such as *Tian Wang Bu Xin Dan* could be translated as 'Heavenly Heart Tonic Elixir' or 'Heavenly Heart Tonic Pill'. The former translation is more literal, the latter sounds better.

Emotion: *Qing Zhi*
Used here to describe the emotions as part of the complex of the human body and mind in TCM physiology and pathology.

The seven emotions mentioned in the '*Huang Di Nei Jing*' are: *Xi, Nu, Si, Bei, Kong* and *Jing*, i.e. joy, anger, worry, pensiveness, sorrow, fear and shock (depending on the translator). In the model of the Five Phases they are ascribed to the following phases (elements): joy = Fire, anger = Wood, pensiveness = Earth, worry = Metal, fear and shock = Water. According to TCM pathology, an excess of any emotion can injure the corresponding organ, for example excessive joy injures the Heart (Fire), excessive anger injures the Liver (Wood) and so on.

In the '*Nei Jing Su Wen*' (Internal Classic, Simple Questions) in the Chapter *Sheng Tong Lun* it is stated concerning the damaging influence of the emotions on the physiological *Qi* and flow of *Qi*:

> *Anger makes the* Qi *surge upwards, joy disperses* Qi, *sorrow withers the* Qi, *fear makes the* Qi *shoot downwards, Cold contracts the* Qi, *Heat makes the* Qi *flow out, shocks bring the flow of* Qi *into disarray, exhaustion consumes* Qi, *pensiveness makes the* Qi *stagnate.*

Emotional stagnation: *Qing Zhi Bu Shu*

Disturbed normal emotional activity resulting in frustration, depression, suppressed anger etc., manifesting as functional or organic disorder. Also see **course**.

Excess and deficiency: *Xu Shi*

Deficiency (*Xu*, Leere in German, Depletion or Inanitas, or asthenia syndrome, vacuity, emptiness, weakness in English), according to the eight parameters of syndrome differentiation, denotes the weakness of the **Upright** *Qi* in contrast to excess (*Shi*, Fülle in German, Repletion, sthenia syndrome, fullness in English), which stands for the strength of the pathogenic factor.

Depending upon which organ is affected, deficiency and excess are characterized by different symptoms; deficiency shows hypofunction, weakness and reduced immunity to pathological factors, whereas excess shows hyperfunction, stagnation (Blood, *Qi*, digestion), inflammatory processes or accumulation of pathogenic substances (Phlegm-rheum, Phlegm, **masses and gatherings, concretions and conglomerations**). Fever, for example, is a typical excess symptom and lack of energy is a typical deficiency symptom.

Exterior, superficial: *Biao* (3rd tone)

Relates to the outermost layer of the human body, opposite to **internal, interior**. Exogenous pathogenic factors first act on the exterior and then proceed further into the interior, unless they are removed by **Wei-Qi (Defensive Qi)** that flows in the superficial layer or by treatment (e.g. diaphoresis).

Exhaustion, taxation: *Lao*

Exhaustion arises from long illness, strong emotional overexertion (see **emotion**) or wrong diet or lifestyle, both of which damage the *Qi* of the *Zang* organs, especially of the Spleen, and can lead to pathogenic *Fire*.

Typical symptoms are general weakness, shortness of breath brought on even by slight exertion, raised temperature, spontaneous sweating without exertion, restlessness and irritability.

External, exogenous: *Wai*

Originating from outside the body. Relates to pathogenic factors that stem from the environment and act on the human body.

Eyes turned upwards: *Dai Yan*

This symptom can suggest a collapse of the *Qi* of the *Tai Yang* channel as well as Wind convulsion in children (*Jing Feng*), or Wind-Phlegm in the *Jue Yin* channel.

Wang Qing-Ren, in his essay on Wind-convulsion, describes this symptom within the following formulas: *Huang Qi Tao Hong Tang* (Astragalus Persica Carthamus Decoction), *Zhu Wei He Rong Tang* (*Wei* and *Ying* Tonifying Decoction), *Ke Bao Li Su Tang* (Guaranteed Resuscitation Decoction).

F

Fen: *Fen*

In today's TCM in China a hundredth of a *liang*, or 0.3 grams. For an overview, see **weights and measurements**.

Fire, pathogenic: *Huo*

In contrast to **ministerial Fire** of the Gate of Vitality *Ming Men*,[3] which is considered a source of life energy, and the Fire of the Five Phases, Fire in TCM pathology is one of the six (pathogenic) excesses (*Liu Yin*). It is regarded as a form of Heat that occurs only as an internal pathogen, as opposed to Wind, Dryness, Dampness and Cold. Nevertheless, exogenous Wind, for example, may transform into 'endogenous' Fire.[4] Pathogenic Fire is, like Wind, Dryness and Summer Heat, a *Yang* pathogenic factor characterized by hyperactivity or inflammation in any organ.

Endogenous pathogenic influences may also lead to Fire: intense emotional stimuli such as the five **emotions** (joy, anger, sorrow, worry and fear) can cause pathogenic Fire. Also see **Heat** and **Heat generation**.

Five palm Heat: *Wu Xin Fan Ri*

(Literally 'heat of the five hearts', heart stands for centre here.) *Yin* deficiency syndrome which often presents as hot soles during the *Yin* time at night.

Five types of exhaustion: *Wu Lao Suo Shang*

Functional disorders of *Qi*, Blood, muscles, bones and sinews caused by overuse and overexertion. Also see **exhaustion**.

Flavour, sapor: *Wei*

Originally the pure taste perception of food and medicinal substances, which was abstracted further in the course of the millennia, and today stands mostly for certain properties of medicinals. For this reason we may not perceive some of the herbs categorized as sweet to actually taste sweet.

---

[3] An extensive discussion of the historical and physiological meaning of the *Ming Men* can be found in an article published in 1962 by Qin Bo-Wei, which was translated into English by Charles Chase and is included in his book *A Qin Bo-Wei Anthology* (see Appendix 7).

[4] 'Endogenous' is in quotation marks because there is no such thing as exogenous Fire, as Nigel Wiseman defines it in *Theoretical Foundations of Chinese Medicine*. Fire is *always* endogenous, even if it can arise from exogenous factors.

Bai Zhu (Rhizoma Atractylodis Macrocephalae) for example is described as bitter and sweet, but as it has a more bitter taste, 'sweet' isn't really the right word. In this case 'sweet' is to be understood as the equivalent of tonifying (*Bu*), as *Bai Zhu* belongs to the group of tonifying medicinals. In total, there are seven flavours, which are also related to the Five Phases.

Pungent (*Xin*): Disperses pathogenic *Qi* (*Xie Qi*) which has invaded the outer layer of the body (*Biao*), improves the circulation of *Qi* and Blood (*Xue*). Therefore it is suitable for the treatment of exterior conditions (e.g. by using *Ma Huang* (Ephedra) or *Gui Zhi* (Cinnamon branch)) as well as *Qi* stagnation (e.g. *Chen Pi* (Orange peel), *Mu Tan* (Sandalwood)) and Blood stasis (e.g. *Hong Hua* (Carthamus)).

Sweet (*Gan*): Strengthens, nourishes and tonifies, especially Stomach and Spleen, which it also harmonizes. Furthermore it calms acute symptoms such as pain and spasms. Therefore it is suitable for most deficiency syndromes, Stomach and Spleen dysfunctions and acute disorders (typical representatives of this group are, for example, Ginseng and Liquorice).

Bland (*Dan*): Removes Dampness and has a diuretic effect, which makes this flavour suitable for the treatment of all syndromes affecting the fluid balance such as urine retention, oedema and so on (*Lai Fu Zi* (dried radish seeds) and *Che Qian Zi* (Plantago seeds) are two of the most common representatives of this flavour).

Sour (*Suan*): Has a gathering and astringing effect, consolidates and maintains a firm stool. Therefore, it is used in the treatment of diarrhoea, chronically increased urine, leukorrhoea, sweating and other types of loss of fluids (e.g. *Rou Dou Kou* (Nutmeg) and *Wu Wei Zi* (Fructus Schisandrae)). Regarding their action, astringing medicinals are almost equal to sour medicinals (e.g. *Wu Bei Zi* (Gallnuts)), but they are used predominantly for loss of Body Fluids.

Bitter (*Ku*): Dries Dampness (*Long Dan Cao* (Chinese Gentian)), purges Heat and Fire (*Shi Gao* (Gypsum) and *Lu Gen* (Reed)), descends rebellious *Qi* (*Xing Ren* (bitter Almond)) and works as a laxative by relaxing the bowels (*Da Huang* (Rhubarb) and *Fan Xie Ye* (Senna leaves)). This group is suitable for the treatment of excess syndromes such as Heat and Cold, for example cough with shortness of breath, vomiting and constipation.

Salty (*Xian*): Softens masses and hardenings like swollen lymph glands and gout (*Hai Zao* (Seaweed) and *Hai Ge Ke* (Clam Shell powder)) and also has a draining action by dissolving and removing abdominal masses (e.g. *Mang Xiao* (Mirabilite)).

Summarized in the Table below are flavour, corresponding organ and Phase (Element) and the therapeutic effect in terms of Chinese pharmacology:

Sour (or astringing)	Bitter	Sweet (or bland)	Pungent	Salty
Liver, Wood	Heart, Fire	Spleen, Earth	Lung, Metal	Kidney, Water
Gathering, consolidating, astringing stool	Drying, cooling	Nourishing, tonifying, (diuretic)	Dispersing	Softening, draining

Fluids: *Ye*

The more concentrated forms of Body Fluids, e.g. nasal secretions, sperm, sputum. Also see **Body Fluids**, **sputum**.

Four masters of the *Jin-Yuan* dynasty: *Si Xue Pai*

The four founders of the Schools of the thirteenth and fourteenth century are:

1. Liu Wan-Su (School of Cooling), who in his work 'San Xiao Lun' criticized the contemporary official prescriptions for being too hot; instead, he recommended cooling and bitter medicinals.
2. In his work 'Rumen Shiqin', Zhang Cong-Cheng (School of Purgation) propounded the use of purgative medicinals for diseases due to emotional problems.
3. Li Dong-Yuan (School of Strengthening Earth), who propounded in the 'Pi Wei Lun' (*Treatise on the Spleen and Stomach*) and other books the method of strengthening the Middle with tonics.
4. Zhu Dan-Xi (School of Nourishing *Yin*), who recommended in the 'Dan-Xi Xinfa' (*Dan-Xi's Best Methods*) and other works a combination of all three Schools. However, he formulated his own theory and argued that *Yin* should be nourished.

Four seasons: *Si Ji*

To promote one's health, Chinese tradition and Taoist philosophy recommend a different lifestyle for every season (see Table).

The *Huang Di Nei Jing*'s advice according to the four seasons:

Activity	Spring	Summer	Autumn	Winter
sleeping/waking up	dusk/early morning	dusk/early	early/early	early/late
recommended clothing	loose, comfortable, preferably light clothing	avoid damp clothing (soaked with perspiration)	no cool or damp underwear	keep head cool, back and feet warm
healthy/unhealthy food and which to avoid	+ sweet/– sour, alcohol – fat, greasy	+ spicy/– sour, – raw, cold, one should not eat one's fill	+ sour/– spicy, – too hot or too dry	+ bitter/– sour, – sour spices
physical exercise	go for gentle walks	go mountain climbing, exercise	moderation	avoid strenuous exercise
mental state	relaxed and cheerful	undaunted, no anger	reflection	calm and meditation

Also see **twenty-four seasonal periods**.

Fu organs: *Fu*

The *Fu* organs or labour organs stand for the six organs attributed to the *Yang* (Gall Bladder, Small Intestine, Stomach, Large Intestine, Urinary Bladder and Triple Burner). Their function is to digest food, to absorb essential constituents and excrete unwanted constituents. One exception is the Gall Bladder, which apart from contributing to digestion also stores bile like the *Zang* organs (storage organs) and thus it belongs to the extraordinary organs.

G

Gan deficiency syndrome: *Gan Ji*

The same factors that in adults lead to exhaustion syndrome (*Lao*) of the Spleen, cause *Gan* deficiency syndrome in children. The signs are a yellow complexion (Earth and Spleen Phase), dry skin and hair, tiredness and dull eyes.

Wang Qing-Ren wrote on this topic:

> . . . *because in most cases the cause of the disease is overfeeding with milk. If too much fatty and sweet food can no longer be absorbed, it will stagnate in the stomach, the transport of food will be impeded and the gastrointestinal tract is gradually damaged. In this way, stagnating Heat is generated. If this Heat becomes greater, the* Gan *deficiency syndrome develops,* Qi *and* Blood *are reduced and Body Fluids (*Jin Ye*) run dry.*

See Chapter 10, Wang Qing-Ren's description in the '*Yi Lin Gai Cuo*', Part 2, of indications for *Tong Qiao Huo Xue Tang* (Orifices Opening Blood Invigorating Decoction), number 14, infantile malnutrition (*Gan* syndrome) (p. 195).

There are overlaps with diseases defined in Western medicine, such as malnutrition and worms in infants.

Gan syndrome of the gums: *Ya Gan*

Swelling, reddening and ulceration of the gums, usually caused by Wind-Heat pathogens. Also see **Gan deficiency syndrome**.

Generate fluids: *Zeng Ye* or *Sheng Jin*

Therapeutic method using a tonifying principle in the treatment of internal Dryness or Body Fluids deficiency.

Globus sensation: *Mei He Qi*

Described as 'globus hystericus' in homeopathy, this is the sensation of a foreign body stuck in one's throat or chest just below the throat, which cannot be moved or dissolved. It occurs most commonly in individuals with Liver-*Qi* depression due to emotional upset. This symptom was first described by Zhang Zhong-Jing in the '*Shang Han Za Bing Lun*' (today's '*Jin Kui Yao Lüe*') and treated with *Ban Xia Hou Po Tang* (Pinellia and Magnolia Decoction).

Grey–white: *Cang Bai*

Coming from *Cang*, black-blue and *Bai*, white: a pale complexion with slight cyanosis. Such a complexion often occurs in unconscious or shock patients.

H

Haematemesis: *Ou Xue*

Vomiting of blood from the stomach or oesophagus. Often a sign of Blood-Heat (*Xue Re*).

Haematuria: *Niao Xue, Sou Xue*

Blood in the urine.

Heart: *Xin*

1. Zang organ which apart from the biomedical functions also incorporates mental functions (see **mind: Shen**).

2. A region below the lower end of the sternum which can include the anatomical organs of the heart and the stomach, as the expression '*Xia Xin*', i.e. 'below the Heart', refers to the epigastrium. For example, this is the case in *Xie Xin Tang* (Heart Relieving Decoction).

3. In established expressions such as '*Wu Xin*' (literally five hearts) the term '*Xin*' denotes centre or meeting point. See **five palm Heat**.

Heat: *Re*

1. Heat can refer to pathogenic factors such as Summer Heat, Wind-Heat and Damp-Heat, but also to endogenous Heat generated by a hyperactivity of *Yang-Qi*, which inside the body can transform into Fire. Generally, the pathogenic factor Heat suggests a raised temperature or fever, inflammations or reddening of the skin or sensations of Heat.

2. Heat in contrast to Cold, in terms of the eight types of syndrome differentiation: here, Heat points to a *Yang* disease and an excess condition as well (except empty Heat due to *Yin* deficiency). Typical symptoms are aversion to heat or hot drinks (also liking for cool temperatures and drinks), a red tongue body with a yellow coating and a rapid pulse, skin erythema and so on.

Heat generation: *Hua Re*

This term refers mostly to the pathogenesis of Fire. For example, Wind or another exogenous pathogenic factor may transform into Heat or Fire inside the body. The latter occurs when a febrile infectious disease (*Wen Re Bing*) invades the *Qi* level and high fever develops. Further symptoms are increased irritability and aversion to heat, dry mouth and lips, thirst, rapid pulse and red tongue body, often with a yellow coating. If the Body Fluids are injured, there is also dark scanty urine and hard, dry stool or constipation.

Hyperactivity of *Yang-Qi* may also lead to endogenous generation of Heat, which mostly manifests as *Fire*. Also see *Heat* and *Fire*.

Hemiplegia: *Ban Shen Bu Sui*

In ancient times it was believed that one side of the body withers (*Ku*) following an apoplexy (see **Wind stroke**) because *Yuan-Qi* cannot nourish one half of the body. Thus, Wang Qing-Ren's famous formula *Bu Yang Huan Wu Tang* (*Yang* Tonifying Five-Tenth Decoction) literally means: *Yang* tonifying, the (lacking) five returning decoction. As Wang points out, hemiplegia is due to the lack of five of the originally ten parts of *Yuan-Qi*.

Holding Blood in the vessels: *She Xue*

The function of holding Blood in the vessels is attributed to *Qi* and the Spleen. From the point of view of haematology, the physiological density of the vessel walls is implicated, which may decrease under the influence of certain infectious diseases and lead to haemorrhaging into the vicinity of the vessel.

Hot to the touch: *Zhuo Re*

Heat that is felt objectively by touch, in contrast to subjective sensations of Heat, for example **five palm Heat** due to *Yin* deficiency, which are only felt by the patient.

Hyperactivity: *Kang*

This is nearly always related to an extreme activity of the *Yang* part of an organ due to a weak *Yin* part lacking control, as in Liver-Fire blazing upwards (*Gan Yang Shang Kang*). It is based on the loss of balance of *Yin* and *Yang*, as explained in the theoretical foundations of TCM.

I

Icterus: *Huang Dan*

The biomedically defined icterus is not absolutely identical with jaundice (*Huang Dan*) in TCM. Jaundice is categorized further into *Yin* and *Yang* jaundice in TCM, but *Yin* jaundice (*Yin Huang Dan*) is not necessarily characterized by a yellow pigmentation but rather by other symptoms in addition (see Table below).

Yang jaundice (*Yang Huang Dan*)	*Yin* jaundice (*Yin Huang Dan*)
Yellow pigmentation of the skin and sclera, fever, no appetite and nausea, dry mouth with bitter taste, pain in the hypochondrium area, yellow and sticky tongue coating (Huang Ni Tai) and a wiry rapid or slippery rapid pulse.	Possible yellow pigmentation of the sclera and dull, sallow yellow pigmentation of the skin (may not be present), raised temperature and easily fatigued, no appetite (still often gaining weight), a pale tongue body with a thick sticky coating, a fine and deep, weak or slow pulse.

While *Yang* jaundice is mostly found in acute cases, for example viral hepatitis, *Yin* jaundice occurs predominantly in cases of chronic hepatitis.

Insufficiency: *Bu Zu*
Absence of a substance or incompleteness of a function, e.g. Spleen-Stomach insufficiency or insufficiency of Defensive *Qi*.

Integrated Chinese Medicine: *Zhong Xi Yi Jie He*
One of the three medical systems in China, where the integration of science and Western medicine with Traditional Chinese Medicine is pursued in order to continue developing and complementing Chinese medicine.

Its aim is to increase the efficiency of diagnosis and treatment by offering a greater choice and mutual complementation of Western and Eastern medical systems. Avoidance of contradictions in the theoretical foundations when employing both systems jointly is achieved by the fact that the practitioner of Integrated Chinese Medicine learns to adopt a flexible attitude, so that a disease or pathological condition can be observed alternately from both perspectives.

Consider the following example: *Lu Rong* (Cornu Cervi Parvum) is the classical *Yang* tonifying medicinal used for male infertility, which is a typical sign of *Yang* deficiency. Is this just superstition or do the horns of the stag in rut in fact have an effect on fertility?

According to various Chinese and Japanese studies the prepared horn contains Mao inhibitors, lysophosphate-1-cholin, chondroitin sulphate A, gangliosides and organic glucoses and also female sex hormones, but no male sex hormones. As Bensky says, preparations of *Lu Rong* did not cause any typical sexual reactions in male rats and mice that had had their gonads removed. Does this mean that *Lu Rong* is perhaps a *Yin* tonic?

The latest Scottish and American studies published in *Nature*[5] have shown that oestrogen is found in high amounts in the efferent spermatic ducts in men. There, it concentrates sperm by reabsorbing the more watery fluids (water = *Yin*) and is probably also responsible for the maturation of sperm. An absence of oestrogen or of its receptors would result in insufficient male fertility (*Yang* deficiency).

If *Lu Rong* or *Yin Yang Huo* (Herba Epimedii), or *Tu Si Zi* (Semen Cuscutae) are prescribed, which are all *Yang* tonics containing phytohormones and substances that stimulate oestrogen, then many infertility disorders in men could be successfully treated. Certainly, the respective symptoms have to be differentiated first, as there are various other types of fertility disorders. Still, this digression from the field of TCM into pharmacology and physiopathology demonstrates how easy it is to relate these different medical systems to each other in Integrated Chinese Medicine.

Internal, interior: *Li*
This term refers to deep layers of the body, such as the *Zang Fu* organs, in contrast to the channels. Within Zhang Zhong-Jing's diagnosis of the six channel stages (*Liu Jing Bian Zhen*) **interior** relates to the *Yang Ming* channel and the three *Yin* channels (*Tai Yin, Shao Yin, Jue Yin*). The *Shao Yang* channel is regarded as half-exterior, half-interior. Also see **exterior**.

Invigorate Blood: *Huo Xue*
To stimulate the flow of Blood. A group of Chinese medicinals that treat slowed or stagnated blood flow. These days, Blood invigorating medicinals are classified into three categories: Blood harmonizing, Blood moving and Blood stasis breaking medicinals.

Invigorate the *Luo* vessels: *Huo Luo*
Mostly used for **Bi-syndrome**, **Blood stasis**, **Wind stroke** and similar conditions with **blockage**. Method for removing obstructions from the vessels and *Luo* vessels, in cases of pain and paralysis. Many Blood invigorating and Blood stasis breaking medicinals are used here, for example *Chong* **medicinals**, and also those of a hot nature.

---

[5] *Nature* (1997; 390;449–450, 509–512)

Example: *Huo Luo Dan* (Pill to Invigorate the Channels).

Irritability: *Xin Fan*
Restlessness or increased irritability due to disease processes that affect the Heart organ, e.g. Heat in the Heart.

L

Latent Heat, hidden Heat: *Fu Re*
When, for example, a febrile disease (*Wen Bing*) can not be cured properly, it hides in the body as residual Heat. Symptoms are irritability, thirst, bad breath, dark urine and hard stools and other typical Heat symptoms. Many kinds of relapses or re-infections come into this category.

Li: li
Unit of weight, today's equivalent would be 0.031 g.

Liang: *liang*, Chinese ounce
Unit of weight, which from the Qing dynasty until today is equivalent to approximately 31.25 g. In the year 1979 during the time of the Chinese reform it was rounded to 30 g. Traditionally, 16 *liang* are equivalent to one *jin* (Chinese pound), which in Taiwan and Hong Kong is 600 g. Due to the rounding off in China, 16 *liang*, which is one *jin*, would be the equivalent of only 480 g; eventually, the *jin* was fixed at 500 g, so now there is no more uniformity. In every case one *liang* has 10 *qian*, 100 *fen* or 1000 *li*. Also see *li*.

Lifting: *Tou*
The therapeutic lifting of a latent pathogen to the exterior or skin layer, for example when promoting the eruptions of measles for quicker healing and prevention of the pathogen progressing into deeper layers.

Limbs, heavy: *Kun*
Physical fatigue or lassitude often occurring in syndromes of Dampness or Spleen deficiency, which arises from insufficient transformation of fluids by the Spleen. Mental capacity remains unaffected, an essential factor for differential diagnosis.

Lin syndrome: *Lin*
This kind of stranguria is characterized by painful and difficult urination and usually develops from Damp-Heat in the Urinary Bladder, from hypo-function and deficiency of Kidney-*Qi*, or partly from descending Middle *Qi*. The term may encompass every kind of dysuria, but it is still a broader expression than **painful urination** and dysuria (also see **anuria**).

Liver–*Qi* depression: *Gan Qi Yu Jie*
The Liver is particularly susceptible to anger, not only according to the Five Phases (Elements), but *Zang Fu* theory also states that stress, anger and emotional pressure can impair the free flow of *Qi*. As the Liver is responsible for the smooth flow of *Qi*, an impairment of its flow may lead to a condition of depressed Liver-*Qi* presenting with pain or pressure in the hypochondrium area (one or both sides) and a wiry pulse.

Several other symptoms may arise from this situation: in the case of **rebellious *Qi*** (*Qi Ni*) a **globus sensation** may develop. In the case of a weak Stomach, Spleen-*Qi* may be attacked by an excessive controlling action of depressed Liver-*Qi* ('Wood suppresses Earth' or 'Spleen deficiency due to Liver depression'), which may also present as pain in the hypochondrium area, and in addition bloatedness, loss of appetite and tiredness. Liver-*Qi* depression over a long period of time may substantiate as *Qi* stagnation or **Blood stasis**, from which in turn abdominal masses, **masses and gatherings**, **concretions and conglomerations** may develop.

Menstrual disorders such as late or early menses may be another direct consequence of Liver-*Qi* depression.

Lochias: *E Lou*
Heavy continuous bleeding of the mother after delivery. Often occurs if Blood stasis

is present prior to delivery. Compare with **metrorrhagia**.

Loss of control: *Bu Gu*

This term relates to the loss of Body Fluids (diarrhoea, spermatorrhoea, vaginal discharge and sweating) or Blood, which can be treated with stabilizing or consolidating medicinals (*Gù Se*). If, for example, *Wei-Qi* is weakened (*Wei Qi Bu Gu*), excessive sweating will deplete the fluids, leading to internal Dryness or *Yin* deficiency.

Also see **Body Fluids**.

M

Maculopapular eruptions: *Ban Zhen*

Macules are flat red skin lesions, papules are raised eruptions of the skin. Both are associated with exogenous Heat conditions (e.g. measles).

Mania and depression: *Dian Kuang*

Mania and depression are both disorders of the Mind. Mania is a *Yang* syndrome because it includes extroverted active symptoms such as aggression, shouting, loud laughing or singing for no reason, whilst depression is a *Yin* syndrome because it has more introverted inactive symptoms such as apathy, quiet talking to oneself, fleeing into dark and secluded rooms, loss of appetite. Although mania is often due to a *Yang-Qi* excess syndrome of the Heart and depression can be due to both a *Qi* deficiency syndrome of the Spleen or the Heart and an excess syndrome like **Liver-*Qi* depression** or Phlegm, when faced with mental disorders one should always think of **Blood stasis**.

Manic agitation: *Kuang Zao*

Agitation or depression with typical manic behaviour. See **mania and depression**.

Masses and Gatherings: *Ji* and *Ju*

Syndromes which refer to abdominal masses or gatherings, especially food in the digestive tract. Masses (*Ji*) denote immovable, hard abdominal masses in contrast to gatherings, which refer to movable and soft abdominal accumulations. The latter are often related to stagnated *Qi* within the *Zang* organs, whereas the former are related to Blood Stasis within the *Fu* organs. Both are accompanied by pain and fullness.

Another form of abdominal masses is **concretions and conglomerations**. These are often confused with masses and gatherings. Both syndromes are related and are often no longer distinguished from each other. Nevertheless, a comparison is shown in the Table below.

Concretions and conglomerations (*Zheng Jia*)		Masses or gatherings (*Ji Ju*)	
Predominantly in the Middle Burner, due to wrong diet		Predominantly in the Lower Burner and due to stagnation caused by **emotional upset** (in women more often following gynaecological disorders)	
Concretions (*Zheng*)	Conglomerations (*Jia*)	Masses (*Ji*)	Gatherings (*Ju*)
In *Zang* organs	In *Fu* organs	Blood stasis between organs and meridians	
More related to Blood	More related to *Qi*	More related to Blood	More related to *Qi*
Hard, immovable	Soft, movable	Fixed place	No fixed place
Fixed pain	Moving pain	Fixed pain	Moving pain
Palpable	Not palpable	Palpable	Not palpable
Remain palpable	Dissipate	Remain palpable	Dissipate after a while

Both syndromes share the same aetiology; they either arise from emotional stagnation and other causes that lead to a stagnation of Liver-*Qi*, or from dietary mistakes which injure the Spleen and impair digestion. The former relates more to accumulations and gatherings (*Ji Ju*), whilst the latter relates more to concretions and conglomerations. Nevertheless, pathogenic Phlegm may also be the cause of all four forms of masses.

Although the initial stagnation of *Qi* cannot be localized and has no substance, it manifests as a changeable gathering or conglomeration, and by its long-term presence will eventually cause Blood stasis. The materializing Blood stasis forms a palpable mass that has a fixed location and a fixed pain, therefore leading to masses and concretions.

This is one of the most characteristic examples in TCM of how functional disorders can turn into organic disorders, and thus diseases that are first only perceived by the patient develop into concrete diseases that can be observed and measured by the physician.

See also **binding** and Tang Zong-Hai's definition within the *Xue Zheng Lun* (Treatise on Blood Syndromes) (see Chapter 11).

Meteorism due to Blood stasis: *Xue Gu*

Heavy abdominal stagnation due to Blood stasis, presenting with black stool, dark urine and caput medusae (distended abdominal veins). As many Blood stasis medicinals show a good effect on liver diseases, a relationship to this syndrome is also acknowledged.

Metrorrhagia: *Beng Lou*

Uterine bleeding (also slight) occurring between periods. Often a sign of Blood stasis. The last character '*Lou*' is also mentioned in '*E Lou*' i.e. lochias, and stands for a continuous slight discharge of blood from the female genital canal. '*Beng*' means 'collapse' and stands for a massive, irregular uterine bleeding. Strictly speaking one should translate '*Beng*' with metrorrhagia and '*Lou*' with metrostaxis, however, in classical literature such a precise differentiation cannot be found, which has resulted in today's modern Chinese literature using both characters together.

Middle: *Zhong*

The Spleen and Stomach, the Middle Burner.

Mind: *Shen*

An abstract principle standing for a healthy physiological performance of the mind, i.e. of consciousness.

In the broader sense, in TCM diagnosis the term *Shen* also stands for the healthy physiological performance of the organs, which for example is reflected in the *Shen* of the tongue and the *Shen* of the pulse.

Ministerial Fire: *Xiang Huo*

The Fire of the Heart (*Jun Huo*) is regarded as imperial Fire. Together with the ministerial Fire from the *Ming Men* (Gate of Vitality) it supports the activities of the *Zang Fu* organs. It also exists in the Liver, Gall Bladder and Triple Burner. Also see footnote[4] for **Fire, pathogenic**.

Miscarriage, prevention of: *An Tai*

Literally meaning 'calming the foetus'. The prevention of habitual miscarriage and the safeguarding of a healthy pregnancy via the use of Chinese medicinals.

Muscles and flesh: *Ji Fu*

The muscles and the flesh surrounding them. They are assessed according to the extent to which they reflect the general health and the physical reserves of the body.

N

Night sweating: *Dao Han*

Spontaneous perspiration during sleep which ends upon waking. Mostly a result of internal Heat due to *Yin* deficiency. Also see **spontaneous sweating**.

Nocturia: *Ye Jian Duo Niao*

Excessive or frequent urination at night. In TCM this symptom occurs mostly in relation to Kidney-*Yang* deficiency. This symptom usually abates after the 'internal body clock' (i.e. the cycle of waking and sleeping in chronobiology) has been synchronized again, which is achieved by prescribing the appropriate astringing and *Yang* strengthening medicinals (e.g. *Yin Yang Huo* (Herba Epimedii), *Sang Piao Xiao* (Ootheca Mantidis) and *Yi Zhi Ren* (Fructus Alpiniae Oxyphyllae)).

Nourish, moisturize: *Zi, Yang*
A tonifying method, used especially for deficiency of *Yin* or Blood (= nourish *Yin*). Also see **tonification**.

Numbness, sensation of: *Ma*
Classical literature defines numbness as 'ants crawling on the skin', a pulsating stabbing sensation and total insensitivity (*Ma Mu*) to sensation or pain. Wang Qing-Ren listed this symptom as one of the prodromal signs of **Wind stroke** (corresponds in the main with our understanding of apoplexy); therefore he contributed a great deal to the diagnosis of stroke. In the '*Yi Lin Gai Cuo*', in the chapter 'The condition before the disease (apoplectic prodromal symptoms)', it is stated: '. . . abruptly their leg went numb or the muscles suddenly twitched and some say they always had a sensation of cold in the tips of their fingers. . .'.

O

Obstruction: *Bi*
Pain and/or numbness caused by an interruption of the flow of *Qi* in the channels. See **blockages** and **block pattern**.

Oliguria: *Niao Shao*
Abnormally small amount of urine.

Oral *Gan*, *Gan* of the mouth: *Kou Gan*
One of the *Gan* deficiency syndromes in children with ulceration of the oral mucosa, Frequently seen in candidiasis (thrush). See *Gan* **deficiency syndrome**.

Orifices: *Qiao*
The seven orifices are external openings of the *Zang Fu* organs, namely eyes (Liver), ears (Kidneys), nose (Lung), mouth (Spleen) and tongue (Heart). They are important pointers for diagnosis (e.g. rhinitis suggests looking to the Lung organ) and treatment (orifices opening medicinals are used to regain consciousness after syncope). Wang Qing-Ren's *Tong Qiao Huo Xue Tang* is effective for Blood stasis affecting the head manifesting in diseases of the orifices, such as tinnitus and sudden deafness.

P

Painful urination, dysuria: *Niao Tong*
Painful urination is often a sign of pathogenic Heat in the Lower Burner or of the so-called **Lin syndrome** (see above).

Pale white: *Dan Bai*
Mostly associated with a pale complexion. Pale stands for Blood deficiency, hence a Blood deficiency syndrome. According to the Five Phases principle, white is related to the Lung organ (functional entity).

Palpitations: *Xin Ji*
A noticeable, evident throbbing of the heart sometimes associated with exhaustion or emotional factors. Also see **panic palpitations**.

Panic palpitations (or fearful throbbing): *Zheng Chong*
Panic palpitations are a clearly noticeable, accelerated throbbing of the heart throughout the chest, which also feels like 'pumping' to the patient. This sensation is stronger than **palpitations** and persists for longer. While palpitations may suggest both excess and deficiency, panic palpitations is a symptom belonging to deficiency syndromes.

Papules: *Ban*
See **maculopapular eruptions**.

Paralysis: *Tan Huan*
Loss of muscular strength and sensitivity.

Pathogen: *Xie*
Every damaging factor that impairs heteropathic (physiological) processes. Pathogenic factors are abstractions of disease-causing influences or structures that act on the body either from the interior or from the exterior.

Pathogenic Qi: *Xie Qi*
See *Qi*.

Phlegm: *Tan*
There is a saying in TCM: 'Phlegm is the mother of all diseases'. In the '*Nei Jing*' only the expression **Phlegm-rheum** syndrome (*Tan Yin Zheng*), 'accumulated rheum', is mentioned. The name 'Phlegm syndrome' did not occur because the '*Nei Jing*' had not yet differentiated it. The term 'Phlegm' was first coined by Zhang Zhong-Jing and has remained in

use since then. Phlegm is a product of the Body Fluids (*Jin Ye*), which are derived from food and drink. As Phlegm is also a transformed product, it cannot be described as an 'untransformed substance'. Normal processes of transformation strengthen the body and result in sufficient *Wei-Qi* and *Ying-Qi* (Defensive *Qi* and Nutritive *Qi*). However, the formation of phlegmy substances has its basis in *Qi* and Blood as well; if transformation becomes abnormal and the Zang Fu organs become diseased, the Body Fluids will also be impaired and thus Phlegm and thick-fluid substances are generated from *Qi* and Blood. Also see **Phlegm-rheum**.

Phlegm–rheum: *Tan Yin*

Phlegm (*Tan*) and Rheum (*Tan Yin*) are generated from a concentration of **Body Fluids** due to the insufficient transporting action of Lung-, Spleen- or Kidney-*Qi* (**Dampness induced generation of Phlegm**), *Yang* deficiency or *Qi* stagnation.

Phlegm is of a more concentrated and turbid nature than Rheum, and it can also lead to physical as well as mental disorders. In the narrow sense, Phlegm is identical with the Western term and is then called exterior Phlegm (*Wai Tan*). In the broad sense however, Phlegm includes a wide range of diseases, whereas Phlegm-rheum manifests merely physically as accumulation of pathogenic water (oedema) in the body cavities, and in the arms and legs.

According to Zhang Zhong-Jing's definition (in the '*Jin Kui Yao Lüe*'), Phlegm-rheum in the narrow sense is water retention in the stomach and intestines, characterized by symptoms such as borborygmi (gurgling intestinal noises), loss of appetite, thin liquid stool, emaciation and retching.

A comprehensive account of the aetiology, pathogenesis, diagnosis and treatment of Phlegm, Phlegm-rheum and pathogenic water accumulation can be found in Steven Clavey's *Fluid Physiology and Pathology in Chinese Medicine* (see Appendix 7).

Pills: *Wan*

A method of preparing medicinals, where either the ground medicinal substances or the extracts of decocted and concentrated medicinals are processed into pills using honey as a binding agent. The so-called 'honey boli' or honeyed pills mostly have a tonifying character and are processed with concentrated honey.

Potency: *You Du*, *Wu Du*

According to the traditional definition, mild medicine is preferable to drastic medicine, so very drastic medicinals should only be used for critical and highly acute syndromes. Consequently, all more or less drastic medicinals were labelled as 'slightly poisonous', 'poisonous' or 'highly poisonous'.

In this case, poisonous does *not* mean 'toxic' as in Western medicine, but in the case of a 'highly poisonous' drug, such as for example Radix Aconiti, it certainly overlaps with the definition of 'toxic'.

As the term 'poisonous' is a very flexible term both in China and in the West, when dispensing medicinals that are labelled 'non-poisonous' one still needs to take into consideration not only the dosage, but also the constitution and age of the patient and the severity of the disease. Furthermore one should discontinue the medicinal as soon as possible after a significant improvement has been achieved, to guarantee the highest degree of safety.

To give an example: in China, the term 'toxicity' is set far lower than in the West, for reasons mentioned above. If modern chemotherapy drugs were to be classified according to Chinese principles, nearly *all* would have to be graded as 'poisonous', as pointed out by Porkert.[6]

Toxicity can be reduced significantly by processing the medicinal. For example, aconite that is properly cooked and prepared as a medicinal is 5000–10 000 times less poisonous than the raw drug.

Polyuria: *Niao Duo*, *Niao Pin*

Excessive urination or frequent scanty urination.

Prescription: *Fang (Fang Zi)*

A composition of medicinals for therapeutic application. Classical prescriptions (*Jing Fang*) and modern prescriptions (*Shi Fang*) are differentiated. Classical prescriptions stem from Zhang Zhong-Jing exclusively and were recorded in the '*Shang Han Za Bing Lun*' (later: '*Shang Han Lun*' and '*Jin Kui Yao Lüe*'); they are now used predominantly in Japan and partly in China. However, the majority of Chinese physicians use modern prescriptions, which is every prescription from the second century up to this day.

---

6 Manfred Porkert, *Klassische Chinesische Pharmakologie*, Heidelberg 1978 (see Appendix 7).

Pulse: *Mai*

Taking the pulse is one of the four foundational diagnostic methods of TCM. The following Table and Box provide an overview of the 28 classical pulses in Chinese medicine.

Purge:

Drain downwards by purgatives like On Huay (Kheum) in order to rid of heat, dampness and other pathogens.

Chinese, English	Quality, characteristics	Main indication
Kou Mai, hollow pulse	Palpable at the superficial and deep level, but hollow in the middle	Loss of Blood (due to bleeding), heavy sweating
Fu Mai, floating pulse	Strongest at the superficial level, less palpable towards the deeper levels	Strong: excess on the exterior. Weak: Blood/*Yin* deficiency
Ge Mai, drum-like pulse	Wiry at the superficial level, hard, big. Hollow in the middle and deep level	Exterior Cold with Middle deficiency, loss of *Qi* or *Yin* (Blood, *Jing*)
Ru Mai, soggy pulse	Can be felt at the superficial level, weak wave, fine and soft	*Yin* deficiency, Kidney-*Jing* exhaustion, pathogenic Dampness
San Mai, scattered pulse	Arrhythmic, only at the superficial level where it is indistinct, no *Chi* pulse, weak	Kidney *Yuan-Qi* scattered, *Yang-Qi* not consolidated; in severe illnesses
Hong Mai, overflowing pulse	Wave arrives powerful and strong, leaves in a long and weak wave	Great Heat, at the superficial level: *Yang*-excess; rapid: pathogenic Fire
Chen Mai, deep pulse	Can only be felt at the deep level	Strong: internal excess. Weak: internal deficiency
Lao Mai, firm pulse	Located at the deep level, where it is long, powerful and wiry	Cold accumulations in the abdomen, heart pain, arteriosclerosis
Ruo Mai, weak pulse	More evident at the deep level, wave is weak, fine and soft	Deficiency of *Qi* or *Yang*, *Yang* sinking, exhaustion, old age
Fu Mai, hidden pulse	Located at the deep bone level, hardly evident even on strong pressure	Excess: blockage of pathogenic energy in the interior, extreme pain

Chinese, English	Quality, characteristics	Main indication
Xuan Mai, wiry pulse	Slim, long and flat (deep), the wave is straight without peak, like a line	Liver-Wind/Fire and *Qi* depression (*Yù*), pain, Phlegm, Stomach deficiency
Chi Mai, slow pulse	Arrives and leaves slowly, less than 70 bpm (up to 3 beats per breath)	Superficial: *Yang* deficiency (*Wei*). Deep: *Ming Men* (*Yang*) deficiency
Jie Mai, knotted pulse	Arrives as if slowed down, missing a beat, arrhythmic	Cold, blockages: *Qi*, Blood, food, Cold Phlegm; *Qi*/Blood deficiency
Se Mai, choppy pulse	Arrives and leaves reluctantly and unsatisfactorily, flat	Weak: chronic conditions, weakness Powerful: *Qi* stagnation, Blood stasis
Huan Mai, slowed-down pulse	Calm and relaxed (pulse), arrives and leaves a little slowed down	Normal, in combination with other pulses pathological (e.g. Dampness), then mostly soggy (*Ruan*)
Shuo Mai, rapid pulse	Rapid pulse, greater than 90 bpm (6–7 beats per breath)	Superficial, weak: *Yin* deficiency. Deep, powerful: internal Heat
Cu Mai, hasty pulse	Fast (>90 bpm), arrhythmic, missing one beat	Pronounced excess of Heat/Fire, blockage of *Qi*, Blood, food or Phlegm
Dong Mai, moving pulse	Powerful, slippery, rapid, only a short peak can be felt but not the wave arriving and leaving	Pain, shock, *Yin/Yang* not harmonized, medication, strong tonics
Wa Mai, hurried pulse	Pulse frequency dashing <140 bpm (7–8 beats per breath)	*Yin* collapse with *Yang* excess, impending collapse of *Yuan-Qi*
Xu Mai, empty pulse	All three positions weak, can only be felt in one level, soggy	All kinds of deficiency syndromes; if weak: *Yang*, if hollow: *Yin*
Wei Mai, minute pulse	Extremely thin and soft; sometimes palpable and then disappears again	Collapse of *Yang*, collapse of Blood and *Qi* (= Ginseng)
Xi Mai, fine pulse	Fine (= slim), soft, like a thread of silk but distinct	*Qi* and Blood deficiency, often Liver/Kidney *Yin*, exhaustion (*Lao*)

hinese, English	Quality, characteristics	Main indication
C*Duan Mai*, short pulse	Does not extend beyond the '*Guan*', flat wave with small peak	Weak: *Qi* deficiency. Powerful: *Qi* stagnation
Dai Mai, intermittent pulse	Missing 1–3 beats regularly: arrhythmias and blockages	*Qi* collapse of the *Zang* organs, Middle Cold, trauma, pain
Shi Mai, full pulse	All levels palpable, long, wave arrives and leaves powerfully	All kinds of excess syndromes
Chang Mai, long pulse	When rolled to and fro it exceeds the normal position of the pulse	Healthy Middle *Qi*; if wiry: Liver-*Yang* Fire

Chinese, English	Quality, characteristics	Main indication
Jin Mai, tight pulse	Feels powerfully elastic like a ball, waves vibrate slightly	Pain, Cold (interior, exterior, *Shang Han*), digestive stagnation
Hua Mai, slippery pulse	Moves smoothly, almost elegantly below the fingers, mostly powerful	Healthy: pregnancy, Blood excess, medication. Ill: Phlegm
Da Mai, big pulse	Broad, long, powerful like *Hong Mai*, wave is even, not surging	Powerful: exogenous Heat. Weak: *Lao* exhaustion (Blood, *Qi*), empty *Yang*

The pathological significance of pulses

Deficiency pulses
Yang deficiency: *Ruo Mai, Chi Mai, Xu Mai, Wei Mai*
Yin deficiency: *Ji Mai, Ru Mai, Fu Mai, Xi Mai, Lao Mai*
Qi deficiency: *Dai Mai, Jie Mai, Duan Mai, Ruo Mai, Ge Mai, Xi Mai, Da Mai*
Blood: *Kou Mai, Jie Mai, Fu Mai, Ge Mai, Xi Mai, Wei Mai, Da Mai*
Other: *Se Mai* = collapse, *Ru Mai* = Kidney-*Jing*, *Ge Mai* = Middle, *Xuan Mai* = Stomach

Excess pulses
Heat: *Hong Mai, Shuo Mai, Cu Mai, Da Mai*
Fire: *Xuan-Chang Mai* (in case of Liver-Fire), *Hong Mai, Cu Mai*
Cold: *Lao Mai, Jin Mai, Jie Mai, Dai Mai*
Dampness: *Ru Mai, Hua Mai*
Phlegm: *Xuan Mai, Hua Mai*
Qi stagnation: *Se Mai, Duan Mai*
Blockage, stasis, *Yù*: *Cu Mai, Jie Mai, Fu Mai, Jin Mai* (Food stagnation), *Se Mai* (Blood, *Qi*), *Xuan Mai*
Pain: *Jin Mai, Fu Mai, Dong Mai, Dai Mai, Xuan Mai*
Other: *Dong Mai* = shock

Definite deficiency pulses
Dai Mai: *Qi*-deficiency
Kou Mai: loss of Blood, Blood deficiency
Ji Mai: *Yin* deficiency
Xuan Mai: Stomach
Se Mai: collapse due to chronic overexertion
Duan Mai (weak): *Qi* deficiency

Definite excess pulses
Lao Mai: Cold accumulation
Ru Mai: Dampness
Duan Mai: *Qi* stagnation
Fu Mai: exterior excess
Chen Mai: interior excess
Shuo Mai: Heat in the interior
Hua Mai: Phlegm
Da Mai: exterior Heat pathogens
Xuan Mai and *Chang Mai*: hyperactive Liver-*Yang*

Deficiency pulses with two indications
Ruo Mai: *Qi* deficiency, *Yang* deficiency
Ru Mai: *Yin* deficiency, Kidney-*Jing* deficiency
Fu Mai: (if weak) *Qi* deficiency, *Yin* deficiency
Xu Mai: (if weak) *Yang* deficiency, *Yin* deficiency
Jie Mai: *Qi* deficiency, Blood deficiency
Da Mai: (if weak) *Qi* deficiency, Blood deficiency in *Xu-Lao* (exhaustion)

Excess pulses with two indications
Se Mai: Blood stasis, *Qi* stagnation
Fu Mai: pain, blockage
Cu Mai: Heat (Fire), one of the six depressions (*Yù*)
Dong Mai: pain, shock
Jie Mai: Cold, one of the six depressions (*Yù*)
Dai Mai: Cold, pain

Q

Qi: *Qi*

This term – pronounced *'chee'* and spelled *ch`i* in the Wade-Giles system – still defies every precise definition. *Qi* is best described as a type of bio-energy, which flows through the entire universe and also the human body in all forms and variations.

However, in today's China *Qi* is described as a substance because it not only possesses energetic but also material properties.[7]

Wiseman and Ellis compare the subgroups of *Qi* essential for the human body – *Yuan-Qi, Jing-Qi, Zhen-Qi* – using the concepts described below.

Tian-Qi (cosmic *Qi*) represents air and its vital oxygen, *Gu-Qi*[8] (Food *Qi*) represents the essential nutrients. *Jing-Qi* (Essence or Sperm-*Qi*) represents the genetic code and the information which is given to children by their parents and facilitates the transformation of *Tian-Qi* and *Gu-Qi* in the

---

[7] For further details regarding modern research on *Qi* the reader is referred to my popular scientific article published in English: '*Qigong, Tai-chi chuan* and encounters of the third kind', Yu Xiang Magazine, Taipei 1993.

[8] This term is often wrongly translated as 'Grain-*Qi*' in English language literature, because the word '*Gu*' means cereal and in the classical sense should be translated as 'staple food'. Taoist fasting '*Bi Gu*', described by Sun Si-Miao in his work '*Qian Jin Yi Fang*' and Ge Hong in his work '*Bao Pu Zi*', means total abstinence from all food, not only from grain. In the '*Nei Jing*', the character is often used together with the character for water (*Shui*), therefore '*Shui Gu*' means food and drink and not food and grain.

The fact that in the People's Republic of China the modern shorthand version uses the character valley (homonym of *Gu*, grain) only causes more confusion, so now out of six translations of the '*Nei Jing*', Section 5, Manifestation of *Yin* and *Yang*, where both characters (valley and grain) appear, I could only find one that is correct. There it is stated: '*The Qi of the valley (Gu) manifests in the Spleen, the Qi of the rain in the Kidney*.' As the Spleen is also called '*Shui Gu Zhi Hai*', i.e. storehouse of food and drink (not 'sea of grain and water') and as both '*Gu*' characters are identical in short form, a correct translation of this section is rarely found, except in the translation of Chinese author Ni Maoshing who grew up in the USA. Also see my article in *Naturheilkunde* 1/2001: '*Pulsdiagnose: Der Atem des Patienten oder der Atem des Therapeuten als Maßstab*' (R. Pflaum Verlag).

cells into a live organism. *Yuan-Qi*, the congenital *Qi* (or more mystically, Pre-Heaven *Qi*), finally combines these three forms of *Qi* that allow the body to live and grow.

Zhen-Qi is the opposite of pathogenic *Qi*, *Xie-Qi*. However, it is identical with the defensive aspect of Upright *Qi* (*Zheng-Qi*). Also see **Upright Qi**, **True Qi**, **Wei-Qi** and **Ying-Qi**.

Qi pain: *Qi Tong*

Pain that was caused by *Qi* stagnation. In contrast to pain due to Blood stasis, which is perceived as stabbing, this type of pain presents as dull and covering a larger area.

Qian: *qian*

Unit of weight, a tenth of one *liang*. From the Qing dynasty to today it was the equivalent of approximately 3.125 g. It was rounded to 3 g after the time of the Chinese reform in 1979, which because of the quality of medicinal drugs in China does not always bring ideal results. However, many people who are not Chinese show a stronger reaction to Chinese prescriptions, so the balance is restored in this case.

Nevertheless, the dosage should always be determined individually for each patient. Also see **liang**.

R

Rebellious Qi (*Ni Qi*), reversal of Qi flow: *Qi Ni*

Apart from deficiency of *Qi*, *Qi* depression and *Qi* stagnation, the flow of *Qi* may also be disturbed, which is then called reversal of the flow of *Qi*. For example. Stomach-*Qi* should normally descend for the transport of food. If it reverses, symptoms such as hiccup or vomiting arise. Lung-*Qi* or Liver-*Qi* may also flow in the wrong direction, causing symptoms such as asthma and shortness of breath (Lung-*Qi*) or headache and dizziness (Liver-*Qi*).

Regulate Blood: *Li Xue*

Therapeutic method where diseases are treated at the Blood level. Although other methods can be implied, such as nourish Blood (*Bu Xue*), cool Blood (*Liang Xue*) and warm Blood (*Wen Xue*), most Chinese texts use this term for stop bleeding (*Zhi Xue*) and invigorate Blood (*Huo Xue*). The latter can be classified into three stages: 1. harmonize Blood (*He Xue*); 2. invigorate Blood (*Huo Xue* or *Hua Yu*); and 3. break Blood stasis (*Po Xue* or *Po Yu*).

Regulate *Qi*: *Li Qi*
Collective term for all therapeutic methods in TCM that concern the *Qi*: strengthen (tonify) *Qi* in *Qi* deficiency, move *Qi* (*Xing Qi*) in *Qi* stagnation, remove obstructions (*Tong Qi*) in Liver-*Qi* depression and harmonize *Qi* (*He Qi*) in **rebellious *Qi*** (*Qi Ni*).

Residual Heat: *Fu Re*
See **latent Heat**, **hidden Heat**.

Running piglet syndrome: *Beng Tun*
This syndrome, first mentioned in the '*Shang Han Lun*' by Zhang Zhong-Jing, mostly points towards Kidney deficiency. It is described as a sensation of a substance or gas ascending from the abdomen to the chest and throat. It also belongs to the five accumulations (*Wu Ji*) which include the *Pi* clumping sensation (see **clumping**).

S

Saliva: *Xian*
The thin-fluid part of the Body Fluids formed in the mouth. According to TCM theory it is regarded as a fluid belonging to the Spleen. Also see **sputum**.

Scrape, *Guasha*: *Gua Sha*
The *Gua-Sha* method (*Gua Sha Fa*) causes a local skin irritation by scraping or scratching with a flat and broad utensil, such as a coin or a spoon, and has an even greater relationship to traditional medicine than the *Ba Guan* method. While cupping is still used in hospitals and clinics in Taiwan and China, the scraping method is only used at home. Nevertheless, in the last few years *Gua Sha* books have boomed in Asia and it has become so popular that now physicians

occasionally prescribe it to their patients as 'homework'.

Using a broad coin or – for reasons of hygiene – a somewhat thick tablespoon (e.g. silver), the sore muscle (mostly in the neck or the shoulder area) is stroked firmly over the skin in *one* direction. When a spoon is used, the convex side faces the skin, so as to avoid cutting into it. This can be continued until a slight reddening of the skin or slight bleeding is visible. In the latter case, the skin should be disinfected afterwards. One may also scrape large areas, for example reflex zones on the skin of the corresponding organs, but for this purpose the *Zou-Guan* method (running cupping) is better as it can encompass a larger area. *Gua Sha* is only recommended for small or uneven areas of skin which cannot be reached with the *Zou-Guan* method.

Seven types of prescriptions: *Qi Fang*
Classical categorization of prescriptions into strong prescriptions (*Da Fang*), mild prescriptions (*Xiao Fang*), quick prescriptions (*Ji Fang*), slow-working prescriptions (*Huan Fang*), even-numbered prescriptions (*Qi Fang*), odd-numbered prescriptions (*Ou Fang*) and compound prescriptions (*Fu Fang*) that combine two or more base formulas. Many modern prescriptions belong to the last category, which – like 'Compound Prescriptions', used for example in the treatment of AIDS – are regarded by the World Health Organization (WHO) as the method of prescription for the twenty first century.

Shortness of breath: *Qi Shao*
Characterized by rapid and shallow breathing. Occurs frequently with *Qi* deficiency.

Sinews: *Jin*
In its anatomical meaning, the word *Jin* sometimes represents sinews, sometimes ligaments and also fasciae. In TCM, these '*Jin*' correspond to the Liver and for this reason present in classical texts in the case of ascites due to Liver disease as caput medusae on the abdominal wall, described as green and protruding sinews (*Jin*). As a matter of fact, in that location they are blood vessels and not sinews, as Wang Qing-Ren had already correctly observed.

On the other hand, it is mentioned in Western *Qi-Gong* literature that the collected *Qi* would be stored in the fasciae (again *Jin*). However, this demonstrates the problem with such translations, as TCM expressions cannot be converted so easily into anatomical terms. The '*Nei Jing*' merely states that 'the *Jin* are the hard', so that the standard work '*Zhong Guo Yi Xue Da Ci Dian*' (*Encyclopaedia of Chinese Medicine*) explains laconically: '*Jin* is the substance that has power in the flesh'.

Six excesses: *Liu yin*
In many English language publications, this term is unfortunately often translated as 'six exogenous pathogenic factors' or 'six environmental factors', which in my opinion is not only a misleading but also a wrong translation.

The word '*Yin*' in today's spelling had already appeared in the '*Li Ji*' (*Classic of Rites*) of the Zhou dynasty, where it indicated negative connotations of exuberance and 'too much'. In the historical records '*Shi Ji*' of Sima Qian it also implied an exuberance of Dampness, after which later generations identified it with a long-lasting rainfall, as in the oldest dictionary of China, the '*Shuo Wen*'. It appears fourteen times in the medical context of the '*Nei Jing*' (*Internal Classic*), solely on its own and not in connection with the number six, where it has the meaning of an exuberance of *Qi* or pathogenic Dampness.

In contrast, the term '*Liu Qi*', i.e. the six *Qi*, is already used in the '*Nei Jing*' and implies firstly six forms of energies in the body, namely *Qi*, Essence (also sperm), Blood, thin-fluid and thick-fluid Body Fluids and the channels. Secondly, it denotes a seasonal classification, namely Wind season (spring), Summer Heat, Fire season (probably late-summer when the farmers burnt their fields), Damp season (Monsoon), Dryness season (autumn) and Cold season (winter).

The '*Nei Jing*' contains many analogies in terms of 'as it is outside, so it is inside' or 'as above, so it is below', where natural phenomena are compared to human physiology.

Today's interpretation of the six excesses (*Liu Yin*) being an excess of the six environmental factors (*Liu Qi*) stems from modern sources and is not acceptable, because the pathogenic factor Fire does not occur as an exogenous factor; it can only develop from other endogenous or exogenous factors inside the body.

The other five of the six excesses are Wind, Summer Heat, Dampness, Dryness and Cold.

Also see **Fire**, **Heat** and **Heat generation**.

Six depressions: *Liu Yu*
As chyme, Blood, *Qi* and Body Fluids are substances that are constantly flowing, every kind of impairment of this flow will thwart physiological processes. When *Qi*, which is responsible for the transportation of all other substances, is in a state of depression (**Liver-Qi depression**), it is the basis of all other depressions, namely **Blood depression**, Dampness depression, Heat depression, Phlegm depression and digestive depression. For this reason, *Qi* should always be treated as well.

The six depressions can mostly be related to an emotional depression, which would equally indicate treatment of the preceding emotion. Also see **Liver-Qi depression** and **emotion**.

Soften, to (of hardenings and masses): *Ruan Jian*
Therapeutic method for treating hardening and clumping such as abdominal masses by using softening and dispelling medicinals. This method is often used for tumours (e.g. lymphomas). Also see **masses and gatherings**, **concretions and conglomerations** and **clumping**.

Soften the Liver: *Rou Gan*
Therapeutic method for treating Liver-*Yin* or Liver-Blood deficiency by using Blood nourishing medicinals. Typical symptoms are dry eyes and mouth, poor sleep with frequent dreams, dizziness and tinnitus and a weak or fine pulse.

Somnolence: *Shi Shui*
Physical tiredness and an excessive need for sleep. Often classified as *Qi* deficiency or excessive Dampness, but it may also suggest *Yin* deficiency Blood stasis.

Spontaneous sweating: *Zi Han*
Spontaneous sweating during the day, also when at rest. In most cases due to a weakness of *Yang* or

a deficiency of *Wei-Qi* (Defensive *Qi*) which fails to regulate the closing of the pores at the superficial layer.

Sputum: *Tuo*
The thick-fluid part of Body Fluids formed in the mouth, which according to TCM theory is regarded as a fluid belonging to the Kidney. Some modern sources also differentiate the site of excretion and ascribe sputum to the sublingual salivary glands but saliva to the other salivary glands. However, this makes no difference for diagnosis or treatment. Also see **saliva**.

Stagnation: *Zhi*
A slowing down or standstill of the flow of a substance. In contrast to 'stasis', which is more related to Blood, this term is mostly used for food stagnation and *Qi* stagnation.

Stasis: *Yu*
A slowing down or standstill of movement, mostly in relation to Blood.

Stasis clot: *Yu Kuai*
Clotting of menstrual flow, mostly indicative of Blood stasis.

Stasis dots: *Yu Dian*
Purple-blue or dark dots on the tongue body which indicate the presence of Blood stasis.

Stasis spots: *Yu Ban*
Purple-blue or dark spots or streaks on the tongue body which indicate the presence of Blood stasis.

Stiffness: *Jiang Zhi*
Difficulty in moving the neck or back, often in the presence of pathogenic Wind.

Strengthen the Spleen: *Jian Pi*
Also called strengthen the Middle, refers to a tonifying therapeutic method using *Qi* strengthening medicinals with a tropism for the Spleen organ (functional entity), e.g. Codonopsitis Pilosulae (*Dang Shen*) and Rhizoma Atractylodis Macrocephalae (*Bai Zhu*) (see **tropism**).

Strengthen the Yang: *Zhu Yang*
A therapeutic method for tonifying *Yang-Qi*.

Strengthening, tonification: *Jian*
Supplementing a *Zang Fu* organ (Stomach, Spleen, Middle etc.). Also see **strengthen the Spleen** and **supplementation**.

Stroke: *Zhong*
Sudden or severe acute disease condition due to pathogenic energy, for example Wind stroke.

Supplementation: *Yi*
Supplementation is a therapeutic method for strengthening the *Zang Fu* organs, *Yang* and *Qi* or for nourishing[9] *Yin* and Blood by using tonifying medicinals.

Syndrome: *Zheng*
In TCM, a syndrome consists of a significant combination of various symptoms, which taken together suggest a certain disease.

Syndrome differentiation and treatment discussion: *Bian Zheng Lun Zhi*
'*Bian Zheng*' means recognizing the disease, whilst '*Lun Zhi*' means finding a treatment method. They are the practical application of the theories of TCM and therefore a fundamental step towards the treatment of diseases.

This consists of theory and treatment principles, which in turn are related to the selection of herbs and prescriptions. These four parts are very closely interrelated; none of them should be missing, or the result will be incorrect. *Bian Zheng Lun Zhi* is derived from the holistic reflection and analysis of the four diagnostic methods (*Si Zhen*) and eight principles (*Ba Gang*); this means that the origin and the development of a disease are used

---

[9] Tonifying, strengthening, nourishing and supplementing basically mean the same. However, it has become the custom in China to use these terms in the following combinations: for supplementing (*Yi*) the organs 'strengthen' (*Jian*) is used, for *Yin* and Blood 'nourish' (*Yang*) or 'moisturize' (*Zi*) and for *Qi* and *Yang* 'tonify' (*Bu*) or build up (*Zhuang*).

as a basis for finding the appropriate treatment, either a composition of medicinals or a combination of acupuncture points. If not the entire condition but only individual aspects of the disease are differentiated, one will fail to recognize the nature of the disease, and thus the treatment and prescription will be used incorrectly.

T

Tonification, to tonify: *Bu (Fa)*
See **supplementation**.

Toxin: *Du*
Toxins are pathogenic or poisonous factors caused by Heat diseases, such as Heat toxins, which give rise to the typical signs of inflammation redness, heat, swelling and pain, as well as serous secretions (pus, lymph). Toxins are treated with Heat cooling and detoxifying medicinals, e.g. Forsythia, Taraxacum etc. According to recent pharmacological findings they show antimicrobial and virustatic effects. In the language of conventional medicine, these toxins can be considered to be pathogenic microorganisms both in their existence and in their effect on the body. However, this is another case in which a TCM term has a broader meaning than its affiliated Western term.

Transformation: *Hua*
'*Hua*' has many meanings in TCM; physiologically it stands for transformation and change, e.g. the transmission of energy from Kidney-*Qi* to the Bladder, which provides it with the power to collect and excrete urine.

Pathologically, it denotes the progressive transformation of one pathogenic energy into another, e.g. 'Phlegm transforming into Fire'.

In treatment, it denotes the regressive transformation of a pathogen into a non-pathogenic state, e.g. 'transformation of Phlegm' (into normal Body Fluids).

Tropism: *Gui Jiang*
A herb's tropism defines its 'site of action' with regard to the TCM organs (functional entities), i.e. how its effect is developed most evidently inside the body, in terms of channels and TCM organs. It should not be forgotten that the holistic 'body system' is always affected in its *entirety* and not selectively (e.g. by treating the Liver, one also affects its interrelated *Fu* organ, the Gall Bladder). Tropism only indicates the area where the main effect takes place. The theoretical foundations and other aspects of the nature of the medicinals should be taken into consideration in this case as well.

For example, ginger, tiger lily bulb, mustard seeds and shallots (*Jiang, Bai He, Bai Jie Zi, Cong Bai*) are all pungent herbs, except lily bulb. Although they all act on the Lung, they do so in totally different ways: ginger warms Cold in the Lung, lily bulb tonifies deficient Lung *Yin*, mustard seeds dissolve Phlegm and shallots balance excess in the Lung.

True *Qi*: *Zhen Qi*
True *Qi* is a synonym for Upright Qi (*Zhen Qi*) which is the body's physiological *Qi* in contrast to pathogenic Qi '*Xie Qi*'. Also see **Qi** and **Upright Qi**.

Turbid: *Zhuo*
According to **Yin Yang** theory, turbid fluids are attributed to *Yin*, whilst clear fluids are attributed to *Yang*. In TCM physiology, the clear parts of food are energetic essences that the Spleen extracts from food. The turbid parts of food are passed on to the intestines for excretion. In TCM pathology, Phlegm and Phlegm-rheum are regarded as the most turbid of all pathogens. Also see **clear** and **Phlegm-rheum**.

Twenty–four seasonal periods (solar seasons): *Jie Qi*
These are periods of 15 days as arranged in the ancient Chinese farmers' almanac, which play an important role in the *Wen-Bing* School (febrile diseases) and in Blood stasis. Also see Chapter 11, Wang Qing-Ren's '*Yi Lin Gai Cuo*': the thirteenth indication for *Tong Qiao Huo Xue Tang* (Orifices Opening Blood invigorating Decoction).

The 24 seasonal periods are:

1. Start of Spring (*Li Chun*), approximately on 5.2.
2. Rain Water (*Yu Sui*), approximately on 20.2.
3. Insect Awakening (*Jing Zhi*), approximately on 7.3.
4. Vernal Equinox (*Chun Fen*), approximately on 22.3.

5. Clear Brightness (*Qing Ming*), approximately on 6.4.
6. Rains of Grain (*Gu Yu*), approximately on 21.4.
7. Start of Summer (*Li Xia*), approximately on 6.5.
8. Small (Grain) Plenty (*Xiao Man*), approximately on 22.5.
9. Grain Ear (*Man Zhong*), approximately on 7.6.
10. Summer Solstice (*Xia Zhi*), approximately on 22.6.
11. Small Summer Heat (*Xiao Shu*), approximately on 8.7.
12. Great Summer Heat (*Da Shu*), approximately on 24.7.
13. Start of Autumn (*Li Qiu*), approximately on 8.8.
14. End of Heat (*Chu Shu*), approximately on 24.8.
15. White Dew (*Bai Lu*), approximately on 8.9.
16. Autumnal Equinox (*Qiu Fen*), approximately on 24.9.
17. Cold Dew (*Han Lu*), approximately on 9.10.
18. Descending Frost (*Shuang Jiang*), approximately on 24.10.
19. Start of Winter (*Li Dong*), approximately on 8.11.
20. Light Snow (*Xiao Xue*), approximately on 23.11.
21. Heavy Snow (*Da Xue*), approximately on 7.12.
22. Winter Solstice (*Dong Zhi*), approximately on 22.12.
23. Little Cold (*Xiao Han*), approximately on 6.1.
24. Severe Cold (*Da Han*), approximately on 21.1.

Tympanites, meteorism: *Gu Zhang*

Contemporary Chinese literature defines 'Gu Zhang', i.e. a drum-like distension, as meteorism and distension of the abdomen due to intestinal gases. However, in classical literature, meteorism and ascites are not so clearly distinguished. Some authors described symptoms of ascites such as protruding veins, but called them 'Gu Zhang'.

Still, ascites was usually referred to as 'Fu Shui', i.e. 'abdominal water'. Therefore, one should always make sure whether 'Gu' or 'Gu Zhang' refers to tympanites or ascites. Also see **ascites**.

U

Upright *Qi*: *Zheng Qi*

Zheng means 'ordered' or 'upright' in Chinese. Upright means normal, in the physiological sense.

When an exogenous pathogenic factor invades the body, it is called pathological *Qi* (*Xie Qi*). According to TCM, fever or a raised temperature are generated from the fight between this pathological *Qi* and the 'ordered', upright *Qi*.

Urinary block: *Niao Bi, Long Bi*

Urinary retention. Being unable to pass urine in spite of a full bladder.

V

Vaginal discharge: *Dai Xia*

In diagnosis, white and yellow discharges are differentiated primarily. The former suggests Cold while the latter suggests Heat. Red or brown discharge indicates intermenstrual bleeding, which may indicate the presence of Blood stasis (one should always think of neoplasms as well). However, based only on this symptom, without any further information, a precise diagnosis or syndrome differentiation cannot be achieved.

Vertigo, dizziness: *Yun*

The sensation of everything revolving around one, in TCM often associated with ascending Liver-*Yang*.

Vessel: *Mai (Mo)*

A vessel in which Blood or *Qi* flows. In another context '*Mai*' can also denote pulse.

Vomit, to: *Ou Tu*

Literally 'retching (*Ou*) and vomiting (*Tu*)' which are respectively: nausea with retching but without vomiting, and vomiting contents of the stomach. As it is used as one in modern Chinese, it is not usually translated separately. In contrast, there is the expression '*Gan Ou*', dry retching, which is used when no substance apart from a little saliva is spat out.

W

Water–rheum: *Shui Yin*

See **Phlegm-rheum**.

Wei and *Ying*: *Wei Ying*

Wei or *Wei-Qi* is the utmost *Yang* aspect of *Qi*: it flows under the epidermis, which is the outermost region of the body. It warms, protects and controls the opening and closing of the pores, which are all functions pertaining to *Yang*.

Ying nourishes and is closely related to Blood (*Yin*); as a result Blood and *Ying* are often not differentiated any further. Also see **Wei-Qi**, **Ying-Qi** and **Ying-Wei disharmony**.

Wei-Qi: *Wei-Qi*

In the same way as *Ying-Qi*, Defensive (or Protective) *Wei-Qi* arises from the extraction of refined food. In comparison to *Ying-Qi* it is more *Yang*, and as *Qi* in comparison to Blood is already of a *Yang*-nature, *Wei-Qi* constitutes one of the strongest *Yang* aspects of the body: it is strong, agile and aggressive, and flows in the outer layers of the body outside the channels. Its main functions are to protect against exogenous pathogenic factors and to control the opening and closing of the pores, in other words thermoregulation by sweating. In addition it warms the *Zang Fu* organs and moisturizes skin and body hair. When it is weakened or disturbed, the body will be more susceptible to pathogens, or there is a tendency to excessive sweating: a so-called *Ying-Wei* disharmony arises.

Also see **Yin and Yang**, **Ying-Qi**, **Ying-Wei disharmony** and **Wei and Ying**.

Weights and measurements

Today in the People's Republic of China (PRC) (market)	China before 1979 and today in TCM	Taiwan today in TCM and in general
1 *Jin* = 500 g = 10 *liang*	1 *Jin* = 500 g = 16 *liang*	1 *Jin* = 600 g = 16 *liang*
1 *liang* = 50 g	1 *liang* = 31.25 g	1 *liang* = 37.5 g
1 *qian* = 5 g	1 *qian* = 3.125 g	1 *qian* = 3.75 g
1 *fen* = 0.5 g	1 *fen* = 0.3125 g	1 *fen* = 0.375 g
1 *li* = 0.05 g	1 *li* = 0.03125 g	1 *li* = 0.0375 g
1 *hao* = 0.005 g	1 *hao* = 0.003125 g	1 *hao* = 0.00375 g

Wind stroke: *Zhong Feng*

The classical meaning of Wind stroke by Zhang Zhong-Jing is a Cold-induced disorder due to pathogenic Wind with symptoms such as fever, headache and a floating pulse. However, this meaning is only valid when referring to the '*Shang Han Lun*'. Present-day meaning defines internal damage due to deficiency of *Qi* and Blood caused by emotions, poor diet or lifestyle, which have led to a disharmony of *Yin* and *Yang* in the *Zang Fu* organs. Middle-aged and elderly men and women are affected.

The consequences and symptoms vary according to the type of Wind stroke, but they mostly match the symptoms of apoplexy.

Causes of Wind stroke may be:

Causes or triggering factors include:

- emotional excesses (anger, stress etc.)
- poor diet (fat, sugar etc.)
- exhaustion, overexertion
- Deficiency/absence of *Zheng-Qi*.

These lead to:

- *Yin/Yang* disharmony, or
- Blood/*Qi* disharmony.

The triggering factor will then lead to:

- Disharmony of the flow of Blood or *Qi*, or to
- Syndromes of Phlegm or Blood stasis.

Vascular/cerebral damage is differentiated as:

1. Mild stroke, TIA, transient sequelae
2. *Jing Luo* stroke (channel and collaterals)
3. *Zang Fu* organ stroke
4. Death.

These have the following symptoms (increasing degree of severity):

1. Problems with speaking and swallowing, paraesthesia, facial paralysis
2. Hemiplegia, impaired consciousness
3. Unconsciousness, spastic or paralytic coma
4. Death

1. Liver-*Yin* deficiency due to pathogenic Wind caused by hyperactivity of Liver-*Yang*, which itself was triggered by emotional upset such as anger.

2. Pathogenic Phlegm due to Excessive consumption of fat, sugar, alcohol and so on, generating pathogenic Heat or Blood stasis. When the body's limits are exceeded, Phlegm may generate pathogenic Wind.

3. Existing deficiency of Blood or *Qi*, which in the presence of a further triggering factor, e.g. sexual overindulgence, may generate deficiency Wind.

4. Existing deficiency of *Zheng-Qi*. If the body is attacked by another pathogenic factor, this may entail a collapse of *Yuan-Qi*.

The resulting Wind stroke is classified according to its degree:

- A *mild Wind stroke* (similar to the clinical picture of TIA or PRIND)[10] with transient sequelae
- A *Luo vessel stroke* with permanent mild paralysis and paraesthesia (equivalent to our degree of severity stage III)
- A *Jing main channel stroke* with hemiplegia (equivalent to stage IV)
- A *Fu organ stroke* with spastic paralysis and unconsciousness, also called block pattern (*Bi-Zheng*)
- A *Zang organ stroke* with total paralysis and unconsciousness, also called desertion pattern (*Tuo Zheng*) (both are equivalent to intracerebral haemorrhaging)
- The last degree, coma and death.

According to the degree of severity, Wind stroke is treated as follows: in the case of unconsciousness, orifices opening medicinals are prescribed, depending on whether Heat or Cold are differentiated, e.g. *An Gong Niu Huang Dan* (Calm the Palace Calculus Bovis Pill), and may be administered via a feeding tube. The unconscious – and in many cases comatose – patient will then regain consciousness and is prescribed (depending on the CT results – either ischemic stroke or intracerebral haemorrhaging) Blood invigorating for-

---

10 PRIND = Prolonged Ischemic Neurological Deficit

mulas, for example *Da Huo Luo Dan*. As the case may be, these formulas may either promote circulation or have a thrombolytic effect; they contain Chinese medicinals that protect brain cells against the damage of ischemia.

Once the patient is out of the acute stage and no longer in danger, a daily acupuncture treatment for paralysis and hemiplegia will be phased in, which, if commenced in time, may lead to a full recovery after 2–3 months.

See also the section 'Foreword to the theory of one-sided paralysis (hemiplegia)' including 'Theory with regard to paralysis and atrophy' in Wang Qing-Ren's '*Yin Lin Gai Cuo*' (Chapter 11, Part 3) and see **block pattern** and **damage**.

Y

Yang, build up: *Zhuang Yang*

A therapeutic method to strengthen Kidney *Yang-Qi* with tonifying or warming medicinals, which often have an effect on the endocrine system and sexual function, e.g. Herba Epimedii (*Yin Yang Huo*). Also see **supplementation**.

Yang, descend: *Qian Yang, Jiang Yang*

Therapeutic method in the case of ascending Liver-*Yang* (*Gan Yang Shang Kang*), usually caused by a deficiency of Kidney-*Yin* (indirectly) or Liver-*Yin* (directly). Symptoms of ascending Liver-*Yang* are dizziness, headache, hearing disorders like tinnitus or deafness, and red eyes. Also see **calm Liver-Wind**.

Yin and *Yang*: *Yin Yang*

Characteristic of *Yin* and *Yang*

Yang	*Yin*
left	right
above	below
exterior	interior
warm, hot	cool, cold
agile	still
bright	dark
male, plus	female, minus
anabolic	catabolic

Corresponding factor of *Yin* and *Yang* in TCM

Yang	*Yin*
Qi	*Xue* (Blood)
Shen (Mind)	*Jing* (Essence)
Wei (Defensive)	*Ying* (Nutritive)
Fu organs (*Yang* functional entities)	*Zang* organs (*Yin* functional entities)
outside the body	inside the body
back	abdomen
midnight to midday	midday to midnight
tonify	drain

In the '*Nei Jing Su Wen*', Chapter 2, it is mentioned:

Yin *and* Yang *and the four seasons are the beginning and end of everything. They are the root of life and death. Anyone living contrary to the principle of* Yin *and* Yang *will damage his life; those living in concordance with this principle will live in harmony.*

Today, there is hardly anyone who has not heard about *Yin* and *Yang*. Nevertheless, this concept is still commonly misunderstood in the West. For example, I often read that the concept of *Yin* and *Yang* is regarded as some kind of 'binary system' as used in computers. This is far from the truth: within a digital electronic system, the flow of current *always* equals 1 (or 'on') or 0 (or 'off'). It is a rigid, unchangeable concept.

Every object, classified according to the concepts of *Yin* and *Yang*, is both *Yin* and *Yang* at the same time. Furthermore, depending on the point of view, it is sometimes more *Yin* and sometimes more *Yang*. This is a flexible and comparative concept.

But how do we visualize such a principle in concrete terms? Let us take sunlight as an example of the principle of *Yin*. It comes from the **sky**, from **above**, is typified as **warm**, **during the day**, **bright**, **light**, and constitutes an **energy** that is not palpable, but nevertheless is tactile and subtle.

Chlorophyll absorbs sunlight and uses its energy to synthesize sugar, which in turn serves as an energy source and a means of storage; it is a vital substance for the plant itself, for all herbivores and indirectly all other creatures. Without

light, there would be no life as we know it. Still, this process requires a substrate, a material counterpart, namely carbon dioxide and water, which are necessary in plant cells for synthesizing light into chemical energy.

Let us take water as an example for the principle of *Yin*. It always flows **downwards**, is **cool** and **dark** out at sea; at **night** it appears in the form of dew and if its density increases, it turns into solid ice. Without water, life would be equally impossible; just as light without water cannot give rise to organic life, neither can water without light. Both need to be balanced in their occurrence, as do *Yin* and *Yang*.

However, these concrete examples always remain relative to each other: water, as an example for *Yin*, may also be interpreted as *Yang* in relation to ice. Ice is more solid, its molecules move slower, it is heavier and cooler than water, which are all qualities pertaining to *Yin*. In short, the concept of *Yin* and *Yang* is a mental construct designed to interpret *relationships*, not to set rigid definitions. This also applies to the Five Phases model and many other abstract concepts used in TCM.

Anatomical aspects of *Yin* and *Yang* in *TCM* are shown in the following Table.

Yang	*Yin*
head	torso and limbs
periphery (skin, muscles)	centre (organs)
back side (occiput, back, pelvis)	front side (face, chest, abdomen etc.)
above the hip	below the hip
lateral aspect of the limbs	medial aspect of the limbs
Fu organs (Small Intestine, Large Intestine, Stomach, Bladder, Gallbladder)	*Zang* organs (Heart, Lung, Spleen, Kidney, Liver)
Yang aspect of the organs	*Yin* aspect of the organs
Qi	Blood, Body Fluids
Wei (defensive aspect)	*Ying* (nutritive aspect)
left side of the body	right side of the body

Research related to *Yin Yang* theory

In 1973, the American researcher L Goldberg proposed the theory, based on findings in cellular physiology, that the fundamental principles of *Yin* and *Yang* would correspond to the relationship of the cyclic nucleotides cAMP and cGMP in terms of mutual dependence, mutual control and mutual balance (but not transformation). According to present-day research, his findings can only meet with qualified assent.

The Second Medical University in Shanghai examined the relationship of cAMP and cGMP in patients with *Yang* deficiency and found that blood values did not change significantly. Nevertheless, it was found that the relative values (normal ratio of cAMP/cGMP approximately 1:5) were reduced by half (1:2.5) in both *Yang* deficiency and *Yin* deficiency patients. Furthermore, due to a change in ratio, a marked tendency towards a predominance of cAMP in *Yin* deficiency and towards a predominance of cGMP in *Yang* deficiency was observed. After the administration of *Yang* tonifying medicinals to *Yang* deficiency patients, the ratio of cAMP/cGMP was normalized.[11]

Chronobiology, which is concerned with the biological clock and circadian rhythms in humans and other creatures, features many systems corresponding to *Yin Yang* theory and its principles. For example, the two 'main clocks' of the human body constitute such a mutually controlling and balancing system (see Table below).

Comparison of functions of the biological clocks

First clock (located in the suprachismatic nucleus of the hypothalamus) regulates	Second clock (probably located in the lateral hypothalamic or ventromedial nucleus) regulates
delta waves, deep sleep (motionless)	REM sleep (eye movements, dreams)
excretion of growth hormone (STH, anabolic effect, 'nourishing')	excretion of cortisol (catabolic effect, stimulates)
excretion of calcium in the urine	excretion of potassium in the urine
skin temperature	core body temperature
similarity to *Ying* (constructive energy, *Yin*)?	similarity to *Wei* (defensive energy, *Yang*)?

[11] 'Clinical and Experimental Studies on *Yang*-Deficiency' in Zhou: *Recent Advances in Chinese Herbal Drugs*. Beijing, Science Press and Brussels, SATAS 1991 (see Appendix 7).

Similarities to the principle of *Yin* and *Yang* are also evident here, although no definite correspondence can be found. Therefore, a universal principle like *Yin Yang* is replicated in many ways in the 'variations of biology'.

Yin–Yang of the Body Fluids: *Xue, Qi, Jin, Ye*

Blood as a moisturizing and nourishing substance pertains to *Yin*. In relation to Blood, *Qi* is *Yang* as it has the functions of warming, protecting against external factors and transforming. The Body Fluids are similar to Blood; they have a more dense substance that has structure and therefore pertains to *Yin*, in contrast to the energetic, ethereal *Qi*.

Similarly to the organs, Body Fluids can be categorized into *Yin* aspects and *Yang* aspects: *Jin*, i.e. clear and thin fluids such as tears and sweat pertain to *Yang*, whilst *Ye*, i.e. turbid and thick fluids such as nasal secretions and synovial fluids pertain to *Yin*. Except for cases where a diagnostic differentiation is necessary, *Jin* and *Ye* are not separated from each other, and are therefore regarded as *Yin*-substances in relation to *Qi*.

Ying–Qi: *Ying-Qi*

Ying-Qi is a *Yin* aspect of *Qi*. Along with Blood, it flows in the vessels as a constructive energy, and is derived from the essences of food (*Shui Gu Zhi Jing*). Also see **Wei-Qi, Wei-Ying, Ying-Wei disharmony** and **Yin and Yang**.

Ying–Wei disharmony: *Ying Wei Bu He*

An exterior syndrome characterized by marked spontaneous sweating. This lack of balance between *Ying* and *Wei* may arise from an either too strong or too weak *Ying* or *Wei*; in the case of *Ying* being too weak and *Wei* being too strong there is sweating and fever at the same time, because *Yang-Qi* forces the sweat (*Yin*) outwards; in the case of *Wei* being too weak and *Ying* being too strong, *Wei-Qi* fails to control the opening and closing of the pores. As a result, there is sweating but no fever. Also see **Wei** and **Ying**.

Yuan Qi: *Yuan Qi*

See **Qi**.

Z

Zang organs: *Zang*

These are the five organs pertaining to *Yin*. Their main function is to store, so they are also called storage organs: Liver, Heart, Spleen, Lung and Kidney. The '*Huang Di Nei Jing*' describes them as 'full, but not filled up' in contrast to the *Fu* organs (labour organs) which take on food or digestive juices (gall) only temporarily, so they are normally hollow and not full. In the '*Nei Jing*', they are described as 'filled up, but not full'.

Zang Fu organs: *Zang Fu*

Collective term for the five *Zang* organs and the six *Fu* organs. Also see **Zang organs** and **Fu organs**.

Appendix 2

Glossary of essential terms in haemorheology

Aggregation, also thrombocyte aggregation, erythrocyte aggregation

A clumping of individual particles massing together is defined as aggregation. Platelet aggregation forming a blood clot (thrombus) is a desired physiological reaction to vessel wall injury, e.g. due to traumata. An excessive aggregation of thrombocytes, for example due to a change in blood composition, is pathological and can lead to embolisms and impaired blood circulation in terms of Blood stasis.

Moreover, erythrocyte aggregation may form a rouleau structure and further branching which are normal in a healthy individual. In certain diseases however, like diabetes mellitus, an unorganized clumping of red blood cells is often observed, which also has a negative effect on blood flow.

Blood flow, properties of blood

The fluidity of blood is composed of its total viscosity (haematocrit), plasma viscosity, erythrocyte aggregation and plasticity of erythrocytes (see below). These factors determine the degree of friction of blood applied to itself and vessel walls. Pathologically, high viscosity can entail slowing down and impediment of blood flow, which results in the tissue being undersupplied with oxygen, nutrients and messenger substances. Such a state is referred to as Blood stasis in TCM.

Fibrinolysis

This is to be understood as the solubilization of fibrin or fibrinogen molecules by streptokinase, urokinase and other enzymes. Fibrinolysis is of major importance in the formation and breakdown of blood clots. Many medicinals for Blood stasis contain fibrinolytic agents.

Haemoconcentration

Loss of body fluids such as blood, sweat, urine (dehydration) etc. can manifest in a lowered amount of essential blood plasma and influence the ratio of solid and liquid substances (cell/plasma) to such a degree that blood 'thickens'. This results in diminished blood flow.

In TCM, such a state of dehydration or exsiccosis is referred to as *Yin* deficiency or Body Fluid deficiency, which can both cause Blood stasis.

Hyperviscosity, high blood viscosity

Viscosity determines the internal friction resistance in gases or fluids. Thus, a high blood viscosity means an increase in friction, and therefore deteriorated fluidity of blood. Fluidity is determined by both the vessels and the composition of blood. Also involved are parameters such as blood pressure, blood vessel diameter, vascular wall properties (smooth, scarred, sclerotic) and vessel architecture (branching, crossing etc.). The ratio of cell/plasma, chemical rejection or tendency to adhesion of erythrocytes, blood cholesterol level and plasticity, amongst other factors, all play a predominant role.

Plasma viscosity is determined principally by the proportion of proteins present, such as fibrinogen.

Plasticity of erythrocytes

Normal erythrocytes can and need to stretch into small elongated forms when passing through capillaries, as these have an even smaller diameter than the erythrocytes. After a lifespan of about 120 days this flexibility decreases and non-deformable erythrocytes are removed by the Spleen and by phagocytosis.

However, if plasticity decreases due to long lifespan or chemical changes in the blood, blood flow to the capillaries will be disturbed, which also leads to Blood stasis syndrome.

Viscosimeter

In the field of haemorheology, this instrument serves for the measurement of blood viscosity (one manufacturer is Hauke in Karlsruhe, Germany). The viscosimeter plays a major role in the diagnosis of Blood stasis in integrated Chinese medicine.

Appendix 3

List of Chinese medicinals with their Western pharmacological actions

This list of Chinese medicinals (in *Pinyin*, as many of the newer or locally known medicinals have no standardized pharmacological name yet) provides a short overview of the already proven pharmacological actions of Chinese medicinals. However, this list is not exhaustive and should only be used as a reference for those practitioners or pharmacists interested in pharmacology, because first there are no indications about potency (which should be looked up in detail), and secondly, prior to prescription of these medicinals, a thorough diagnosis and syndrome differentiation according to the principles of TCM needs to be made. **Medicinals that invigorate Blood stasis are in bold**. This facilitates quick referencing of the pharmacological effects of Blood invigorating and other medicinals.

Also see Chapter 1, 'Introduction: thought models in Chinese medicine'.

LIST OF CHINESE MEDICINALS WITH THEIR WESTERN PHARMACOLOGICAL ACTIONS

(with Blood invigorating medicinals in bold)
© 1997 Gunter Neeb

Adrenocortical stimulating effect
Ren Shen, Gan Cao, **Sheng Di Huang** (Rehmannia), He Shou Wu, Chuan Xin Lian, Chai Hu

AIDS therapy relevant medicinals or HIV inhibiting effect
Tian Hua Fen, Wu Zhen Song, Xiang Xun, Gan Cao, Mian Hua Gen, Zi Hua Di Ding, Niu Bang Zi, Chuan Xin Lian, Zi Cao, Kung Xin Lian Zi Cao, Jin Yin Hua, Chuang Lian, Yin Yang Huo, Guo Ji Jue Guan Zhong, Xia Ku Cao, Qian Li Guang, Di Er Cao, Huang Qin, Da Qing Ye, **Hu Zhang** (Polygonum Cuspidati), Yun Zhi, Bai Hua She She Cao, Qing Dai, Chang Chun Hua, Zhen Zhu Cai, Xi Shu, Zhong Jie Feng, **E Zhu** (Curcuma Ezhu), Ya Dan Zi

Anti–aging effect (free radical scavengers and others)
Ren Shen, **San Qi** (Notoginseng), Shan You, Wu Mei, Dong Chong Xia Cao, **Sheng Di Huang** (Rehmannia), Xiang Ri Hui Zi, Hong Qi, He Shou Wu, Ci Shen Ren, Luo Bu Ma, Cha Ye, Jiao Gu Lan, Hai Ma, Tu Si Zi, Ju Hua, Yin Er, Yin Yang Huo, Ge Jie, Ji Li, Shou Di

Anti–allergic, antihistaminic effect
Ba Jiao Hui Xiang, Da Zao, Shan Nai, Mao Gen, Wu Yao, Wu Mei, Mu Ju, Di Long, Xi He Liu, Bai He, Fang Feng, Du Heng, Lian Qiao, Xin Yi, Chen Xiang, Qiang Huo, Ling Zhi, E Wei, Chi Lao Ya, Yu Xing Cao, Xi Xin, Zhi Shi, Jing Jie, Bi Cheng Qie, Qing Jiao, Qing Pi, **Tao Ren** (Persica), Xu Chang Qing, Fen Fang Ji, Huang Jing Jie, Zhu Dan, Ma Huang, Bo Luo Hui, E Bu Shi Cao, Chan Tui, She Xiang

Anti–amoebic effect
Da Suan, Ba Dou, Bai Tou Weng, Ya Dan Zi, Chan Shan

Anti–arteriosclerotic effect
Wen Jing, **Chi Shao** (Paeonia Rubra), Mu Dan Pi (Moutan), He Shou Wu, Gui Ban, Chen Pi, Kun Bu, Nan Tian Zhu Zi, Gu Sui Bu, Xiang Xun, Chuan Shan Long, Jiao Gu Lan, Xu Chang Qing, Nian Bi Xie

Anti–arrhythmic effect on the heart
San Qi (Notoginseng), San Ke Zhen, Shan Dou Gen, Guang Zao, Tian Xian Zi, Shui Qing, Gan Song, Gan Cao, Shi Suan, Bei Dou Gen, Gua Lou, Di Long, Xi Yang Shen, Yang Jiao Ao, Mai Men Dong, **Mu Dan Pi** (Moutan), He Shou Wu, Sha Ji, Qiang Huo, Ling Zhi, Fu Zi, Ku Shen, Ku Dou Zi, Luo Bu Ma, Nao Yang Hua, Shi Di, Bi Bo, Bi Cheng Qie, Gou Teng, Du Huo, Yang Jing Hua, Lian Zi Xin, Tang Song Cao, Fen Fang Ji, Huang Lian, Huang Bai, She Chuang Zi, Yin Yang Huo, Ge Gen, Fu Shou Cao, Jie Cao, Hu Ji Shen

Anti–asthmatic effect
Shan Dou Gen, Xiao Hui Xiang, Xiao Ye Pi Pa, Ma Qian Zi, Ma Dou Ling, Yun Zhi, Che Qian Cao, Ai Ye, Shi Diao Lan, Shi Chang Pu, Bai Song Ta, Bai Qu Cai, Di Long, Lao Guan Cao, Bai He, Bai Bu, **Dang Gui** (Angelica Sinensis), Hua Shan Shen, **Si Gua Luo** (Luffa), Mu Jing Zi, Mu Jing Ye, Fo Shou, Han Xiu Cao, Ling Zhi, Chen Pi, Ren Dong Teng, Qing Pi, Pi Pa Ye, Ku Xing Ren, Yun Xiang Cao, **Hu Zhang** (Polygonum Cuspidati), Kun Bu, Ye Jiao Teng, Pao Tong Guo, Hu Tui Zi, Jing Jie, Jing Tiao, Bi Chen Qie, Gou Teng, Qing Pi, Hua Mu Pi, Huang Jing Zi, She Chuang Zi, Zhu Dan, Mao Yan Cao, Xuan Fu Hua, Shang Lu, Ma Huang, Mian Hua Gen, Guang Dong Hua, Zi Su Ye, Ge Jie, E Bu Shi Cao, Zao Shan Bai, Jin Ji Er, Ai Di Cha, Han Cai, Zang Hui Xiang, Gao Ben, Can Su

Anti-carcinogenic effect

Ren Shen, Er Cha, Dao Dou, **San Qi** (Notoginseng), San Jian Shan, San Ke Zhen, Da Zao, **Da Huang** (Rheum), Da Suan, Da Ma Yao, San Dou Gen, Shan You Gan, Qian Jin Zi, Chuan Wu, Nü Zhen Zi, Xiao Hui Xiang, Ma Qian Zi, Ma Lin Zi, Tian Dong, Tian Hua Fen, Tian Nan Xing, Wu Hua Guo, Yun Zhi, **Yunnan Baiyao**, Mu Gua, Niu Bang Zi, Mao Gen, Chang Chun Hua, Gan Cao, Gan Sui, Shi Suan, Long Yan Rou, Xian He Cao, Bai Ji, Bai Zhu, Bai Qu Cai, Bai Xian Pi, Gua Lou, Dong Ling Cao, Dong Chong Xia Cao, Di Long, Di Yu, Di Er Cao, Lao Guan Cao, Dang Gui (Angelica Sinensis), Deng Xin Cao, Nong Ji Li, Xun Gu Feng, Hong Qi, Hong Dou Kou, Hong Che Zhou Cao, Yuan Zhi, Ling Mian Zhen, Lu Hui, Lu Sun, **Su Mu** (Sappan), **Chi Shao** (Paeonia Rubra), Gui Ban, Bu Gu Zhi, Ling Zhi, Pi Pa Ye, Ci Wu Jia, Ku Shen, Ku Xing Ren, **Hu Zhang** (Polygonum Cuspidati), Kun Bu, Kun Ming Shan Hai Tang, Jing Qiao Mai, Jin Qian Bai Hua She, Zhong Jie Feng, Yu Xing Cao, Ye Jiao Teng, Guan Zhong, Nan She Teng, Cao Wu, Fu Ling, Cha Ye, Ya Dan Zi, Gou Wen, Qiu Shui Xian, Xiang Xun, Xiang Jia Pi, Gui Jiu, Du Huo, Chuan Xin Lian, Mei Deng Mu, **Jiang Huang** (Curcuma Longa), Luo Tuo Peng Zi, Jiao Gu Lan, Can Sha, **Tao Ren** (Persica), Tao Er Qi, **E Zhu** (Curcuma Ezhu), Chai Hu, Dang Shen, Chou Cao, Lang Du, Tang Song Cao, Hai Long, Hai Shen, Fen Fang Ji, Yi Zhi, Ba Qia, Tu Si Zi, Ju San Qi, Xue Lian, Chang Shan, Ying Er, Zhu Ling, Zhu Ya Zao, Lu Rong, Ban Mao, Mian Hua Gen, Zong Lü Tan, Lü Cao, Cong Bai, Xi Shu, Zi Shan, Zi Cao, Zi Wan, Ge Qiao, Bi Ma Zi, Lei Gong Teng, Feng Du, Xi Sheng Teng, Chan Tui, Fu She, Jiang Can, Jie Cao, Yi Yi Ren, Teng Huang, Can Su, Bie Jia

Anti-cholinesterase-like effect

Yi Ye Qiu, Gan Cao, Shi Suan

Anti-cholinergic effect

Jing Zhi, Yang Jin Hua, Huang Qin

Anti-emetic effect

Gan Jiang, Sheng Jiang, Ban Xia, Fu Long Gan, Lian Qiao, Huo Xiang

Anti-ischemic effect on heart musculature

Ren Shen, **San Qi** (Notoginseng), San Ke Zhen, **Chuan Xiong** (Ligusticum), Guang Zao, **Yuan Hu** (Corydalis), Yunnan Baiyao, **Mao Dong Qing** (Ilex Pubescens), Gan Song, Bei Dou Gen, Gua Lou, **Dang Gui** (Angelica Sinensis), Rou Gui, Bing Pian, **Hong Hua** (Carthamus), Mai Men Dong, **Mu Dan Pi** (Moutan), He Shou Wu, Qiang Huo, Mei Gui Hua, CiWu Jia, Ci Lao Ya, Ku Shen, Gou Ji, Bi Bo, Bi Cheng Qie, Xia Ye Hong Jing Tian, **Jiang Huang** (Curcuma Longa), Zhu Shi Ma, Jiao Gu Lan, Dang Shen, Tang Song Cao, Fen Fang Ji, **Yi Mu Cao** (Leonurus), Huang Jing, Ye Ju Hua, Yin Yang Huo, Ge Gen, Rei Xiang

Anti-convulsive effect

Ding Xiang, Qi Ye Lian, Tian Ma, Tian Nan Xing, Niu Huang, Shen Ma, Shi Chang Pu, Long Chi, Long Gu, Sheng Jiang, Xian Mao, Di Long, Xi Yang Shen, Zhu Sha, Quan Xie, Qing Cai, **Chi Shao** (Paeonia Rubra), **Mu Dan Pi** (Moutan), Ling Zhi, Ji Shi Teng, Hu Jiao, Gou Teng, Yu Bai Fu, Qing Pi, Gui Zhi, Dang Shen, Sang Bai Pi, Ju San Qi, Ling Yang Jiao, Peng Sha, Wu Gong, Suan Zao Ren, Can Tui, Xiong Dan, Jiang Can, Jie Cao, Bi Hu

Antibody production inhibiting

Dang Gui (Angelica Sinensis), Gan Cao, Da Zao, Bu Gu Zhi

Antibody production stimulating

Huang Qi, Yin Yang Huo, Xiang Xun, Ren Shen, Zi He Che, He Shou Wu, **Sheng Di Huang** (Rehmannia)

Anti-malarial effect

Ma Bian Cao (Verbena), Qing Hao, Kun Ming Shan Hai Tang, Wei Ling Xian, Ya Dan Zi, Chang Shan, He Chao Ya

Anti-microbial effect

Ding Xiang, Ba Jiao Hui Xiang, Er Cha, Jiu Xiang Chong, Gan Jiang, Tu Mu Xiang, Xing Pi, Tu Jing Jie, **Da Huang** (Rheum), Da Suan, Da Ji, Da Feng Zi, Da Qing Ye, Shan Nai, Shan Zha (Crataegus), Shan Dou Gen, Chuan Bei Mu, Chuan Lian Zi, Guang Zao, Xiao Ji, Xiao Hui Xiang, Xiao Ye Pi Pa, Ma Qian Zi, Ma Dou Ling, Ma Ti Jin, Lü Ti Cao, **Ma Bian Cao** (Verbena), Tian Dong, Tian Hua Fen, **Yunnan Baiyao**, Mu Gua, Mu Xiang, Mu Zei, Mu Fu Rong Ye, Wu Wei Zi, Wu Bei Zi, Niu Bang Zi, **Mao Dong Qing** (Ilex Pubescens), Sheng Yao, Shen Ma, **Dan Shen** (Salvia Miltiorrhiza), Wu Yao, Wu Mei, Ai Ye, Gan Song, Shi Wei, Shi Diao Lan, Shi Liu Pi, Long Dan, Long Yan Rou, Si Ji Qing, Sheng Jiang, Bai Ji, Bai Zhu, Bai Shao, Bai Zhi, Bai Fan, Bai Guo, Bai Tou Weng, Bai Jie Zi, Bai Song Ta, Bai Mao Gen, Bai Qu Cai, Bai Bian Dou, Bai Xian Pi, Gua Lou, Dong Ling Cao, Xuan Shen, Di Jiao, Di Yu, Di Er Cao, Di Fu Zi, Di Gu Pi, Di Jing Cao, Lao Guan Cao, Xi He Liu, Bai Bu, **Dang Gui** (Angelica Sinensis), Rou Gui, Rou Dou Kou, Zhu Ru, **Xue Jie** (Sanguis Draconis), Xue Yu Tan, He Huan Pi, Jue Ming Zi, Bing Pian, Yang Ti, Guan Mu Tong, Xun Gu Feng, Fang Feng, Hong Mao Qi, Hong Dou Kou, Hong Ci Teng, Hong Che Zhou Cao, **Si Gua Luo** (Luffa), Mai Dong, Yuan Zhi, Wu Yi, Hua Jiao, Cang Er Zi, Lu Hui, **Su Mu** (Sappan), Su He Xiang, **Chi Shao** (Paeonia Rubra), Chi Xiao Dou, Lian Qiao, Bian Qian Cao, Wu Zhu Yu, **Mu Dan Pi** (Moutan), He Shou Wu, Han Xiu Cao, Xin Yi, Qiang Huo, Bu Gu Zhi, Ling Zhi, E Wei, Ren Dong Teng, Ji Shi Teng, Ji Guan Gua, Qing Hao, Qing Mu Xiang, Pi Pa Ye, Ban Lan Gen, Song Luo, Ku Mu, Ku Shen, Ku Xing Ren, Yun Xiang Cao, Qing Ma Zi, Qi Ning, Zhu Ma Gen, Mao Mei, **Hu Zhang** (Polygonum Cuspidati), Zhi Mu, Jing Qian Cao, Jin Yin Hua, Zong Jie Feng, Yu Xing Cao, Ye Jiao Teng, Lu Gan Shi, Pao Tong Guo, Ze Qi, Xi Xin, Guan Zhong, Wu Tui Zi, Jing Jie, Nan She Teng, Nan Tian Zhu Zi, Bi Bo, Bi Cheng Qie, Yin Cheng, Fu Ling, Cha Ye, Pi Shi, Hou Po, Wei Ling Xian, Gu Sui Bu, Xiang Mao, Xiang Fu, Xiang Ru, Yang Cong, Chuan Xin Lian, Mei Deng Mu, **Jiang Huang** (Curcuma Longa), Luo Tuo Peng Zi, Qing Jiao, Qing Pi, Can Sha, Gui Zhi, Hua Mu Pi, He Tao Ren, An Ye, Lian Fang, **E Zhu** (Curcuma Ezhu), Yan Fu Mu, Gan Feng Cai, Xia Ku Cao, Chai Hu, Dang Shen, Qian Dan, She Gan, Chao Cao, Xu Chang Qing, Gao Liang Jiang, Hai Zao, Hai Jin Sha, Fen Fang Ji, Yu Zhi Zi, Sang Ye, Shan Ji Sheng, Ji Mu, Ba Qie, Tu Si Zi, Ju Hua, Huang Qin, Huang Lian, Huang Bai, Huang Jing Zi, Huang Jing Ye, Huang Yao Zi, Pi Jiu Hua, Ye Ju Hua, Ye Dong Qing Guo, Zhu Ling, Zhu Dan, Zhu Ya Zao, Mao Yan Cao, Xuan Fu Hua, Ma Huang, Lu Xian Cao, Yin Yang Huo, Duan Xue Liu, Xu Duan, Bo Luo Hui, Mian Hua Gen, Lü Cao, Cong Bai, Bian Xu, Xiong Huang, Liu Huang, Zi Cao, Zi Zhu, Zi Qi, Zi Wan, Zi Jin, Zi Su Zi, Zi Su Ye, Zi Du Juan, Jing Tian San Qi, Fan Xie Ye, Hua Shi, Rei Xiang, Huai Hua, Pu Gong Ying, Peng Sha, Feng Fang, Feng Du, Wu Gong, Jing Ji Er, Ai Di Cha, Man Jing Zi, Han Cai, La Jiao, Mo Han Lian, He Shi, Xie Bai, Shu Liang, Bo He, Zang Hui Xiang, Gao Ben, Qu Mai, She Xiang Cao

Anti-mycotic effect

San Qi (Notoginseng), **Da Huang** (Rheum), Da Suan, Wu Bei Zi, Sheng Ma, Wu Mei, Bai Zhi, Bai Xian Pi, Xuan Shen, Mu Ju, **Sheng Di Huang** (Rehmannia), Qing Cai, Lu Sun, Qing Hao, Ci Ren Shen, Ku Shen, Ku Lian Pi, Shi Jun Zi, Hu Huang Lian, Nan Sha Shen, Hai Shen, Zhi Zi, Ju Hua, Huang Lian, Huang Bai, Ban Mao, Cong Bai, Zi Su Ye, Fan Qie, Bin Lang, Zhang Nao, Jie Cao, Huo Xiang

Antioxidant effect

Ren Shen, Da Zao, Da Suan, **Shan Zha** (Crataegus), Nü Zhen Zi, Wu Wei Zi, Wu Bei Zi, Gan Cao, Lao Guan Cao, Xi Yang Shen, **Dang Gui** (Angelica Sinensis), Zhu Ye Shen Ren, Lu Sun, Chen Pi, Ci Lao Ya, **Hu Zhang** (Polygonu Cuspidati), Hu Sui, Cha Ye, An Ye, Chai Hu, Xu Chang Qing, Gao Shan Hong Jing Tian, Zi Shi, Huang Jing, Lu Rong, Zi Su Zi, Huai Hua, Hu Ji Shen

Anti-parasitic (intestinal parasites) effect

Ding Xiang, Tu Mu Xiang, Tu Jing Jie, Shan Dao Nian Hao, Chuan Lian Zi, Wu Mei, Shi Liu Pi, Sheng Jiang, Xian He Cao, Lü Song Jiu Mao, He Huan Pi, Hua Jiao, Ku Lian Pi, Shi Jun Zi, Guan Zhong, Hu Lu Ba, Nan Gua Zi, Yin Chen, Ya Dan Zi, Qian Dan, Hai Ren Cao, Lei Wan, Fei Zi, Bin Lang, He Shi, He Cao Ya, Ze Gu Cai

Anti-schistosomal effect

Gan Jiang, Ba Dou, Xian He Cao, Qing Hao, Ku Lian Pi, Nan Gua Zi, Hai Zao, Xuan Cao Gen, Xiong Huang, He Cao Ya, Qu Mai

Anti-trichomonal effect

Da Suan, Bai Fan, Bai Tou Weng, Bai Xian Pi, Ku Shen, Bi Cheng Xie, Lei Wan, He Cao Ya

Antitussive effect

*Da Zao, Chuan Bei Mu, Xiao Ye Pi Pa, Ma Qian Zi, Ma Dou Ling, **Ma Bian Cao** (Verbena), Che Qian Cao, Ai Ye, Gan Cao, Shi Wei, Shi Diao Lan, Shi Chang Pu, Bai Song Ta, Ba Qu Cai, Ban Xia, Lao Guan Cao, Xi He Liu, Bai He, Bai Bu, Hua Shan Shen, An Hui Bei Mu, **Si Gua Luo** (Luffa), Mu Jing Zi, Mu Jing Ye, Ren Dong Teng, Qing Feng Teng, Pi Pa Ye, Pi Pa He, Ku Xing Ren, Yun Xiang Cao, **Hu Zhang** (Polygonum Cuspidati), Kun Bu, Jin Qiao Mai, Pao Tong Guo, Jing Tiao, Bi Chen Qie, Qing Pi, Tie Gen, Hua Mu Pi, **Tao Ren** (Persica), Tao Er Qi, Du Xian Zi, Chai Hu, Zhe Bei Mu, Sang Bai Pi, Zhu Dan, Mao Yan Cao, Xuan Fu Hua, Shang Lu, Mian Hua Gen, Guang Dong Hua, Zi Wan, Zi Su Ye, Zi Du Juan, E Bu Shi Cao, Zhao Shan Bai, Ai Di Cha, Man Shan Hong, Xian Zhu Li, Xiong Dan, Zang Hui Xiang, Can Su*

Anti-ulcerative effect

*Ding Xiang, Ren Shen, Gan Jiang, **Da Huang** (Rheum), Shan Dou Gen, Xiao Hui Xiang, **Yuan Hu** (Corydalis), Yun Zhi, Mu Xiang, Wu Jia Pi, Wu Wei Zi, Gan Cao, Sheng Jiang, Bai Ji, Bai Zhu, Gua Lou, Mu Ju, Rou Gui, Hong Dou Kou, Hua Jiao, Cang Zhu, Lian Qian Cao, Wu Zhu Yu, Ku Shen, Zhong Jie Feng, Bi Bo, Bi Cheng Qie, Qi Cai, Hou Po, Ya Dan Zi, Luo Tuo Peng Zi, Jiao Gu Lan, Chai Hu, Dang Shen, Hai Piao Xiao, Huang Bai, Ying Er, Lu Rong, Huai Hua, Pu Gong Ying, Fu She, She Xiang*

Antiviral effect

***San Qi** (Notoginseng), **Da Huang** (Rheum), Da Suan, Da Qing Ye, Yun Zhi, Wu Bei Zi, Hua Ju Hong, Gan Cao, Shi Liu Pi, Lao Guan Cao, Xi Yang Shen, Bai Bu, Hong Mao Qi, Lian Qiao, Wu Zhu Yu, Han Xiu Cao, Chen Pi, Qing Hao, Ban Lan Gen, Jin Yin Hua, Guan Zhong, Hu Tui Zi, Nan She Shen Teng, Bi Bo, Bi Cheng Xie, Yin Chen Hao, Xiang Ru, **Jiang Huang** (Curcuma Longa), Can Sha, Gui Zhi, Chai Hu, Gao Shan Hong Jing Tian, Hai Shen, Sang Ji Shen, Huang Lian, Huang Yao Zi, Chang Shan, Ye Ju Hua, Shang Lu, Ma Huang, Yin Yang Huo, Ban Mao, Mian Hua Gen, Zi Cao, Ai Di Cha, Bin Lang, Man Jing Zi, Bo He, Teng Huang*

Calming effect

*Qi Ye Lian, Xiao Ji, Xiao Ye Pi Pa, Tian Ma, Tian Nan Xing, **Yuan Hu** (Corydalis), Yun Zhi, Mu Zei, Wu Wei Zi, Niu Huang, Sheng Ma, Yu Mi Xu, Ai Ye, Gan Song, Shi Suan, Shi Diao Lan, Shi Chang Pu, Lung Chi, Lung Gu, Sheng Jiang, Xian Mao, Bai Shao, Bai Tou Weng, Bai Song Ta, Dong Chong Xia Cao, Di Long, Bai He, Zhu Sha, Hua Shan Shen, He Huan Hua, Wen Jing, Yang Jiao Ao, Fang Feng, **Hong Hua** (Carthamus), Hong Qi, Mai Jiao, Yuan Zhi, Du Zhong, Du Heng, Liang Mian Zhen, Qing Cai, **Chi Shao** (Paeonia Rubra), **Mu Dan Pi** (Moutan), Mu Jing Zhi, Gui Ban, Ling Zhi, Ji Shi Teng, Ching Mu Xiang, Qing Feng Teng, Chi Wu Jia, Ku Dou Zi, Luo Bu Ma, Nao Yang Hua, Xi Xin, Shi Di, Hu Jiao, Nan She Teng, Fu Ling, Gou Teng, Yu Bai Fu, Zhu Shi Ma, Jiao Gu Lan, Zhu Zi Shen, Qing Pi, Gui Zhi, Du Xian Zhi, Chai Hu, Dang Shen, Chou Wu Tong, Xu Chang Xing, Gao Shan Hong Jing Tian, Shang Bai Piu, Zhi Zi, Ju San Qi, Huang Qin, Pi Jiu Hua, Ling Yang Jiao, Zi Cao, Zi Su Ye, Jing Tian San Qi, Rei Xiang, Ai Di Cha, Suan Zao Ren, Chan Tui, Xiong Dan, Jiang Can, Bi Hu, Gao Ben*

Blood pressure reducing effect
Ba Li Ma, Ren Shen, Er Cha, **San Qi** (Notoginseng), San Ke Zhen, Da Ji, **Shan Zha** (Crataegus), Shan Dou Gen, Chuan Wu, Chuan Bei Mu, Xiao Ye Pi Pa, Tian Ma, Mu Zei, Che Qian Zi, Niu Huang, Niu Bang Zi, Chang Chun Hua, Huo Ma Ren, Shui Niu Jiao, Yu Zhu, Yu Mi Xu, Gan Song, Shi Suan, Shi Diao Lan, Bei Dou Gen, Tian Xuan Hua, Shen Jiang, Bai Guo, Bai Qu Cai, Xuan Sheng, Di Long, Di Yu, Di Gu Pi, Yi Bei Mu, Wen Jing, Jue Ming Zi, Hong Mao Qi, Nai Jiao, Yuan Zhi, Du Zhong, Hua Sheng Yi, Qing Cai, **Chi Shao** (Paeonia Rubra), Fu Shan Hua, Wu Zhu Yu, **Mu Dan Pi** (Moutan), Mu Jing Ye, Fo Shou, Xing Yi, Sha Yuan Zi, Chen Xiang, Ling Zhi, Ren Dong Teng, Ji Shi Teng, Qing Hao, Qing Mu Xiang, Qing Feng Teng, Chi Wu Jia, Ku Mu, Ku Lian Pi, Lun Huan Teng, **Hu Zhang** (Polygonum Cuspidati), Kun Bu, Luo Bu Ma, Nao Yang Hua, Bi Bo, Bi Cheng Qie, Cha Ye, Gou Teng, Xiang Fu, Pang Da Hai, Liang Jun, Yang Jin Hua, Zhu Shi Ma, Zhu Zi Shen, He Tao Ren, Du Xian Zi, Lai Fu Zi, Lian Zi Xin, Xia Ku Cao, Chou Wu Tong, Xu Chang Qing, Tang Song Cao, Hai Zhe, Sang Bai Pi, Sang Ji Sheng, Tu Si Zi, Huang Qin, Huang Lian, Huang Bai, Chang Shan, Ye Ju Hua, Lu Rong, Yin Yang Huo, Ling Yang Jiao, Duan Xue Liu, Ge Gen, Jin Tian San Qi, Huai Hua, Ji Li, Feng Du, Zhao Shan Bai, Jin Ji Er, Suan Zao Ren, Man Jing Zi, Xi Qian Cao, La Jiao, Hu Ji Shen, Fu She, Jie Cao, Ze Gu Cai, Gao Ben

Blood pressure raising effect
Han Xiu Cao, Chen Pi, Qing Pi, Ze Xie, Zhi Ke, Zhi Shi, Ying Yu, Ma Huang, Kuan Dong Hua, Can Su

Blood fat reducing effect
Da Suan, **Shan Zha** (Crategus), Shan Dou Gen, Nü Zhen Zi, Yun Zhi, Sheng Ma, **Dan Shen** (Salvia Miltiorrhiza), Yue Jian Cao Zi, Huo Ma Ren, **Shui Zhi** (Hirudo), Shui Fei Ji, Shui Niu Jiao, Yu Zhu, Di Gu Pi, Xi Yang Shen, **Dang Gui** (Angelica Sinensis), Hui Hui Dou, Wen Jing, Jue Ming Zi, **Hong Hua** (Carthamus), Hong Che Zhou Cao, Du Zhong, Du Heng, Lu Sun, He Shou Wu, Gui Ban, Sha Ji, Sha Yuan Zi, Ren Dong Teng, Chi Lao Ya, Ku Dou Zi, Mu Su, **Hu Zhang** (Polygonum Cuspidati), Kun Bu, Luo Bu Ma, Jin Yin Hua, Ye Jiao Teng, Ze Xie, Gou Qi Zi, Bi Bo, Cha Ye, Yang Cong, **Jiang Huang** (Curcuma Longa), Zhu Shi Ma, Jiao Gu Lan, He Tao Ren, Xu Chang Qing, Hai Zao, Huang Qin, Huang Lian, Huang Jing, Yin Er, **Yin Xing Ye** (Ginkgo), Ying Yang Huo, Ge Gen, Zi Su Zi, Ha Ma You, Hei Zhi Ma, Huai Hua, Suan Zao Ren, Xiong Dan, Fu She

Blood clotting and blood thrombus formation enhancing effect
San Qi (Notoginseng), Tu Jing Pi, **Da Huang** (Rheum), Da Ji, Xiao Ji, **Ma Bian Cao** (Verbena), Yunnan Bai Yao, Ai Ye, Shi Liu Pi, Long Chi, Long Gu, Xian He Cao, Bai Ji, Bai Mao Gen, Di Yu, Di Jing Cao, Xi Yang Shen, Fu Long Gan, Xue Yu Tan, Yang Ti, Hong Ci Teng, Hua Sheng Yi, Hua Rei Shi, **Su Mu** (Sappan), Song Hua Fen, Qi Cai, Zhu Ma Gen, Mao Mei, **Hu Zhang** (Polygonum Cuspidati), Jin Yin Hua, Guan Zhong, Lian Fan, Gan Feng Cai, Ji Mu, Ju San Qi, Yin Yang Huo, Duan Xue Liu, Zong Lü, Zong Lü Tan, Zi Cao, Zi Zhu, Jing Tian San Qi, Huai Hua, Feng Fan, Muo Han Lian, Shu Liang, Ou Jie

Blood clotting and blood thrombus formation inhibiting effect
Ding Xiang, Jiu Li Xiang, San Ke Zhen, Gan Jiang, Da Fu Pi, **Chuan Xiong** (Ligusticum), Xiao Hui Xiang, Tian Zhu Huang, Mu Xiang, Mu Zei, **Mao Dong Qing** (Ilex Pubescens), Shen Ma, **Dan Shen** (Salvia Miltiorrhiza), Wu Yao, **Shui Zhi** (Hirudo), Bai Zhu, Bai Bian Dou, Di Long, **Dang Gui** (Angelica Sinensis), **Xue Jie** (Sanguis Draconis), Deng Zhan Xi Xin, **Hong Hua** (Carthamus), Hua Jiao, Su He Xing, **Chi Shao** (Paeonia Rubra), **Mu Dan Pi** (Moutan), Xin Yi, Ling Zhi, Fu Zi, Kun Bu, Jin Qian Baqi Hua She, Nan Sha Shen, Bi Cheng Qie, Cha Ye, Gou Teng, Du Huo, Zhu Shi Ma, Gui Zhi, **Tao Ren** (Persica), **E Zhu** (Curcuma Ezhu), Yan Fu Mu, Xia Tian Wu, Dang Shen, Gao Liang Jiang, Hai Zao, **Yi Mu Cao** (Leonurus), Ma Huang, Feng Du, Wu Gong, Man Jing Zi, Xi Qian Cao, Xiong Dan, Fu She, Bi Hu

Blood sugar reducing effect
Ren Shen, San Bai Cao, Tu Mu Xiang, Da Suan, Shan Yao, Chuan Wu, Liu Bang Zi, Chang Chun Flower, Yu Zhu, Gan Cao, Bai Zhu, Di Gu Pi, Mai Ya, Cang Zhu, Cang Er Zi, Ling Zhi, Ku Xing Ren, **Hu Zhang** (Polygonum Cuspidati), Zhi Mu, Ze Xie, Gou Qi Zi, Li Zhi He, Yang Cong, Du Xian Zi, Xia Ku Cao, Gao Shan Feng Jing Tian, Sang Ye, Huang Lian, Huang Jing, Ye Dong Qing Guo, Yin Er, Yin Yang Huo, Ge Gen, Zi Cao, Ge Jie, Yi Yi Ren

Blood sugar elevating effect
Xuan Shen, Xia Ye Hong Jing Tian, Qing Jiao, Chai Hu, Dang Shen, Zi Su Ye, She Xiang Cao

Cholagogue effect
Ding Xiang, Gan Jiang, **Da Huang** (Rheum), Guang Zao, Xiao Hui Xiang, Niu Huang, Ai Ye, Long Dan, Sheng Jiang, Yang Ti, Cang Zhu, Jin Qian Cao, Jin Yin Hua, Bu Huang Lian, Bi Cheng Xie, Yin Chen, Wei Ling Xian, Liang Jun, Mei Ren Jiao, **Jiang Huang** (Curcuma Longa), Hai Jin Sha, Zhi Zi, Bian Xu, Pu Gong Ying, Xiong Dan, Bo He

Cholinergic effect
Shi Suan, Xiang Jia Pi, Bin Lang

Diuretic effect
Da Ma Yao, Chuan Mu Tong, Ma Ti Jin, Che Qian Zi, Che Qian Cao, Yu Mi Xu, Shi Wei, Bai Zhu, Bai Mao Gen, Di Fu Zi, Wen Jing, Yang Jiao Ao, Guan Mu Tong, Du Zhong, Lian Qian Cao, Wu Zhu Yu, **Mu Dan Pi** (Moutan), Qing Ma Zi, Qi Cai, Luo Bu Ma, Jin Qian Cao, Jin Bian Long She Lan, Ze Xie, Fu Ling, Hai Jing Sha, Fu Ping, Sang Bai Pi, Sang Ji Shen, Zi Shi, Huang Qi, Zhu Ling, Shang Lu, Ma Huang, Hu Lu, Ting Li Zi, Bian Xu, Feng Fang, Lou Gu, Qu Mai

Emetic effect
Shi Suan, Qing Mu Xiang, Chang Shan

Detoxifying effect
Wu Wei Zi, Wu Bei Zi, Gan Cao, Bai Bian Dou, Ban Xia, Di Jin Cao, Cang Zhu, Mei Gui Hua, Song Ruo, Jin Ying Hua, Lai Fu Zi, Gao Shan Hong Jing Tian, Huang Qi, Ge Gen

Inflammation inhibiting effect
Ding Gong Teng, Jiu Li Xiang, **San Qi** (Notoginseng), Gan Jiang, **Da Huang** (Rheum), Da Qing Ye, Shan Dou Gen, Chuan Wu, Guan Zao, Guan Jin Qian Cao, Nü Zhen Zi, Xiao Ji, Ma Dou Ling, **Ma Bian Cao** (Verbena), Tian Ma, Yun Zhi, **Yunnan Baiyao**, Mu Fu Rong Ye, Wu Jia Pi, Liu Huang, **Niu Xi** (Achyranthis Bidentata), **Mao Dong Qing** (Ilex Pubescens), Sheng Ma, Hua Jie Hong, **Dan Shen** (Salvia Miltiorrhiza), Ba Ji Tian, Shi Suan, Shi Diao Lan, Long Dan, Bei Dou Gen, Tian Xuan Hua, Si Ji Qing, Sheng Jiang, Xian Mao, Xian He Cao, Bai Shao, Bai Zhi, Bai Song Ta, Dong Ling Cao, Mu Ju, Di Yu, **Dang Gui** (Angelica Sinensis), Zhu Jie Ren Shen, **Xue Jie** (Sanguis Draconis), Xue Yu Tan, Bing Pian, Xun Gu Feng, Fang Feng, **Hong Hua** (Carthamus), Hong Qi, Hong Mao Qi, Du Zhong, Cang Er Zi, Ru Hui, **Su Mu** (Sappan), **Chi Shao** (Paeonia Rubra), Lian Qiao, **Mu Dan Pi** (Moutan), Xin Yi, Sha Yuan Zi, Jiang Huo, Fu Zi, Ren Dong Teng, Qing Feng Teng, Pi Pa Ye, Ci Ren Shen, Ci Lao Ya, Ku Mu, Ku Shen, Ku Dou Zi, Qi Cai, **Hu Zhang** (Polygonum Cuspidati), Kun Ming Shan Hai Tang, Jin Qiao Mai, Jin Qian Cao, Jin Yin Hua, Yu Xing Cao, Ze Xie, Xi Xin, Jing Jie, Cao Wu, Gu Sui Bu, Qiu Sui Xian, Xiang Fu, Xiang Jia Pi, Yui Bai Fu, Du Huo, Chuan Xin Lian, **Jiang Huang** (Curcuma Longa), Zhu Shi Ma, Zhu Zi Shen, Qing Jiao, Qing Pi, Jie Geng, **Tao Ren** (Persica), He Tao Ren, An Ye, Du Xian Zi, Lai Fu Zi, Xia Ku Cao, Chai Hu, Dang Shen, She Gan, Chou Wu Tong, Xu Chang Qing, Gao Shan Hong Jing Tian, Fen Fang Ji, Sha Luo Zi, Zhi Zi, Ba Qi, Ju San Qi, Huang Qin, Huang Qi, Huang Lian, Huang Jing Ye, Xue Lian, She Tui, Ye Ju Hua, Yin Er, Shang Lu, Ma Huang, Lu Rong, Ying Yang Huo, Duan Xue Liu, Kuan Dong Hua, Liu Huang, Zi Cao, Zi Du Juan, Ge Qiao, Ge Jie, He Zhi Ma, Fan Qie, Rei Xiang, Huai Hua, Shuo Diao, Lei Wan, Lei Gong Teng, Feng Fang, Feng Du, Jing Ji Er, Man Shan Hong, Man Jing Zi, Xi Qian Cao, Xiong Dan, Fu She, Gao Ben, Can Su, She Xiang

Exhaustion and tiredness counteracting effect
Ren Shen, Wu Mei, Xi Yang Shen, Lu Sun, E Jiao, Ci Wu Jia, Xia Ye Hong Jing Tian, Gao Shan Hong Jing Tian, Ma Huang, Bie Jia

Fever reducing effect
Gan Jiang, Da Qing Ye, San Dou Gen, Niu Huang, Sheng Ma, Shi Suan, Shi Gao, Bei Sha Shen, Sheng Jiang, Bai Zhi, Di Long, Di Gu Pi, Xi He Liu, Rou Gui, Fang Feng, **Chi Shao** (Paeonia Rubra), Lian Qiao, **Mu Dan Pi** (Moutan), Qiang Huo, Qing Hao, Ku Mu, Ku Shen, Ku Dou Zi, Qi Cai, Kun Ming Shan Hai Tang, Zhi Mu, Jin Qiao Mai, Jin Ying Hua, Ze Qi, Xi Xin, Jing Jie, Yin Chen, Xiang Fu, Chuan Xing Lian, Gui Zhi, Du Xian Zi, Chai Hu, She Gan, Xu Chang Qing, Fu Ping, Sang Bai Pi, Chang Shan, Ye Ju Hua, Ma Huang, Ling Yang Jiao, Ge Gen, Zi Cao, Zi Su Ye, Suan Zao Ren, Chan Tui, Xiong Dan, Gao Ben, Ma Huang

Uterus stimulating effect
Jiu Li Xiang, Wu Wei Zi, **Niu Xi** (Achyranthis Bidentata), Di Long, Yang Jiao Ao, **Hong Hua** (Carthamus), Hong Mao Qi, Mai Jiao, Yuan Zi, Du Zhong, Gui Ban, Xin Yi, Qi Cai, Guan Zhong, Chong Lou Pai Cao, **Tao Ren** (Persica), Chou Cao, Hai Long, **Yi Mu Cao** (Leonurus), Ji Mu, Xue Lian, Chang Shan, Duan Xue Liu, Xu Duan, Fei Zi, Shu Liang, Bo He, Qu Mai

Smooth muscle inhibiting, anti-spasmodic effect
Ding Xiang, Qi Ye Lian, Gan Jiang, Shan Yao, Shan Dou Gen, Chuan Bei Mu, Guang Zao, Xiao Ye Pi Pa, Tian Xian Zi, Mu Xiang, Niu Huang, Sheng Ma, Wu Mei, Gan Song, Bai Zhi, Mu Ju, Di Jiao, Yi Bei Mu, Hua Shan Shen, Du Heng, Liang Mian Zhen, **Chi Shao** (Paeonia Rubra), Fu Sang Hua, Fo Shou, Chen Xiang, Ling Zhi, Chen Pi, Ren Dong Teng, Qing Pi, Yun Xiang Cao, Xi Xin, Zhi Ke, Bi Bo, Zhi Wei Ling Xian, Xiang Mao, Xiang Ru, Mei Ren Jiao, Xia Tian Wu, Chou Cao, Hai Shen, Yi Zhi, Huang Yao Zi, Xue Lian, She Chuang Zi, **Yin Xing Ye** (Ginkgo), Ma Huang, Guang Dong Ye, Guang Dong Hua, Ge Gen, Zi Du Juan, Rei Xiang, Huai Hua, Zhao Shan Bai, Xiong Dan, Bo He, Zang Gui Xiang, Gao Ben, Huo Xiang, Can Su

Smooth stomach and intestine musculature stimulating effect
Ba Jiao Feng, Shan Yao, Chuan Lian Zi, Xiao Ji, Xiao Hui Xiang, Ba Dou, Shi Suan, Lü Song Jiu Mao, Ji Nei Jin, Hu Lian Pi, Qi Cai, Luo Han Guo, Nao Yang Hua, Chien Niu Zi, Gan Feng Chai, Ya Dan Zi, Lai Fu Zi, Gao Shan Hong Jing Tian, Sang Bei Pi, Zhi Zi, Zi Su Ye, Suo Yang, Feng Du, Xi Sheng Teng, Zang Hui Xiang, Qu Mai

Haematopoiesis enhancing effect
Niu Huang, **Dang Gui** (Angelica Sinensis), He Shou Wu, E Jiao, Chan Sha, Dang Shen, Shang Shen, Yin Er, Ma Huang, Xi Su

Hepatoprotective effect (preventing liver cells from damage)
Er Cha, **San Qi** (Notoginseng), **Da Huang** (Rheum), Da Suan, Shan Dou Gen, Nü Zhen Zi, Xiao Ji, Mu Gua, Wu Wei Zi, Sheng Ma, **Dan Shen** (Salvia Miltiorrhiza), Shui Qing, Shui Fei Ji, Gan Cao, Long Dan, Sheng Jiang, Bai Zhu, Bai Shao, Di Er Cao, Lao Guan Cao, Xi He Liu, **Dang Gui** (Angelica Sinensis), Dang Yao, Wen Jing, Hua Jiao, Lu Hui, Lian Qiao, Wu Zhu Yu, He Shou Wu, Sha Ji, Sha Yuan Zi, Ling Zhi, Qing Hao, Qing Ye Dan, Ci Lao Ya, **Hu Zhang** (Polygonum Cuspidati), Chui Pen Cao, Jing Yin Hua, Ze Xie, Gou Qi Zi, Yin Chen, Fu Ling, Yang Jin Hua, Chuan Xin Lian, Mei Ren Jiao, **Jiang Huang** (Curcuma Longa), Chai Hu, Dang Shen, Zhi Zi, Zi Shi, Zhu Ling, Pu Gong Ying, Mo Han Lian, Jie Cao, Bie Jia

Coronary arteries dilating effect
Ba Li Ma, **San Qi** (Notoginseng), Shan Za, **Chuan Xiong** (Ligusticum), **Yuan Hu** (Corydalis), Wu Wei Zi, **Shui Zhi** (Hirudo), **Dan Shen** (Salvia Miltiorrhiza), Shi Chang Pu, Si Ji Qing, Xuan Sheng, **Hong Hua** (Carthamus), Su He Xiang, **Chi Shao** (Paeonia Rubra), Mu Jing Zi, He Shou Wu, Bu Gu Zhi, Ling Zhi, Fu Zi, Mao Mei, Zhi Shi, Ying Yu, Hai Feng Teng, **Yi Mu Cao** (Leonurus), Ju Hua, Huang Jing, Ying Xing Ye, Lu Xian Cao, Ying Yang Huo, Jing Tian San Qi, Ji Li, Hu Ji Shen, Jie Cao, She Xiang

Heart tonifying effect
Ren Shen, **Shan Zha** (Crategus), Chuan Wu, **Chuan Xiong** (Ligusticum), Ma Li Jing, Niu Huang, Shui Fei Ji, Yu Zhu, Tian Xuan Hua, Sheng Jiang, Jia Zhu Tao, Yang Jiao Ao, Hong Qi, Mai Men Dong, Du Zhong, **Chi Shao** (Paeonia Rubra), He Shou Wu, Fo Shou, Ling Zhi, Fu Zi, Qing Pi, Ci Lao Ya, Xi Xin, Zhi Ke, Zhi Shi, Nan Sha Shen, Xiang Fu, Xiang Jia Pi, Chuan Shan Long, Gui Zhu Tang Jie, Gao Shan Hong Jing Tian, Yi Zhi, Huang Qi, Huang Jin, Huang Hua Jia Zhu Tao, Xue Lian, Ma Huang, Yin Yang Huo, Ling Yang Jiao, Ting Li Zi, Feng Fang, Feng Du, Wu Gong, Fu Shou Cao, Suan Zao Ren, Hu Ji Shen, Zhang Nao, Can Su, She Xiang

Histamine secretion stimulating effect
Wu Jiu, Qing Feng Teng, Feng Du, Xi Sheng Teng

Hypoxia tolerance enhancing effect (general)
Ding Xiang, Ren Shen, Gan Jiang, Guang Zao, Nü Zhen Zi, Tian Ma, **Dan Shen** (Salvia Miltiorrhiza), Gan Song, Si Ji Qing, Bai Shao, Bai Song Ta, Gua Lou, Xi Yang Shen, Bai He, **Dang Gui** (Angelica Sinensis), Deng Zan Xi Xin, Hong Qi, Mai Men Dong, Gui Ban, Ling Zhi, Er Jiao, Ci Wu Jia, Ci Lao Ya, Bi Bo, Gao Liang Jiang, Gao Shan Hong Jing Tian, Hai Long, Hai Feng Teng, Yin Yang Huo, Ge Gen, Suan Zao Ren, Mo Han Lian, Bie Jia

Immune-suppressive effect
San Jian Shan, Shan Dou Gen, Chuan Wu, Tian Dong, Tian Hua Fen, Wu Jia Pi, Wu Wei Zi, Gan Sui, Shi Diao Lan, Bei Sha Shen, **Hong Hua** (Carthamus), Ku Shen, Ku Dou Zi, Kun Ming Shan Hai Tang, Chui Pen Cao, Zhong Jie Feng, Ze Xie, Xiang Xun, Chuan Shan Long, Chuan Xin Lian, Zu Shi Ma, Luo Tuo Peng Zi, Xia Ku Cao, Chai Hu, Huang Qin, She Chuang Zi, Pi Ma Zi, Lei Gong Teng, Chan Tui, **Shou Di** (Rehmannia)

Immune-stimulating effect
Ren Shen, San Qi (Notoginseng), Da Suan, Shan Yao, **Shan Zha** (Crategus), Guang Zao, Nü Zhen Zi, Tian Ma, Yun Zhi, **Yunnan Baiyao**, Wu Mei, Ba Ji Tian, Gan Cao, Shi Gao, Long Dan, Long Yan Rou, Xian Mao, Bai Shao, Bai Bian Dou, Dong Chong Xia Cao, An Di Jiao, Di Er Cao, **Dang Gui** (Angelica Sinensis), Fang Feng, Hong Qi, Mai Dong, Du Zhong, Lu Sun, Mu Jing Ye, He Shou Wu, Gui Ban, Sha Ji, Sha Yuan Zi, Ling Zhi, E Jiao, Fu Zi, Qing Jiao, Qing Mu Xiang, Ban Lan Gen, Ci Wu Jia, Ci Lao Ya, Ku Xing Ren, Luo Bu Ma, Jin Yin Hua, Yu Xing Cao, Gou Qi Zi, Fu Ling, Qi Cai, Xiang Ru, Jiao Gu Lan, Zhu Zi Shen, Dang Shen, Hai Shen, Sang Shen, Tu Si Zi, Huang Qi, Huang Lian, Huang Jing, Hung Jing Ye, Yin Er, Zhu Ling, Lu Rong, Lu Xian Cao, Yin Yang Huo, Zi He Che, Ge Jie, Ge Qiao, Suo Yang, Ge Shan Xiao, Pu Gong Ying, Feng Du, Jing Ji Er, Suan Zao, Wu Ji Sheng, Yi Yi Ren, Can Su, Bie Jia, She Xiang

Immunoglobulin stimulating
Huang Qi, Ling Zhi, Yin Yang Huo, Zi He Che, He Shou Wu, **Sheng Di Huang** (Rehmannia)

Insecticidal, anti-exoparasitic effect
Mu Fu Rong Ye, Zhi Xie Mu Pi, Bai Bu, Wu Yi, Bu Gu Zhi, Yu Teng, Hu Jiao, Pi Shi, Gui Jiu, Yang Cong, Chu Chong Ju, Luo Tuo Peng Zi, Buo Luo Hui, Liu Huang, La Jiao

Interferon production stimulating
Huang Qi, Bai Dou

Contraceptive with abortive effect
Jiu Li Xiang, Tu Jing Pi, Ma Dou Ling, **Wang Bu Liu Xing** (Vaccaria), Mu Jing Pi, Wu Bei Zi, **Niu Xi** (Achyranthis Bidentata), **Shui Zhi** (Hirudo), Gan Sui, Ban Xia, Di Long, He Huan Pi, Bing Pian, Xun Gu Feng, Fu Shan Hua, **Mu Dan Pi** (Moutan), Mu Jing Zi, E Wei, Kun Ming Shan Hai Tang, Jing Ying Hua, Jin Bian Long She Lan, Guan Zhong, Cha Ye, Wei Ling Xian, Chuan Xing Lian, Luo Tuo Peng Zi, **E Zhu** (Curcuma Ezhu), Chou Cao, Huang Jing Zi, Xue Lian, Lu Xian Cao, Mian Hua Gen, Zhong Lü Tan, Xiong Huang, Zhi Cao, Lei Gong Teng, Xi Qian Cao, She Xiang

Learning and memory enhancing effect
Ren Shen, Qing Cai, Ling Zhi, Dang Shen, Lu Rong

Leukocyte formation enhancing effect
San Ke Zhen, Nü Zhen Zi, Di Yu, Bai He, Rou Gui, Bu Gu Zhi, **Hu Zhang** (Polygonum Cuspidati), Liang Jun, Sang Shen, Ban Mao, Muo Han Lian, Can Su

Local anaesthetic effect
Chuan Wu, Tian Zhu Huang, Bai Qu Cai, Di Jiao, Du Heng, Hua Jiao, Fo Shou, Xin Yi, Ji Chi Teng, Xi Xin, Cao Wu, Xiang Fu, An Ye, Ju San Qi, Xue Shang Yi Zhi Hao, She Chuang Zhi, Bo Luo Hui, Can Su

Lymphoblast–transformation enhancing effect
Dang Gui (Angelica Sinensis), Huang Qi, Bai Zhu, Dang Shen, Yi Yi Ren, Yin Yang Huo, Ling Zhi, E Jiao, Nü Zhen Zi, Ren Shen, Bai Dou, He Shou Wu, Huang Jing

Mutation inhibiting effect
Da Zao, Niu Bang Zi, Sheng Jiang, Lao Guan Cao, Xi Yang Shen, Xiang Ri Kui Zi, Ku Xing Ren, Cha Ye, Xiang Xun, **Jiang Huang** (Curcuma Longa), Chai Hu, She Chuang Zi, Zhu Ling, E Bu Shi Cao

Peripheral blood vessel dilating effect
Ren Shen, Chuan Wu, **Chuan Xiong** (Ligusticum), Mu Zei, Shui Fei Ji, Bai Shao, Gua Lou, **Dang Gui** (Angelica Sinensis), Du Zhong, Xin Yi, Shi Wu Jia, Luo Bu Ma, Mei Ren Jiao, Zhu Shi Ma, Zhu Zi Shen, Gui Zhi, **Tao Ren** (Persica), Yan Fu Mu, Hai Feng Teng, Sang Ji Shen, Ji Mu, **Yin Xing Ye** (Ginkgo), Ge Gen, Fu She, Jie Cao

Peripheral blood vessel constricting effect
Yi Zhi, Ma Huang, Duan Xue Liu, Xi Sheng Teng

Phagocytosis enhancing effect
Wu Jia Pi, **Dang Gui** (Angelica Sinensis), Huang Qi, Bai Zhu, Dang Shen, Yin Yang Huo, Du Zhong, Ling Zhi, Xiang Xun, Ren Shen, Fu Ling, **Sheng Di Huang** (Rehmannia), Bu Gu Zhi, Shan Yao, Gan Cao

Purgative or draining effect
Da Huang (Rheum), Qian Jin Zi, Wu Hua Guo, Huo Ma Ren, Gan Sui, Gua Lou, Mang Xiao, Yang Ti, Lu Hui, Jin Bian Long She Lan, Qian Niu Zi, Pang Da Hai, **Tao Ren** (Persica), Liu Huang, Fan Xie Ye, Bi Ma Zi

Skeletal muscles relaxing effect
Ba Jiao Feng, Xin Yi, Lun Huan Teng, Nan Tian Zhu Zi, Feng Fang Ji, Xi Sheng Teng

Expectorant effect
Da Zao, Shan Gen Cai, Shan Zi Wan, Chuan Bei Mu, Guan Zao, Xiao Hui Xiang, Xiao Ye Pi Pa, Ma Qian Zi, Ma Dou Ling, Tian Nan Xiang, Che Qian Cao, Ai Ye, Gan Cao, Shi Wei, Shi Diao Lan, Bai Jie Zi, Bai Song Ta, Bai Qu Cai, Gua Lou, Ban Xia, Lao Guan Cao, Bai Bu, Hua Shan Shen, An Hui Bei Mu, Hong Dou Kou, **Si Gua Luo** (Luffa), Yuan Zhi, Hua Rei Shi, Mu Jing Zi, Mu Jing Ye, Fo Shou, Han Xiu Cao, Ling Zhi, Chen Pi, Ren Dong Teng, Ji Shi Teng, Qing Pi, Pi Pa Ye, Pi Pa He, Mu Ma Dou, Jing Qiao Mai, Pao Tong Guo, Ze Qi, Jing Jie, Jing Tiao, Di Cheng Qie, Yu Bai Fu, Qing Pi, Jie Geng, Hua Mu Pi, Tao Er Qi, Ye Dong Qing Guo, Zhu Dan, Zhu Ya Zao, Mao Yan Cao, Shang Lu, Mian Hua Gen, Guang Dong Ye, Guang Dong Hua, Liu Huang, Zhi Wan, Zi Su Ye, Zi Du Juan, Er Bu Shi Cao, Zao Shan Bai, Ai Di Cha, Man Shan Hong, Han Cai, Xian Zhu Li, Bo He, Chan Su, She Xiang Cao

Pain relieving effect

Ding Xiang, Qi Ye Lian, Ba Li Ma, **San Qi** (Notoginseng), Gan Jiang, Chuan Wu, Xiao Hui Xiang, Tian Ma, Tian Zhu Huang, **Yuan Hu** (Corydalis), Yun Zhi, Mu Zei, **Niu Xi** (Achyranthis Bidentata), Sheng Ma, Shi Suan, Bei Dou Gen, Bei Sha Shen, Sheng Jiang, Bai Shao, Bai Zhi, Bai Tou Weng, Dong Ling Cao, Bai Bu, **Dang Gui** (Angelica Sinensis), Rou Gui, Quan Xie, Bing Pian, Xun Gu Feng, Fang Feng, **Hong Hua** (Carthamus), Hong Qi, Mai Jiao, Du Zhong, Du Heng, Liang Mian Zhen, Hua Jiao, **Chi Shao** (Paeonia Rubra), Wu Zhu Yu, **Mu Dan Pi** (Moutan), Xin Yi, Qiang Huo, Ling Zhi, Fu Zi, Ji Shi Teng, Qing Feng Teng, Ku Dou Zi, Kun Ming Shan Hai Tang, Jin Qian Cao, Jin Qian Bai Hua She, Nao Yang Hua, Xi Xin, Jing Jie, Bi Cheng Jing, Cao Wu, Yin Yu, Wei Ling Xian, Gou Wen, Xiang Fu, Du Huo, Yang Jing Hua, Zhu Shi Ma, Jiao Gu Lan, Zhu Zi Shen, Qing Pi, Gui Zhi, Chai Hu, Dang Shen, Chou Wu Tong, Xu Chang Qing, Lang Du, Gao Liang Jiang, Hai Shen, Fen Fang Ji, Sang Bai Pi, Bi Qi, Ju San Qi, Xue Lian, Xue Shang Yi Zhi Hao, Liu Huang, Ruei Xiang, Feng Fang, Feng Du, Ai Di Cha, Suan Zao Ren, Man Jing Zi, Chan Tui, La Jiao, Gao Ben, Can Su, She Xiang

Shock abating effect

Tian Xian Zi, Fo Shou, E Jiao, Fu Zi, Qing Pi, Nao Yang Hua, **San Qi** (Notoginseng)

Sex hormone effect

Xiao Hui Xiang, Wu Jia Pi, Ba Ji Tian, Xian Mao, Hong Che Zhou Cao, Gui Ban, Bu Gu Zhi, Guan Zhong, Xiang Fu, Hai Ma, Tu Si Zi, Huan Jing Zi, Pi Jiu Hua, She Chuang Zi, Lu Rong, Ying Yang Huo, Ban Mao, Ge Jie, Ha Ma You, Suo Yang, Ji Li, She Xiang

Stone disintegration and stone expulsion enhancing effect

Shi Wei, Chen Pi, Jin Qian Cao, Hai Jin Sha, Xiong Dan

Metabolism enhancing effect

Ren Shen, **San Qi** (Notoginseng), Wu Jia Pi, Wu Wei Zi, **Niu Xi** (Achyranthis Bidentata), Long Yan Rou, Bai Zhu, Xi Yang Shen, Gui Ban, Ci Wu Jia, Gou Qi Zi, Huang Qi, Yin Er, Lu Rong, Ha Ma You

Radiation tolerance enhancing effect

Ren Shen, **San Qi** (Notoginseng), **Chuan Xiong** (Ligusticum), Wu Mei, Shui Fei Ji, **Dang Gui** (Angelica Sinensis), Rou Gui, Ling Zhi, E Jiao, Kun Bu, Mu Ma Dou, Cha Ye, Xiang Jia Pi, Liang Jun, Can Sha, He Tao Ren, Chai Hu, Gao Shan Hong Jing Tian, Hai Shen, Hai Piao Xiao, Zi Shi, Yin Er, Zhu Ling, Huai Hua, Feng Du, Can Su

Stress tolerance enhancing effect

Ren Shen, **San Qi** (Notoginseng), Wu Wei Zi, Ba Ji Tian, Long Yuan Rou, Dong Chong Xia Cao, Xi Yang Shen, Hua Jiao, Guo Ji Zi, Huang Qi, Lu Rong, Ha Ma You

T-lymphocyte production enhancing effect

Tian Men Dong, Bai Zhu, Yi Yi Ren, Yin Yang Huo, Ling Zhi, Nü Zhen Zi, Ren Shen, Bai Xiao Dou, Huang Jing

Thrombocyte aggregation inhibiting effect

Ding Xiang, Ren Shen, San Bai Cao, Gan Jiang, Da Suan, San Geng Cai, Guang Zao, Tian Xian Zi, Niu Huang, Hua Ju Hong, Shui Fei Ji, Ai Ye, Bei Dou Gen, Si Ji Qing, Sheng Jiang, Gua Lou, **Dang Gui** (Angelica Sinensis), Rou Gui, **Xue Jie** (Sanguis Draconis), Fang Feng, Su He Xiang, **Chi Shao** (Paeonia Rubra), Xin Yi, Ling Zhi, Ban Lang Gen, **Hu Zhang** (Polygonum Cuspidati), Luo Bu Ma, Zhi Mu, Cha Ye, Gou Teng, Xiang Xun, Du Huo, Chuan Xin Lian, **Jiang Huang** (Curcuma Longa), Jiao Gu Lan, Gui Zhi, Xia Tian Wu, Dang Shen, Gao Liang Jiang, Fen Fang Ji, Huang Lian, Ye Ju Hua, Ge Gen, Suan Zao Ren, Hu Ji Shen, Xie Bai

Thrombolytic effect

Yuan Zhi, Feng Du, Qu Mai, **Yunnan Baiyao**

Adaptogenic effect
Ren Shen, Wu Jia Pi, Xian Mao, Dang Shen, Gao Shan Hong Jing Tian

Wound and burn injuries healing effect
Shan Yao, Si Ji Qing, Lu Hui, Di Yu, Gu Sui Bu, Lu Rong

CNS exciting effect
Yi Ye Qiu, Ba Jiao Feng, San Geng Cai, Ma Sang, Ma Qian Zi, Wu Wei Zi, Bai Zhi, Xin Yi, Ci Lao Ya, Mu Ma Dou, Bi Bo, Xiang Jia Pi, Xia Tian Wu, Ma Huang, Zhang Nao, She Xiang

Appendix 4

Index of medicinals and formulas

Regarding translations of formula names, it is sometimes difficult to decide whether to laugh or to cry. Apart from erroneous translations like Bensky's 'Eight Treasure Pill to Benefit Mothers', where the characters for Leonuris (*Yi Mu Cao*) in Chinese contain the word mother, there are also clumsy expressions like the German formula name: 'Sclerotium Poria Cocos, Ramulus Cinnamomi Cassiae, Rhizoma Atractylodes Macrocephalae and Radix Glycyrrhizae Uralensis fried in honey Decoction'. Other translations become unintentionally humorous, for example: 'Pill of the Fifth and Sixth Heavenly Stalk', 'Ten Half-Charred Medicinals Powder' or 'Decoction Which Can Erect Roof Tiles' and so on.

In general, I do not agree with English speaking authors such as Flaws et al on the point that it is essential to be able to speak Chinese in order to study Chinese medicine. But I do hold the opinion that it is necessary to know a language and its applications in practice when translating formula names.

The following table lists both Bensky's and Maciocia's translations together with my own, which I have added, firstly in order to make the formula names more accessible for the reader, and also in order not to reproduce partially wrong translations.

My translations are based on the criteria of systematics and logic, brevity and pithiness, and semantic relationship.

Systematics and Logic

According to the functional translation theory (Reiß/Vermeer 1984), a purpose-directed translation can be regarded as the foundation of TCM professional practice; i.e. practical usefulness of the translation is the predominant goal. For the native reader, the translation should be easy to understand, easy to remember, methodical and logical.

I followed these principles, for example, in the translation of Wang Qing-Ren's formulas. As they all contain the words '... *Zhu Yu Tang*' (which means 'Eliminate Blood stasis ... Decoction'), I decided to translate them all as 'Anti-Stasis ... Decoction'. I have deliberately created the new word 'anti-stasis' in order to differentiate from the physics term 'antistatic', which relates to electricity, but not to Blood stasis. According to Wang's anatomical differentiation, we get:

Xue Fu Zhu Yu Tang = Anti-Stasis Chest Decoction
Ge Xia Zhu Yu Tang = Anti-Stasis Abdomen Decoction
Shao Fu Zhu Yu Tang = Anti-Stasis Lower Abdomen Decoction
Shen Tong Zhu Yu Tang = Anti-Stasis Pain Decoction
Hui Yan Zhu Yu Tang = Anti-Stasis Epiglottis Decoction

Tong Jing Zhu Yu Tang = Anti-Stasis Exanthema
Decoction
Gu Xia Yu Xue Tang = Anti-Stasis Ascites
Decoction.

When encountering related formulas, e.g. in variations of 'Rehmannia Six Ingredients Decoctions' (. . . *Wei Di Huang Tang*), I gave them names which indicated their relationship if this relationship was also evident in the Chinese name.

Brevity and Pithiness

As one can see in the following Table, my translations are always as short as possible. For example, the complete botanical name with its Latin adjectives has been replaced by its main genus name. It is a matter of semantic information (i.e. which formula is meant) and not about the exact ingredients and their preparation (raw, heated, carbonized etc.), which often cannot be derived from the name anyway. Even in Chinese, long names are often abbreviated by reducing them to one syllable. For example the formula *'Ma (Huang) Xing (Ren) Shi (Gao) Gan (Cao) Tang'*, which, with the even longer botanical name should be called 'Herba Ephedrae, Semen Armeniacae Armarum, Gypsum Fibrosum, Radix Glycyrrhizae Uralensis Decoction' is renamed 'Ephedra, Prunus, Gypsum, Glycyrrhiza Decoction'.

Semantic Relationship

My translation depends on the information conveyed by the Chinese name. When the word *Tang* (Decoction) is used, it is different from *Yin* (Drink), as the latter is mostly administered cold. On the other hand, a Chinese person will always understand that *Jin* (gold, metal) alludes to the functional concept of the Lung in Chinese medicine. I prefer to translate the Chinese metaphor with an informative word, such as Lung, instead of a literal rendition.

Nevertheless, I have tried to preserve the historical context as much as possible. For example old formulas that contain the term *'Zi Gong'* (e.g. in *'Ai Fu Nuan Gong Wan'*), which means 'palace of the child' were translated with the older English word 'womb' instead of uterus. Of course, they meant the uterus, but in those days, the anatomical understanding of what we know now as the uterus was different. I was able to translate the same word *'Gong'* in the modern formula *'Gong Wai Huai Yun Fang'* (Extra Uterine Pregnancy Formula) with uterus, because this formula was created in the context of anatomical knowledge of the 1970s.

Perfection?

Unfortunately not. I am still dissatisfied with some of my translations, e.g. with Sudden Smile Powder (*Shi Xiao San*), which does not quite reflect the meaning of the Chinese original. For this reason I am open to suggestions and will happily integrate them into new developments of the translation. I have rarely chosen to change a formula's name into something completely different from the literal translation. However, this was done in the case of *Si Ni San*, which I interpreted as 'Cold Limbs Powder', and *Si Ni Tang*, interpreted as 'Collapse Decoction'. A literal translation would be 'Four Rebellious Powder' and 'Four Rebellious Decoction' (German edition uses the word 'Kontravektionen' instead of 'rebellious' – Translator's note). Their similar characters in Chinese but completely dissimilar indications have led to many misunderstandings and accidents in China. I think the problem can be solved by employing different translations.

If in doubt, the practitioner should look up the formula's names in *Pinyin*. Together with *Pinyin* names of acupuncture points, they form an international standard, which an English or German translation cannot guarantee.

Llist of Formulas: English – Chinese with Their other English Translations

I have used the following formula names in this book and other publications. As a reference, two other English translations from Bensky's and Maciocia's books are given.

Formula name (Neeb)	Formula name (*Pinyin*)	Formula name (Bensky)	Formula name (Maciocia)
Achyranthis Powder	Xi Jiao San	Rhinocerus Horn Decoction	Cornu Bisontis Decoction
Aconite Centre Regulating Decoction	*Fu Zi Li Zhong Tang*		
Analgesic Myrrh Powder With Additions	*Zhi Tong Mo Yao San*		
Ancient Bone Expanding Powder	*Gu Kai Gu San*		
Ancient Myrrh Draconis Powder	*Gu Mo Jie San*		
Antelopis Uncaria Drink	*Ling Jiao Gou Teng Yin*	Antelope Horn and Uncaria Decoction	Cornu Antelopis-Uncaria Decoction
Anti-Diarrhoea Centre Regulating Decoction	*Zhi Xie Tiao Zhong Tang*		
Anti-Itching *Yang* Tonifying Decoction	*Zhu Yang Zhi Yang Tang*		
Anti-Stasis Abdomen Decoction	*Ge Xia Zhu Yu Tang*	Drive Out Blood Stasis Below the Diaphragm Decoction	Eliminating Stasis Below the Diaphragm Decoction
Anti-Stasis Ascites Decoction	*Gu Xia Yu Xue Tang*		
Anti-Stasis Chest Decoction	*Xue Fu Zhu Yu Tang*	Drive Out Stasis in the Mansion of Blood Decoction	Blood Mansion Eliminating Stasis Decoction
Anti-Stasis Epiglottis Decoction	*Hui Yan Zhu Yu Tang*		
Anti-Stasis Exanthema Decoction	*Tong Jing Zhu Yu Tang*		
Anti-Stasis Lower Abdomen Decoction	*Shao Fu Zhu Yu Tang*	Drive Out Blood Stasis in the Lower Abdomen Decoction	Lower Abdomen Eliminating Stasis Decoction
Anti-Stasis Pain Decoction	*Shen Tong Zhu Yu Tang*	Drive Out Blood Stasis from a Painful Body Decoction	Body-Pain Eliminating Stagnation Decoction
Aquilaria Directing *Qi* Downwards Decoction	*Chen Xiang Jiang Qi San*		Aquilaria Subduing *Qi* Powder
Arrest Coughing and Wheezing Powder	*Ding Chuan Tang*	Arrest Wheezing Powder	Stop Breathlessness Powder
Astragalus Decoction	*Huang Qi Tang*		Astragalus Decoction
Astragalus Cinnamomum Five Ingredients Decoction	*Huang Qi Gui Zhi Wu Wu Tang*		
Astragalus Four Ingredients Decoction	*Huang Qi Si Wu Tang*		
Astragalus Ledebouriella Decoction	*Huang Qi Fang Feng Tang*		

Formula name (Neeb)	Formula name (*Pinyin*)	Formula name (Bensky)	Formula name (Maciocia)
Astragalus Liquorice Decoction	*Huang Qi Gan Cao Tang*		
Astragalus Persica Carthamus Decoction	*Huang Qi Tao Hong Tang*		
Astragalus Red Wind Decoction	*Huang Qi Chi Feng Tang*		
Biota Decoction	*Bai Ye Tang*		
Black Gold Pill	*Wu Jin Tang*		Black Gold Pill
Blocked Kidney Decoction	*Shen Zhuo Tang*		
Blood Invigorating Angelica Decoction	*Dang Gui Huo Xue Tang*		
Blood Invigorating Recovery Decoction	*Fu Yuan Huo Xue Tang*		
Blood Stasis Purging Decoction	*Xia Yu Xue Tang*		
Buddha's Hands Powder	*Fo Shou San*		
Caryophyllus Persimmon Decoction	*Ding Xiang Shi Di Tang*		
Cinnamon and Poria Pill	*Gu Zhi Fu Ling Wan*	Cinnamon Twig and Poria Pill	Ramulus Cinnamomi-Poria Pill
Citrus Aurantium Allium Cinnamomum Decoction	*Zhi Shi Xie Bai Gui Zhi Tang*		Citrus Allium Cinnamomum Decoction
Citrus Reticulata Bambusa Decoction	*Chen Pi Zhu Ru Tang*		
Cock Crow Powder	*Ji Ming San*		
Codonopsis and Perilla Drink	*Shen Su Yin*	Ginseng and Perilla Leaf Decoction	Ginseng Perilla Decoction
Cold Limbs Powder	*Si Ni San*	Frigid Extremities Powder	Four Rebellious Powder
Collapse Decoction	*Si Ni Tang*	Frigid Extremities Decoction	
Cooling Detoxifying Powder	*Qing Re Xiao Du San*		
Coptidis Gallbladder Warming Decoction	*Huang Lian Wen Dan Tang*	Coptis Decoction to Warm the Gallbladder	Coptis Warming the Gall-Bladder Decoction
Corium Erinacei Powder	*Ci Wei Pi San*		
Cyperus Citrus Powder	*Xiang Ke San*		
Detoxifying, Blood Invigorating Decoction	*Jie Du Huo Xue Tang*		
Detoxifying, Blood Tonifying Decoction	*Du Huo Xue Tang*		

Formula name (Neeb)	Formula name (*Pinyin*)	Formula name (Bensky)	Formula name (Maciocia)
Dragon Horse Pastilles	*Long Mai Zi Lai Dan*		
Earth Dragon Tiger Decoction	*Fu Fang Di Hu Tang*		
Easygoing Walk Powder	*Xiao Yao San*	Rambling Powder	Free and Easy Wanderer Powder
Eight Immortals Longevity Pill	*Ba Xian Chang Shou Wan*	Eight-Immortal Pill for Longevity	Eight Immortals Longevity Pill
Eight Treasures Decoction	*Ba Zhen Tang*	Eight-Treasure Decoction	Eight Precious Decoction
Emergency *Yang* Recovery Decoction	*Ji Qiu Hui Yang Tang*		
Euphorbia Heart Pill	*Sui Xin Dan*		
Extra Uterine Pregnancy Formula	*Gong Wai Huai Yu Fang*		
Fennel Tincture	*Xiao Hui Xiang Jiu*		
Five Accumulations Powder	*Wu Ji San*	Five-Accumulation Powder	Five-Accumulation Powder
Five Seeds Conceiving Pill	*Wu Zi Yan Zong Wan*		Five-Seed Developing Ancestors Pill
Four Ingredients Decoction	*Si Wu Tang*	Four-Substance Decoction	Four Substances Decoction
Four Wonderful Powder	*Si Miao San*		Four Wonderful Powder
Gallbladder Warming Decoction	*Wen Dan Tang*	Warm the Gallbladder Decoction	Warming the Gall-bladder Decoction
Gastrodia Uncaria Drink	*Tian Ma Gou Teng Yin*	Gastrodia and Uncaria Decoction	Gastrodia-Uncaria Decoction
Generate Change Decoction	*Sheng Hua Tang*		
Gentiana Liver Venting Decoction	*Long Dan Xie Gan Tang*	Gentiana Longdancao Decoction to Drain the Liver	Gentiana Draining the Liver Decoction
Gentiana Powder	*Qin Jiao San*		
Ginseng Lung Relieving Decoction	*Ren Shen Xie Fei Tang*		
Glehnia Ophiopogonis Decoction	*Sha Shen Mai Dong Tang*	Glehnia and Ophiopogonis Decoction	Glehnia-Ophiopogon Decoction
Gourd Extract	*Chou Hu Lu Jiu*		
Great Chest Relieving Decoction	*Da Xian Xiong Tang*		
Great Comprehensive Ten Tonics Pill	*Shi Quan Da Bu Tang*	All-Inclusive Great Tonifying Decoction	Ten Complete Great Tonification Decoction
Great *Yin* Strengthening Decoction	*Da Bu Yin Wan*	Great Tonify the *Yin* Pill	Big Tonifying the *Yin* Pill
Great *Yuan* Tonic	*Da Bu Yuan Jian*		

Formula name (Neeb)	Formula name (*Pinyin*)	Formula name (Bensky)	Formula name (Maciocia)
Guaranteed Resuscitation Decoction	*Ke Bao Li Su Tang*		
Guide Out Phlegm Decoction	*Dao Tan Tang*	Guide Out Phlegm Decoction	Conducting Phlegm Decoction
Gushing Spring Powder	*Yong Quan San*		
Hand-made Pill	*Shou Nian Wan*		
Harmony Pill	*Bao He Wan*	Preserve Harmony Pill	Preserving and Harmonizing Pill
Heart Relieving Decoction	*Xie Xin Tang*	Drain the Epigastrium Decoction	Draining the Heart Decoction
Heavenly Heart Tonic Pill	*Tian Wang Bu Xin Dan*	Emperor of Heaven's Special Pill to Tonify the Heart	Heavenly Emperor Tonifying the Heart Pill
Hematite Inula Decoction	*Dai Zhe Xuan Fu Tang*		
Inula Decoction	*Xuan Fu Hua Tang*		
Invigorating Drink of the Immortals	*Xian Fang Huo Ming Yin*		
Jade Dragon Paste	*Yu Long Gao*		
Jade Windscreen Powder	*Yu Ping Feng San*	Jade Windscreen Powder	Jade Wind Screen Powder
Jade Woman Decoction	*Yu Nu Jian*	Jade Woman Decoction	Jade Woman Decoction
Kidney *Yang* Drink	*You Gui Yin*	Restore the [Right] Kidney Decoction	Restoring the [Right] Kidney Decoction
Kidney *Yang* Pill	*You Gui Wan*	Restore the [Right] Kidney Pill	Restoring the [Right] Kidney Pill
Kidney *Yin* Drink	*Zuo Gui Yin*	Restore the [Left] Kidney Decoction	Restore the [Left] Kidney Decoction
Kidney *Yin* Pill	*Zuo Gui Wan*	Restore the [Left] Kidney Pill	Restoring the [Left] Kidney Pill
Lepidium and Jujube Decoction	*Ting Li Da Zao Tang*		
Linking Decoction	*Yi Guan Jian*	Linking Decoction	One Linking Decoction
Lonicera Forsythia Powder	*Yin Qiao San*	Honeysuckle and Forsythia Powder	Lonicera-Forsythia Powder
Lung Cooling, Phlegm Resolving Decoction	*Qing Jin Hua Tan Tang*		Clearing Metal and Resolving Phlegm Decoction
Lung Relieving Powder	*Xie Bai San*	Drain the White Powder	Draining Whiteness Powder
Lycium, Chrysanthemum Rehmannia Eight Decoction	*Qi Ju Di Huang Wan*	Lycium Fruit, Chrysanthemum and Rehmannia Pill	Lycium-Chrysanthemum-Rehmannia Pill
Menses Warming Decoction	*Wen Jing Tang*	Warm the Menses Decoction	Warm the Menses Decoction

Formula name (Neeb)	Formula name (*Pinyin*)	Formula name (Bensky)	Formula name (Maciocia)
Middle Regulating Decoction	*Li Zhong Wan*	Regulate the Middle Pill	Regulating the Centre Pill
Middle Strengthening the *Qi* Tonic	*Bu Zhong Yi Qi Tang*	Tonify the Middle and Augment the *Qi* Decoction	Tonifying the Centre and Benefitting *Qi* Decoction
Morus Armeniaca Decoction	*Sang Xing Tang*	Mulberry Leaf and Apricot Kernel Decoction	Morus-Prunus Decoction
Morus Chrysanthemum Decoction	*Sang Ju Yin*	Mulberry Leaf and Chrysanthemum Decoction	Morus-Chrysanthemum Decoction
Morus Decoction	*Sang Bai Pi Tang*		Cortex Mori Decoction
Mother-of-Pearl Pill	*Zhen Zhu Mu Wan*	Mother-of-Pearl Pill	Concha Margaritiferae Pill
Nine *Qi* Pill	*Jiu Qi Wan*		
Onion, Honey and Pig's Gallbladder Decoction	*Mi Cong Zhu Dan Tang*		
Ophicalcitum Powder	*Hua Rui Shi San*		
Orifices Opening, Blood Invigorating Decoction	*Tong Qiao Huo Xue Tang*	Unblock the Orifices and Invigorate the Blood Decoction	Opening the Orifices and Invigorating Blood Decoction
Origin Protecting Anti-Dysentery Decoction	*Bao Yuan Hua Chi Tang*		
Overcoming Stagnation Pill	*Yue Ju Wan*	Escape Restraint Pill	Gardenia-Ligusticum Pill
Patchouli *Qi* Rectifying Powder	*Huo Xiang Zheng Qi San*	Agastache Powder to Rectify the *Qi*	Agastache Upright *Qi* Powder
Peony Decoction	*Shao Yao Tang*	Peony Decoction	Paeonia Decoction
Peony Liquorice Decoction	*Jia Ji Hua TuTang*		
Persica Carthamus Drink	*Tao Hong Yin*		Prunus-Carthamus Decoction
Persica Carthamus Four Ingredients Decoction	*Tao Hong Si Wu Tang*	Four-Substances Decoction with Safflower and Peach Pit	Persica Carthamus Four Substances Decoction
Persica Paeonia Decoction	*Tao Ren Shao Yao Tang*		
Phlegm Expelling Pill	*Gun Tan Wan*	Vaporize Phlegm Pill	Chasing Away Phlegm Pill
Pinellia-Atractylodes-Gastrodia Decoction	*Ban Xia Bai Zhu Tian Ma Tang*	Pinellia, Atractylodes Macrocephala, and Gastrodia Decoction	Pinellia-Atractylodes-Gastrodia Decoction
Polyporus Decoction	*Zhu Ling Tang*	Polyporus Decoction	Polyporus Decoction
Protecting the Source Decoction	*Bao Yuan Tang*		
Providing Faithfully Three-Seeds Decoction	*San Zi Yang Qin Tang*	Three-Seed Decoction to Nourish one's Parents	Three-Seed Nourishing the Parents Decoction
Psychosis Decoction	*Dian Kuang Meng Xing Tang*		

Formula name (Neeb)	Formula name (*Pinyin*)	Formula name (Bensky)	Formula name (Maciocia)
Pueraria Decoction	*Ge Gen Tang*		
Pulsatilla Decoction	*Bai Tou Weng Tang*	Pulsatilla Decoction	Pulsatilla Decoction
Pulse Generating Powder	*Sheng Mai San*	Generate the Pulse Powder	Generating the Pulse Powder
Qi Passage Powder	*Tong Qi Tang*		
Qi Rectifying Persica Carthamus Decoction	*Tao Hong Cheng Qi Tang/Tad He Cheng Qi Tang*	Peach Pit Decoction to Order the *Qi*	Persica Conducting *Qi* Decoction
Rehmannia Six Pill	*Liu Wei Di Huang Wan*	Six-Ingredient Pill with Rehmannia	Six-Ingredient Rehmannia Pill
Relaxing the Vessels Decoction	*Shu Jing Huo Xue Tang*		
Resistance Decoction	*Di Dang Tang*		
Rheum Eupolyphaga Pill	*Da Huang Zhe Chong Wan*		
Rhino-Rehmannia Decoction	*Xi Jiao Di Huang Tang*	Rhinocerus Horn and Rehmannia Decoction	Cornu Bufali-Rehmannia Decoction
Sal Ammoniac Pill	*Nao Sha Wan*		
Salvia Drink	*Dan Shen Yin*	Salvia Decoction	Salvia Decoction
Seven *Li* Powder	*Qi Li San*		
Shen's Rehmannia Decoction	*Sheng Di Huang Tang*		
Six Gentlemen Decoction	*Liu Jun Zi Tang*	Six-Gentlemen Decoction	Six Gentlemen Decoction
Small Bupleurum Decoction	*Xiao Chai Hu Tang*	Minor Bupleurum Decoction	Small Bupleurum Decoction
Small Channel Invigorating Pill	*Xiao Huo Luo Dan*		
Small Chest Relieving Decoction	*Xiao Xian Xiong Tang*	Minor Sinking Into the Chest Decoction	Small Sinking [*Qi* of the] Chest Decoction
Small Green Dragon Decoction	*Xiao Qing Long Tang*	Minor Bluegreen Dragon Decoction	Small Green Dragon Decoction
Small Menses Regulating Decoction	*Xiao Tiao Jing Tang*		
Spinosa Decoction	*Suan Zao Ren Tang*	Sour Jujube Decoction	Ziziphus Decoction
Spleen and Kidneys Tonifying Decoction	*Pi Shen Shuang Bu Tang*		Decoction Tonifying Both Spleen and Kidneys
Spleen Recovering Decoction	*Gui Pi Tang*	Restore the Spleen Decoction	Tonifying the Spleen Decoction
Spleen Warming Decoction	*Wen Pi Tang*	Warm the Spleen Decoction	Warming the Spleen Decoction
Stomach Calming Powder	*Ping Wei San*	Calm the Stomach Powder	Balancing the Stomach Powder

Formula name (Neeb)	Formula name (*Pinyin*)	Formula name (Bensky)	Formula name (Maciocia)
Stomach Refreshing Powder	*Qing Wei San*	Clear the Stomach Powder	Clearing the Stomach Powder
Stop Coughing Powder	*Zhi Sou San*	Stop Coughing Powder	Stopping Cough Powder
Styrax Pill	*Su He Xiang Wan*	Liquid Styrax Pill	Styrax Pill
Substitute Resistance Powder/Pill	*Dai Di Dang San/Wan*		Surrogate Keeping Out Powder
Sudden Smile Powder	*Shi Xiao San*	Sudden Smile Powder	Breaking into a Smile Powder
Sudden Smile Powder with Angelica and Ligusticum	*Gui Xiong Shi Xiao San*		
Ten Tonics Pill	*Shi Bu Wan*	Ten-Tonic Pill	
Three *Bi* Decoction	*San Bi Tang*		
Three Break-throughs Decoction	*San Ao Tang*	Three Unbinding Decoction	Three Break Decoction
Three Wonders Medicine Pill	*San Miao San*	Three Marvel Pill	Three Wonderful Powder
Trauma Pill	*Die Da Wan*		
Trichosanthes Allium Pinellia Decoction	*Gua Lou Xie Bai Ban Xia Tang*	Trichosanthes Fruit, Chinese Chive and Pinellia Decoction	Trichosanthes-Allium-Pinellia Decoction
Trichosanthes Allium Rice Wine Decoction	*Gua Lou Xie Bai Bai Jiu Tang*	Trichosanthes Fruit, Chinese Chive and Wine Decoction	Trichosanthes-Allium-White Wine Decoction
True Warrior Decoction	*Zhen Wu Tang*	True Warrior Decoction	True Warrior Decoction
Two Deities Pill	*Er Shen San*		Two Spirits Powder
Two '*Di*' Decoction	*Liang Di Tang*		Two '*Di*' Decoction
Two Old Decoction	*Er Chen Tang*	Two-Cured Decoction	Two Old Decoction
Wei and Ying Strengthening Decoction	*Zhu Wei He Rong Tang*		
White Tiger Decoction	*Bai Hu Tang*	White Tiger Decoction	White Tiger Decoction
Will Reinforcing and Calming Decoction	*An Shen Ding Zhi Wan*		Calming the Mind and Settling the Will-Power Pill
Wind Allaying Decoction	*Xi Feng Tang*		
Wise Healing Decoction	*Sheng Yu Tang*	Sage-Like Healing Decoction	Sage-Like Healing Decoction
Womb Warming Artemisia Cyperus Pill	*Ai Fu Nuan Gong Wan*	Mugwort and Prepared Aconite Pill for Warming the Womb	Artemisia-Cyperus Warming the Uterus Pill
Wondrous Pill to Invigorate the Channels	*Huo Luo Xiao Ling Dan*	Fantastically Effective Pill to Invigorate the Collaterals	Miraculously Effective Invigorating the Connecting Channels Pill

Formula name (Neeb)	Formula name (*Pinyin*)	Formula name (Bensky)	Formula name (Maciocia)
Wood Fungus Powder *Yang* Tonifying Five-Tenth Decoction	*Mu Er San Bu Yang Huan Wu Tang*	Tonify the *Yang* to Restore Five Tenths Decoction	Tonify *Yang* and Restoring Five Tenths Decoction
Yin Nourishing Bi Dissolving Decoction	*Yang Yin Tong Bi Tang*		
Yellow Rhino Pills (without rhinoceros)	*Xi Huang Wan*		
Zingiber Heart Relief Decoction	*Sheng Jiang Xie Xin Tang*		

Appendix 5

List of formulas in this book, Chinese–English with quantities

Some of the listed formulas are rarely mentioned in the book, as they are obsolete these days and scarcely used in practice. Formulas of this type often contain self-made medicinals and act as a reference. Therefore they sometimes do not have their dosages specified.

AI FU NUAN GONG WAN (Womb Warming Artemisia Cyperus Pill)

9 g	Folium Artemisiae Argyi (*Ai Ye*)
18 g	Rhizoma Cyperi (*Xiang Fu*)
9 g	Fructus Evodiae (*Wu Zhu Yu*)
9 g	Radix Ligustici Wallichii (*Chuan Xiong*)
9 g	Radix Paeoniae Lactiflorae (*Bai Shao*)
9 g	Radix Astragali (*Huang Qi*)
4.5 g	Radix Dipsaci (*Xu Duan*)
3 g	Radix Rehmanniae (*Sheng Di Huang*)
1.5 g	Cortex Cinnamomi (*Rou Gui*)
9 g	Radix Angelicae Sinensis (*Dang Gui*)

BA ZHEN TANG (Eight Treasures Decoction)

9 g	Radix Angelicae Sinensis (*Dang Gui*)
9 g	Radix Ginseng (*Ren Shen*)
9 g	Radix Paeoniae Albae (*Bai Shao*)
9 g	Rhizoma Atractylodis Macrocephalae (*Bai Zhu*)
9 g	Sclerotium Poria Cocos (*Fu Ling*)
12 g	Radix Rehmanniae Praeparatae (*Shu Di Huang*)
6 g	Radix Ligustici Wallichii (*Chuan Xiong*)
3 g	Radix Glycyrrhizae Praeparatae (*Zhi Gan Cao*)

BAI HU TANG (White Tiger Decoction)

9 g	Rhizoma Anemarrhenae (*Zhi Mu*)
30 g	Gypsum Fibrosum (*Shi Gao*)
3 g	Radix Glycyrrhizae (*Gan Cao*)
9 g	Semen Oryzae Nonglutinosae (*Jing Mi*)

BAI TOU WENG WANG (Pulsatilla Decoction)

15 g	Radix Pulsatillae Chinensis (*Bai Tou Weng*)
12 g	Cortex Phellodendri (*Huang Bai*)
12 g	Rhizoma Coptidis (*Huang Lian*)
12 g	Cortex Fraxini (*Qin Pi*)

BAI YE TANG (Biota Decoction)

30 g	Folium Biotae Orientalis (*Ce Bai Ye*)
30 g	Rhizoma Zingiberis (*Gan Jiang*)
30 g	Folia Artemisia Sinensis (*Ai Ye*)

BAO YUAN HUA CHI TANG (Origin Protecting Anti-Dysentery Decoction)

80 g	Radix Astragali (*Huang Qi*) and 40 g Talcum (*Hua Shi*) to be taken in the evening with 20 g of sugar.

BAO YUAN TANG (Protecting the Source Decoction)

20 g	Radix Astragali (*Huang Qi*)
20 g	Radix Panax Ginseng (*Ren Shen*)
8 g	Cortex Cinnamomi Cassia (*Rou Gui*)
5 g	Radix Glycyrrhizae Uralensis (*Gan Cao*)

BU YANG HUAN WU TANG (Yang Tonifying Five-Tenth Decoction)

20 g	Radix Astragali (*Huang Qi*)
6 g	Radix Angelicae Sinensis (*Dang Gui Wei*)
3 g	Radix Ligustici Wallichii (*Chuan Xiong*)
6 g	Radix Paeoniae Rubrae (*Chi Shao Yao*)
3 g	Semen Persicae (*Tao Ren*)
3 g	Flos Carthami (*Hong Hua*)
3 g	Lumbricus (*Di Long*)

CHEN PI ZHU RU TANG (Citrus Reticulata Bambusa Decoction)

15 g	Pericarpium Citri Reticulatae (*Chen Pi*)
15 g	Glycyrrhiza Uralensis (*Gan Cao*)
15 g	Bambusa in Taeniam (*Zhu Ru*)
7.5 g	Radix Panax Ginseng (*Ren Shen*)
3 slices	Zingiberis Recens (*Sheng Jiang*)
1 piece of	Fructus Zizyphi Jujubae (*Da Zao*)

CHEN XIANG JIANG QI SAN (Aquilaria Directing Qi Downwards Decoction, after Shen)

One part of each, ground into powder:
Lignum Aquilariae (*Chen Xiang*)
Radix Aucklandia Lappa (*Mu Xiang*)
Herba Bupleurum (*Chai Hu*)
Radix Paeoniae Lactiflorae (*Bai Shao*)
Radix Asari (*Xi Xin*)
Pericarpium Citri Reticulatae Viride (*Qing Pi*)
Fructus Perillae Fructescentis (*Zi Su Zi*)
Pour down with a decoction of ginger.

CHOU HU LU JIU (Gourd Extract)

A dry gourd (Lagenaria Siceraria, *Ku Hu Lu*) is roasted until it can be pulverized. Mix powder with 12 ml of ricewine and drink.

CI WEI PI SAN (Corium Erinacei Powder)

The dry-roasted skin of Erinaceum europaeus or Dauricus (*Ci Wei*) is pulverized and administered in the morning together with rice wine.

DA HUANG ZHE CHONG WAN (Rheum Eupolyphaga Pill)

40 g	Rhizoma et Radix Rhei (*Da Huang*)
80 g	Radix Scutellaria (*Huang Qin*)
120 g	Radix Glyzhyrriza (*Gan Cao*)
80 g	Semen Persicae (*Tao Ren*)
80 g	Semen Pruni Armeniacae (*Xing Ren*)
160 g	Radix Paeoniae Lactiflorae (*Bai Shao Yao*)
400 g	Radix Polygoni (*He Shu Wu*)
40 g	Lacca Sinica Exsiccatae (*Gan Qi*)
80 g	Tabanus (*Mang Chong*)
80 g	Hirudo (*Shui Zhi*)
80 g	Holotrichia (*Qi Cao*)
40 g	Eupolyphaga (*Tu Bie Chong*)

DA XIAN XIONG TANG (Great Chest Relieving Decoction)

10 g	Radix et Rhizoma Rhei (*Da Huang*) – boil and reduce to 1/3 of the liquid
10 g	Mirabilitum (*Mang Xiao*) – add at the end of the cooking process
1 g	Euphorbia Kansui (*Gan Sui*) – pulverize and wash down together with decoction.

DAI DI DANG TANG (Substitute Resistance Decoction)

12 g	Radix et Rhizoma Rhei (*Da Huang*)
3 g	Mirabilitum (*Mang Xiao*)
3 g	Radix Angelicae Sinensis (*Dang Gui*)
3 g	Radix Rehmanniae Glutinosae (*Sheng Di Huang*)
3 g	Squama Manitis (*Chuan Shan Jia*)
1.5 g	Ramulus Cinnamomi Cassiae (*Gui Zhi*)
6 pieces	Semen Persicae (*Tao Ren*)

DAN SHEN YIN (Salvia Drink)

30 g	Radix Salviae Miltiorrhizae (*Dan Shen*)
5 g	Lignum Santali Albi (*Tan Xiang*)
5 g	Fructus Amomi (*Sha Ren*)

DANG GUI HUO XUE TANG (Blood Invigorating Angelica Decoction)

9 g	Radix Angelicae Sinensis (*Dang Gui*)
4.5 g	Radix Paeoniae Rubrae (*Chi Shao*)
4.5 g	Radix Rehmannia Glutinosae (*Sheng Di Huang*)
4.5 g	Ramulus Cinnamomi Cassia (*Gui Zhi*)
2.5 g	Sclerotium Poriae Cocos (*Fu Ling*)
2.5 g	Fructus Citri Aurantii (*Zhi Ke*)
2.5 g	Radix Bupleuri (*Chai Hu*)

1.5 g	Radix Glycyrrhizae Uralensis (*Gan Cao*)
1.2 g	Rhizoma Zingiberis Officinalis (*Gan Jiang*)
0.6 g	Flos Carthami (*Hong Hua*)
20 pc	Semen Persicae (*Tao Ren*)

To be taken with rice wine.

DI DANG TANG (Resistance Decoction)

30 pc	Hirudo (*Shui Zhi*)
30 pc	Tabanus (*Meng Chong*)
20 pc	Semen Persicae (*Tao Ren*)
48 g	Rhizoma et Radix Rhei (*Da Huang*)

DIAN KUANG MENG XING TANG (Psychosis Decoction)

32 g	Semen Persicae (*Tao Ren*)
12 g	Radix Bupleuri (*Chai Hu*)
8 g	Rhizoma Cyperi (*Xiang Fu*)
12 g	Caulis Akebiae Mutong (*Mu Tong*)
12 g	Radix Paeoniae Rubrae (*Chi Shao*)
8 g	Rhizoma Pinelliae (*Ban Xia*)
8 g	Pericarpium Arecae (*Da Fu Pi*)
8 g	Pericarpium Citri Reticulatae (*Chen Pi*)
12 g	Pericarpium Citri Reticulatae Viride (*Qing Pi*)
12 g	Cortex Mori Lactiflorae (*Sang Bai Pi*)
16 g	Fructus Perillae (*Su Zi*)
20 g	Radix Glycyrrhizae Uralensis (*Gan Cao*)

DIE DA WAN (Trauma Pill)

Wine-prepared Rhizoma Rhei (*Jiu Jun*)
Wine-prepared Rhizoma Cyperi (*Jiu Xiang Fu*)
Radix Notoginseng (*San Qi*)
Flos Carthami (*Hong Hua*)
Eupolyphaga (*Tu Bie Chong*)
Pyritum (*Zi Ran Tong*)
Wine-prepared Radix Angelicae (*Jiu Dang Gui*)
Radix Paeoniae Rubrae (*Chi Shao*)
Lignum Sappan (*Su Mu*)
Radix Rehmanniae (*Sheng Di Huang*)

To be ground in equal parts and formed into honey balls of 3 g each.

DING XIANG SHI DI TANG (Caryophyllus Persimmon Decoction)

6 g	Flos Caryophylli (*Ding Xiang*)
9 g	Calix Kaki (*Shi Di*)

3 g	Radix Ginseng (*Ren Shen*)
6 g	Rhizoma Zingiberis Recens (*Sheng Jiang*)

DU QI WAN (Pathogenic Qi Decoction)

15 g	Radix Rehmanniae Praeparatae (*Shu Di Huang*)
9 g	Radix Dioscoreae Oppositae (*Shan Yao*)
9 g	Sclerotium Poria Cocos (*Fu Ling*)
9 g	Cortex Moutan Radicis (*Mu Dan Pi*)
9 g	Fructus Corni Officinalis (*Shan Yu Rou*)
9 g	Rhizoma Alismatis Orientalis (*Ze Xie*)
3 g	Fructus Schisandrae (*Wu Wei Zi*)

ER CHEN TANG (Two Old Decoction)

6 g	Pericarpium Citri Reticulatae (*Chen Pi*)
6 g	Rhizoma Pinelliae (*Ban Xia*)
9 g	Sclerotium Poriae Cocos (*Fu Ling*)
1.5 g	Radix Glycyrrhizae Praeparatae (*Zhi Gan Cao*)

ER SHEN WAN (Two Deities Pill)

120 g	Fructus Psoralea (*Bu Gu Zhi*)
60 g	Semen Myristicae Fragrantis (*Rou Dou Kou*)
120 g	Rhizoma Zingiberis Officinalis (*Gan Jiang*)
49 pc	Fructus Zizyphi Jujubae (*Da Zao*)

To be made into pea-sized pills.

FO SHOU SAN (Buddha's Hands Powder)

9 g	Radix Ligustici Wallichii (*Chuan Xiong*)
15 g	Radix Angelicae Sinensis (*Dang Gui*)

FU FANG DI HU TANG (Earth Dragon Tiger Decoction)

Lumbricus (*Di Long*)
Radix et Rhizoma Polygoni Cuspidati (*Hu Zhang*)
Caulis Akebiae (*Mu Tong*)
Herba Plantaginis (*Che Qian Zi*)
Semen Raphani Sativi (*Lai Fu Zi*)
Radix Astragali (*Huang Qi*)
Squama Manitis (*Chuan Shan Jia*)
Radix Glycyrrhizae Uralensis (*Gan Cao*)

(No dosage recommendations could be found.)

FU YUAN HUO XUE TANG (Blood Invigorating Recovery Decoction)

30 g	Rhizoma et Radix Rhei (*Da Huang*)
15 g	Radix Bupleuri (*Chai Hu*)
9 g	Radix Angelicae Sinensis (*Dang Gui*)
9 g	Semen Persicae (*Tao Ren*)
6 g	Flos Carthami (*Hong Hua*)
6 g	Squama Manitis (*Chuan Shan Jia*)
9 g	Radix Trichosanthis (*Tian Hua Fen*)
6 g	Radix Glycyrrhizae (*Gan Cao*)

FU ZI LI ZHONG TANG (Aconite Centre Regulating Decoction)

6 g	Radix Aconiti Lateralis Praeparata (*Zhi Fu Zi*)
7.5 g	Rhizoma Zingiberis Officinalis (*Gan Jiang*)
7.5 g	Rhizoma Atractylodis Macrocephalae (*Bai Zhu*)
7.5 g	Radix Ginseng (*Ren Shen*)
7.5 g	Radix Glycyrrhizae Uralensis Praeparatae (*Zhi Gan Cao*)

GE GEN TANG (Pueraria Decoction)

12 g	Radix Puerariae (*Ge Gen*)
6 g	Herba Ephedrae (*Ma Huang*)
6 g	Ramulus Cinnamomi Cassia (*Gui Zhi*)
6 g	Radix Paeoniae Lactiflorae (*Shao Yao*)
6 g	Radix Glycyrrhizae Uralensis (*Gan Cao*)
9 g	Rhizoma Zingiberis Recens (*Sheng Jiang*)
3 pc	Fructus Zizyphi Jujubae (*Da Zao*)

GE XIA ZHU YU TANG (Anti-Stasis Abdomen Decoction)

9 g	Faeces Trogopteri (*Wu Ling Zhi*)
9 g	Radix Angelicae Sinensis (*Dang Gui*)
6 g	Radix Ligustici Wallichii (*Chuan Xiong*)
9 g	Semen Persicae (*Tao Ren*)
6 g	Cortex Moutan Radicis (*Mu Dan Pi*)
6 g	Radix Paeoniae Rubrae (*Chi Shao Yao*)
6 g	Radix Linderae (*Wu Yao*)
3 g	Rhizoma Corydalis (*Yan Hu Suo*)
6 g	Radix Glycyrrhizae Uralensis (*Gan Cao*)
3 g	Rhizoma Cyperi (*Xiang Fu*)
9 g	Flos Carthami (*Hong Hua*)
5 g	Fructus Citri Aurantii (*Zhi Ke*)

GONG WAI HUAI YUN FANG (Extra Uterine Pregnancy Formula)

15 g	Radix Salviae Miltiorrhizae (*Dan Shen*)
9 g	Radix Paeoniae Rubrae (*Chi Shao*)
9 g	Semen Persicae (*Tao Ren*)
9 g	Resinum Olibani (*Ru Xiang*)
9 g	Myrrha (*Mo Yao*)

GUAN XIN ER HAO FANG (Coronary Decoction No. 2)

15 g	Radix Ligustici Wallichii (*Chuan Xiong*)
15 g	Radix Paeoniae Rubrae (*Chi Shao*)
30 g	Radix Salviae Miltiorrhizae (*Dan Shen*)
15 g	Flos Carthami (*Hong Hua*)
15 g	Lignum Dalbergiae Odiferae (*Jiang Xiang*)

GU KAI GU SAN (Ancient Bone Expanding Powder)

40 g	Radix Angelica Sinensis (*Dang Gui*)
20 g	Radix Ligustici Wallichii (*Chuan Xiong*)
64 g	Plastrum Testudinis (*Gui Ban* Xue)
8 g	Crinis Carbonisatus hominis (*Xue Yu Tan*)
160 g	Radix Astragali (*Huang Qi*)

GU MO JIE SAN (Ancient Myrrh Draconis Powder)

12 g	Myrrha (*Mo Yao*)
12 g	Sanguis Draconis (*Xue Jie*)

To be taken with boiled water.

GU XIA YU XUE TANG (Anti-Stasis Ascites Decoction)

32 g	Semen Persicae (*Tao Ren*)
2 g	Radix et Rhizoma Rhei (*Da Huang*)
6 g	Eupolyphaga (*Tu Bie Chong*)
4 g	Euphorbia Kansui (*Gan Sui*)

GUA LOU XIE BAI BAI JIU TANG (Trichosanthis Allium Ricewine Decoction)

15 g	Fructus Trichosanthis (*Gua Lou*)
9 g	Bulbus Allii Macrostemi (*Xie Bai*)
~300 ml	Vinum (rice wine or dry white wine)

GUA LOU XIE BAI BAN XIA TANG (Trichosanthis Allium Pinellia Decoction)

12 g	Fructus Trichosanthis (*Gua Lou*)
9 g	Bulbus Allii Macrostemi (*Xie Bai*)
12 g	Pinellia (Rhizoma Pinelliae Ternatae (*Ban Xia*)
~300 ml	Vinum (rice wine or dry white wine)

GUI PI TANG (Spleen Recovering Decoction)

9 g	Radix Astragali (*Huang Qi*)
9 g	Rhizoma Atractylodis Macrocephalae (*Bai Zhu*)
9 g	Sclerotium Poriae Cocos (*Fu Ling*)
9 g	Arillus Longan (*Long Yan Rou*)
9 g	Semen Zizyphi Spinosae (*Suan Zao Ren*)
9 g	Radix Codonopsitis Pilosulae (*Dang Shen*)
3 g	Radix Aucklandiae (*Mu Xiang*)
3 g	Radix Glycyrrhizae Uralensis Praeparata (*Zhi Gan Cao*)

GUI XIONG SHI XIAO SAN (Sudden Smile Powder with Angelica and Ligusticum)

Pollen Typhae (*Pu Huang*)
Faeces Trogopteri (*Wu Ling Zhi*)
Angelicae Radix Sinensis (*Dang Gui*)
Ligustici Radix Wallichii (*Chuan Xiong*)

Take equal parts and make into a powder.

GUI ZHI FU LING WAN (Cinnamon and Poria Pills)

9 g	Ramulus Cinnamomi (*Gui Zhi*)
9 g	Sclerotium Poriae Cocos (*Fu Ling*)
9 g	Cortex Moutan Radicis (*Mu Dan Pi*)
9 g	Semen Persicae (*Tao Ren*)
9 g	Radix Paeoniae Rubrae (*Chi Shao*)

HUA RUI SHI SAN (Ophicalcitum Powder)

120 g	Ophicalcitum (*Hua Rui Shi*)
30 g	Calculus Bovis (*Niu Huang*)

To be taken in small portions with alcohol and infant's urine (*Tong Niao*).

HUANG QI CHI FENG TANG (Astragalus Red Wind Decoction)

80 g	Radix Astragali (*Huang Qi*)
4 g	Radix Paeoniae Rubrae (*Chi Shao*)
4 g	Radix Ledebouriellae (*Fang Feng*)

HUANG QI FANG FENG TANG (Astragalus Ledebouriella Decoction)

120 g	Radix Astragali (*Huang Qi*)
4 g	Radix Ledebouriellae (*Fang Feng*)

HUANG QI GAN CAO TANG (Astragalus Liquorice Decoction)

80 g	Radix Astragali (*Huang Qi*)
32 g	Radix Glycyrrhizae (*Gan Cao*)

HUANG QI GUI ZHI WU WU TANG (Astragalus Cinnamomum Five Ingredients Decoction)

9 g	Radix Astragali Praeparatae (*Zhi Huang Qi*)
9 g	Radix Paeoniae Lactiflorae (*Shao Yao*)
9 g	Ramulus Cinnamomi Cassia (*Gui Zhi*)
18 g	Rhizoma Zingiberis Recens (*Sheng Jiang*)
12 pc	Fructus Zizyphi Jujubae (*Da Zao*)

HUANG QI SI WU TANG (Astragalus Four Ingredients Decoction)

Radix Astragali (*Huang Qi*)
Radix Ginseng (*Ren Shen*)
Rhizoma Atractylodis Macrocephalae (*Bai Zhu*)
Sclerotium Poria Cocos (*Fu Ling*)
Radix Paeoniae Lactiflorae (*Shao Yao*)
Radix Glycyrrhizae Uralensis (*Gan Cao*)
Rhizoma Zingiberis Recens (*Sheng Jiang*)
Radix Angelicae Sinensis (*Dang Gui*)
Radix Rehmanniae Glutinosae (*Sheng Di Huang*)
Radix Ligustici Wallichii (*Chuan Xiong*)
Flos Lonicerae Japonicae (*Jin Yin Hua*)

HUANG QI TAO HONG TANG (Astragalus Persica Carthamus Decoction)

320 g	Radix Astragali (*Huang Qi*)
12 g	Semen Persicae (*Tao Ren*)
12 g	Flos Carthami (*Hong Hua*)
8 g	Radix Astragali (*Huang Qi*)

8 g   Semen Persicae (*Tao Ren*)
8 g   Flos Carthami (*Hong Hua*)

HUI YAN ZHU YU TANG (Anti-Stasis Epiglottis Decoction)

15 g   Semen Persicae (*Tao Ren*)
15 g   Flos Carthami (*Hong Hua*)
9 g   Radix Glycyrrhizae Uralensis (*Gan Cao*)
12 g   Radix Platycodi (*Jie Geng*)
12 g   Rhizoma Rehmanniae (*Sheng Di*)
6 g   Radix Angelicae (*Dang Gui*)
3 g   Radix Scrophularia (*Xuan Shen*)
3 g   Radix Bupleuri (*Chai Hu*)
6 g   Fructus Citri Aurantii (*Zhi Ke*)
6 g   Radix Paeoniae Rubrae (*Chi Shao*)

HUO LUO XIAO LING DAN (Wondrous Pill to Invigorate the Channels)

15 g   Radix Angelicae Sinensis (*Dang Gui*)
15 g   Radix Salviae Miltiorrhizae (*Dan Shen*)
15 g   Resina Olibani (*Ru Xiang*)
15 g   Myrrha (*Mo Yao*)

HUO XIANG ZHENG QI SAN (Patchouli *Qi* Rectifying Powder)

90 g   Herba Agastachis (*Huo Xiang*)
30 g   Folium Perillae (*Zi Su Ye*)
30 g   Radix Angelicae Dahuricae (*Bai Zhi*)
30 g   Pericarpium Arecae (*Da Fu Pi*)
30 g   Sclerotium Poriae (*Fu Ling*) Cocos
60 g   Rhizoma Atractylodis Macrocephalae (*Bai Zhu*)
60 g   Rhizoma Pinelliae Praeparatae (*Zhi Ban Xia*)
60 g   Pericarpium Citri Reticulatae (*Chen Pi*)

JI MING SAN (Cock Crow Powder)

30 g   Radix et Rhizoma Rhei (*Da Huang*)
9 g   Radix Angelicae Sinensis (*Dang Gui*)
27 pc   Semen Persicae (*Tao Ren*)

JI QIU HUI YANG TANG (Emergency *Yang* Recovery Decoction)

32 g   Radix Aconiti Lateralis Praeparatae (*Fu Zi*)
16 g   Rhizoma Zingiberis (*Gan Jiang*)

16 g   Rhizoma Atractylodis Macrocephalae (*Bai Zhu*)
12 g   Radix Glycyrrhizae Uralensis (*Gan Cao*)
8 g   Semen Persica (*Tao Ren*)
8 g   Radix Ginseng (*Ren Shen*)
8 g   Flos Carthami (*Hong Hua*)

JIA JI HUA TU TANG (Peony Liquorice Decoction)

Radix Glycyrrhizae Uralensis (*Gan Cao*)
Radix Paeoniae Lactiflorae (*Bai Shao*)

JIE DU HUO XUE TANG (Detoxifying, Blood Invigorating Decoction)

8 g   Fructus Forsythiae (*Lian Qiao*)
8 g   Radix Puerariae (*Ge Gen*)
12 g   Radix Bupleuri (*Chai Hu*)
8 g   Radix Angelicae Sinensis (*Dang Gui*)
20 g   Radix Rehmanniae (*Sheng Di Huang*)
12 g   Radix Paeoniae Rubrae (*Chi Shao*)
32 g   Semen Persicae (*Tao Ren*)
20 g   Flos Carthami (*Hong Hua*)
4 g   Fructus Citri Aurantii (*Zhi Ke*)
8 g   Radix Glycyrrhizae (*Gan Cao*)

JIU QI WAN (Nine *Qi* Pill)

9 g   Rhizoma Curcumae Longae (*Jiang Huang*)
12 g   Rhizoma Cyperi Rotundi (*Xiang Fu*)
6 g   Radix Glycyrrhizae Uralensis (*Gan Cao*)

KAI GU SAN (Bone Expanding Powder)

See *Gu Kai Gu San*

KE BAO LI SU TANG (Guaranteed Resuscitation Decoction)

60 g   Radix Astragali (*Huang Qi*)
12 g   Radix Ginseng (*Ren Shen*)
8 g   Rhizoma Atractylodis Macrocephalae (*Bai Zhu*)
8 g   Radix Glycyrrhizae Uralensis (*Gan Cao*)
8 g   Radix Angelicae Sinensis (*Dang Gui*)
8 g   Radix Paeoniae Lactiflorae (*Shao Yao*)
12 g   Semen Zizyphi Spinosae (*Suan Zao Ren*)
8 g   Fructus Lycii (*Gou Qi Zi*)

4 g   Fructus Psoralea (*Bu Gu Zhi*)
4 g   Fructus Corni Officinalis (*Shan Zhu Yu*)

LIU WEI DI HUANG WAN (Rehmannia Six Pill)

24 g   Radix Rehmanniae Praeparatae (*Shu Di Huang*)
12 g   Fructus Corni (*Shan Zhu Yu*)
12 g   Rhizoma Dioscoreae (*Shan Yao*)
9 g   Rhizoma Alismatis (*Ze Xie*)
9 g   Cortex Moutan (*Mu Dan Pi*)
9 g   Sclerotium Poria (*Fu Ling*) Cocos

LONG MA ZI LAI DAN (Dragon Horse Pastilles)

320 g Semen Strychni (*Ma Qian Zi*)
8 pc   Lumbricus (*Di Long*)
600 ml sesame oil (*Xiang You*)

Quoting Wang Qing-Ren:

Pour the sesame oil in pan and heat it until it boils. Now fry the nux-vomica seeds until they make loud cracking noises.[1] If you take a seed, open the gap on its side with a knife and split it into two halves, the inner part should look reddish-purple when done. After that it should be ground into a fine powder and mixed with the pulverized Lumbricus. Then, with a little liquid it is formed into pills the size of green soy beans (mung beans).

MI CONG ZHU DAN TANG (Onion, Honey and Pig's Gallbladder Decoction)

120–132 g   Mel (*Bai Mi*)
4 pc   Alium Fistulosum (*Cong Tou*)
~300 ml   rice wine (*Huang Jiu*)
One pig's gallbladder (*Zhu Dan*)

---

[1] Today Nux-vomica seeds are heated together with sand in a pan in order to eliminate their toxicity. This process is explained on page 13 of Philippe Sionneau's 'Pao Zhi' (see Appendix 7). Whilst at university, I also prepared Nux-vomica seeds in this way, but noticed that only top quality seeds produce the cracking noise described by Wang. If they are moist or even mouldy, they will char slowly without a sound. However today, preparation of raw medicinals is not incumbent on doctors but on pharmacologists and drug experts. This is to maintain standards in potency and prevent poisoning if prepared by non-professionals. Therefore, I strongly discourage any layperson from carrying out the preparation method described above.

MU ER SAN (Wood Fungus Powder)

40 g   Auricularia Auricula (*Mu Er*) or Tremella Fuciformis (*Bai Mu Er*)
20 g   granulated sugar (*Bing Tang*)

NAO SHA WAN (Sal Ammoniac Pill)

8 g   Sal Ammoniac, pulverized (*Nao Sha*)
~100 seeds of Fructus Gleditsiae (*Zao Jiao*)
~600 ml vinegar (*Gan Cu*)

The first two ingredients are added to the vinegar to steep for three days. Subsequently, the mixture is boiled in an earthenware pot until dry. The ammonium chloride crystals on the bottom of the pot are turned over with a spatula and are scooped on top of the Gleditsia seeds until everything is dried (on a low flame). It can also be dried slowly close to the hob.

NIU XI SAN (Achyranthis Powder)

30 g   Radix Achyranthis Bidentatae (*Niu Xi*)
23 g   Radix Paeoniae Rubrae (*Chi Shao*)
23 g   Semen Persicae (*Tao Ren*)
23 g   Ramulus Cinnamomi Cassia (*Gui Zhi*)
23 g   Rhizoma Corydalis Yanhusuo (*Yuan Hu*)
23 g   Radix Angelicae Sinensis (*Dang Gui*)
23 g   Cortex Moutan Radicis (*Mu Dan Pi*)
23 g   Radix Aucklandiae Lappae (*Mu Xiang*)

Take in small portions (3 g) with warm rice wine.

QI LI SAN (Seven Li Powder)

30 g   Sanguis Draconis (*Xue Jie*)
5 g   Flos Carthami (*Hong Hua*)
5 g   Resina Olibani (*Ru Xiang*)
5 g   Myrrha (*Mo Yao*)
0.4 g Moschus (*She Xiang*)
0.4 g Borneolum (*Bing Pian*)
7.5 g Catechu (*Er Cha*)
4 g   Cinnabaris (*Zhu Sha*) (obsolete in modern formulas)

QIN JIAO SAN (Gentiana Powder)

30 g   Radix Gentianae Qinjiao (*Qin Jiao*)
30 g   Radix Glycyrrhizae Uralensis (*Gan Cao*)
15 g   Herba Menthae Haplocalycis (*Bo He*)

QING RE XIAO DU SAN (Cooling Detoxifying Powder)

Dosage for children:

1.5 g	Rhizoma Coptidis (*Huang Lian*)
1.5 g	Fructus Gardeniae Jasminoidis (*Zhi Zi*)
1.5 g	Fructus Forsythia (*Lian Qiao*)
1.5 g	Radix Angelicae Sinensis (*Dang Gui*)
1.8 g	Radix Ligustici Wallichii (*Chuan Xiong*)
1.8 g	Radix Paeoniae Lactiflorae (*Shao Yao*)
1.8 g	Radix Rehmannia Glutinosae (*Sheng Di Huang*)
0.5 g	Radix Glycyrrhizae Uralensis (*Gan Cao*)
3 g	Flos Lonicerae Japonicae (*Jin Yin Hua*)

REN SHEN XIE FEI TANG (Ginseng Lung Relieving Decoction)

Radix Ginseng (*Ren Shen*)
Radix Scutellariae Baicalensis (*Huang Qin*)
Fructus Gardenia Jasmin. (*Zhi Zi*)
Fructus Citri Aurantii (*Zhi Ke*)
Herba Menthae Haplocalycis (*Bo He*)
Radix Glycyrrhizae Uralensis (*Gan Cao*)
Fructus Forsythiae (*Lian Qiao*)
Semen Pruni Armeniacae (*Xing Ren*)
Cortex Mori Albae Radicis (*Sang Bai Pi*)
Radix et Rhizoma Rhei (*Da Huang*)
Radix Platycodi Grandiflori (*Jie Geng*)
(No dosage recommendations could be found.)

SAN BI TANG (Three Bi Decoction)

3 g	Radix Ginseng (*Ren Shen*)
3 g	Radix Astragali (*Huang Qi*)
3 g	Rhizoma Atractylodis Macrocephalae (*Bai Zhu*)
3 g	Radix Angelicae Sinensis (*Dang Gui*)
3 g	Radix Ligustici Wallichii (*Chuan Xiong*)
3 g	Radix Paeoniae Lactiflorae (*Shao Yao*)
3 g	Sclerotium Poriae Cocos (*Fu Ling*)
1.5 g	Radix Glycyrrhizae Uralensis (*Gan Cao*)
1.5 g	Ramulus Cinnamomi Cassia (*Gui Zhi*)
1.5 g	Radix Stephaniae Tetrandrae (*Fang Ji*)
1.5 g	Radix Ledebouriellae Divaticata (*Fang Feng*)
1.5 g	Radix Aconiti (*Wu Tou*)
1.5 g	Herba et Radix Asari (*Xi Xin*)
3 slices	Rhizoma Zingiberis Recens (*Sheng Jiang*)
2 pc	Fructus Zizyphi Jujubae (*Da Zao*)

SHAO FU ZHU YU TANG (Anti-Stasis Lower Abdomen Decoction)

3 g	Fructus Foeniculi (*Xiao Hui Xiang*)
6 g	Rhizoma Zingiberis (*Gan Jiang*)
9 g	Rhizoma Corydalis (*Yan Hu Suo*)
6 g	Myrrha (*Mo Yao*)
6 g	Radix Angelicae Sinensis (*Dang Gui*)
6 g	Radix Ligustici Wallichii (*Chuan Xiong*)
3 g	Cortex Cinnamomi (*Rou Gui*) Cassiae
9 g	Radix Paeoniae Rubrae (*Chi Shao*)
9 g	Pollen Typhae (*Pu Huang*)
9 g	Faeces Trogopteri (*Wu Ling Zhi*)

SHEN FU TANG (Ginseng Aconite Decoction)

12 g	Radix Ginseng (*Ren Shen*)
9 g	Radix Aconiti Lateralis Praeparatae (*Fu Zi*)

SHEN SU YIN (Codonopsis and Perilla Drink)

7.5 g	Radix Ginseng (*Ren Shen*)
7.5 g	Folium Perillae Frutescentis (*Zi Su Ye*)
7.5 g	Radix Puerariae (*Ge Gen*)
7.5 g	Radix Peucedani (*Qian Hu*)
7.5 g	Rhizoma Pinelliae Ternatae (*Ban Xia*)
7.5 g	Sclerotium Poriae Cocos (*Fu Ling*)
5 g	Pericarpium Citri Reticulatae (*Chen Pi*)
5 g	Radix Glycyrrhizae Uralensis (*Gan Cao*)
5 g	Radix Platycodi Grandiflori (*Jie Geng*)
5 g	Fructus Citri Aurantii (*Zhi Ke*)
5 g	Radix Aucklandiae Lappae (*Mu Xiang*)
3 pc	Fructus Zizyphi Jujubae (*Da Zao*)
3 slices	Rhizoma Zingiberis Recens (*Sheng Jiang*)

SHEN TONG ZHU YU TANG (Anti-Stasis Pain Decoction)

4 g	Radix Gentiana Qinjiao (*Qin Jiao*)
8 g	Radix Ligustici Wallichii (*Chuan Xiong*)
12 g	Semen Persicae (*Tao Ren*)
12 g	Flos Carthami (*Hong Hua*)
8 g	Radix Glycyrrhizae (*Gan Cao*)
4 g	Radix Notopterygii (*Qiang Huo*)
8 g	Myrrha (*Mo Yao*)
12 g	Radix Angelicae Sinensis (*Dang Gui*)
8 g	Faeces Trogopteri (*Wu Ling Zhi*)
4 g	Rhizoma Cyperi (*Xiang Fu*)
12 g	Radix Achyrantis (*Niu Xi*)
8 g	Lumbricus (*Di Long*)

SHEN ZHUO TANG (Blocked Kidney Decoction)

6g	Radix Glycyrrhizae Uralensis (*Gan Cao*)
6g	Rhizoma Atractylodis Macrocephalae (*Bai Zhu*)
12g	Sclerotium Poriae Cocos (*Fu Ling*)
12g	Rhizoma Zingiberis (*Gan Jiang*)

SHENG DI HUANG TANG (Shen's Rehmannia Decoction)

6g	Rhizoma Rehmanniae Exsiccatae (*Gan Di Huang*)
1.5g	Lacca Sinica Exsiccatae (*Gan Qi*)
~30ml	*Ou Zhi* (lotus root juice)
~30ml	*Shen Lan Ye* (juice of folium Isatidis)
3pc	Tabanus (*Mang Chong*)
2pc	Hirudo (*Shui Zhi*)
3g	Radix et Rhizoma Rhei (*Da Huang*)
1.5g	Semen Persicae (*Tao Ren*)

SHENG HUA TANG (Generate Change Decoction)

25g	Radix Angelicae Sinensis (*Dang Gui*)
9g	Radix Ligustici Wallichii (*Chuan Xiong*)
6g	Semen Persicae (*Tao Ren*)
2g	Rhizoma Zingiberis (*Gan Jiang*)
2g	Radix Glycyrrhizae Praeparatae (*Zhi Gan Cao*)

SHENG JIANG XIE XIN TANG (Zingiber Heart Relief Decoction)

12g	Rhizoma Zingiberis Recens (*Sheng Jiang*)
9g	Radix Glycyrrhizae Uralensis (*Gan Cao*)
9g	Radix Ginseng (*Ren Shen*)
3g	Rhizoma Zingiberis (*Gan Jiang*)
9g	Radix Scutellaria Baicalensis (*Huang Qin*)
6g	Rhizoma Pinelliae Ternatae (*Ban Xia*)
3g	Rhizoma Coptidis (*Huang Lian*)
2pc	Fructus Zizyphi Jujubae (*Da Zao*)

SHENG MAI TANG (Pulse Generating Powder)

10g	Radix Ginseng (*Ren Shen*)
15g	Radix Ophiopogonis (*Mai Dong*)
6g	Fructus Schisandrae (*Wu Wei Zi*)

SHENG YU TANG (Wise Healing Decoction)

6g	Radix Rehmanniae Recens (*Sheng Di Huang*)
6g	Radix Rehmannia Praeparatae (*Shu Di Huang*)
6g	Radix Astragali (*Huang Qi*)
6g	Radix Ginseng (*Ren Shen*)
3g	Radix Angelicae Sinensis (*Dang Gui*)
3g	Radix Ligustici Wallichii (*Chuan Xiong*)

SHI XIAO SAN (Sudden Smile Powder)

Pollen Typhae (*Pu Huang*)
Faeces Trogopteri (*Wu Ling Zhi*)

To be mixed in equal parts and pulverized, 6g per preparation.

SHOU NIAN WAN (Hand-made Pill)

6g	Rhizoma Corydalis (*Yan Hu Suo*)
6g	Faeces Trogopteri (*Wu Ling Zhi*)
6g	Fructus Tsaoko (*Cao Guo*)
6g	Myrrha (*Mo Yao*)

SHU JING HUO XUE TANG (Relaxing the Vessels Decoction)

5g	Radix Angelicae Sinensis (*Dang Gui*)
4g	Radix Paeoniae Lactiflorae (*Bai Shao*)
4g	Radix Rehmanniae (*Sheng Di Huang*)
3g	Radix Ligustici Wallichii (*Chuan Xiong*)
4g	Semen Persicae (*Tao Ren*)
3g	Sclerotium Poria Cocos (*Fu Ling*)
4g	Rhizoma Atractylodis (*Cang Zhu*)
4g	Pericarpium Citri Reticulatae (*Chen Pi*)
3g	Rhizoma et Radix Notopterygii (*Qiang Huo*)
3g	Radix Angelicae Dahuricae (*Bai Zhi*)
4g	Radix Clematidis (*Wei Ling Xian*)
3g	Radix Stephaniae Tetrandrae (*Fang Ji*)
3g	Radix Ledebouriellae (*Fang Feng*)
3g	Radix Gentianae (*Long Dan Cao*)
4g	Radix Achyranthis Bidentatae (*Niu Xi*)
2g	Radix Glycyrrhizae Uralensis (*Gan Cao*)

SI NI SAN (Cold Limbs Powder)

Radix Bupleuri (*Chai Hu*)
Radix Paeoniae Albae (*Bai Shao*)

Fructus Citri Aurantii Immaturus (*Zhi Shi*)
Radix Glycyrrhizae Praeparatae (*Zhi Gan Cao*)

To be mixed in equal parts and pulverized, up to 12 g per administration.

SI NI TANG (Collapse Decoction)

12 g	Radix Glycyrrhizae Praeparatae (*Zhi Gan Cao*)
9 g	Rhizoma Zingiberis (*Gan Jiang*)
9 g	Radix Aconiti Lateralis Praeparatae (*Fu Zi*)

SI SHEN WAN (Four Deities Pill)

200 g	Semen Myristicae (*Rou Dou Kou*)
400 g	Fructus Psoralae (*Bu Gu Zhi*)
200 g	Fructus Schisandrae (*Wu Wei Zi*)
100 g	Fructus Evodiae (*Wu Zhu Yu*)

To be mixed, pulverized and made into pills, with Chinese dates (200 g) and fresh ginger juice (200 g), 6–9 g twice daily.

SI WU TANG (Four Ingredients Decoction)

12 g	Radix Rehmanniae Praeparatae (*Shu Di Huang*)
9 g	Radix Angelicae Sinensis (*Dang Gui*)
6 g	Radix Ligustici Wallichii (*Chuan Xiong*)
9 g	Radix Paeoniae (*Shao Yao*)

SUI XIN DAN (Euphorbia Heart Pill)

9 g	Euphobia Gansui Pulveratae (*Gan Sui*)
~100 ml	Sanguis Suis (Pig's blood) (*Zhu Xue*)

TAO HONG SI WU TANG (Persica Carthamus Four Ingredients Decoction)

9 g	Radix Angelicae Sinensis (*Dang Gui*)
9 g	Semen Persicae (*Tao Ren*)
9 g	Radix Paeoniae Rubrae (*Chi Shao*)
6 g	Radix Ligustici Wallichii (*Chuan Xiong*)
6 g	Flos Carthami (*Hong Hua*)
15 g	Radix Rehmanniae (*Sheng Di Huang*)

TAO HONG CHENG QI TANG (Qi Rectifying Persica Carthamus Decoction)

12 g	Semen Persicae (*Tao Ren*)
12 g	Rhizoma et Radix Rhei (*Da Huang*)

6 g	Ramulus Cinnamomi Cassiae (*Gui Zhi*)
6 g	Mirabilitum Depurati (*Mang Xiao*)
6 g	Radix Glycyrrhizae Uralensis Praeparatae (*Zhi Gan Cao*)

TAO REN SHAO YAO TANG (Persica Paeonia Decoction)

7.5 g	Semen Persicae (*Tao Ren*)
6 g	Radix Paeoniae Lactiflorae (*Shao Yao*)
6 g	Radix Ligustici Wallichii (*Chuan Xiong*)
6 g	Radix Angelicae Sinensis (*Dang Gui*)
6 g	Ramulus Cinnamomi Cassiae (*Gui Zhi*)
6 g	Lacca Sinica Exsiccatae (*Gan Qi*)
6 g	Radix Glycyrrhizae Uralensis (*Gan Cao*)

TAO REN CHENG QI TANG (Qi Rectifying Persica Decoction)

15 pc	Semen Persicae (*Tao Ren*)
12 g	Radix et Rhizoma Rhei (*Da Huang*)
9 g	Radix Glycyrrhizae Uralensis (*Gan Cao*)
9 g	Ramulus Cinnamomi Cassiae (*Gui Zhi*)
9 g	Mirabillitum (*Mang Xiao*, to be added after boiling)

TING LI DA ZAO TANG (Lepidium and Jujube Decoction)

15 g	Semen Lepidii (*Ting Li Zi*)
5 pc	Fructus Zizyphi Jujubae (*Da Zao*)

TONG JING ZHU YU TANG (Anti-Stasis Exanthema Decoction)

32 g	Semen Persicae (*Tao Ren*)
16 g	Flos Carthami (*Hong Hua*)
12 g	Radix Paeoniae Rubrae (*Chi Shao*)
16 g	Squama Manitis (*Chuan Shan Jia*)
12 g	Spina Gleditsiae Sinensis (*Zao Jiao Ci*)
12 g	Fructus Forsythiae (*Lian Qiao*)
12 g	Lumbricus (*Di Long*)
4 g	Radix Bupleuri (*Chai Hu*)
0.3 g	Moschus (*She Xiang*)

TONG QI SAN (Qi Passage Powder)

38 g	Radix Bupleuri (*Chai Hu*)
38 g	Rhizoma Cyperi (*Xiang Fu*)
38 g	Radix Ligustici Wallichii (*Chuan Xiong*)

TONG QIAO HUO XUE TANG (Orifices Opening, Blood Invigorating Decoction)

3 g	Radix Paeoniae Rubrae (*Chi Shao Yao*)
3 g	Radix Ligustici Wallichii (*Chuan Xiong*)
9 g	Semen Persicae (*Tao Ren*)
9 g	Flos Carthami (*Hong Hua*)
3 g	Herba Allii Fistulosi (*Lao Cong*)
5 g	Fructus Ziziphi Jujubae (*Da Zao*)
0.15 g	Moschus (*She Xiang*)
250 ml	wine (*Huang Jiu*)

WEN JING TANG (Menses Warming Decoction)

9 g	Fructus Evodiae (*Wu Zhu Yu*)
6 g	Ramulus Cinnamomi Cassiae (*Gui Zhi*)
9 g	Radix Angelicae Sinensis (*Dang Gui*)
6 g	Radix Ligustici Wallichii (*Chuan Xiong*)
6 g	Radix Paeoniae Lactiflorae (*Bai Shao*)
6 g	Cortex Moutan Radicis (*Mu Dan Pi*)
9 g	Colla Corii Asini (*E Jiao*)
9 g	Radix Ophiopogonis (*Mai Men Dong*)
6 g	Radix Ginseng (*Ren Shen*)
6 g	Rhizoma Pinelliae (*Ban Xia*)
6 g	Radix Glycyrrhizae (*Gan Cao*)
6 g	Rhizoma Zingiberis Recens (*Sheng Jiang*)

WU JIN WAN (Black Gold Pill)

120 g	Rhizoma Cyperi (*Xiang Fu*)
15 g	Radix Aucklandiae Lappae (*Mu Xiang*)
15 g	Olibanum (*Ru Xiang*)
15 g	Myrrha (*Mo Yao*)
15 g	Ramulus Cinnamomi Cassia (*Gui Zhi*)
30 g	Faeces Trogopteri (*Wu Ling Zhi*)
30 g	Semen Persicae Pulveratae (*Tao Ren Fen*)
30 g	Rhizoma Corydalis (*Yan Hu Suo*)
30 g	Radix Linderae Strychnifoliae (*Wu Yao*)
30 g	Rhizoma Curcumae Ezhu (*E Zhu*)
90 g	Radix Angelicae Sinensis (*Dang Gui*)

To be made into a pill with 90 g of Lignum Sappan (*Su Mu*), 60 g Flos Carthami (*Hong Hua*), approximately 1 litre of black beans (*Hei Dou*). Take in small portions with warm rice wine.

WU ZI YAN ZONG WAN (Five Seeds Conceiving Pill)

24 g	Semen Cuscutae (*Tu Si Zi*)
24 g	Fructus Lycii (*Gou Qi Zi*)
3 g	Fructus Schisandrae (*Wu Wei Zi*)
12 g	Fructus Rubi Chingii (*Fu Pen Zi*)
6 g	Herba Plantaginis Majoris (*Che Qian Zi*)

XI FENG TANG (Wind Allaying Decoction)

9 g	Radix Achyranthis Bidentatae (*Huai Niu Xi*)
9 g	Haematitum (*Dai Zhe Shi*)
6 g	Os Draconis (*Long Gu*)
6 g	Concha Ostrae (*Mu Li*)
6 g	Plastrum Testudinis (*Gui Ban*)
6 g	Radix Scrophulariae Ningpoensis (*Xuan Shen*)
6 g	Tuber Asparagi Cochinchinensis (*Tian Men Dong*)
6 g	Radix Paeoniae Lactiflorae (*Bai Shao*)
3 g	Herba Artemisiae Yinchenhao (*Yin Chen Hao*)
3 g	Fructus Meliae Toosendan (*Chuan Lian Zi*)
3 g	Fructus Hordei Vulgaris Germinantus (*Mai Ya*)
3 g	Radix Glycyrrhizae Uralensis (*Gan Cao*)

XI HUANG WAN (Yellow Rhino Pills (without rhinoceros)

1 g	Calculus Bovis (*Niu Huang*)
4.5 g	Moschus (*She Xiang*)
30 g	Olibanum (*Ru Xiang*)
30 g	Myrrha (*Mo Yao*)
30 g	Millet (*Huang Mi*)

XI JIAO DI HUANG TANG (Rhino–Rehmannia Decoction)

10–30 g	Cornu Bufali (*Shui Niu Jiao*)
24 g	Radix Rehmanniae Glutinosae (*Sheng Di Huang*)
9 g	Radix Paeoniae (*Shao Yao*)
6 g	Cortex Moutan Radicis (*Mu Dan Pi*)

XIA YU XUE TANG (Anti-Stasis Ascites Decoction)

See *Gu Xia Yu Xue Tang*

XIA YU XUE TANG (Blood Stasis Purging Decoction)

9 g	Radix et Rhizoma Rhei (*Da Huang*)
9 g	Semen Persicae (*Tao Ren*)
9 g	Eupolyphaga (*Bie Chong*)

XIAN FANG HUO MING YIN (Invigorating Drink of the Immortals)

3 g	Radix Angelicae Dahuricae (*Bai Zhi*)
3 g	Bulbus Fritillariae Thunbergii (*Zhe Bei Mu*)
3 g	Radix Ledebouriellae Divaricata (*Fang Feng*)
3 g	Radix Paeoniae Rubrae (*Chi Shao*)
3 g	Radix Angelicae (*Sheng Gui Wei*)
3 g	Radix Glycyrrhizae Uralensis (*Gan Cao*)
3 g	Spina Gleditsiae Sinensis (*Zao Jiao Ci*)
3 g	Squama Manitis (*Chuan Shan Jia*)
3 g	Radix Trichosanthis (*Tian Hua Fen*)
3 g	Olibanum (*Ru Xiang*)
3 g	Myrrha (*Mo Yao*)
9 g	Flos Lonicerae Japonicae (*Jin Yin Hua*)
9 g	Pericarpium Citri Reticulatae (*Chen Pi*)

XIANG KE SAN (Cyperus Citrus Powder)

9 g	Rhizoma Cyperi (*Xiang Fu*)
6 g	Fructus Citri Aurantii (*Zhi Ke*)
3 g	Pericarpium Citri Reticulatae Viride (*Qing Pi*)
3 g	Pericarpium Citri Reticulatae (*Chen Pi*)
3 g	Radix Linderae Strychnifoliae (*Wu Yao*)
3 g	Radix Paeoniae Rubrae (*Chi Shao*)
3 g	Rhizoma Curcucmae Ezhu (*E Zhu*)
9 g	Radix Angelicae Sinensis (*Dang Gui Wei*)
1.5 g	Flos Carthami (*Hong Hua*)
1.5 g	Radix Glycyrrhizae Uralensis (*Gan Cao*)

XIAO CHAI HU TANG (Small Bupleurum Decoction)

12 g	Radix Bupleuri (*Chai Hu*)
9 g	Radix Scutellariae (*Huang Qin*)
9 g	Rhizoma Pinelliae (*Ban Xia*)
9 g	Radix Codonopsitis Pilosulae (*Dang Shen*)
6 g	Radix Glycyrrhizae Uralensis Praeparatae (*Zhi Gan Cao*)
9 g	Rhizoma Zingiberis Recens (*Sheng Jiang*)
4 pc	Fructus Zizyphi Jujubae (*Da Zao*)

XIAO HUI XIANG JIU (Fennel Tincture)

40 g	Semen Foeniculi (*Xiao Hui Xiang*)

Pulverize coarsely, then douse with approximately 300 ml of rice wine which has been briefly boiled up. Steep for 15 minutes, then filter and administer.

XIAO HUO LUO DAN (Small Channel Invigorating Pill)

180 g	Radix Aconiti Carmichaeli (*Chuan Wu*)
180 g	Radix Aconiti Kusnezoffii (*Cao Wu*)
180 g	Lumbricus (*Di Long*)
180 g	Rhizoma Arisaematis (*Tian Nan Xing*)
66 g	Olibanum (*Ru Xiang*)
66 g	Myrrha (*Mo Yao*)

To be made into pills of 3 g each, taken in portions.

XIAO TIAO JING SAN (Small Menses Regulating Decoction)

3 g	Myrrha (*Mo Yao*)
3 g	Succinium (*Hu Po*)
3 g	Ramulus Cinnamomi Cassiae (*Gui Zhi*)
3 g	Radix Paeoniae Lactiflorae (*Shao Yao*)
3 g	Radix Angelicae Sinensis (*Dang Gui*)
1.5 g	Radix Asarum (*Xi Xin*)
1.5 g	Moschus (*She Xiang*)

Take the powder with warm rice water.

XIAO XIAN XIONG TANG (Small Chest Relieving Decoction)

12 g	Rhizoma Pinelliae Ternatae (*Ban Xia*)
6 g	Rhizoma Coptidis (*Huang Lian*)
30 g	Fructus Trichosanthis (*Gua Luo Shi*)

XIAO YAO SAN (Easygoing Walk Powder)

9 g	Radix Bupleuri (*Chai Hu*)
9 g	Radix Angelicae Sinensis (*Dang Gui*)
9 g	Radix Paeoniae Lactiflorae (*Bai Shao*)
9 g	Rhizoma Atractylodis Macrocephalae (*Bai Zhu*)
9 g	Sclerotium Poriae Cocos (*Fu Ling*)
6 g	Radix Glycyrrhizae Uralensis (*Zhi Gan Cao*)
6 g	Rhizoma Zingiberis Officinalis Recens (*Sheng Jiang*)
3 g	Herba Menthae Haplocalycis (*Bo He*)

XIE XIN TANG (Heart Relieving Decoction)

9 g	Radix et Rhizoma Rhei (*Da Huang*)
6 g	Rhizoma Copitidis (*Huang Lian*)
9 g	Radix Scutellariae (*Huang Qin*)

XUAN FU DAI ZHE TANG (Hematite Inula Decoction)

9 g	Flos Inulae (*Xuan Fu Hua*)
6 g	Radix Ginseng (*Ren Shen*)
10 g	Rhizoma Zingiberis Recens (*Sheng Jiang*)
9 g	Haematitum (*Dai Zhe Shi*)
6 g	Radix Glycyrrhizae Uralensis (*Zhi Gan Cao*)
9 g	Rhizoma Pinelliae Ternatae (*Ban Xia*)
10 pc	Fructus Zizyphi Jujubae (*Da Zao*)

XUAN FU HUA TANG (Inula Decoction)

90 g	Flos Inulae (*Xuan Fu Hua*)
14 stalks of Allium (*Cong*)	
2–3 slices of Ginger (Zingiberis Recens, *Sheng Jiang*)	

XUE FU ZHU YU TANG (Anti-Stasis Chest Decoction)

9 g	Radix Angelicae Sinensis (*Dang Gui*)
9 g	Radix Rehmanniae (*Sheng Di Huang*)
12 g	Semen Persicae (*Tao Ren*)
9 g	Flos Carthami (*Hong Hua*)
6 g	Fructus Aurantii (*Zhi Qiao*)
6 g	Radix Paeoniae Rubra (*Chi Shao*)
3 g	Radix Bupleuri (*Chai Hu*)
3 g	Radix Glycyrrhizae (*Gan Cao*)
5 g	Radix Ligustici Wallichii (*Chuan Xiong*)
5 g	Radix Platycodi (*Jie Geng*)
9 g	Radix Achyranthis Bidentatae (*Niu Xi*)

YANG YIN TONG BI TANG (Yin Nourishing Bi Dissolving Decoction)

9 g	Semen Persicae (*Tao Ren*)
9 g	Flos Carthami (*Hong Hua*)
12 g	Radix Rehmanniae (*Sheng Di Huang*)
15 g	Semen Ligustri (*Nü Zhen Zi*)
30 g	Semen Trichosanthis (*Gua Lou*)
9 g	Radix Codonopsitis (*Dang Shen*)
9 g	Rhizoma Cyperi (*Xiang Fu*)
9 g	Tuber Ophiopogonis (*Mai Men Dong*)
9 g	Rhizoma Corydalis (*Yuan Hu*)

YONG QUAN SAN (Gushing Spring Powder)

9 g	Semen Vaccaria (*Wang Bu Liu Xing*)
4.5 g	Radix Trichosanthis (*Tian Hua Fen*)
9 g	Radix Glyzyrrhizae (*Gan Cao*)
4.5 g	Radix Angelicae (*Dang Gui*)
9 g	Squama Manitis (*Chuan Shan Jia*)

YOU GUI YIN (Kidney Yang Drink)

8–50 g	Radix Rehmanniae Praeparatae (*Shu Di Huang*)
3 g	Fructus Corni (*Shan Zhu Yu*)
6 g	Rhizoma Dioscoreae (*Shan Yao*)
6 g	Fructus Lycii (*Gou Qi Zi*)
5 g	Radix Glycyrrhizae (*Gan Cao*)
6 g	Cortex Eucommiae (*Du Zhong*)
4 g	Cortex Cinnamomi Cassiae (*Rou Gui*)
7 g	Radix Aconiti Lateralis Praeparatae (*Fu Zi*)

YU LONG GAO (Jade Dragon Paste, also called Shen Yu Gao)

16 g	Radix Ampelopsis Japonicae (*Bai Lian*)
16 g	Rhizoma Cimicifugae (*Sheng Ma*)
16 g	Radix Angelicae Sinensis (*Dang Gui*)
16 g	Fructus Forsythiae (*Lian Qiao*)
16 g	Flos Lonicerae (*Yin Hua*)
16 g	Squama Manitis (*Chuan Shan Jia*)
16 g	Radix Aconit. Car. (*Chuan Wu*)
16 g	Corium Aconiti Carmichaeli Elephantis (*Xiang Pi*)
6 g	Gummi Olibanum (*Ru Xiang*)
6 g	Myrrha (*Mo Yao*)
12 g	Calomelas (*Qing Fen*)
1 g	Borneol (*Bing Pian*)
1 g	Moschus (*She Xiang*)
80 g	white vinegar (*Bai Zhan*)
800 ml	sesame oil (*Xiang You*)

YU ZHU SAN (Poligonatum Odoratum Powder)

Si Wu Tang (Four Ingredients Decoction) plus *Yiao Wei Cheng Qi Tang* (Stomach Regulating *Qi* Rectifying Decoction)

12 g	Radix Rehmanniae Praeparatae (*Shu Di Huang*)
9 g	Radix Angelicae Sinensis (*Dang Gui*)
6 g	Radix Ligustici Wallichii (*Chuan Xiong*)
9 g	Radix Paeoniae (*Shao Yao*)

12 g   Radix et Rhizoma Rhei (*Da Huang*)
12 g   Mirabillitum (*Mang Xiao*)
6 g   Radix Glycyrrhizae Uralensis (*Gan Cao*)

ZHEN WU TANG (True Warrior Decoction)

9 g   Radix Paeoniae (*Shao Yao*)
9 g   Rhizoma Zingiberis Recens (*Sheng Jiang*)
6 g   Rhizoma Atractylodis Macrocephalae (*Bai Zhu*)
9 g   Radix Aconiti Lateralis Praeparatae (*Fu Zi*)

ZHI SHI XIE BAI GUI ZHI TANG (Citrus Aurantium Allium Cinnamomum Decoction)

12 g   Fructus Citri Aurantii (*Zhi Ke*)
12 g   Cortex Magnoliae Officinalis (*Hou Po*)
9 g   Bulbus Allii Macrostemi (*Xie Bai*)
6 g   Ramulus Cinnamomi Cassiae (*Gui Zhi*)
12 g   Fructus Trichosanthis (*Gua Lou*)

ZHI TONG MO YAO SAN (Analgesic Myrrh Powder With Addition)

9 g   Myrrha (*Mo Yao*)
9 g   Sanguis Draconis (*Xue Jie*)
6 g   Radix et Rhizoma Rhei (*Da Huang*)
6 g   Mirabillitum (*Mang Xiao*)
9 g   Concha Haliotidis (*Shi Jue Ming*)

ZHI XIE TIAO ZHONG TANG (Anti-Diarrhoea Centre Regulating Decoction)

32 g   Radix Astragali (*Huang Qi*)
12 g   Radix Codonopitis (*Dang Shen*)

8 g   Radix Glycyrrhizae Uralensis (*Gan Cao*)
8 g   Radix Angelicae Sinensis (*Dang Gui*)
8 g   Radix Atractylodis Macrocephalae (*Bai Zhu*)
8 g   Rhizoma Paeoniae Albae (*Bai Shao*)
4 g   Radix Ligustici Wallichii (*Chuan Xiong*)
12 g   Flos Carthami (*Hong Hua*)
4 g   Radix Aconiti Lateralis Praeparata (*Fu Zi*)
2 g   Rhizoma Alpiniae Officinalis (*Gao Liang Jiang*)
2 g   Cortex Cinnamomi (*Guan Gui*)

ZHU WEI HE RONG TANG (Wei and Ying Strengthening Decoction)

80 g   Radix Astragali (*Huang Qi*)
8 g   Radix Glycyrrhizae Uralensis (*Gan Cao*)
8 g   Rhizoma Atractylodis Macrocephalae (*Bai Zhu*)
12 g   Radix Ginseng (*Ren Shen*)
8 g   Radix Paeoniae Lactiflorae (*Shao Yao*)
4 g   Radix Angelicae Sinensis (*Dang Gui*)
8 g   Semen Zizyphi Spinosae (*Suan Zao Ren*)
6 g   Semen Persicae (*Tao Ren*)
6 g   Flos Carthami (*Hong Hua*)

ZHU YANG ZHI YANG TANG (Anti-Itching Yang Tonifying Decoction)

40 g   Radix Astragali (*Huang Qi*)
8 g   Semen Persicae (*Tao Ren*)
8 g   Flos Carthami (*Hong Hua*)
4 g   Spina Gleditsiae Sinensis (*Zao Jiao Ci*)
4 g   Radix Paeoniae Rubrae (*Chi Shao*)
4 g   Squama Manitis (*Chuan Shan Jia*)

Appendix 6

Epilogue: Inspector White Coat

Do you know Inspector White Coat? No? He is the investigator, the sleuth, the criminologist inside every one of us. Whenever you have encountered some unknown disease, and you have felt challenged to find all the relevant literature and information on it, to track the disease down, to investigate all suspicious facts and to finally face it and say: 'There it is, I've got it, the culprit is evident and that's how to arrest him!' Well, that's Inspector White Coat in you. Let's follow him on one of his exciting cases.

Inspector White Coat is called to the hospital to investigate three alleged murders. A thrombotic apoplexy, an ischemic myocardial infarction and a liver carcinoma following viral hepatitis. At first there was no apparent connection; however, the laboratory's medical assistant was able to provide a clue, according to which all three cases were sought out by the same visitor, who had previously been observed sneaking about the hospital. The night warden also reported that this chap would show up in the evening hours especially; at night he would sneak about the hospital corridors against regulations.

Inspector White Coat started his investigations right away, asked a few questions and then suddenly he spotted someone in dark red clothing disappearing round a corner. He examined the list of visitors of the three victims: someone had signed up for apoplexy and infarction, someone described by the nurse as a phlegmatic guy in a yellow suit, a certain Mr A Sclerosis. For a long time this chap had been wanted for his criminal

activities. When he and the chap in the red clothing show up you know they're up to no good. For carcinoma there was another signature, reading H Viscosity. The laboratory's medical assistant recalled his name, too.

White Coat traced these clues but they only proved to be false leads: the Viscosity Brothers were part of a big family, and they all had an alibi. The oldest of the brothers, whose name was Plasma, showed the Inspector the door, saying: 'You can come back when you've found something, there's no one called Hyper living here.'

When White Coat returned home to his mother Mel – a short form of the old-fashioned name Mellitus – she told him of a nice young man in purple clothing who had come for a visit. However, after he had gone her leg suddenly started to turn black. Inspector White Coat was alarmed, because it looked like gangrene. He asked her whether there had been anything unusual about the visitor. 'He moved very slowly and wanted to poke around the whole house, but I did not allow that of course,' said Mel. At that moment, White Coat's baby sister Mense came in holding her tummy in pain. 'Well, what's the matter?' White Coat and his mother asked. 'Oh, don't worry, it's just that a friend of mine called Stasis always used to visit me once a month, but today he hurt me, I don't know why. It's a pain as if someone stabbed me with a knife. . . .'

After they had thought it over for a while, it became obvious that the chap who had visited Mel was the same man who had given Mense this pain.

White Coat concluded: 'I see, now that I am hard on his heels, that this scoundrel is threatening my family!'

But White Coat had an idea: he drove back to the hospital and began systematically to ask everyone about the ominous visitor. He had already found some clues in cardiology, neurology and oncology anyway, but then he went on to gynaecology, traumatology, dermatology and immunology; even on the locked ward he found entries in the guestbook. He added two and two together and in conclusion came up with the following description: the criminal, known as either Stasis or Viscosity, used many masks; he always wore purple or dark red clothing, moved very slowly and sometimes showed up with shady characters like Slerosis or Rheuma. White coat hung up this rather paltry 'Wanted' poster, and he was lucky: a nurse from the urogenital department on her way home had seen him run off over the bridge into China Town.

The old guard at the bridge, Ragune, confirmed the nurse's observation: 'That's right, this gentleman crosses this bridge every day; maybe he's visiting someone in China Town.' White Coat crossed over and enquired for a man answering the suspect's description in the small grocery stores, but to no avail. 'Many people go in and out of here every day, how are you supposed to spot anyone?' All of a sudden, as he was standing in front of one of the impressive Chinese pharmacies, where there was a good smell of herbs and any number of little drawers inside, he had an idea: 'Why not?' he wondered. 'A person who goes into hospitals might also go into pharmacies.'

White Coat delivered his usual description of the suspect, but this was greeted by the unexpected laughter of the old pharmacist: 'That chap goes everywhere, except to our place.'

'You *know* him then?'

'Indeed. His name is *Yu Xue*, or the other way round *Xue Yu*, an ancient demon who has been making trouble in China for over 2000 years.' White Coat smiled to himself about the Chinaman's superstition.

'And why does he never come here?'

'Because here we have the only thing that scares him off: herbs and acupuncture.'

'May I have a few samples of these herbs?'

'Well, yes . . . why not? How about haematite, mastix and myrrh?[1]'

'What? Look, I'm not an exorcist. Don't you have any proper herbs?'

'I surely do. Whitethorn fruits, red peony leaves and vaccaria seeds.[2]'

'Yes, yes, I can get that in any park around here. I was thinking of something more oriental.'

'Certainly, here you are, Mister, that's saffron from Tibet, peach kernels from Persia and verbena from Eastern France.[3]'

'Oh,' said White Coat, disappointed. 'I had expected something of a more exotic nature.'

'No problem at all. You can gladly have some earthworms, cockroaches and leeches.[4] These help a lot in removing obstructions from the vessels.'

'Ahem, I'd rather take the herbs then. . . . The peach kernels, you know?'

'Or why not try scorpions, centipedes[5] and. . . .'

'Don't bother! I will take the saffron and peaches and the rest. Could you wrap them up for me?'

The old pharmacist shrugged his shoulders. 'Well, as you please. . . .'

'What's the meaning of yüü sh-ee-ye anyway?'

'I'm sorry?'

'Well you just said his name: yüü sh-ee-ye or sh-ee-ye yüü?'

The Chinaman gave a wide (but polite) grin: 'Ah, you mean *Yu Xue*?' In your language, that's depression of Blood or Blood stasis.'

'Blood . . . stasis . . . hmm . . .' White Coat pondered.

Afterwards, White Coat came back several times to get advice and medicinals from the Chinese pharmacy (rumour has it he got leeches as well . . .). He gave them to his mother and sister, who would never see the mysterious visitor come

---

[1] *Zi Ran Tong* (Pyritum), *Ru Xiang* (Pistatia Lentisus, DAB), *Mo Yao* (Myrrha).
[2] *Shan Zha* (Fructus Crategi), *Chi Shao* (Herba Paeoniae Rubrae), *Wang Bu Liu Xing* (Semen Vaccariae).
[3] *Hong Hua* (Flos Carhami), *Tao Ren* (Semen Persicae), *Ma Bian Cao* (Herba Verbenae Offic inalis).
[4] *Di Long* (Lumbricus), *Tu Bie Chong* (Eupolyphaga), *Shui Zhi* (Hirudo).
[5] *Quan Xie* (Scorpio), *Wu Gong* (Scolopendra).

to their house again. White Coat composed the following 'Wanted' poster according to the pharmacist's description.

Wanted – Blood Stasis, aka Hyper Viscosity, aka Blood depression, aka Yu Xue or Xue Yu for suspected serial murder and violence.

The culprit is characterized by his various masks; however, he prefers to wear purple or dark red and has a rough temper. He prefers showing up in the evening and at night and visits middle-aged and elderly citizens, but also women at certain times. What remains after his visit is a stabbing pain (always in the same spot) or dry skin or haemorrhaging. Of particular significance is his secret sign which can be found under the tongue. He prefers showing up in the company of other known criminals, such as A Sclerosis, T Rauma, C Hronic or the Chinese scoundrels known as Heat, Qi stagnation, Cold, Dryness and Phlegm. His crimes are committed in all places where there is Blood.

This 'Wanted' poster was also circulated in the hospital, and White Coat distributed the medicinals everywhere Stasis had shown up. In his free time he learned some acupuncture as well, although he had his doubts about this demon whom one could scare off with needles. After all, this chap was known to prefer haunting middle-aged and elderly people. And for White Coat was no teenager anymore.

At any rate, since those days he has been able to help a lot of people to get rid of this dangerous imp, who was under the gravest suspicion of murder. However, there are still many hospitals and private clinics where B Stasis is sneaking about and causing damage without being discovered. Therefore, the following advice is to be given to the population: 'Take care! You and your Blood should always keep moving, Blood Stasis lurks everywhere!'

For any information leading to the ultimate arrest of this criminal there is a reward offered by the International Nobel Prize Committee.

Appendix 7

Bibliography

Listed are only those publications that are either mentioned or used in this book, of which I have one copy each in my personal library. Due to the restricted space and scope further reading material cannot be mentioned here. To the interested reader I recommend the extensive bibliography and author index in Steven Clavey's book *Fluid Physiology and Pathology in Traditional Chinese Medicine*.

CHINESE LANGUAGE PUBLICATIONS

Publications about Chinese medical theories and clinical practice

Ge, Hong (Jin dynasty).
Bao Pu Zi Nei Pian.
Zhong Guo Chuantong Wen Hua Du Ben, Beijing, Beijing Yan Shan Press 1995

Ge, Hong (Jin dynasty).
Zhou Hou Lue Ji Fang.
Beijing, People's Health Publishing 1963, 1996

Guo, Ai-Chun (modern edn).
Huang Di Nei Jing Su Wen Yu Yi.
Beijing, People's Health Publishing 1992, 1995

Ha, Li-Tian, (today's China).
Fu Ke Yi An Yi Hua Xuan.
Tianjin, Science & Technology Press Tianjin 1982

Li, Dong-Yuan (Jin dynasty).
Pi Wei Lun and *Hou Fa Ji Yao* in *Dong Yuan Yi Ji.*
Beijing, People's Health Publishing 1993, 1996

Lin, Pei-Qin (Qing dynasty).
Lei Zheng Zhi Cai.
Beijing, People's Health Publishing 1988, 1996

Tang, Zong-Hai (Qing dynasty).
Xue Zheng Lun in *Zhuan Shi Cang Shu – Zi Ku – Yi Bu* vol 3.
Hainan, Hainan International News Press Center 1995

Wang, Ken-Tang (Ming dynasty).
Zheng Zhi Zhun Sheng vol 1 – *Za Bing.*
Shanghai, Science & Technology Press 1959, 1995

Wang, Qing-Ren (Qing dynasty).
Yi Lin Gai Cuo.
1. *Zhong Guo Yi Xue Da Cheng* vol 22. Shanghai, Science & Technology Press 1937, 1990, 1992
2. *Zhuan Shi Cang Shu – Zi Ku – Yi Bu*, vol 6. Hainan, Hainan International News Press Center, 1995
3. *Ming Ching Zhong Yi Lin Zheng Xiao Cong Shu.* Beijing, China, Chinese Medicine Press 1995

Ye, Tian Shi (Qing dynasty).
Lin Zheng Zhi Nan Yi An. Edited by Xu Ling Tai.
Shanghai, Shanghai People's Publishing 1959, 1976

Zhang, Lu (Qing dynasty).
Zhang Shi Yi Tong.
Beijing, China, Chinese Medicine Press 1995

Zhang, Xi-Chun (1860–1933).
Yi Xue Zhong Zhong Can Xi Lu.
Shijiazhuang, Hebei Science & Technology Press 1985, 1994

Zhang, Jie-Bin (Ming dynasty).
Jing Yue Chuan Shu.
Beijing, Chinese Medical Press 1994, 1996

Zhang, Zhong-Jing (Han dynasty).
Shang Han Za Bing Lun. Edited later by Wang Su-He in *Shang Han Lun* and *Jin Kui Yao Lüe.* These were used for the (traditional script) edition *Gao Deng Zhong Yi Yan Jiu Can Kao Cong Shu,* vols 11 and 12. Taipei, Zhi Yin Publishers 1990

Zhang, Zi-He (Jin dynasty).
Ru Men Shi Qin in *Zi-He Yi Ji.* Beijing, People's Health Publishing 1994, 1996

Zhu, Dan-Xi (Yuan dynasty).
Ge Zhi Yu Lun and *Ju Fang Fa Hui,* both in *Dan Xi Yi Ji.*
Beijing, People's Health Publishing 1993, 1995

Books on blood stasis

Chen, Ke-Ji, et al.
Huo Xue Hua Yu Yao Hua Xue Yao Li Yu Lin Chuang. Jinan, Shan Dong Science & Technology Press 1995

Nei, Long-Dao (Gunter Neeb).
Man Xing Xue Yu Zheng Tu Mo Xing De Zhi Lüe Ji Gong Neng Xing Tai Xue De Guan Cha Yan Jiu. (Experimental long-term study on chronic Blood stasis/hyperviscosity syndrome – pathomorphology and functional impairment of internal organs.) Doctoral thesis in Chinese. Tianjin, International College for Traditional Chinese Medicine and Pharmacology Tianjin, Research Division 1998

Zhong Guo Yi Yao Xue Yuan (Taiwan) and Zhong Gou Zhong Xi Yi Jie He Xue Hui (China).
Hai Xia Liang An: Huo Xue Hua Yu Yu Chuan Zheng Fang Yao Yan Jiu.
Beijing, Chinese Medicine & Pharmacy Technology Publishing 1994

Zhong Guo Zhong Xi Yi Jie He Xue Hui (Society for Integrated Chinese and Western Medicine), Huo Xue Hua YuYan Jiu Xue Hui (Society for Research of Blood invigorating and Blood stasis).
Huo Xue Hua Yu Yan Jiu.
Beijing, Chinese Medicine & Pharmacy Technology Publishing 1995

Books on Chinese medicinals

Li, Yi-Kui et al.
Zhong Yao vol 2 *Xian Dai Zhong Yi Yao Ying Yong Yu Yan Jiu Da Xi.*
Shanghai, Shanghai University of TCM Press 1995

Li, Shi-Zhen.
Ben Cao Gang Mu. In *Bai Hua Ben Cao Gang Mu* vols 1–3.
Beijing, Xue Yuan Press 1994

Shen Nong (attributed to).
Shen Nong Ben Cao Jing.
Beijing, Science & Technology Press 1996

Xu, Zheng-Hua et al.
Zhong Yao Xue vol 1–3 (Taiwan edition). *Gao Deng Zhong Yi Yan Jiu Can Kao Cong Shu* vols 14 and 15. Taipei, Zhi Yin Publishers 1991

Yin, Jian et al.
Zhong Yao Xian Dai Yan Jiu Yu Lin Chuang Ying Yong
vol 1. Beijing, Xue Yuan Press 1993, 1995, vol 2. Beijing, Chinese Medical Classical Works Press 1995

Yin, Jian et al.
Zhong Yi Yao Da Ci Dian vols 1–3.
Jiang Su New Medical College, Shanghai, Shanghai Science & Technology Press 1977, 1995

Zhang, Ben-Xiang et al.
Xian Dai Zhong Yao Yao Li Xue.
Tianjin, Science & Technology Press 1997

Other modern books

Nei, Long-Dao (Gunter Neeb).
Gu Jin Yi Xue Dui Bai He Bing Zhi Yan Jiu. In *Zhong Yi Chuan Tong Yi Yao Yan Jiu* vol 1, p. 94 ff. Beijing, Chinese Medical Classics Press 1997

Qin, Bo-Wei.
Qian Zhai Yi Xue Jiang Gao.
Shanghai, Shanghai Science & Technology Press 1964

Ren, Ying-Chiu.
Shang Han Lun Zheng Zhi Lei Quan.
Hong Kong, Hong Kong Won Yit Publishing 1980

Tang, Wen-Hua (ed).
Huo Xue Hua Yu Wen Xian Zhuan Ji (1949–1986).
Shanghai, University of Medical Science
Shanghai Publishing 1989

Wu, Yu-Xiang et al.
Shi Yong Zhong Yi Xue Ye Xue.
Shanghai, Shanghai College of TCM Press 1989

Wu, Min-Yu et al.
Yi Xue Mian Yi Xue vol 2.
Hefei, Chinese Science & Technology University
Press 1995

Wang, Wen-Jian et al.
Shi Yan Yan Jiu vol 20 *Xian Dai Zhong Yi Yao Ying
Yong Yu Yan Jiu Da Xi.*
Shanghai, Shanghai University of TCM Press
1995

Wang, Yong-Yan et al.
Lin Chuang Zhong Yi Nei Ke Xue vols 1–2.
Beijing, Beijing Press 1994

Yang, Si-Shu et al.
Zhong Yi Lin Chuang Da Chuan.
Beijing, Science & Technology Press 1991, 1994

Yang, Yu-Zhou.
Shang Han Lun Liu Zheng Bing Bian.
Beijing, People's Health Publishing 1991

Zhan, Jian-Fei et al.
Xian Dai Zhong Yi Nei Fen Mi Bing Xue.
Shanghai, Medical Science University Press
1994

Zong, Chuan-He (ed) et al.
Zhong Yi Fang Ji Tong Ze.
Hebei, Science and Technology Publishing 1995

German language publications

Bensky D, Barolet R.
*Chinesische Arzneimittelrezepte und
Behandlungsstrategien.*
Kötzting, Verlag für Ganzheitliche Medizin Dr.
Erich Wühr GmbH 1996

Maciocia G.
Die Grandlagen der Chinesischen Medizin.
Kötzting, Verlag für Ganzheitliche Medizin Dr.
Erich Wühr GmbH 1994

Maciocia G.
Die Praxis der Chinesischen Medizin.
Kötzting, Verlag für Ganzheitliche Medizin Dr.
Erich Wühr GmbH 1997

Maciociz G.
*Die Gynäkologie in der Praxis der Chinesischen
Medizin.*
Kötzting, Verlag für Ganzheitliche Medizin Dr.
Erich Wühr GmbH 2000

Nover A.
*Der Augenhintergrund – Untersuchungstechnik und
typische Befande.*
Stuttgart, Schattauer Verlag 1964, 1987

Paulus E, Ding, Yu-He.
*Handbuch der traditionellen Chinesischen
Heilpflanzen.*
Heidelberg, Haug Verlag 1987

Porkert M.
Klinische Chinesische Pharmakologie.
Heidelberg, Verlag für Medizin Fischer 1978

Porkert M.
*Die theoretischen Grandlagen der Chinesichen
Medizin.*
Stuttgart, S. Hirzel Verlag 1982

Porkert M.
Klassische Chinesische Rezeptur.
Zug, Acta Medicinae Sinensis 1984

Porkert M.
Neues Lehrbuch der Chinesischen Diagnostik.
Dinkelscherben, Phainon Editions & Media
GmbH 1993

Shang Xianmin, et al.
*Praktische Erfahrungen mit der Chinesischen
Arzneimitteltherapie.*
Kötzting, Verlag für Ganzheitliche Medizin Dr.
Erich Wühr GmbH 1993

Schnorrenberger CC.
*Lehrbuch der Chinesischen Medizin für westliche
Ärzte, Die theoretischen Grandlagen der
Chinesischen Akupunktur and Arzneiverordnung.*
Stuttgart, Hippokrates Verlag 1979, 1985

English language publications

Bensky D, Barolet R.
Chinese herbal medicine: formulas and strategies.
Seattle, Eastland Press 1990

Bensky D, Gamble A.
Chinese herbal medicine: materia medica,
Revised Edn.
Seattle, Eastland Press 1986, 1993

Chase C (translator), Zhang Ting Liang.
A Qin Bo-Wei anthology.
Brookline, Paradigm Publications 1997

Clavey S.
Fluid physiology and pathology in Traditional
Chinese Medicine.
Melbourne, Churchill Livingstone 1995

Ehrly AM.
Therapeutic hemorheology.
Berlin, Springer Verlag 1991

Kaptschuk TJ.
Chinese medicine: the web that has no
weaver.
London, Rider 1983, London, Random Century
Group 1991

Maciocia G.
The foundations of Chinese medicine.
London, Churchill Livingstone 1989

Maciocia G.
The practice of Chinese medicine.
London, Churchill Livingstone 1994

Maciocia G.
Obstetrics and gynecology in Chinese
medicine.
London, Churchill Livingstone 1998

Nanjing College of TCM.
Concise traditional Chinese gynecology.
Nanjing, Jingsu Science & Technology Publishing
House 1988

Needham J.
Science and civilization in China vols 2 and 4.
(Taiwan edition)
Taipei, Caves Books 1985/86, original edition
Cambridge University Press 1983

Shao, Nian-Fang.
The treatment of knotty diseases.
(*Zhong Guo Zhen Jiu Zhong Yao Zhi Liao Yi Nan
Bing Zheng.*)
Jinan, Shandong Science and Technology Press,
1990

Sionneau P.
Pao Zhi: an introduction to the use of processed
Chinese medicinals.
Boulder, Blue Poppy Press 1995

Unschuld PU.
Medicine in China – a history of ideas. (Taiwan
edition)
Taipei, Southern Materials Center 1987

Vangermeersch L, Sun PL.
Bi-syndromes or rheumatic disorders treated by
TCM.
Brussels, SATAS s.a. 1994

Ware JR (translator).
Alchemy, medicine, religion in the China of AD
320. (Taiwan edition)
Taipei, Southern Materials Center 1984, original
edition Cambridge, MA, MIT Press 1966

Yang, Shou-Zhong, Flaws B.
The heart and essence of Dan-Xi's methods of
treatment.
Boulder, Blue Poppy Press 1993

Zhou, Jinhuang et al.
Recent advances in Chinese herbal drugs –
actions and uses.
Beijing, Science Press and Brussels, SATAS
1991

French language publications

Granet M.
La pensée chinoise.
Paris, Albin Michel 1934

Maspero H.
Le taoïsme et les religions chinoises.
Paris, Gallimard 1971

Schipper K.
Le corps taoïste.
Paris, Librairie Arthème Fayard 1982

Dictionaries used for this book

An English-Chinese medical dictionary (*Ying Han Yi Xue Ci Dian*).
Shanghai, Science & Technology 1984, 1996

Chinese-English dictionary of Traditional Chinese Medicine. Ou Ming et al.
Hong Kong, Joint Printing Co 1988

Chinese – English manual of commonly-used drugs in Chinese medicine. Ou Ming et al.
Hong Kong, Joint Printing Co 1989

Dictionary of Traditional Chinese Medicine.
Hong Kong, Commercial Press, Joint Printing Co 1984

English – Chinese Chinese – English dictionary of Traditional Chinese Medicine.
Nigel Wiseman. Hunan, Science and Technology Press 1996

Er Ya Jin Zhu. Xu Chao Hua. Tianjin, Nan Kai University Press 1987, 1994

Gu Jin Yu Chang Yung Zi Zi Dian. Beijing, Commercial Publishing House 1993, 1995

Huang Di Nei Jing Ci Dian. Guo, Ai-Chun et al.
Tianjin, Science and Technology Publishers 1991, 1995

Shuo Wen Jie Zi Zhu. (Han dynasty)
Shanghai, Shanghai Publisher for Classical Works 1981, 1995

The Chinese – English medical dictionary. (*Han Ying Yi Xue Da Ci Dian*.)
Beijing, Ren Min Wei Sheng Chu Ban She 1987, 1993, 1996

Western names for Chinese disease classes. Hung-Yen Hsu.
Taiwan, Oriental Healing Arts Institute 1990

Yeong Dah concise medical dictionary. (*Yong Da Jian Ming Dao Min Yi Xue Ci Dian*.)
Taipei 1992

Zhongguo Yixuedacidian. Xie Guan et al. Beijing, Zhong Guo Zhong Yi Yao Chu Ban She 1994

Zhong Hua Ben Cao. Guo Jia Zhong Yi Yao Guan Li Ju.
Shanghai, Shanghai Ke Xue Ke Ji Chu Ban She 1998

Appendix 8

Eminent Chinese physicians and their works

The eminent famous physicians named in this book are listed here in alphabetical order. The family name, mentioned first in Chinese, is printed in capitals. After each title follows an entry of the modern reprint (if still available).

CHEN Shi-Duo (Qing dynasty)
Bian Zheng Lu, Beijing, People's Health Publishing 1989, 1996
A great theoretical book describing extensively all types of syndrome differentiation along with diagnosis and treatment.

CHEN Shi-Gong (Ming dynasty, 1555–1636)
Wai Ke Zheng Zong, Tianjin, Science & Technology Press 1993, 1996
One of the most influential books about surgery compiled by the author after 40 years of experience. It includes diagnosis, treatments, operations, case studies and formulas.

CHENG Guo-Peng (Qing dynasty)
Yin Xue Xin Wu, Chinese Beijing, Publisher for Chinese Medicine and Herbs 1996
Cheng Zhong-Ling brings together 30 years of clinical practice succinctly and practically in this valuable piece of work.

FU Qing-Zhu (Ming/Qing dynasty, 1607–1684)
Fu Qing-Zhu Nü Ke, Fu Qing-Zhu Nan Ke and *Bian Zheng Lu*
The Taoist Fu Shan was surely the most famous gynae-cologist in Chinese. He wrote so extensively that even
after his death his manuscripts were still being published, for example Bian Zheng Lu, Yu Shi Mi Lu *and* Dong Tian Ao Zhi, *edited and published by Chen Shi-Duo.*

GE Hong (Jin dynasty, 281–341)
Bao Pu Zi Nei Pian, Zhong Guo Chuantong Wen Hua Du Ben, Beijing, Beijing Yan Shan Press 1995
Taoist-medical book relating to Nei-Dan and Wai-Dan practices, dietetics and magic.
Zhou Hou Lue Ji Fang, Beijing, People's Health Publishing 1963, 1996
Simple formulas and commonly used medicinals. The first vaccination method was developed by Ge Hong.

GONG Yan-Shen (Ming dynasty)
Shou Shi Bao Yuan, Shenyang, Liao Ning Science & Technology Publishers 1997
The Taoist author to some extent founded TCM geriatrics and gerontology in his work. He emphasizes the preservation and strengthening of Yuan Qi, *similar to many other Taoist authors, and describes many syndromes and diseases and their treatment.*

HA Li-Tian (today's China)
Fu Ke Yi An Yi Hua Xuan, Tianjin, Science & Technology Press Tianjin 1982
An excellent piece of work for clinical practice by a doctor whose family has been practising Chinese medicine for generations.

HUA TUO (attributed to)
Zhong Zang Jing, Beijing, Hua Xia Publishers
Beijing 1995
This book, attributed to the legendary physician Hua Tuo, in fact comes from the period of the Six Kingdoms (4th–7th century). Apart from 49 articles about diagnosis and treatment it contains an exact analysis of disease signs from which a favourable or unfavourable prognosis can be derived.

HUANG-FU Mi (Han dynasty)
Zhen Jiu Jia Yi Jing (259 AD), Beijing, People's Health Publishing 1994, 1996
Taoist Huang-Fu Shi-An wrote this first detailed acupuncture monograph.

LI Dong-Yuan (Jin dynasty, 1180–1251)
Pi Wei Lun, *Yong Yao Fa Xiang* and *Hou Fa Ji Yao* in *Dong Yuan Yi Ji*, Beijing, People's Health Publishing 1993, 1996
These are the works of Li Gao, one of the four masters of the thirteenth century, founder of the 'School of Spleen and Stomach Tonification'. In the Yong Yao Fa Xiang, *medicinals were categorized according to the four qualities, i.e. lifting, sinking, descending and ascending.*

LI Shi-Zhen (Ming dynasty, 1518–1655)
Ben Cao Gang Mu in *Bai Hua Ben Cao Gang Mu*, vols 1–3, Beijing, Xue Yuan Press 1994
The monumental work of Li Yan-Wen, which was compiled over 30 years, partly with the aid of field studies, partly during his travels throughout China. Due to its authority, it has remained unrivalled for a long time.
Bin Hu Mai Xue Beijing, Xue Yuan Press 1997
The pulse classic, which has most forcefully shaped pulse diagnosis as it is practised today, and to this day is still in use, remaining almost unchanged. Li lists 27 pulse variations in this book.

LI Zong-Zi (Ming dynasty, 1588–1655)
Yi Zong Bi Du, Beijing, People's Health Publishing 1995, 1996
Li Shi-Cai combined his own experience with the knowledge of the early classics. He described medicinals, medical theories and several syndromes, to which he added the corresponding context from the 'Nei Jing', 'Shang Han Lun' and other texts.

LIN Pei-Qin (Qing dynasty)
Lei Zheng Zhi Cai (1851), Beijing, People's Health Publishing 1988, 1996
Outstanding expert in the classics who put his practical experience and case studies into writing.

QIN Bo-Wei (Qing dynasty until middle of 20th century.)
Qian Zhai Yi Xue Jiang Gao (collection of lectures), Shanghai, Shanghai Science & Technology Publishers 1964
The most famous physician of the first part of the twentieth century, who made contributions to the development of modern TCM up to the 1960s. He passed on his extensive knowledge to numerous students in Chinese universities.

SHEN NONG (attributed to)
Shen Nong Ben Cao Jing, Beijing, Science & Technology Press 1996
The oldest herbal medicine classic dating from the first century AD listing 365 medicinals that are categorized into three classes (valuable, common and less valuable). It assessed the efficacy and mildness of the medicinals.

SUN Si-Miao (Tang dynasty, 581–682)
Qian Jin Fang, Beijing, Hua Xia Press 1994
The famous Taoist doctor of the Tang dynasty who is said to have lived to the age of 141 years. In this book he compiled the entire medical and dietary knowledge of his time in two volumes. The second volume was started when he was in his nineties. The Taoist influence is very evident.
Yin Hai Jing Wei, Shanghai, Gu Ji Publishers 1991, 1994
Although this important work about ophthalmology is attributed to Sun Si-Mo, it probably stems from Gao Bao-Wei, thirteenth century.

TANG Zong-Hai (Qing dynasty, 1862–1918)
Xue Zheng Lun, Beijing, Chinese Publisher for Chinese Medicine and Herbs 1996
Diagnosis and therapy of all kinds of haemorrhagic illnesses including 170 diseases. Tang Rong-Chuan developed a new area in TCM.

WANG Ken-Tang (Ming dynasty, 1549–1613)
Zheng Zhi Zhun Sheng vols 1–6, Shanghai, Science & Technology Press 1959, 1995

A comprehensive work including a good deal of personal experience and detailed descriptions in 6 volumes, covering various internal diseases, Shang Han, formulas, traumatology, paediatrics and gynaecology.

WANG Qing-Ren (Qing dynasty, 1768–1831)
Yi Lin Gai Cuo
1. *Zhong Guo Yi Xue Da Cheng*, vol 22, Shanghai, Science & Technology Press 1937, 1990, 1992
2. *Zhuan Shi Cang Shu – Zi Ku – Yi Bu*, vol 6, Hainan, Hainan International. News Press Center, 1995
3. *Ming Ching Zhong Yi Lin Zheng Xiao Cong Shu*, Beijing, China Chinese Medicine Press 1995
This book contains anatomical studies and practical experience in the treatment of all diseases caused by Blood stasis including apoplexies and post-apoplectic hemiplegia. A daring piece of work.

WANG Shu-He (Han dynasty, 3rd century)
Mai Jing, Beijing, Science & Technology Press 1996
This is the first pulse classic that Wang derived from the 'Nei Jing'.

WU Ju-Tong (Qing dynasty, 1758–1836)
Wen Bing Tiao Bian, Zhong Guo Yi Xue Da Cheng, Shanghai, Science & Technology Press 1937, 1990, 1992
The most renowned classic of the 'Febrile Disease School'. Wu Tang brought together the works of his predecessors, amongst whom are Wu You-Ke , Ye Tian-Shi and Xue Xue, and further developed the 'Triple Burner' theory in the event of invading pathogens.

WU Zhi Wang (Ming dynasty)
Ji Yin Gang Mu, Beijing, Science & Technology Press 1996
Wu Shu-Qing's gynaecological work is based on wang Ken-Tang's earlier work but takes it further, likewise with the description of the diagnosis and treatment of gynaecological diseases.

XU Da-Chun (Qing dynasty, 1693–1771)
Yi Xue Yuan Liu Lun, Hui Xi Bing An, Yi Guan Bian etc. in *Xu Dan-Chun Yi Shu Quan Ji*, Beijing, People's Health Publishing 1988, 1996
Xu Ling-Tai (also known as Xu Da-Ye) was a universal genius who apart from medicine studied astronomy, water and engineering crafts, poetry and literature. He advocated his own often original ideas about TCM, such as, for example, the sparing usage of medicinals and the reduction of classic formulas to those medicinals that correspond directly with syndrome differentiation. He was strongly opposed to the use of warm or purgative medicinals, which he demonstrated quite controversially in his critique Yi Guan Bian. After 50 years of medical practice he retired of his own accord and, according to typical Taoist etiquette, retreated to the mountainside. He was an extraordinary man.*

XUE Xue (Qing dynasty, 1681–1770)
Shi Re Lun, Beijing, Chinese Medicine Press 1995
Xue Sheng Bai, also known as Yi Piao, was a contemporary of Ye Tian-Shi. He also contributed to the theory of febrile disease, and concerned himself especially with diseases due to Damp-Heat.

YANG Ji-Zhou (Ming dynasty, 1522–1620)
Zhen Jiu Da Cheng, Tianjin, Science & Technology Press 1993, 1995
The last great classic on acupuncture that clarified and standardized divergent views on channels and points. To this day this system has remained unchanged.

YE Tian Shi (Qing dynasty, 1667–1746)
Lin Zheng Zhi Nan Yi An, edited by Xu Ling Tai, Shanghai, Shanghai People's Publishing 1959, 1976
Diagnosis and treatment of febrile diseases. Ye Gui established the four stages theory: the pathogenic factor successively invades the Wei, Qi, Ying and Xue stages.

ZHANG Jie-Bing (Ming dynasty, 1563–1640)
Jing Yue Chuan Shu, Beijing, Chinese Medical Press 1994, 1996
A comprehensive work of the great scholar Zhang Jing-Yue in 64 volumes. Being a Taoist, Zhang belonged to the school of 'There is never too much Yang – there is never too little Yin', which emphasizes the use of warm and tonifying medicinals. He invented many new formulas and wrote in a very learned and literate style.
Lei Jing, Beijing, People's Health Publishing 1964, 1995
This is one of the best reference books for the 'Huang Di Nei Jing'. Zhang classified the entire 'Nei Jing' into Yin-Yang, organs, pulse, channels, theories, acupuncture and so on, which facilitates their comparison.

ZHANG Lu (Qing dynasty, 1617–1700)
Zhang Shi Yi Tong, Beijing, Chinese Medicine
Press 1995
*Zhang Lu-Yu spent 50 years composing the 16 volumes
of his work which, amongst other things, describes vaccination methods. He was a follower of the School of
warming and invigoration, and outlined its strengths.*

ZHANG Xi-Chun (1860–1933)
Yi Xue Zhong Zhong Can Xi Lu, Shijiazhuang,
Hebei Science & Technology Press 1985, 1994
*Zhang was one of the early supporters of the integra-
tion of Chinese and Western medicine. He developed
many new formulas, also combining aspirin with
Chinese medicinals. Zhang Shou-Fu lived into the
twentieth century.*

ZHANG Zhong-Jing (Han dynasty, middle of
2nd century – beginning of 3rd century)
Shang Han Za Bing Lun, edited later by Wang Su-
He as *Shang Han Lun* and *Jin Kui Yao Lue*. The
Taiwan edition (traditional script) was used: *Gao
Deng Zhong Yi Yan Jiu Can Kao Cong Shu*, vols 11
and 12, Taipei, Zhi Yin Publishers 1990
*The Shang Han is concerned predominantly with infec-
tions and developed the 'Six Stages' theory, according
to which a pathogenic factor can travel from the
outermost level* (Tai Yang) *to the innermost level* (Jue

Yin). *The* Jin Kui, *however, describes the treatment of
various diseases and is thus the first book on internal
medicine.*

ZHANG Zi-He (Jin dynasty, 1156–1228)
Ru Men Shi Qin in *Zi-He Yi Ji*, Beijing, People's
Health Publishing 1994, 1996
*Zhang Cong-Zheng founded the 'Purgative School' for
attacking pathogenic factors, as he was probably influ-
enced by Indian healing methods and their use of purga-
tive, diaphoretic and emetic medicinals. He also stressed
the importance of pathogenesis and emotional therapy.
He thus laid the foundation for the development of
TCM psychology.*

ZHU Dan-Xi (Yuan dynasty, 1281–1358)
Ge Zhi Yu Lun and *Ju Fang Fa Hui*, both in *Dan
Xi Yi Ji*, Beijing, People's Health Publishing 1993,
1995
*Zhu Zhen-Heng, a moralist advocate of Neoconfucian-
ism, founded the 'Nourishing Yin School', nevertheless,
he maintained the point of view of his older contemporaries Li Gao, Zhang Yuan-Su and Zhang Zi-He, who
were collectively known as 'the four masters of the*
Jin-Yuan *period'. In* Ju Fang Fa Hui *he criticized the
current popular but improper usage of the* Ju *collection
of formulas, which was applied without syndrome
differentiation.*

Appendix 9

Short bibliography of author's publications (in chronological order)

CHINESE

Nei, Long-Dao (Gunter Neeb). Traditional and modern methods of treating the Lily-syndromes. (*Gu Jin Yi Xue Dui Bai He Bing Zhi Yan Jiu.*) In: *Zhong Yi Chuan Tong Yi Yao Yan Jiu* vol 1, p 94 ff., Beijing, Chinese Medical Classics Press 1997, ISBN 7-80013-741-4/R737

Nei, Long Dao (Gunter Neeb). Experimental long-term study of the chronic Blood stasis/hyperviscosity syndrome – pathomorphology and functional disorders of the internal organs. (Thesis for Master's degree in Chinese.) International College for Traditional Chinese Medicine and Pharmacology Tianjin, Research Division, Tianjin, China 1998

Nei, Long-Dao (Gunter Neeb). Experimental animal studies of chronic Blood stasis syndrome. (*Man Xing Yu Xue Zheng Dong Wu Mo Xing de Zhi Zuo ji Shi Yan Yan Jiu.*) In: Congress Papers of the 2nd International Congress of TCM in Tianjin, China, 1998, p 351 ff.

Nei, Long-Dao (Gunter Neeb). Investigation of chronic Blood stasis as an experimental model for studies – its functional and organic and pathomorphological findings in hares. (*Man Xing Xue Yu Zheng Tu Mo Xing de Zhi Bei ji Gong Neng Xing Tai Xue de Guan Zha Yan Jiu.*) In: Thesis and Research Papers of Lecturers at the 5th Chinese Congress of the Society of Integrated Chinese Medicine, September 1999, Beijing, China, p 47 ff.

Nei, Long-Dao (Gunter Neeb). Comparison of two therapeutic systems in history, cell culture, in animals and 200 Chinese and German patients in clinical expression, results of diagnosis and treatment. (*Chuantong Yixue zai Zhongguo he Ouzhou de Tongyidian yu Bingli Biaoshi, Zhenduan, Zhiliao Fanying he Tongji.*) Doctoral thesis in Chinese. International College for Traditional Chinese Medicine and Pharmacology Tianjin, Research Division, Tianjin, China, January 2001

ENGLISH:

Trick or treat? Westerners encounter Traditional Chinese Medicine. In: TCM Quarterly 2/1994, Taipei, Taiwan, p 23 ff.

The geomedicine of TCM. In: Orientation. The Magazine of the Anglo-Dutch Institute of Oriental Medicine. 11/1999, Amsterdam, Netherlands, p 42 ff.

The TCM-model: defining the profession for the 21st Century. In: Orientation. The Magazine of the Anglo-Dutch Institute of Oriental Medicine 1/2000, Amsterdam, Netherlands

Non-linear medicine: prospects of a future medicine and the role of TCM in its development. In: Congress papers of the Congress of TCM in The Netherlands, June 2000, Maastricht, Netherlands

2000 Years of medical exchange; Part 1–4, in 'The Lantern – A Journal of Chinese Medicine' Issue 1–4, Carlton, Australia 2005

GERMAN

TV documentary

Schlaf als Schlüssel des Alterungsprozesses. In: Archimedes, ARTE on 24th August 2000

Interview: Deutschlandfunk, Studenten-forum 1.2.2001

Wunschbox: Thema TCM (Mai 2002)

Books

Cooperated on *Leitfaden Traditionelle Chinesische Medizin.* (Hg. Claudia Fockes, Norman Hillenbrand, Chapter 1 and 6 and Glossary, Verlag Urban & Fischer, München 2000)

Das Blutstasesyndrom – Chinas klassisches Konzept in der modernen Medizin. Verlag für Ganzheitliche Medizin Dr. Erich Wühr GmbH, Kötzting, 2001

Zweitausend Jahre Erfahrung: Klassische Texte aus der chinesischen Medizin. Verlag für Ganzheitliche Medizin Dr. Erich Wühr GmbH, Kötzing, expected publication 2002

Wen Bing – Infektionskrankheiten in der traditionellen Chinesischen und Neuen Humanmedizin. Verlag für Ganzheitliche Medizin Dr. Erich Wühr GmbH, Kötzing, expected publication 2003

In Claudia Focks, Praktischer Leitfaden TCM, Kapitel 1 und 8 (Arzneikräuter), Verlag Urban & Fischer Mai/2003

Articles

Schlaf als Schlüssel des Alterungsprozesses. In: *Zeitschrift für Traditionelle Chinesische Medizin* 1/1998, Verlag für Ganzheitliche Medizin Dr. Erich Wühr GmbH, Kötztting, p 55 ff.

Wie man chinesische Medizin studiert und dennoch ein sturer Hesse bleibt. In: *Zeitschrift für Traditionelle Chinesische Medizin* 2/1998, Verlag für Ganzheitliche Medizin Dr. Erich Wühr GmbH, Kötzting, p 129 ff.

Adressen und Angebote von TCM-Hochschulen oder Universitäten in China. In: *Zeitschrift für Traditionelle Chinesische Medizin* 2/1998, Verlag für Ganzheitliche Medizin Dr. Erich Wühr GmbH, Kötzting, p 132 ff.

Praktische Anwendung chinesischer Arzneimittel, Teil 1. In: *Zeitschrift für Traditionelle Chinesische Medizin* 1/98, Verlag für Ganzheitliche Medizin Dr. Erich Wühr GmbH, Kötzting, p 43 ff.

Praktische Anwendung chinesischer Arzneimittel, Teil 2. In: *Zeitschrift für Traditionelle Chinesische Medizin* 2/1998, Verlag für Ganzheitliche Medizin Dr. Erich Wühr GmbH, Kötzting, p 120 ff.

Praktische Anwendung chinesischer Arzneimittel, Teil 3. In: *Zeitschrift für Traditionelle Chinesische Medizin* 3/1998, Verlag für Ganzheitliche Medizin Dr. Erich Wühr GmbH, Kötzting, p 187 ff.

Zusammenhänge in der Diagnose von TCM-Blutstase-Syndromen und schulmedizinisch definierten Laborparametern. With Bi-Hsia Yeh. In: *Zeitschrift für Traditionelle Chinesische Medizin* 2/1999, Verlag für Ganzheitliche Medizin Dr. Erich Wühr GmbH, Kötzting, p 107 ff.

Experimentelle Erzeugung des chronischen Blutstase-Syndroms und Erforschung seiner pathologischen Folgen am Tiermodell. In: *Zeitschrift für Traditionelle Chinesische Medizin* 1/1999, Verlag für Ganzheitliche Medizin Dr. Erich Wühr GmbH, Kötzting, p 48 ff.

Praktische Anwendung chinesischer Arzneimittel, Teil 4. In: *Zeitschrift für Traditionelle Chinesische Medizin* 3/1999, Verlag für Ganzheitliche Medizin Dr. Erich Wühr GmbH, Kötzting, p 177 ff.

Zur Frage der Blutstase. In: *Die Volksheilkunde/Der Heilpraktiker* April 2000

'Akupunktur bei Blutstase', 'Kleine Geschichte der Blutstase' and *'Taoisten in der chinesischen Medizin'.* In: *Kongreßheft des 31. Internationalen Kongresses für Akupunktur und Traditionelle Chinesische Medizin*, Rothenburg, June 2000

Akupunkturtechniken und Nadeltechniken. In: *Naturheilkunde, Spezialthema TCM August 2000*, Richard Pflaum Verlag, München

Pulsdiagnose – Atem des Arztes oder des Patienten. In: *Naturheilkunde* 1/2000, Richard Pflaum Verlag, München

Die Terra incognita der modernen Medizin: Mykosen – Nässe-Krankheiten der TCM. In: *Zeitschrift für*

Traditionelle Chinesische Medizin 1/01, Verlag für Ganzheitliche Medizin Dr. Erich Wühr GmbH, Kötzting, p 51 ff.

Praktische Anwendung chinesischer Arzneimittel, Teil 5. Expected publication in: *Zeitschrift für Traditionelle Chinesische Medizin* 4/2001, Verlag für Ganzheitliche Medizin Dr. Erich Wühr GmbH, Kötzting

Articles between 2000–2005:
ca. 50 in: Zeitschrift für traditionelle chinesische Medizin, VGM-Wühr-Verlag, Kötzting, Die Volksheilkunde/Der Heilpraktiker, Zeitschrift Naturheilkunde, Richard Pflaum Verlag, München (3) Natur-Heilkunde-Journal, Wahrlich Verlag, Meckenheim (1)

Index